The British Columbia

Atlas of Wellness

2nd Edition

Leslie T. Foster
C. Peter Keller
Brian McKee
Aleck Ostry

with contributions from Analisa Blake, Pat Bluemel, Diane Braithwaite, John Fowler,
Ian Macek, and Noëlle Virtue

Western Geographical Press

Department of Geography, University of Victoria
P.O. Box 3060, Victoria BC, Canada V8W 3R4
phone: 250-721-7357 email: dbraith@uvic.ca

Library and Archives Canada Cataloguing in Publication

The British Columbia atlas of wellness / Leslie T. Foster ... [et al.]. -- 2nd ed.
Includes bibliographical references.
ISBN 978-0-919838-34-5

1. British Columbia--Statistics, Medical--Maps. 2. Health status indicators--British Columbia--Maps.
3. Public health--British Columbia--Statistics--Maps. I. Foster, Leslie T., 1947-

RA407.5.C3F68 2011   614.4'2711   C2011-905725-5

The reader is invited to use the maps and tables from this report in support of their work. The Atlas, maps, and tables can be downloaded from the University of Victoria Department of Geography website at www.geog.uvic.ca/wellness, or hard copies can be ordered from the Department of Geography at:

Western Geographipcal Press, Department of Geography, University of Victoria,
PO Box 3060 STN CSC, Victoria, BC V8W 3R4

Telephone: 1-250-721-7357   Fax: 1-250-721-6216   Email: dbraith@uvic.ca

Printed in Canada

In Memory

Harold (Harry) D. Foster

(1943 - 2009)

Medical Geographer extraordinaire, colleague, and friend, as well as
founder and series editor of the Western Geographical Series from its inception in 1970.

Thank you for all you have done to push the frontiers of knowledge
and to challenge us to always look at all perspectives, and
for working so tirelessly to get new ideas published.

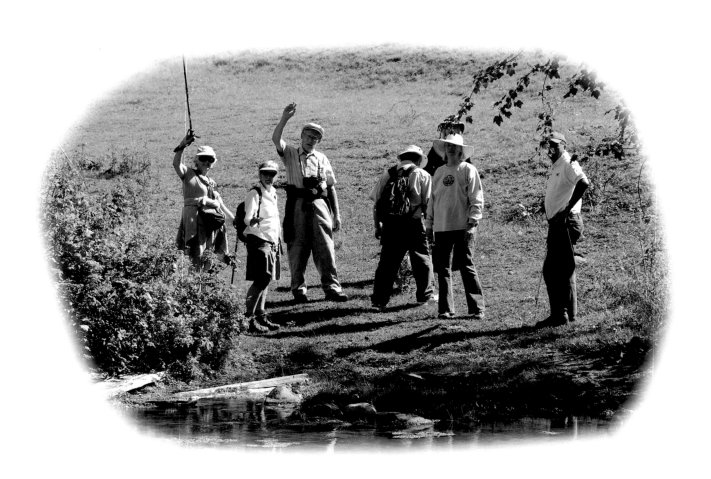

Contents

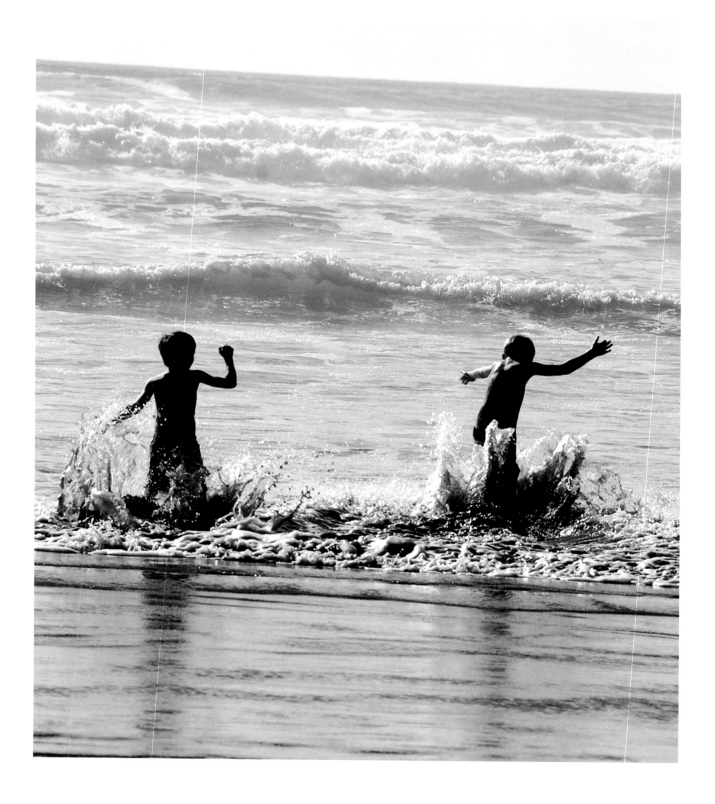

Acknowledgements

As mentioned in the original atlas, the final publication of a product like this is indeed the result of the efforts of many individuals and groups acting as a formal or informal team. Many people and organizations—too numerous to mention them all—have had important input to this edition of the BC Atlas of Wellness. We would like to take this opportunity to recognize the contributions and ideas of our colleagues who were involved in the original atlas publication. Although they had no formal input to this second edition, their ideas remained and need to be acknowledged. These include: Jack Boomer, Michael Hayes, Perry Hystad, Patti Jensen, Ken Josephson, Gord Miller, David Weicker, and Martin Wright.

We also would like to acknowledge the financial support from both the Ministry of Health and the Michael Smith Health Research Foundation, without which this new edition of the Atlas would not have been possible. Andrew Hazlewood of the Ministry of Health has been an important sponsor of the project from the start, and arranged for the initial funding and support for the project. He also must be credited with the original idea for such a publication as the BC Atlas of Wellness, and provided us with access to many other resources, including data, information, and people. In particular, we would like to recognize the sterling work undertaken by one of Andrew's staff members. Richard Mercer provided us with major support, and with data from the Canadian Community Health Surveys (3.1 and 4.1) that make up a large number of the indicators and maps in the Atlas.

Special thanks go to the following: from the Ministry of Health, Cathy Arbour, Rosemary Armour, Shelley Canitz, Ron Duffell, Lisa Forster-Coull, Susan Garvey, Tom Gregory, Trevor Hancock, Matt Herman, Lorie Hrycuik, Perry Kendall, Del Nyberg, Sergio Pastrana, Marilyn Shinto, Laurie Woodland and Margaret Yandel; from the Ministry of Education, Karlic Ho, and Janet Powell; from the Ministry of Community, Sport and Cultural Development, David Galbraith and Margo Ross; from the Ministry of Children and Family Development, Martin Wright; from the Ministry of Community and Rural Development, Doug Bourhill; from the McCreary Centre Society, Maya Peled, Colleen Poon, and Annie Smith; from the BC Healthy Living Alliance, Noëlle Virtue; and from 2010 Legacies Now, Michelle Hohne.

In working on the Atlas, we engaged in a very productive partnership with BC Stats, Ministry of Labour and Citizens' Services which resulted in, among other things, the development of an interactive wellness mapping product. We would like to recognize Pat Bluemel, Jennifer Hansen, Don McCrae, Dave O'Neil, Shannon Pendergast, Cathy Stock and Natalie Work for their work, cooperation, ideas, and support for the project.

Photo credits go to Les Foster, Betty Honsinger, Peter Keller, Brian McKee and Mary Virtue,

As part of the redevelopment of the Atlas, we developed a series of supplements to the original Atlas so that we might try out different ways of presenting data. We would like to thank Analisa Blake, Denise Cloutier-Fisher and Noëlle Virtue, who each contributed to one or more of the supplements. We would also like to thank colleagues in the Department of Geography and the School of Child and Youth Care at the University of Victoria for their encouragement and support for our work. In particular, Diane Braithwaite, as usual, did an outstanding job of copyediting, and Betty Honsinger, Alastair McKee and Chris Virtue provided us with important assistance in data checking and proof reading. However, any errors or omissions remain ours.

Leslie T. Foster, C. Peter Keller,
Brian McKee and Aleck Ostry
Victoria, June, 2011

Preface

The genesis of the British Columbia Atlas of Wellness came after a brief meeting with Andrew Hazlewood, then Assistant Deputy Minister of Population, Health and Wellness in the Ministry of Health. The topic of discussion was the concept of a wellness approach to mapping health in BC. Mapping health-related data in the province was initiated in the late 1980s, but it looked at mortality, morbidity, or system use, not the actual "health" or wellness of British Columbians. The concept of taking a wellness approach had not been tried before. Hence, the beginning of the first edition of the Atlas.

The Atlas was developed in response to the BC government's ActNow BC initiative. The overall goal of ActNow BC was to help make BC the healthiest jurisdiction to host a modern day Olympic and Paralympic games. The Atlas assisted in focusing the attention of diverse ministries and their funded agencies on ways to contribute to ActNow BC, and to ensure that actions to support the initiative would recognize the geographical diversity of the province. It was well known that achieving the provincial goals of ActNow BC would require attention to the fact that health, wellness, illness, and health system infrastructure varied substantially throughout the province. As such, it was important to get a broad geographical baseline of these variations so that differences, and anticipated improvements, could be measured over time.

This second edition of the Atlas goes well beyond the key goals established by ActNow BC. Of the more than 400 maps included in this edition, approximately half are updates to maps presented previously, but the other half are new, reflecting interests expressed by users of the first edition, and the discovery of new data sources.

Like health, wellness is multi-faceted and is a term that is used in everyday discourse without much thought to what it entails. There is an assumption that everyone knows what it is. Achieving some definition of wellness, and agreement around what influences it, was a major issue in developing and organizing the Atlas. A second issue was defining an appropriate geographical unit for mapping purposes. Within the province, there are myriad geographical administrative units for which data are collected. This makes both measuring and mapping wellness a challenging prospect.

We have not collected any primary data for inclusion in the Atlas. Rather, our approach has been to use existing data, albeit from a variety of sources, for different time periods and for well used geographical administrative units such as Health Service Delivery Areas, School Districts, Regional Districts, and Economic Development Regions. To enable comparisons among geographies, averages, means, rates, or percentages have been used. There is also a limited number of what we refer to as "custom maps" that are not based on any of these geographical units, but use the boundary of BC as a whole. These use unique indicators that relate to the key components of ActNow BC.

The second edition of this Atlas is roughly divided into four parts. The first part provides background and context, instructions on "how to use and read" the maps, and a demographic summary of the province. The next group of chapters provides the geography of health determinants and wellness assets and uses indicators that describe the key "pillars" of the ActNow BC initiative: smoke-free environments and behaviour; food security and nutrition; physical activity; healthy weights; and healthy pregnancies. The third part focuses on chronic-free conditions and wellness outcomes. The final part provides a summary of the geography of wellness within BC, and suggests opportunities for developing geographical wellness benchmarks.

Throughout the Atlas, a "half-full" or asset approach to mapping indicators is taken, rather than a "half-empty" or deficit approach. Put simply, this involves using indicators such as healthy weight rather than overweight status or obesity, non-smoking behaviour rather than smoking behaviour, activity-related indicators rather than those related to inactivity and sedentary behaviour, healthy pregnancies and birth outcomes rather than maternal and perinatal complications, chronic-free conditions rather than prevalence of conditions such as diabetes, cancers, and heart disease, and good health indicators rather than morbidity and mortality measures. This is our way of using the wellness concept in the Atlas.

It is not our intent to explain the variations in the many indicators that we map. The aim of this edition of the BC Atlas of Wellness is to present data in a useful and understandable manner. We want the maps "to speak for themselves," and our job is to construct them and describe the key points that emerge from the maps and accompanying tables and graphs as a basis for discussion by interested groups, researchers, policy and decision makers, and individuals. By opening the Atlas at any page, there is a geographical "story" to be told about the wellness indicator on that page. Each colour map shows those areas that are doing the "best" as measured by key indicators, and those that may require improvements in wellness. It is our hope that users will ask questions of themselves, and others in their community and region, about the "whys and wherefores" of the patterns that emerge.

We anticipate that the half-full rather than half-empty approach we use— mapping the positive rather than the negative, mapping assets rather than deficits—will result in fuller discourse on why variations exist, and what can be achieved from a wellness perspective. This can only help improve the overall health and wellness of the province and its residents' food security and nutrition, physical activity, healthy weights, healthy pregnancy, reduction in chronic conditions, and wellness outcomes.

As with any publication of this nature, new events and data often overtake what has been presented. As the Atlas goes to press, there have been developments in a variety of areas contained within its pages. For example, additional Strong Start Centres have been announced and smokers will be provided with free nicotine-replacement therapies to reduce smoking. But the most important development involves ActNow BC itself. The initiative has been replaced by a much broader Healthy Families BC strategy. This change, we believe, mirrors the broader approach to health and wellness that we demonstrate throughout this Atlas and our work on wellness mapping. No doubt there will be new initiatives implemented as part of Healthy Families BC to improve the health and wellness of BC citizens, and at the same time reduce the geographical inequities in health and wellness throughout the province.

Leslie T. Foster, C. Peter Keller,
Brian McKee and Aleck Ostry
Victoria, June, 2011

Foreword

Health geomatics has made great strides in the last few years because of improved geographic information systems, and the use of mapping in the public health arena is steadily increasing. But health and wellness mapping has a long history. John Snow is viewed by many as the first modern-day epidemiologist and health "mapper." In 1854, Snow studied the locations of cholera victims in London and was able to identify how the disease was transmitted and thus make recommendations to prevent future outbreaks. As I noted in the *Foreword* to the 1st Edition of the *British Columbia Atlas of Wellness*, this publication follows a long tradition in public and population health mapping, and shows geographical variations and inequities for a variety of wellness-related indicators. While many previous atlases have focused on health system use and public health problem areas, this 2nd Edition of the *BC Atlas of Wellness* remains unique in that it focuses on assets rather than deficits. This focus was recognized as an innovative approach to knowledge development and transfer by the Public Health Agency of Canada (2009) in its *Report on the Integrated Healthy Living Strategy*.

Having wellness as its focus, this Atlas provides a diversity of indicators that reflect the multi-faceted concept of wellness. These indicators are based on administrative data, and also on key surveys such as the Canadian Community Health Surveys (CCHS). These surveys have become an important source of information for public health practitioners and policy makers over the past decade, and have enabled us to gauge how individuals feel about a variety of issues that may influence their health and well-being, and also how they rate their own health and important life matters.

While the original *BC Atlas of Wellness* had a major focus on the province's health promotion ActNow BC strategy, this edition has been expanded. It contains updated indicators that focus on the determinants of health and wellness, but now includes comparisons to both earlier data and Canadian averages for, smoke-free environments and behaviours, food security and healthy nutrition, physical activity, healthy weights, and healthy pregnancies and births. Additional material has been added, with a specific emphasis on food security and being free of chronic conditions, as a result of requests from users of the original Atlas. In total, over 400 separate maps along with supporting tables are included that provide data related to indicators of various facets of wellness.

The material presented provides the user with visualizations of regional differences, as well as variations based on gender and age groupings and, where appropriate, statistical testing shows whether or not differences are significant. The information can be used to generate questions and discussions among community groups, public health policy makers and decision makers, school boards, and local governments on why one region does better than other regions on one or more indicators. Are regional inequalities in wellness indicators important enough to warrant local action to target health promotion initiatives both geographically and demographically? If so, what can be done to improve wellness? What can be learned from the regions that are the best or excel on certain aspects of wellness?

The maps and tables have also been created from a variety of somewhat scattered existing data sources, some of which may not be well known to policy makers and others interested in wellness. The information provided can be used to help target health promotion initiatives both geographically and demographically. The Atlas adds value to raw data so that rates can be compared among regions, and by providing them in this manner, makes them available to any one who wishes to use the data for their own purposes. Further, the Atlas and a series of supplements that focus on seniors, women, and inter-provincial comparisons are available to all through the website http://www.geog.uvic.ca/wellness.

By focusing on assets and taking a wellness approach, the *BC Atlas of Wellness* provides a unique and most interesting look at health and wellness in the province. It can assist communities and regions to learn more about their health and wellness relative to other parts of the province, and it complements reports that have been produced through my office.

P.R.W. Kendall, OBC, MBBS, MSc, FRCPC
Provincial Health Officer
British Columbia
May, 2011

1

Introduction to the Second Edition of the British Columbia Atlas of Wellness

The first edition of the *BC Atlas of Wellness* was published in 2007 in response to the government of British Columbia's health promotion initiative called ActNow BC, which was established in 2005. The initiative was introduced to encourage British Columbians to make healthy lifestyle choices to improve their quality of life, reduce the incidence of preventable chronic disease, and reduce the burden on the health care system. ActNow BC was an integrated, whole-of-government approach that involved contributions from a variety of partners, including municipalities, non-governmental organizations, schools, communities, and the private sector, to develop and deliver programs and services that would assist individuals to quit or never start smoking, to be more physically active, to eat healthier foods, to achieve and maintain a healthy weight, and to make healthy choices in pregnancy.

The rationale for the Atlas was to visually communicate data and information about key and novel wellness indicators for BC. A secondary purpose was to highlight patterns that emerged from these data in an interesting and informative way, and where possible to show changes over time at the provincial level while also providing comparisons at the national level. The objective was not only to help people recognize and understand why certain geographical patterns might occur, but also to encourage questions provincially, regionally, and locally as to the reasons for the patterns, why wellness varied over space, and what could or should be done about it. These remain the key components of this second edition.

Rarely does a day go by without maps being featured in the media to help locate an issue, to understand geographical relationships, or to demonstrate a geographical variation. The common expression that "a picture is worth (or can save) a thousand words" certainly also holds true for a map. But a map also can generate a hundred questions. Why do geographical patterns exist

and what is causing them? What can be learned from these patterns and are these differences a good thing, and if not, what can be done to improve matters? Research has shown that the public wants maps packaged in the form of atlases to allow them to browse their community and region, to understand regional variation, and to allow for relative comparison—i.e., How am I doing in my region or community compared to other regions or communities? (Keller, 1995; Mitton et al., 2009). Further, decision makers and policy makers have also indicated the need to have data provided to them in map form to help inform decisions (Mitton et al., 2008).

This chapter provides a recent history of the ActNow BC initiative and its key goals. The background is important as a context for understanding how the *BC Atlas of Wellness* is put together in terms of its framework and in terms of the indicators that are mapped. This is followed by a brief discussion of the usefulness of maps and atlases for the purpose of displaying wellness and health initiatives. A review of the changes incorporated into the second edition of the *BC Atlas of Wellness* is also provided, followed by a description of the chapters of the Atlas.

A Brief History of ActNow BC

There were a couple of motivations that led to the establishment of ActNow BC. First was the July 2003 announcement that British Columbia would host the 2010 Winter Olympic and Paralympic Games, and that the legacy was to be a healthier population (Geneau et al., 2009). Second, in 2004, the Select Standing Committee on Health was asked, among other things, to investigate successful health promotion campaigns in other jurisdictions with a view to assessing their usefulness for BC. The Committee was also asked to look at how to promote "healthy lifestyles," and to consider savings that might result from the improved fitness of the population (BC Select Standing Committee on Health, 2004). The Committee noted that 40% of the commonest chronic diseases resulted from one or more of the following: smoking, poor diet, physical inactivity, obesity, and irresponsible alcohol consumption. The Committee felt that the whole population could respond to the excitement of hosting the Games and become healthier as a result.

The government's strategic plan published in 2005 indicated that BC was not only to lead the way in North America in healthy living and physical fitness, but was to be the healthiest jurisdiction to host the Olympic and Paralympic Games (Government of British Columbia, 2006). Five key goals were established, around which the *BC Atlas of Wellness* is primarily, but not exclusively, organized. The key 2010 targets for ActNow BC were:

1. Increase by 20% the proportion of the BC population (aged 12+ years) that is physically active or moderately active during leisure time from the 2003 prevalence of 58.1% to 69.7%.

2. Increase by 20% the proportion of the BC population (aged 12+ years) that eats the daily recommended level of fruits and vegetables from the 2003 prevalence of 40.1% to 48.1%.

3. Reduce by 10% the proportion of the BC population (aged 15+ years) that uses tobacco, from the 2003 prevalence of 16% to 14.4%.

4. Reduce by 20% the proportion of the BC population (aged 18+ years) that is currently classified as overweight or obese from the 2003 prevalence of 42.3% to 33.8%.

5. Increase by 50% the number of women counselled regarding alcohol use during pregnancy, and have focused strategies for the prevention of fetal alcohol spectrum disorder (ActNow BC, 2010).

ActNow BC was initially coordinated through the Ministry of Health. In August 2006, the stewardship role was transferred to the Ministry of Tourism, Sport and the Arts (MTSA), and the BC government appointed a Minister of State for ActNow BC under MTSA and established an ActNow BC Branch to provide the whole-of-government and cross-sector stewardship, coordination, strategic communications/marketing guidance, and evaluation support. In June 2008, the BC government announced the creation of the Ministry of Healthy Living and Sport, moved the coordinating function of ActNow BC to this new Ministry, and eliminated the position of Minister of State for ActNow BC. In June 2009, a new cabinet was established and ActNow BC remained part of the Ministry of Healthy

Living and Sport, and a Minister of State for the Olympics and ActNow BC was appointed. In late July of 2010, the then Minister of Healthy Living and Sport indicated a strategic change in ActNow BC activities. While the four pillars of physical activity, healthy eating, living tobacco-free and consuming alcohol responsibly remained as important components of government's chronic disease prevention strategy, ActNow BC became largely focused on physical activity and community engagement. Further programming was to become tailored to reach under served populations as well as the general public. The Ministry of Healthy Living and Sport was disbanded in October 2010 and ActNow BC transferred to the Ministry of Health.

In implementing the ActNow BC initiative, government recognized that success in achieving these goals needed long-term changes in beliefs, values, and behaviours, and while government could be the leader, it could not do it alone. There was a need for influential community partners, and four key partners were singled out: BC Healthy Living Alliance (BCHLA), 2010 Legacies Now, BC Recreation and Parks Association (BCRPA), and the Union of BC Municipalities (UBCM).

The BCHLA was formed in 2003, before the introduction of ActNow BC, and worked to promote chronic disease prevention and alliance building. It consisted of a variety of key organizations with interests in chronic disease prevention. Voting members of the BCHLA include the BC Lung Association, BC Pediatric Society, BCRPA, Canadian Cancer Society, BC and Yukon Division, Canadian Diabetes Association, Dietitians of Canada, BC Region, Heart and Stroke Foundation of BC and Yukon, Public Health Association of BC, UBCM. Other key organizations involved included the Health Authorities, the Centre on Aging at the University of Victoria, Directorate of Agencies for School Health BC and the Arthritis Society of BC/Yukon to name a few. Collectively, BCHLA at one time represented nearly 40 organizations, 40,000 volunteers, 4,300 health and recreation professionals, and close to 200 local governments (Geneau et al., 2009).

BCHLA produced several important documents in early 2005 that have been significant in terms of giving publicity to ActNow BC goals (BCHLA, 2005a), as well as providing an analysis of the risk factors associated with chronic disease and an effectiveness analysis of interventions (BCHLA, 2005b). This Alliance received more than $25 million in one-time funding in 2006 to help government achieve its ActNow BC goals and developed 15 initiatives in healthy eating, tobacco smoking cessation/prevention, physical activity, and community capacity building (http://www.bchealthyliving.ca). These are described and analysed later in the Atlas.

2010 Legacies Now was first created in 2000 to assist with the Olympic bid, and to help ensure that the benefits of the 2010 Olympics were shared throughout the province. It became an independent society in 2002, with a mandate to ensure "a strong and lasting sport system for the province that increased participation and supported safe, healthy, and vibrant communities." Its mandate was expanded in early 2004 to include the arts, volunteerism, and literacy, and to develop a network of community committees throughout the province to support these areas. These were all important initiatives that helped to develop assets for wellness , and in 2006, Legacies Now was provided with nearly $5 million to support ActNow BC initiatives (http://www.2010legaciesnow.com). In February 2011, 2010 Legacies Now became LIFT Philanthropy Partners with a mandate to "accelerate the growth and impact of selected not-for-profit organizations to create positive and lasting social change through sport and healthy living, and literacy and lifelong learning. The overall aim is to enhance social well-being and economic prosperity in communities across Canada" (http://www.liftpartners.ca).

The BCRPA, like 2010 Legacies Now, is a non-profit society and, as its name suggests, it is "dedicated to building and sustaining active healthy lifestyles and communities in BC." It also has a role in helping to increase sports and recreation activity in the province (http://www.bcrpa.bc.ca).

The fourth key organization was the UBCM, which has represented the interests of municipalities in the province for more than a century. The UBCM was provided $5 million in government funding in 2005 to establish a Community Health Promotion Fund that provided grants, on a competitive basis, to local government to support health promotion focusing on healthy living and chronic disease prevention in support of ActNow BC goals.

The Ministry of Health was aware that all ministries within government had the ability to influence the achievement of ActNow BC goals. To help focus on the ActNow BC initiative, a cross-ministry group of assistant deputy ministers from each ministry in government was created, and $15 million over 3 years was made available for projects brought forward that supported the ActNow BC goals. Ministries, or their funded agencies, needed to match these funds in order to qualify for funding. In 2006, ministries were expected to include within their respective service plans a set of initiatives that demonstrated how they would contribute to ActNow BC. Just as the Atlas was going to press in May 2011, ActNow BC as a name was dropped by the BC government following the release of the new Premier's Healthy Families BC initiative. This

initiative was called "the most comprehensive health-promotion program anywhere in Canada" and "will support British Columbians in managing their own health, reducing chronic disease and ensuring that pregnancy and support programs target the province's most vulnerable families. Additionally, the strategy will continue to focus on healthy eating initiatives, including a public awareness campaign around sodium and sweetened beverage reduction" (Office of the Premier, 2011). The ActNow BC branch has since changed its name to Health Promotion Supports and Engagement, and the new strategy will be supported by a committee of Assistant Deputy Ministers on Chronic Disease Prevention.

We believe that this shift to a broader approach to health promotion and chronic disease prevention especially for the province's vulnerable families gives more weight to the mapping approach that we have taken as it helps to identify those regions which are doing well, and those regions which are vulnerable to poorer health and wellness outcomes.

Mapping Wellness and Health

Maps have been used as a form of communication in health and wellness studies for over 150 years. The origin of modern spatial epidemiology and health geography was the 1854 mapping of cholera victims in London, when descriptive statistics and maps were used by John Snow to identify how cholera was transmitted, making recommendations for prevention of future outbreaks (Keller & Hystad, 2007). Today, health and wellness researchers use geographic information systems (GIS) and web-based mapping to expand beyond disease mapping to examine a number of scientific hypotheses, such as disease etiology, equitable access to health services, or the social determinants of health. Contemporary GIS is recognized as a powerful information technology to facilitate convergence of disease-specific information and its analysis in relation to population settlements, surrounding social and health services, and the natural environment (WHO, 2007).

Increasingly, health-related maps are valued by decision makers and policy makers. The visual depiction of data in maps has a particular appeal also for non-experts (e.g., board or senior-management decision makers). They are often viewed as a relatively quick and easy method to get information to groups and individuals that are pressed for time and unable or unwilling to read lengthy material because of time commitments. In particular, as noted earlier, maps are valuable in presenting comparisons because data are on one page and represent a useful way to make a point (Mitton et al., 2009).

Our review of health mapping and health-related atlases in the first edition of the Atlas noted that the vast majority focused on mapping negative (e.g., mortality and morbidity) rather than positive factors, "deficits" rather than "assets," and "illness" rather than "wellness." This was not meant as criticism, as focusing on problem areas and issues helps to get attention so that improvements can be achieved. What we provided in the *BC Atlas of Wellness* was a unique focus on the positive rather than the negative. This second edition of the Atlas uses over 140 pages of maps which present a large variety of indicators that provide a wide ranging picture of wellness in BC. We take the optimist's half-full approach rather than the pessimist's half-empty approach and map wellness, or assets that can help determine, maintain, and improve wellness at the population level within the province. Instead of mapping obesity, we map healthy weights; instead of mapping smoking rates, we map smoke-free rates; instead of mapping physical inactivity, we map physical activity, and many more such indicators.

In health mapping, the tradition has been to compare communities and regions using maps that communicate degrees of something wrong. This atlas instead facilitates comparison by focusing on what is right, and hopefully what can be learned by others from this comparison. Examining the "best" area with a specific wellness indicator may help others learn what characteristics are at work in that area and can be used or adopted elsewhere.

The conditions we have selected, with one or two exceptions, show assets for wellness, just as obesity or smoking are risk factors for illness, poor development, and premature mortality. Focusing on wellness indicators and those areas that achieve high values on particular wellness assets can help provide some understanding of what is achievable, and those regions that feel they need to make improvements can learn from the "best." The best values can become benchmarks for others to achieve, as these values have already been attained by one or more regions or communities in the province. And the ones who are doing the best can strive to do even better, thus raising the wellness bar or benchmark. One area can learn from another area in terms of what works, and adopt some of the strategies used by the communities that demonstrate high levels of "wellness." Communities can also evaluate which of the indicators we provide in the Atlas are important ones to them, and decide whether to focus on improving them over time.

In the first edition of the Atlas, we expressed some concern that our focus on wellness could lead to the conclusion that all was "well" in the province, thus potentially undermining the need to focus attention on problem issues. This was clearly not our intent. A quick glance at many of the maps and tables will show that there are major "gradients" or differences in wellness between various areas in the province, and between different groups within the province. There are certainly areas that need improvement, and can be improved. Studying the areas or regions that appear to be the "best" on a particular wellness indicator may assist others to try to emulate their results by finding out what they are doing "right" to achieve these results. These areas will become clear when using the Atlas.

Our concerns have been largely unfounded, and we have been gratified by the local, national, and international response to our approach of mapping wellness. Within the province, the release of the Atlas was met with a lot of positive media interest, while at the national level the Atlas was described as an innovative approach to knowledge development and transfer by the Public Health Agency of Canada (2009a). Internationally, it has been recognized as setting the benchmark for Atlases of this nature (Exeter, 2009), and publicized by the Measuring the Progress of Societies organization (Giovannini & Hall, 2009). Further it has become clearer that others are looking to the positive approach rather than focusing in on problems. For example, the salutogenic model, which looks at health and wellness generating factors, is being used increasingly by health promotion researchers. Rather than disease prevention, the focus has moved to the assets that promote health and wellness (see Chapter 2).

It is also interesting to note that, since we started work on wellness mapping, several others have been doing similar work, and mapping has become much more interactive, based on improvements to GIS software. A couple of examples are provided here. Statistics Canada allows individuals to map nearly 90 health-related variables by health regions across the country. While actual values for health regions are not provided, information is given that shows whether values are significantly higher or lower than the Canadian average (Statistics Canada, 2008). Indicators are based on a variety of sources, and cover the period 1996 to 2006. Further, in 2007, Health Canada introduced the interactive Food and Nutrition Atlas of Canada, based on results from CCHS 2.2 (Nutrition) 2004 data. Information was only available at the provincial level for approximately 40 indicators, but some were wellness oriented, although only significant differences with the Canada-wide survey were provided (Health Canada, 2007).

Within Canada, a project that has been recommended by the Standing Senate Committee on Social Affairs, Science and Technology of the Canadian parliament is

Newfoundland and Labrador's system of Community Accounts, which "allows users to access information on key economic and social indicators, organized by geography and data topic, providing users with information on the status and progress of their communities and their regions from an economic and social perspective" (Government of Newfoundland and Labrador, 2009).

A good example, elsewhere, of a project that focuses on mapping wellness and well-being at the community level is the CIV Community Indicators Victoria from Australia (Institute of Community Engagement and Policy Alternatives, 2006). Data and reports are presented on the well-being of the population by providing an integrated set of community well-being indicators. These indicators include a broad range of measures designed to identify and communicate economic, social, environmental, democratic, and cultural trends and outcomes. Approximately 60 wellness and well-being indicators can be mapped interactively.

At the global level, the Sustainable Society Foundation (2010) has developed an interactive mapping project that allows comparisons among nations based on a series of indicators. Overall "well-being indices" based on human, environmental, and economic well-being have been developed. More recently, the Organisation for Economic Cooperation and Development (2011a) has introduced a Well-being index as part of its new Better Life Initiative.

Advancements and Changes

Since the original Atlas was completed in 2007, work continued to experiment with data and formatting based on preliminary responses to the Atlas. As part of this approach, we have developed several supplements to support the original Atlas. All of the supplements used data from the Canadian Community Health Surveys (CCHS). The first supplement focused on seniors using 2005 CCHS data, while the second provided Canada-wide maps that allowed comparisons of BC with all other provinces and territories with data from 2007. Subsequent supplements used 2007/8 CCHS data and provided information about BC wellness, while the fourth supplement had a focus on women's wellness (McKee et al., 2008; 2009a,b; Virtue et al., 2010). These supplements helped us improve the format for this edition of the BC Atlas of Wellness.

Between 2008 and 2010, we also entered into a partnership with BC Stats which allowed us to develop some new interactive products related to our wellness project. Data have been made available so that variables from the original Atlas, as well as this one, can be compared two at a time and graphed to see the type of relationships that might be evident. Further, more detailed, data are also made available through this arrangement (BC Stats, 2010a).

Format Changes

For those indicators that are derived from CCHS data, comparisons between the 2005 and 2007/8 samples are provided at the provincial level on the tables accompanying the maps. This allows the reader to see whether or not there has been a significant change between the two samples. Further, a graph has been added that gives a comparison with the Canada-wide average for a given indicator for key age cohorts as well as by gender.

It should be noted that the 2005 CCHS averages may be slightly different than those recorded in the original Atlas. This relates to the fact that Statistics Canada now reports the CCHS data differently. The denominator previously was based on the total sample size, while now it only includes those who answered the question. Consequently, the denominator is smaller than the total sample size, often resulting in a slightly higher value for 2005 than previously reported. In examining this issue, we are satisfied that the relative values and geographic patterns previously reported for Health Service Delivery Areas (HSDA) have not changed in any significant manner, and the comparisons between 2005 and 2007/8 use consistent denominators to ensure correct comparisons.

Further, sport membership data that had previously been reported at the Economic Development region geography is now reported at the HSDA level.

The number of chapters has been increased. Previously, all the wellness indicators were included in one chapter, which comprised most of the Atlas. We have changed this so that each domain (e.g., smoke-free issues, healthy weights) are now single chapters for ease of use. We have also added a new chapter, Free of Chronic Conditions. Free of chronic conditions had previously been included with Wellness Outcomes.

A new administrative boundary for mapping certain indicators has been introduced. This is based on the province's Regional District model, and provides more detailed geographic coverage of certain new indicators.

Indicator Changes

There has been an expansion of the number of indicators mapped. While the first edition of the Atlas had approximately 120 different indicators and over 270 maps, this edition has approximately 160 indicators contained in over 400 maps. While many of the indicators reported in the first edition have been updated in this new edition, some have been dropped for a variety of reasons. First, several have shown no change from the original Atlas, particularly those related to the physical environment. Second, some were removed because there were no new data for them. These included several of the community assets indicators (e.g., community centres, playing fields) and some CCHS indicators (e.g., health utilities index). Third, some of the ActNow BC related program data (e.g., Active Communities) have not been renewed because much of the population had access to this initiative and so little change would have occurred. Fourth, some indicators were removed because legislative changes were implemented, which meant there would be total coverage of the province of a certain wellness characteristic (e.g., municipal smoking restriction bylaws, smoking restrictions in schools, nutrition policies in schools). Overall, approximarely 40 indicators were dropped.

New indicators have replaced some of the ones removed. For example, six individual indicators that helped to make up the CCHS Health Utilities Index have been added, while more indicators related to younger children (particularly those in grades 3/4 in schools) have also been included. Additional indicators related to a variety of wellness assets have been included, such as those related to housing, improving health, employment composition, arts and culture, income equity, volunteerism, nutrition, food supply and food security, new ActNow BC-related programs, and leisure time physical activities, to mention a few. In total, over 80 new indicators have been added.

Organization of the Atlas

Along with this introductory chapter, the Atlas consists of a total of 13 chapters. Chapter 2 provides a summary description of recent wellness and well-being frameworks and key wellness indicators, while Chapter 3 describes the key databases used for constructing our wellness maps. In addition, a guide is provided to help the user read the maps and tables that follow throughout the rest of the Atlas. Chapter 4 provides maps and tables on some key demographic variables that describe the make-up of the BC population in order to provide a context for the maps that follow.

Chapter 5 is the largest chapter in the Atlas, and provides information describing various components of wellness assets. These include families and income, housing characteristics, social connections, aspects of improving

health, education, culture and arts, volunteerism, and safety.

The next five chapters cover key components of the original ActNow BC initiative. Chapter 6 looks at issues related to tobacco-free conditions. Chapter 7 provides indicators related to nutrition and food security, and includes food growing environments, farming, alcohol consumption, healthy eating, and food safety. Chapter 8 includes a variety of factors related to physical activity, while Chapter 9 provides maps and tables on issues of healthy weights. Chapter 10 illustrates items concerning healthy pregnancy and birth.

The next two chapters cover issues that reflect being free of chronic conditions (Chapter 11) and overall wellness outcomes (Chapter 12). The concluding discussion is contained in Chapter 13, and summarizes a variety of key patterns that emerge from the maps and tables presented in the Atlas.

2

Wellness Frameworks and Indicators: An Update

As noted in the first edition of the Atlas, wellness is not easily defined. It implies more than just the absence of disease or illness; wellness is generally viewed from a holistic perspective, and represents the positive aspects of physical, mental, social, and spiritual health (Foster & Keller, 2007; Kindig, 2007; Panelli & Tipa, 2007; Miller, 2005; Larson, 1999). This notion is supported by the World Health Organization's definition of human health as "a state of complete physical, mental and social well-being and not merely the absence of disease and infirmity" (WHO, 1948). It can be argued that wellness is subjective and has a value judgment about what it is and what it isn't (Miller & Foster, 2010). This chapter provides a brief update to the literature that was included in the original *BC Atlas of Wellness,* and describes many of the frameworks and indicators that have more recently been developed to measure wellness and its broad attributes.

The Broadening of Wellness Concepts

Historically, health was focused on disease and illness, or negative attributes rather than positive factors (Millar & Hull, 1997; Foster & Keller, 2007); however, the last half-century has seen a shift to view health from a more positive perspective. It has also seen health used interchangeably with well-being and wellness (Miller & Foster, 2010; cited in Edmunds, 2010), which are holistic in nature, encompassing more than just the physical aspects of an individual, but also the mental, spiritual, emotional, and social dimensions. In some cases, wellness includes a much broader range of dimensions that will be discussed later in the chapter. While this concept of health is being 'rediscovered' by most western societies, it was never truly lost to indigenous populations who have always defined health from a holistic viewpoint (Elliott & Foster, 1995).

The modern use of the word "wellness" dates to the mid-

twentieth century from the work by Halbert Dunn and his book *High-Level Wellness,* in which Dunn defined wellness as "an integrated method of functioning which is oriented to maximizing the potential of which an individual is capable. It requires that the individual maintain a continuum of balance and purposeful direction within the environment where he is functioning" (Dunn, 1961, pp 4-5). Although the book and use of the term wellness received little attention at the time, his ideas were later embraced and expanded upon in the 1970s (SRI International, 2010).

Current literature reveals additional terms corresponding and interrelating to the concept of wellness, such as well-being, life satisfaction, quality of life, human development, flourishing, and happiness. The following represents just a few of the many parameters and dimensions found in the literature to describe aspects of wellness and its close component, well-being.

High levels of wellness involve "progress toward a higher level of functioning, an optimistic view of the future and one's potential" (Larson, 1999, p. 129), and this involves the "integration of the total individual – body, mind and spirit – in the functioning process" (Neilson, 1988, p. 4, as quoted in Larson, 1999). Travis and Callander (2010) argue that to understand the underlying causes of disease we must recognize the levels of disconnection around us. They state "full-spectrum wellness is a multidimensional approach to health and well-being that extends from the individual to the collective and ultimately planet itself" (p. 8). It is about the connections between our state of well-being and our:

- Body, emotions, mind, and spirit;

- Earliest life experiences and our health over our entire lifespan;

- Family, friends, and community;

- Personal and work life; and,

- Environment – from our internal space, to our home, our neighbourhood, and the entire planet.

Another way to consider wellness is by using Antonovsky's salutogenic (or origins of health) model that focuses on factors that support and increase well-being rather than on factors that merely prevent disease (Antonovsky, 1996; Eriksson & Lindstrom, 2008; Lindstrom & Eriksson, 2009). Salutogenesis assumes that illness rather than health is perhaps the norm for people, and looks at factors that enable people to remain healthy despite being bombarded by disease and illness. Two key factors are seen to promote salutogenesis. The first refers to so-called "Generalised Resistance Factors," which consist of such components as: social support, knowledge, experience, intelligence, financial resources, and traditions. The second is a "Sense of Coherence," which is a positive way of viewing life and the ability to manage the stresses of living. Increasingly, salutogenesis is gaining acceptance as a useful model for promoting health and wellness and addressing health inequities (Billings & Hassem, 2009). In a similar context, the BC Atlas of Wellness looks at positive approaches to health, and views key influencers as wellness assets that enable people to stay well and lead happy, satisfying lives. Indeed, the idea of health or wellness assets that we used in the first edition of the Atlas is also being used more often (Morgan & Ziglio, 2007).

Copestake (2007, p.5) sees well-being as "a state of being with others in society where (a) people's basic needs are met, (b) they can act effectively and meaningfully in pursuit of their goals, and (c) they feel satisfied with their life." Well-being has also been defined as "the presence of the highest possible quality of life in its full breadth of expression, focused on but not necessarily exclusive to: good living standards, robust health, a sustainable environment, vital communities, an educated populace, balanced time use, high levels of civic participation, and access to and participation in dynamic arts, culture and recreation" (Institute of Well-being, 2009, p.i). More recently, Brown and Alcoe (2010) define well-being as essentially how we relate *inwards* to ourselves and come to understand ourselves through the physical, mental, spiritual, and emotional levels, and how we relate *outwards* to others, our community, and our environment.

It is quite apparent that wellness and well-being are indeed often used and defined interchangeably.

Wellness and Well-being Framework Dimensions

Measuring wellness is an inexact and changing science (Millar & Hull, 1997) made up of both objective and subjective indicators. In some cases, emphasis is placed entirely on subjective indicators, from both a personal (health, relationships, safety, standard of living, achieving, and community connectedness) and national perspective (the economy, the environment, social conditions, governance, business, and national security) (Cummins et al., 2008).

Most models of wellness include many dimensions (SRI International, 2010). In exploring wellness related frameworks from around the world, it is clear that there is no specific formula for measuring wellness, but there are many recurring dimensions that have been included in various frameworks. It is also interesting to note that while some frameworks have begun to use the terminology 'wellness' or 'well-being,' others have remained with an overall health perspective yet include many subjective wellness indicators. A recent example of this is *Population and Public Health Indicators for British Columbia* (Provincial Health Services Authority, 2008a).

In the past couple of decades, wellness and well-being frameworks have been viewed internationally on quite a broad scale, and especially in the last decade, the indicators they have used have been both objective (quality of life) and subjective (happiness or life satisfaction as self-reported by individuals) (Lepper & McAndrew, 2008). Such frameworks are taking the place of, or complementing, as a key indicator, Gross Domestic Product (GDP), which was routinely used to approximate a country's standard of living, and also considered an equivalent to the population's well-being (Ferdjani, 2010; Hamilton & Redmond, 2010). A few international and Canadian examples are described in the following paragraphs, along with one from BC.

International examples

In Holland, the Institute for Social Research has used the 'life situation index' (*leefsituatie-index*) to present an overview of life of the Dutch population since 1974. The index has indicators in eight domains: housing, health, sports, social participation, socio-cultural leisure activities, ownership of durable consumer goods, holidays, and mobility; and all focus on outcomes, not inputs (Boelhouer, 2010).

In 1989, more than 260 benchmark well-being indicators were approved by the Oregon State legislature, and the first *Oregon Benchmark Progress Report* was published in

1991 and contained nearly 160 separate indicators related to Oregon's well-being. The key domains were related to people, quality of life, and economy (Oregon Progress Board, 1991). Benchmark reports have been published every 2 years, and over time the number of indicators reported has been refined to approximately 90. The last report (2009) had indicators focused on the following: economy, education, civic engagement, social support, public safety, built environment, and natural environment (Oregon Progress Report, 2009). While funding for the Oregon Progress Board was eliminated in 2009, the indicators are being maintained by the state government (State of Oregon, 2009).

The United Nations Development Programme published its first *Human Development Report* with its new Human Development Index (HDI) in 1990. "The premise of the HDI, considered radical at the time, was elegantly simple: national development should be measured not simply by national income, as had long been the practice, but also by life expectancy and literacy" (United Nations Development Programme, 2010, p. iv). The 2010 report contained numerous sub-indices that measure issues of inequality, including gender inequality, multi-dimensional poverty, empowerment, sustainability and vulnerability, human security, perceptions of individual well-being and happiness, civic and community well-being, demographic trends, decent work, education, health, financial flows and commitments, economy and infrastructure, and access to information and communication technology.

The Australian Bureau of Statistics (2010) released the first issue of *Measures of Australia's Progress* (MAP), then called Measuring Australia's Progress, in April 2002. A suite of social, economic, and environmental indicators was developed that aimed to measure the country's progress. Social indicators included: health; education and training; work; crime; family, community, and social cohesion; and democracy, governance, and citizenship. Economic indicators included: national income; national wealth; household economic well-being; housing; and productivity. Environmental indicators included: biodiversity; land; inland waters; oceans and estuaries; atmosphere; and waste.

The New Economics Foundation (NEF) launched the *Happy Planet Index* in 2006. The Index "identified health and a positive experience of life as universal human goals, and the natural resources that our human systems depend upon as fundamental inputs. A successful society is one that can support good lives that don't cost the Earth. The index measures progress towards this target – the ecological efficiency with which happy and healthy lives are supported" (NEF, 2009a, p. 3). It includes factors such as: community, technology, healthcare, economy, values, family and friends, education, governance, employment, consumption, and leisure time. More recently, NEF has introduced a National Accounts of Well-being which included indicators related to personal well-being (e.g., self-esteem, positive feelings, emotional well-being, satisfying life, competence, meaning, and purpose), social well-being (e.g., supportive relationships, trust, and belonging), and well-being at work (e.g., job satisfaction, satisfaction with work-life balance, the emotional experience of work, and assessment of work conditions) (NEF, 2009b).

Also established in 2006 was the *Sustainable Society Index* (SSI) (van der Kerk & Manuel, 2010). The objective of developing this index "was to have an easy and transparent instrument at hand to measure the level of sustainability of a country and to monitor progress to sustainability" (van der Kerk & Manuel, 2010, p. 12). Initially, the SSI was comprised of 22 indicators, but the most recent SSI has 24 indicators. These indicators are rolled up into three major indices: the first, Human Well-being, consists of 9 indicators divided among human sanitation, personal development, and well-balanced society; the second, Environmental Well-being, also consists of 9 indicators divided among healthy environment, climate and energy, and natural resources; the third, Economic Well-being, consists of 6 indicators divided among preparation for the future and economy. For 2010, Canada had a rank of 42 out of 151 countries.

New frameworks have been developed in the past couple of years, such as the *Melbourne Charter* (2008), which focuses on assets and risks related to mental health and well-being, while the *Genuine Progress Index* (GPI) values natural, social, and human capital as well as equity, environmental quality, security, and population health (Canadian Population Health Initiative, 2009). In the US, a well-being index was created that has been calculated on a monthly basis nationally by Gallup since January 2008 (Gallup & Healthways, 2011). Gallup and Healthways also produce a biannual report on the well-being of each of the US states and their respective cities, as well as an annual report on each of the 435 US congressional districts' overall well-being composite score and a score in each of six sub-indices, including life evaluation, emotional health, physical health, healthy behaviour, work environment, and basic access.

In early February, 2008, France established *The Commission on the Measurement of Economic Performance and Social Progress* (Stiglitz, Sen, & Fitoussi, 2009a,b) because of dissatisfaction with current indicators of economy and society. A key message and unifying theme emerging from the report of the Commission was the need to "*shift emphasis from measuring economic production to measuring people's well-being.* And measures of well-being should be put in a context of sustainability" (Stiglitz, Sen, & Fitoussi, 2009a p.12). The report went on to note that well-being is multi-dimensional, and the following should be considered simultaneously: material living standards (income, consumption, wealth); health; education; personal activities including work; political voice and governance; social connections and relationships; environment (present and future conditions); and insecurity, of an economic as well as physical nature. Further "Quality-of-life indicators in all the dimensions covered should assess inequalities in a comprehensive way" (Stiglitz, Sen, & Fitoussi, 2009a, p.15).

One of the more novel frameworks has been constructed to develop the *Gross National Happiness Index*, developed by the Centre for Bhutan Studies and launched in late 2008 to account for many more dimensions than are included in traditional GDP figures. The index consists of factors in nine key domains: psychological well-being, time use, community vitality, culture, health, education, environmental diversity, living standard, and governance (The Centre for Bhutan Studies, 2008).

More recently, the UK government has become interested in measuring well-being (Thomas & Evans, 2010; Waldron, 2010). Initially, an All-Party Parliamentary Group on Well-being Economics was established in 2009 to: promote the enhancement of well-being as an important government goal; encourage the adoption of well-being indicators as complementary measures of progress to GDP; and promote policies designed to enhance well-being. Through the Office for National Statistics (ONS), the new UK Conservative government launched a debate on national well-being. It started in November 2010 and ended in April 2011. The consultation document notes no fewer than 25 indicators that the literature has described as being important in measuring well-being, and has established a Well-being Knowledge Bank (ONS, 2010).

Just as the Atlas was going to press, the Organization for Economic Cooperation and Development (OECD), announced that it was developing comparative information on the conditions of the lives of people in developed market economies. The result, to be published in late 2011 will allow the comparisons of well-being across OECD countries based on material living conditions and quality of life (OECD, 2011a). The index is comprised of the following topics: housing, income, jobs, community, education, environment, governance, health, life satisfaction, safety, and work-life balance, and includes a total of 21 indicators. The index currently covers 34 member countries of the OECD, and data are provided in such a manner that users can develop their own weighting of the indicators, similar to the manner suggested in the our original Atlas, to develop their own index (OECD, 2011b).

Some Canadian examples

Within Canada, several wellness/well-being frameworks have been developed. In 1999, the Federation of Canadian Municipalities (FCM) introduced the *Quality of Life Reporting System* (QOLRS) (FCM, 1999; 2010). Starting with 16 municipalities, the QOLRS now has 24 communities in 7 provinces that report indicators. Only Vancouver and Surrey are included from BC. Eight domains of indicators were included: population resources; community affordability; quality of employment; quality of housing; community stress; health of community; community safety; and community participation. Soon after, the Toronto Community Foundation published Toronto's first *Vital Signs* report in 2001, and has published periodic reports on key quality of life issues in the community. Since that time, 16 communities, including Vancouver and Victoria in BC, now provide similar reports. Each community chooses its own indicators, but every year there are a set of common issues and core indicators that all foundations include in their reports, and upon which Community Foundations of Canada bases its national report. Community foundations consult with a wide range of local groups to ensure their indicators capture their area's unique issues and attributes (Toronto Community Foundation, 2010).

In January 2007, May identified 13 domains of well-being: production; infrastructure and production capital; knowledge capital; natural resource capital; ecosystems; social relationships; income consumption leisure; employment and working conditions; education, literacy, skills, and training; society, culture, politics, and justice; community safety and social vitality; demographics; and health. Later that year, the Conference Board of Canada published its *Report Card on Canada*, which was designed "to identify relative strengths and weaknesses in Canada's socio-economic performance," and has provided annual updates since that time. Although earlier reports had been issued, this new report card covered six key domains: economy, society, innovation, environment, health, and education and skills. The Conference Board of Canada indicated that a high, sustainable quality of life for Canadians was dependent on high and sustainable performances in these six domains. Canada's performance is regularly compared with 17 other "peer" nations based on population size, land mass, and income per capita (Conference Board of Canada, 2011).

Human Resources and Skills Development Canada (2010) developed a series of indicators to measure well-being starting in 2008. "Individual Canadians and their families interact with each other and with social institutions over the course of their lives, building up and expending resources of different kinds (such as time, finances, goods and services, and social networks). Resources can be personal assets such as health and skills. Resources can also be the goods and services provided by social institutions. Finally, resources can be societal assets such as the environment and social order." Ten key domains have been recognized: learning; financial security; environment; security; health; leisure; social participation; family life; housing; and work.

More recently, the *Canadian Index of well-being* (CIW) has started to measure well-being from the perspective of quality of life, including items such as: standard of living, health, the quality of our environment, education and skill levels, the way we use time, the vitality of communities, participation in the democratic process, and the state of leisure and culture (Canadian Index of Well-being, 2010a).

A BC example

Within BC, perhaps the best known group that measures issues of well-being on a regular basis is the BC Progress Board, which was established in 2001 to measure and benchmark BC's performance over time and relative to other jurisdictions. This approach was to help to determine if competitiveness and quality of life are improving, and to advise on strategies, policies, and actions that could enhance BC's economic and social well-being regardless of whether government, business, or individual actions are required (BC Progress Board, 2002). Key areas that are measured include economic growth, standard of living, jobs, environmental quality, health outcomes, and social condition, and the number of key indicators have been increased over time (BC Progress Board, 2010). BC is ranked on its "performances" relative to other Canadian provinces, neighbouring jurisdictions, and certain OECD countries.

Key Wellness Dimensions for the BC Atlas of Wellness

In the first edition of the *BC Atlas of Wellness* the following dimensions were identified, based on an extensive review of the literature: physical, psychological/emotional, social, intellectual, spiritual, occupational, and environmental (Miller & Foster, 2006). Key works included those by Adams et al. (1997), Anspaugh et al. (2004), Crose et al. (1992), Durlak (2000), Hales (2005), Helliwell (2005),

Hettler (1980), Leafgren (1990), Renger et al. (2000), Ryan and Deci (2001), and Ryff and Singer (2006), among others. As noted above, recent developments have centred on the importance of these established dimensions and added new dimensions into the framework. These new dimensions include economic, cultural, climate, as well as governance and social justice. What follows is a brief update to the material discussed in the first edition of the *BC Atlas of Wellness*.

Physical wellness

Physical wellness is probably the most common dimension included in health and wellness frameworks, and generally refers to an individual's physical health, physical activity level, nutrition, self-care, and vitality or longevity (Miller & Foster, 2006; Alcoe, 2010; Brown & Alcoe, 2010). Physical wellness can relate specifically to an individual's physical fitness, such as one's strength and flexibility, amount and type of physical fitness, or intent to participate in physical activities. It can also relate to whether or not there are organized sports, activities, or facilities available (Active Healthy Kids Canada, 2010). Physical wellness incorporates such things as diet and whether or not an individual has access to healthy food, whether they are a healthy weight, or whether their consumption of fat, salt, and sugar are at healthy levels.

Physical wellness can also relate specifically to an individual taking specific actions and avoiding potentially harmful behaviours such as smoking, illicit drug use, and excessive alcohol consumption. In addition, physical health includes both objective indicators such as life expectancy at birth (Veenhoven, 2008), and subjective indicators like self-reported health, which can often be a good predictor of objective health outcomes (OECD, 2008). However, physical wellness does not always correlate with a sense of well-being; a person can have poor health and at the same time experience positive well-being, or vice versa (Anspaugh, Hamrick, & Rosato, 2004).

Psychological /emotional wellness

Psychological/emotional wellness can include feelings, behaviour, relationships, goals, and personal strengths (Hamilton and Redmond, 2010). It encompasses indicators such as happiness, life satisfaction, and positive mental health. Happiness "incorporates a sense of individual vitality, opportunities to undertake meaningful, engaging activities which confer feelings of competence and autonomy, and the possession of a stock of inner resources that helps one cope when things go wrong" (New Economics Foundation, 2009a, p.10). A feeling of happiness can also help to heal the sick, and acts as a protector against getting ill for people in good health (Veenhoven, 2008).

Psychological wellness includes having an element of control over one's life and the ability to deal with the demands and stresses experienced as part of our everyday lives, which evidence has shown can have a positive effect on our health and well-being (McEwan et al., 2008).

Psychological and emotional wellness include experiencing curiosity and enjoyment in life, having an optimistic outlook on life and the future, a feeling of fulfillment and self-esteem and self-acceptance, and the ability to bounce back from setbacks and failures, often referred to as resiliency (Foster & Keller, 2007). Psychological and emotional wellness can also reduce anxiety and distress, and give one the ability to stand back from difficult situations and react in a more resourceful way (Alcoe, 2010; Brown & Alcoe, 2010).

Social wellness

Social wellness relates to the relationships and interactions one has with others, the community, and nature (Foster and Keller, 2007). Included in social wellness is how an individual engages with and supports the community and environment in everyday actions such as volunteer work (May, 2007) or belonging to a community or social group (New Economics Foundation, 2004). "Giving time or money voluntarily to help others is seen by sociologists as a marker of cohesiveness in a society" (Charities Aid Foundation, 2010, p.1). Trust is also an important aspect of social wellness, and has been shown to increase well-being in communities (Drabsch, 2010; May, 2007).

Social support networks are important for social wellness – having the support of family and friends "results in improved sense of well-being and is important in helping people to manage stress and the adverse impacts of challenging life events and circumstances" (Lightman, Mitchell, & Wilson, 2008, p.5). Supportive environments are also essential for social wellness, such as the types of supports available and the existence of networks and community organizations – all permit people to build connections with others and form relationships of trust (Lightman, Mitchell & Wilson, 2008; May, 2007).

Indicators for social wellness include one's sense of belonging, whether an individual has social, emotional, and informational support, and how connected they feel to their family, friends, and community.

Intellectual wellness

Intellectual wellness includes both a personal commitment to lifelong learning and an interest in sharing one's knowledge with others. Intellectual wellness can help with positive thinking and decision-making, and enable an individual to use creative problem-solving to overcome barriers and difficulties (Brown & Alcoe, 2010). It "is the degree to which one engages in creative and stimulating activities, as well as the use of resources to expand knowledge and focus on the acquisition, development, application, and articulation of critical thinking" (Foster & Keller, 2007, p.13). As such, education and literacy are important elements to achieving intellectual wellness, and are routinely shown to influence an individual's health and well-being as they enable coping mechanisms and other life skills (Lightman, Mitchell & Wilson, 2008; Field, 2009). Education and literacy can also help with the ability to function in various societal contexts and plan for and adapt to future situations (Institute of Well-being, 2009), and have been shown to have a strong correlation with future personal prosperity and well-being (BC Progress Board, 2008).

Education is particularly important during childhood, and is one of the major indicators used by *Save the Children* for their child well-being and development index (Save the Children, 2008). Other indicators that can be used to measure intellectual wellness include a child's readiness to learn, library use, awareness of cultural events, and an interest in future learning.

Spiritual wellness

Spiritual wellness includes an increased contentment and a sense of connection with something 'greater' than oneself, and involves learning more about "who you are" and recognizing inner values and resources (Alcoe, 2010; Brown & Alcoe, 2010). It can provide a feeling of fulfillment, giving one meaning in life and connection to other human beings (Canadian Institute for Health Information, 2008). Spiritual wellness can give a sense of purpose and help to create a personal set of beliefs and values to be used in everyday conduct and actions.

It is important to note that spiritual wellness is not synonymous with religion; however, religious beliefs can be included within the concept of spiritual wellness. Indigenous groups have recognized spirituality as a key element of health for a long time, while the relationship between spirituality, religion, and health has been an emerging issue in western research (McEwan et al., 2008). The Australian Unity well-being Index Survey 19 (Cummins et al., 2008) found that people who have a weak level of satisfaction with their spiritual/religious beliefs have low subjective well-being.

Occupational wellness

Occupational wellness includes the level of satisfaction one achieves from work, and the extent to which one's occupation allows for the expression of skills and values. It includes working conditions and whether or not the workplace is safe or stressful – all of which can contribute to one's health and well-being (Lightman, Mitchell & Wilson, 2008). Occupational wellness can include a sense of fulfillment in one's work, and the balance of work and leisure time (Foster & Keller, 2007).

More recently, occupational wellness has been associated with the workplace environment and the availability of wellness programs as it is recognized that people spend a large portion of their day in the workplace. Environments that prohibit tobacco use, serve healthy food in the canteen, offer physical activities or facilities to employees, and provide employees with a sense of control over their work can all contribute to occupational wellness.

Environmental wellness

Previous definitions of environmental wellness focused on the interaction of individuals to their home, work, community, and nature (Miller & Foster, 2006), however more recent literature defines it from an ecological perspective, focusing on the built, or physical, environment and the natural environment (Institute of well-being, 2009; May, 2007).

The built environment refers to how an area or neighbourhood is designed, and has been shown to have a significant effect on population health (Canadian Population Health Initiative, 2006; Provincial Health Services Authority, 2008b). A built environment that is conducive to wellness would include such things as adequate green space for recreation, areas built for walking and cycling, a safe environment to encourage outdoor pursuits, areas of vegetation to help improve air quality, good public transportation, and smoke-free public areas including parks and beaches (Provincial Health Services Authority, 2008b; Lightman, Mitchell & Wilson, 2008; May, 2007).

The environment might include the exposure to pollutants and safe water and food supplies, which all have a direct impact on health and wellness (Lightman, Mitchell & Wilson, 2008). Also included could be the ecosystem as a whole, and in some cultural contexts where people live in close harmony to the land, the well-being of herds or wild species can have a direct effect on the overall wellness of the people living within that ecosystem (May, 2007).

Economic wellness

Economic wellness was historically linked to Gross Domestic Product (GDP). The Index of Economic well-being (IEWB) looks at a much broader definition of economic wellness, such as average current consumption flows, aggregate wealth accumulation for future consumption, economic equality, and economic security (Osberg, 2009).

Income is obviously an important indicator in economic wellness as it determines living conditions and access to important things such as safe housing and neighbourhoods, food security, and aids individuals and families to purchase their basic needs. Increased income can, in some cases, help to alleviate stress (Lightman, Mitchell & Wilson, 2008); however, increased income past the point where those basic needs are attained has increasingly less influence on wellness (May, 2007).

Income can have a direct impact on the wellness and health of individuals and families, but it can also affect the overall health of a society. It has been shown that societies with a more equal income distribution have better overall health than those societies with a wider variation in the distribution of income (Mikkonen & Raphael, 2010).

Other indicators to measure economic wellness include the relative distribution of wealth, poverty rates, income volatility, and economic security, including the security of jobs, food, housing, and the social safety net (Institute of Well-being, 2009).

Cultural wellness

UNESCO has defined culture as "the set of distinctive spiritual, material, intellectual and emotional features of a society or a social group that encompasses not only art and literature, but lifestyles, ways of living together, value systems, traditions, and beliefs" (UNESCO, 2009, p.1).

Culture is deeply embedded within one's personal identity (Torjman, 2004), and thus cultural wellness has become a particularly important factor in measuring wellness in societies where there are substantial differences in cultural backgrounds. Many wellness and well-being frameworks out of Australia and New Zealand place an emphasis on cultural wellness (Hamilton & Redmond, 2010; Grieves, 2009; Ministry of Social Development, 2008).

Participation in cultural events or programs has "been found to promote social connectedness in communities and shape civic behaviour later in life" (Torjman, 2004, p.6). On the flip side, cultural groups that feel excluded or stigmatized can be associated with greater risks and poorer health outcomes (Lightman, Mitchell & Wilson, 2008).

Cultural wellness can include: acceptance of different cultures and having society accept one's own cultural identity (Lightman, Mitchell & Wilson, 2008); freedom from discrimination and feelings of exclusion due to ethnicity, race, religion, or values; the ability to participate in cultural events; access to and participation in the arts (Canadian Index of Well-being, 2010b; Pennock, 2009; Institute of Well-being, 2009); and such things as speaking an indigenous language and having the ability to retain that language (Ministry of Social Development, 2008).

The *Canadian Index of Well-being* (CIW) embraces leisure time and cultural participation and the significant contributions they make to the well-being of individuals, communities, and society at large (Canadian Index of Well-being, 2010b). In fact, Torjman (2004, p.5) found that "culturally based programs in the areas of art, drama, music and dance provide a different, but equally important, means of building skills in creative thinking, decision-making and problem-solving. They foster social skills including co-operative work, negotiation, conflict resolution and tolerance for difference as well as personal skills such as individual responsibility, perseverance, self-management and integrity," thus contributing to individual and community well-being.

Indicators for the CIW include engagement in arts and culture activities, volunteering for culture and recreation, attendance at performing arts performances, visitation to parks and historic sites, nights away on vacation, and household expenditures on culture and recreation.

Climate wellness

It is not surprising that extreme weather and climate variations can have an unfavourable effect on well-being of both individuals and societies. While the dimension of climate wellness is not found in many frameworks as yet, it is an area that is likely to have a greater impact as extreme weather events such as heat waves, floods, snowstorms, and droughts increase in many parts of the world. Major changes in climate will necessitate adjustments for individuals, communities, and societies as a whole.

These effects of climate change have been shown to cause emotional distress and negatively impact on mental health (Miller & Foster, 2010). Extreme weather can also cause disruptions to social and economic activities within households, communities, or entire nations. The Australian Unity well-being Index found a decrease from 2007 to 2008 in Australians' satisfaction with the natural environment due to the effects of climate change in Australia (Cummins et al., 2008).

Governance/social justice wellness

Governance and social justice wellness is also a dimension found in only a few wellness frameworks, however the political environment in which one lives can greatly affect one's well-being (May, 2007). Rights and freedoms can also have an enormous impact on well-being (Pennock, 2009). Social justice includes such aspects as the distribution of resources, the application of the law, and the treatment by others as individuals and as members of society (May, 2007).

The Legatum Institute (2009, p.14) found that "countries in which sound governance leads to satisfied citizens are most likely to have the healthiest economic fundamentals and the most entrepreneurial societies. Accountable political institutions, protections for civil liberties, predictability in contracts, and reliable regulatory structures all help promote prosperity."

Indicators for governance and social justice wellness include satisfaction with the electoral process, access to information, and the openness, transparency, effectiveness, fairness, and equity of governments (Helliwell, 2005; Pennock, 2009; Institute of Well-being, 2009).

Health determinants – wellness assets

In keeping with the WHO definition of health, the so-called "determinants of population health" can be viewed as assets for wellness. By assets we mean that possession of certain characteristics results in greater likelihood of a higher level of wellness. They do not "determine" wellness, but rather provide an increased potential for wellness.

While the Lalonde Report (1974) developed the framework related to important factors that determined health status (lifestyle, environment, human biology, and health services), research evidence now shows that the following are key "determinants" of health, or wellness assets: income and social status; social support networks; education; employment/working conditions; social environments; physical environments; personal health practices and coping skills; early child development; biology and genetic endowment; health services; gender; and culture (PHAC, 2003;Canadian Population Health Initiative, 2004, 2006, 2008a, b; Keon & Pepin, 2009). To these can be added: income distribution/equity; unemployment and job security; food security; aboriginal status; race; and disability (Mikkonen & Raphael, 2010).

But while these assets are individually important, many also act in concert with each other, and the Commission on the Social Determinants of Health (CSDH) (2008) takes a broad holistic view of the social determinants of health: "The poor health of the poor, the social gradient in health within countries, and the marked health inequities between countries are caused by the unequal distribution of power, income, goods, and services, globally and nationally, the consequent unfairness in the immediate, visible circumstances of peoples lives – their access to health care, schools, and education, their conditions of work and leisure, their homes, communities, towns, or cities – and their chances of leading a flourishing life" (p. 1).

More recently, the issues of determinants and inequities have been raised by the Standing Committee on Social Affairs, Science and Technology of the Canadian Parliament. The Committee noted that at least half of the health of Canada's population could be attributed to socioeconomic factors that are complex and intertwined, and also noted the importance of these assets at different life stages of individuals. Finally, where an individual resides was viewed as being very important for health (Keon & Pepin, 2009). Further, Hayes (2007) has noted that the influence of social factors on health status has been known for over 150 years in Britain, and many studies have shown how certain of these assets (e.g., income and education) show consistent health- and wellness-related gradients, such that the higher the income or educational achievements, the greater the health and wellness status of the population (Keon & Pepin, 2009; Mikkonen & Raphael, 2010). Hayes has also described the importance of place on health and wellness (Hayes, 2007), and increasingly place, neighbourhood, and community are viewed as important because of their assets in health promotion and wellness generation, while differences among countries are often a result of differing policies related to wellness dimensions.

Summary

It is clear from the recent wellness-related frameworks developed around the globe and in Canada that wellness is viewed from an holistic perspective and represents a positive state of being rather than just the absence of disease. Although there are many different models and frameworks, they are all based upon similar core dimensions that include the attributes discussed above. Many of the components contribute to wellness through a series of complex and interacting mechanisms, but many of the factors are subjective in nature and involve perceptions by individuals. As frameworks continue to evolve, so too will indicators and dimensions of wellness, but the vast majority of the indicators included in this Atlas are included in one or more of the frameworks and studies discussed above, or relate to the original ActNow BC initiatives. However, it is important to note that while the

ActNow BC framework is still important for this Atlas, we have moved far beyond that initiative and incorporated additional dimensions that have been discussed in both the academic and grey literature.

3

Data, Information, and Map Interpretation

Introduction

This chapter provides a summary of the data sources we have utilized in the Atlas, along with the key map outlines that are used to map the geographical variations in wellness indicators and assets. A brief guide on how to analyse the maps, tables, and graphs used in the following chapters is also provided.

In producing the wellness maps, several key data sets and information sources were used. Criteria for including data are as follows:

- Data provide measures related to wellness dimensions and assets for wellness.

- Data have been collected on an ongoing or periodic basis. This allows an opportunity to measure changes and trends over time.

- Data can be analysed on a geographical basis, primarily for the 16 Health Service Delivery Areas (HSDAs) of the province. This ensures that geographical differences can be measured, and patterns detected. For some maps, depending on the data source, School Districts (59), Economic Development Regions (8), or Regional Districts (29) are used (see following pages). In some cases, "custom" maps are presented, based on a single, novel indicator.

- Data are readily available and can be accessed inexpensively. No new data have been specifically collected for the analyses included in the Atlas. Rather, existing data are brought together from a variety of different sources in order to develop the maps. However, some of the data that we use have been modified to add value so that comparisons can be made. For example, raw data are often converted into percentages or rates so that standard comparisons can be made between geographical regions.

- Data have not been mapped and published elsewhere in the way we have developed. Certain indicators, or their derivatives, may have been previously mapped, but in a different manner. This is often related to the wellness approach, or "half-full" approach we have taken, rather than the "half-empty" approach that other health-related atlases often employ. In large part, the maps included in the Atlas are unique, and have been constructed specifically for the purposes of this Atlas. In just a couple of instances this is not the case, as key maps and data are necessary to provide context for the maps that follow.

Some of the key data sources we use are based on survey data. Information collected through surveys is very useful for measuring dimensions and assets related to wellness. As previously noted, wellness is not an easy thing to define, and it can be argued that wellness is subjective and has a value judgment about what it is and what it isn't (Miller & Foster, 2010). Using individuals' responses to specific questions captures this subjectivity around wellness.

A major challenge that a project of this nature faces is the issue of having current information. It may take a couple of years for data to be checked and verified from survey data, and surveys such as the Canada Census occur only every 5 years. Many of the indicators in this chapter are based on survey data, so may be several years old. However, in most cases they were the latest that were readily available for geographical analyses at the time of writing. Where appropriate, comparisons with the last previous survey are made so that changes can be assessed.

Several administrative data sets are also included. The following are the key data sources that were used for mapping purposes, and limitations and cautions are noted.

The Canadian Community Health Survey

The Canadian Community Health Survey (CCHS) is undertaken by Statistics Canada, in partnership with Health Canada, on a regular basis across the country. Because CCHS is a national survey, it allows geographical comparisons to be made not only within the province, but also between provinces and with overall Canadian averages (McKee et al., 2009). This data set was used prominently in the original BC Atlas of Wellness, and is again a mainstay of this second edition: approximately 50 indicators and close to 250 maps are derived from this data set. There is a standard set of questions asked of all participants, whose ages range from 12 years and up. Provinces can buy extra modules of questions dealing with a variety of different health- and wellness-related factors. BC, for example, purchased additional modules related to such areas of interest as social and emotional supports, food security, food content, and injuries in the 2007/8 survey (CCHS 4.1), which is the latest full survey data set available for BC at the time of writing.

The CCHS was initially undertaken every second year, and the original Atlas reported wellness indicators based on the 2005 CCHS 3.1 data set. Since then, a change in procedure has taken place so that surveys are undertaken every year, and it is possible to report a half sample on an annual basis. This is certainly very useful for making comparisons year-to-year and for comparisons among provinces, but because the annual sample is only one-half of a full sample as was collected in 2005, the sample size for examining within-province differences is not as useful for our purposes.

The data collection for the full sample for CCHS 4.1, which can be reasonably compared with the 2005 sample, took place over the 24-month period of January 2007 to December 2008 inclusive. Approximately 50% of the respondents were sampled in both years. The total combined sample size (N) was approximately 14,650. Data collection varied throughout the months of the year, with over 1,800 being sampled in March and May of both years, and less than 700 sampled in each of June and December of both years. Accordingly, some caution is required in interpreting the results of the maps and supporting tables, especially for those questions that might be related to seasonal activities. Further, over that time period, there were major changes in the economy which

may have affected some of the responses occurring late in 2008.

As noted above, respondents are limited to those 12 years of age and older and, as the title suggests, the survey collects information from respondents living in the general community. Therefore data are limited, in that individuals living in institutions (e.g., care or health institutions, jails) or living on Indian reserves or Crown lands, full-time members of the Canadian Armed Forces, and residents of very remote regions are not included. Some of these groups, particularly Aboriginal peoples, are known to have, on average, generally poorer health and wellness status than the remainder of the population (Kendall, 2009); those in care facilities are often there because of poor health or disability factors, and those in correctional facilities also have much poorer health status than the general population (Møller et al., 2007). As a consequence, the data presented from the survey may be biased toward more positive values of wellness, although approximately 98% of the Canadian population aged 12 and older are covered. However, given the relatively large numbers of remote communities, particularly Indian reserves, in the province, it is likely that the coverage for BC may be lower than the national average.

As with any survey data, although best attempts are made to ensure clarity of questions, honesty of responses, and randomness in the selection of respondents, these criteria may not always be fully met, and caution should always be practiced when studying the data and making conclusions based on the resulting analyses.

The Share File data set has been used for our analysis. Only responses from those individuals who agreed to share their data with Statistics Canada's partners (e.g., provincial/territorial health departments) are included in the Share File. Reporting of the data follows the guidelines suggested by Statistics Canada (Statistics Canada, 2009).

Indicators from samples of less than 10 individuals, or those with a coefficient of variation greater than 33.33% are not reported in this analysis, while those with a coefficient of variation between 16.67% and 33.33% are noted because of potential instability in results. This instability is usually related to smaller sample sizes.

Selected characteristics of the BC CCHS 4.1 respondents were as follows:

- Nearly 97% of interviews were conducted in English, 2% were conducted in Chinese languages, and 1% in other languages.

- 52% were married or living common law, 27% were

single or never married, and 21% were widowed, divorced, or separated.

- 54% were females.

- Median annual family income was just under $60,000.

- 74% were born in Canada, 11% in Europe, 10% in Asia, and 5% elsewhere.

- Approximately 5% self-identified as Aboriginal.

- Approximately 60% of the total sample had paid work, and for those between the ages of 15 and 74 years, more than 74% of men and over 59% of women respondents were in the paid work force.

- Over 19% had at least a bachelor degree.

For BC, survey data are available at the HSDA level, and numerous indicators based on the survey are mapped in this Atlas. In most cases, indicators are mapped using the five map model introduced in the first edition of the *BC Atlas of Wellness*, and most are based on the following demographic cohorts:

- Respondents age 12 years and over

- Male respondents age 12 years and over

- Female respondents age 12 years and over

- Respondents age 12 to 19 years

- Respondents age 65 years and over

Data are also provided for the age group 20 to 64 years (mid-age cohort), but maps are not provided because in most, but not all, instances, patterns and results are very similar to the age 12 years and over group. In some instances, different age groups are used as the standard age groups are not appropriate. This occurs primarily for indicators related to questions concerning working, or being free of chronic conditions. For example, all indicators related to working and work settings use the following age groups: 15 to 75 years; 15 to 24 years; 25 to 44 years; 45 to 75 years. These groups better reflect the working age population. The free of chronic disease indicators in Chapter 11 have the following age cohorts: 12 years and over; 35 to 49 years; 50 to 64 years; and 65 years and over. These reflect the fact that most chronic diseases are age-related.

Another difference involves the stress-related indicator in Chapter 12, which uses the age cohort 15 years and over, rather than 12 years and over, to reflect the fact that the question was only asked of respondents aged 15 years and older. Finally, the Body Mass Index (BMI) indicator

uses these age groups: 18 years and over; 20 to 34 years; 35 to 64 years; and 65 years and over. A different BMI calculation was used for the under 18 age group, and we were not confident that comparisons with the younger age group would be entirely valid. A separate set of maps has been developed for the younger age cohort, and this allows us to give gender comparisons.

The values of the indicators are given as percentages (%) of respondents answering a question in a manner that is positive from a wellness perspective (e.g., percent non-smoker, rather than percent smoker is used). Provincial values from the 2005 CCHS 3.1 sample are compared for the majority of the variables so that changes between 2005 and 2007/8 can be observed – have things become better, or worse – and a graph is provided that allows comparisons between the BC and Canadian samples for the 2007/8 CCHS data set, so that differences between BC and Canada can be analysed – is BC doing better or worse than Canada as a whole. In some cases, not all provinces/territories participated in certain modules of the CCHS, and so "Canada" values are only the average of those who did participate. Therefore, caution in making comparisons is necessary in these cases. Cautions are noted in the text where this occurs.

A brief discussion of sample size, confidence intervals, and significance levels is important so that users can understand the meaning of the term "*significant*" when used with sample survey data in the Atlas. Sample survey data only give an estimate of the actual value, and so it is useful to provide confidence intervals for each value. The intervals provide the range that the actual value of the population will fall within, and we have used a confidence interval of 95%. What this means is that, if the survey was repeated, the point value would occur within this interval 95 times out of 100. For example, if the point estimate of an indicator is 80%, and the standard error of the estimate yields a 3% error either side of 80%, then the point value estimated by repeated sampling of the population will be in the interval from 77% to 83%, 95 times out of 100. If a larger sample is collected, the confidence interval will be narrower, giving a clearer picture of the true value of the response. For example, if the sample size is doubled, the confidence interval either side of the estimated value may shrink to say 2%, so that the estimate of the value will fall within 2% either side of 80%, that is, 78% to 82%. As the sample size increases, the confidence interval gets narrower, giving a closer approximation of the true value.

For our purposes, confidence intervals have been calculated using the "bootstrap" methodology provided by Statistics Canada. To determine if two sample estimates are *significantly different*, their confidence intervals are compared. If one sample (A) has a value of 80% with a confidence interval of 6%, its real value lies within the range of 77% to 83%, or 3 percentage points either side of 80%. If another sample (B) has a value of 76% and a confidence interval of 4%, the real value falls within the range of 74% to 78%. Because the lowest value (77%) of sample A is less than the highest value (78%) of sample B, we cannot say that the two values are *statistically significantly different* from one another. If a third sample (C) has a value of 88% with a confidence interval of 8%, then its true value falls within the range of 84% to 92%. Because the lowest value of sample C (84%) is higher than the highest confidence interval values of both samples A and B, then we can say with 95% confidence that sample C is *statistically significantly different* (higher) than both samples A and B. Use of the term *"significantly different"* in the Atlas means there is a *statistically significant difference* between two values.

McCreary Centre Society Adolescent Health Survey (AHS)

Over the past decade or so, the McCreary Centre Society (MCS), a non-profit agency in Vancouver, BC, focused on youth health and behaviour, has undertaken four major surveys of students in grades 7 to 12 in BC. The most recent survey (AHS IV), which included over 29,315 BC public school students in 1,760 classrooms across 50 of BC's 59 school districts, was completed between February and June 2008. It was the largest survey of its kind in Canada, and provided a comprehensive picture of the physical and emotional health of BC youth, including risk and protective factors. There were nearly 150 questions in the survey instrument, which was administered in randomly selected classes throughout most school districts. Participation was voluntary, and parental consent procedures were determined at the school district level.

Selected characteristics of the AHS IV respondents are as follows (note, not all students identified their grade level):

- 48.5% were males and 51.5% were females
- 19% were in grade 7 (5,496 students)
- 17% were in grade 8 (4,890 students)
- 18% were in grade 9 (5,195 students)
- 16% were in grade 10 (4,743 students)
- 16% were in grade 11 (4,805 students)
- 14% were in grade 12 (4,114 students)

Public health nurses, nursing students, and other trained personnel administered the confidential and anonymous survey in English. This may have affected those youth who were new immigrants and/or those who did not have the language or literacy skills to complete the questionnaire, so some caution in interpreting results is needed. While this is a very rich and robust data set, not all school districts in the province elected to be included in the survey, leaving several areas of the province without data. Data, while collected at the school level, were sampled and weighted by Statistics Canada based on the characteristics of the school population in each HSDA, so that the samples were representative of all BC youth in grades 7 to 12. For 2008, data gaps occurred for Northeast, and data for Fraser South and Fraser East were combined and weighted accordingly. More information about the MCS survey, along with numerous reports based on their surveys, can be found on the McCreary Centre Society website (McCreary Centre Society, 2010). As with the CCHS indicators, those from AHS IV have 95% confidence intervals, calculated by staff at MCS, so that *significant differences* could be noted.

School District Data

There is a variety of data related to wellness indicators available from school districts, including survey and administrative data. For several years, the BC Ministry of Education has undertaken annual satisfaction surveys of students in selected grades, canvassing various issues, including: achievement, human and social development, safety, preparation for the future, school environment, and health. The survey also canvasses parents and teachers and is known as the School Satisfaction Survey. We only use the Students Satisfaction Survey results in the Atlas. The survey is delivered online, takes about 10 minutes to complete, and is available 24/7 from January to mid-April. These data are readily available at the school district level (Ministry of Education, 2010c). Some key characteristics of the student respondents in 2008/9 are as follows:

- 90% of grade 3/4 participated (33,968 students)
- 88% of grade 7 participated (36,539 students)
- 72% of grade 10 participated (33,489 students)
- 59% of grade 12 participated (26,031 students)
- 49% were females and 51% were males

A number of indicators have been mapped at this geographic level, including physical activity, nutrition, learning how to stay healthy, learning about art and music, school safety, bullying, and smoke-free behaviours.

Although a survey instrument was used only for grades 3/4, 7, 10, and 12, all students in those grades were surveyed, eliminating the need for developing confidence intervals, as was necessary for the CCHS and McCreary AHS data. Given the young age of some of the respondents, and the fact that the response rate drops off as grade increases, caution should be exercised when interpreting results.

Educational achievement data are also available. Key indicators include Foundation Skills Assessments for Grades 4 and 7 in reading, writing, and numeracy. There has been controversy about the use of these assessments, and not all students participate. Approximately 17 to 18% of potential respondents did not participate in the 2009/10 school year, so some caution in interpreting the results is necessary.

The Human Early Learning Partnership (HELP) at the University of British Columbia continues to collect "readiness to learn" data on entry level kindergarten students throughout the province of BC using the Early Development Instrument (EDI). Only a limited number of maps are included in this Atlas, as others are available elsewhere (HELP, 2010).

2006 Canada Population Census

The Government of Canada undertakes a general census of the total population and its characteristics every 5 years. The 2011 census data will not be available for some time, and so the 2006 census data were used in the Atlas as they represent the latest available. Key assets of wellness and determinants of health are available from this data source, and several are mapped to provide a sense of the "assets" or "positives" available at the population level to support wellness. The data for our purposes were publicly available through BC Stats, which has been an important partner in working with us and providing advice on this Atlas. One caution with respect to census data is that several of the population characteristics depend on self-identification, such as "Aboriginal heritage." This may be underestimated as a result.

The format for the 2011 census has been changed, so that a majority of questions have become voluntary rather than mandatory, as was previously the case. Only a limited number of questions will be mandatory, and these are related to numbers living in a household, names, age, sex, language, and marital status. The so called "long form" census, which is given to 20% of households, provides a lot of key socioeconomic data, much of which is related to wellness assets. This component of the census is now voluntary, and will be collected as part of the National Household Survey. This change was introduced by the

Federal Government because of stated privacy concerns. While this does not affect the quality of data in the current edition of this Atlas, it may be compromised for any future editions. Questions to be included in the voluntary survey include a variety of factors such as activity limitations, citizenship and immigration, ethnic origin, religion, mobility, place of birth of parents, education, labour market activities, place of work, work activity, child care and support payments, income, and housing (Statistics Canada, 2011a). For the 2006 census, these questions were mandatory for 20% of households.

2006 Canada Agricultural Census

This is a new data source introduced to this edition of the Atlas to reflect an increased interest in wellness related to nutrition and food security. The agricultural census runs concurrently with the population census. The agricultural census uses the word "operator" to define a person responsible for the management and/or financial decisions made in the production of agricultural commodities, and an agricultural operation is defined as a farm, ranch, or other operation that produces agricultural products intended for sale, and includes small operations sometimes known as "hobby farms." The census collects data such as number of farms and farm operators, farm areas, business operating arrangements, land management practices, livestock, and crop inventories (Statistics Canada, 2011b). For the purposes of this Atlas, we map a variety of food- and nutrition-related indicators at the Regional District administrative level, such as organic farming, greenhouse production, and main farming types.

BC Vital Statistics

The BC Vital Statistics Agency collects a variety of data on births, deaths, and marriages. Important wellness data on maternal conditions, perinatal conditions, and outcomes for newborns and infants (first year of life) are collected through the Notice of Birth (NOB) registration. A healthy beginning for a child is related to healthy development through to adulthood. Important vital statistics data used in this Atlas include, among others, age of mother giving birth, birth weight, and length of pregnancy before delivery—all key wellness factors for newborns. Some caution is required with the use of the NOB data, as they rely on individual birthing professionals to complete all of the required components of the form, and data were not always complete. Also, the data presented in the Atlas only cover events that occurred in the province. Events occurring to BC residents elsewhere are not included, and this is potentially problematical for the northeast and southeast of the province, where difficult or risky births may occur in the neighbouring province of Alberta. Again, caution is required when analysing the maps.

2010 Legacies Now

2010 Legacies Now, as noted in Chapter 1, is an independent entity that recently changed its name to LIFT Philanthropy Partners with a mandate to "accelerate the growth and impact of selected not-for-profit organizations to create positive and lasting social change through sport and healthy living, and literacy and lifelong learning".

Over the past few years, 2010 Legacies Now has received data from Sports BC, a non-profit agency that represents more than 80 sports organizations, including over 60 designated provincial sports organizations. Membership registration has been collected for numerous sports and games activities. Key rates of sport club membership, as measured by registration in different sports activities, have been used in the Atlas based on the data provided through 2010 Legacies Now. There is a new system in place that can provide the data at the HSDA level. In the first edition of the Atlas, data were only available at the Economic Development Region level. These data do not include sports activities undertaken through schools and, as such, participation rates are likely an underestimate of actual sports participation in the province.

BC Healthy Living Alliance

As part of the ActNow BC initiative, BC Healthy Living Alliance (BCHLA) introduced a series of initiatives to support smoke-free living, healthy nutrition, physical activity, and community capacity building. Based on these program initiatives, we have been able to develop a series of custom maps by working in partnership with BCHLA to show the geography and reach of the various programming initiatives.

Other Data Sources

There is a variety of other data sources used to map different indicators. These include, among others, agricultural land reserve, public library statistics, climatic features related to agriculture, housing data, and a variety of custom maps based on key website available data related to wellness factors and ActNow BC.

Geographical Units Used for Mapping

Throughout the Atlas, there are several different administrative geographical units that we use for mapping purposes. The most common one is the Health Service

Delivery Area (HSDA) unit. While there are five geographical Health Authorities in the province, each is made up of separate HSDAs that number 16 in total. This administrative unit has been chosen as the base geographical unit for the Atlas primarily because it is the most detailed geographical breakdown we could get for the key data source that we use, the CCHS. Using a common mapping unit enables an examination of the values of different indicators for any HSDA, thus allowing the ability to build an overall wellness picture of that HSDA based on numerous indicators.

The school district administrative unit, of which there are 59 geographical units in the province (an additional school district, Ecole Scolaire Francophone, is not geographically based, but is generally included in the total values for the provincial school population), is the next most common geographical administrative unit used. The Regional District, of which there are 29, is a new administrative unit used in this Atlas. Finally, we also use the Economic Development region unit for one key series of indicators related to lifelong learning.

Finally, a number of what we call "custom maps" have been produced. These have only the outline of the province as the geographical unit used. These maps tend to show specific locations within BC (e.g., Farmers Markets), or isolines of a particular feature (e.g., Growing Degree Days).

Maps are related to one or more of the following: wellness determinants and assets, smoke-free environments, nutrition and food security, physical activity, healthy weights, and healthy pregnancy and birth. These are the key components of the original ActNow BC initiative. In addition, indicators related to being free of chronic conditions, and overall wellness outcomes, are included.

Interpreting the Maps, Tables, and Graphs

Most data are divided into quintiles for mapping purposes. A quintile represents one-fifth or 20% of the administrative units being mapped for any particular indicator. Different colours differentiate the quintile groupings. Most range from GREEN for those geographical units with indicator wellness values in the highest or best quintile (or top 20%) through colour gradations to RED for the lowest quintile (or bottom 20%) value areas. For indicators that are neutral, in the sense that a high or low value does not denote better or poorer wellness, neutral colours are used, such as shades of BLUE, and quintiles are still used for these indicators for mapping purposes.

Cautions and Caveats in Map Interpretation

When using maps to view information and data, the user should be aware of a couple of major cautions, especially for many of the maps presented in this Atlas. While we are able to show variations in indicator values *between* different HSDAs, or school districts, we do not show variations *within* HSDAs. In some instances, such as Vancouver, with a high population density, and large variations in many socioeconomic characteristics, the variations in the indicator values within the HSDA may be greater than those between Vancouver and all other HSDAs.

The population in BC is very much concentrated in the southwest of the province and southern part of Vancouver Island. Much of the interior, north, and southeast of the province is sparsely populated, but contains large tracts of land mass (see Chapter 4).

Users must be cautioned against coming to a conclusion that much of the province has high or low values related to a certain indicator. While technically that may be correct from the perspective of land mass covered, it would not be correct to say those values occur to most of the population in the province.

The following four pages provide base maps for HSDAs, School Districts, Regional Districts, and Economic Development Regions, along with the names of the individual administrative units. They are followed by a brief guide on how to interpret and analyse the maps and tables used in the Atlas.

The CCHS sample data provide an example of the most frequent map page format, along with a supporting table. Only the CCHS map model is described here, but the majority of other maps are of a similar nature for presentation and analysis purposes. For CCHS data only, a graph is also presented so that comparisons can be made between BC and Canada for specific cohorts.

Two pages are devoted to each indicator so that the user can read and see at a glance a summary of what is happening geographically within the province for that indicator, as well as how provincial values compare with Canadian values. Comparisons can be made as follows, and in each case *statistically significant differences* are noted:

- Age cohorts can be compared both at the provincial and individual HSDA levels. Specifically, youth (12 to 19 years) and seniors (65 years and over) are compared with the mid-age cohort (20 to 64 years).

- Differences between sexes at the provincial level and at the individual HSDA level can be noted.

- Provincial values for 2005 and 2007/8 can be compared to show differences over time.

- Provincial results can be compared with Canadian results for each age cohort and by sex for the 2007/8 sample data, to show differences.

- Geographical patterns can be viewed within BC.

The maps on the page 29 plot sample data to illustrate the presentation methodology used throughout the Atlas. The values in percent (%) for HSDA respondents who answered the question in a positive way from a wellness perspective are listed in the table opposite the maps. The algorithm that was used places each of the highest and lowest three HSDAs in the best and worst category respectively, while the next best and next worst three HSDAs are set in the second and fourth groups respectively, with the remaining four placed in the middle group. The algorithm is designed to highlight the highest (best) and lowest (worst) performing HSDAs. Where two or more units share the same score and fall into overlapping groups, they are placed in the least extreme category of the overlap (i.e., the bias is toward the middle group rather than to the extremes). The colour index at the side of the maps provides the range of values of the five (quintile) groups used for mapping.

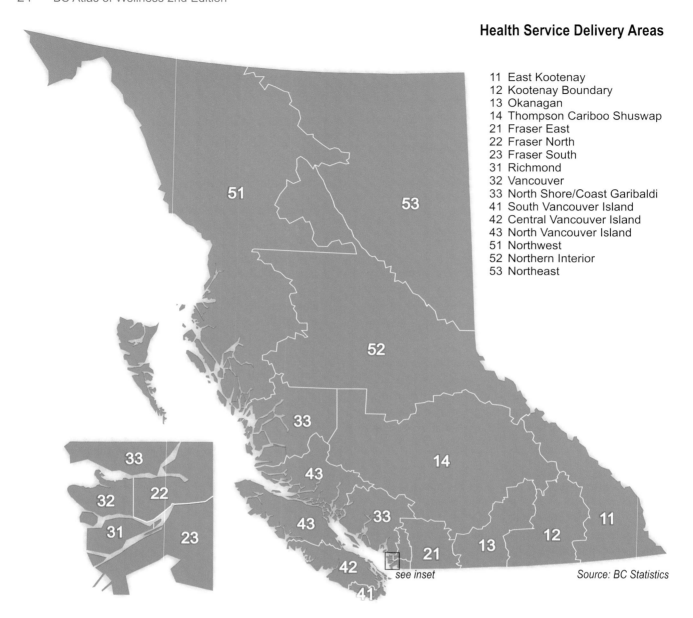

Health Service Delivery Areas

11 East Kootenay
12 Kootenay Boundary
13 Okanagan
14 Thompson Cariboo Shuswap
21 Fraser East
22 Fraser North
23 Fraser South
31 Richmond
32 Vancouver
33 North Shore/Coast Garibaldi
41 South Vancouver Island
42 Central Vancouver Island
43 North Vancouver Island
51 Northwest
52 Northern Interior
53 Northeast

Source: BC Statistics

School Districts

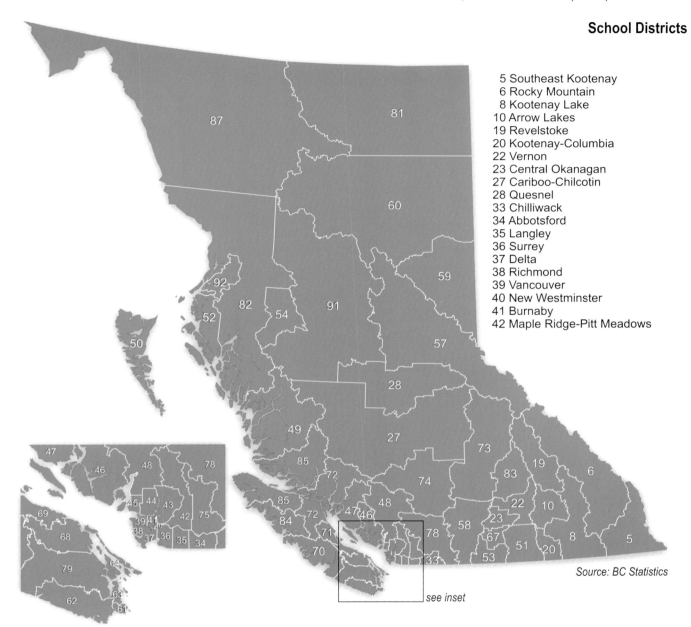

5 Southeast Kootenay
6 Rocky Mountain
8 Kootenay Lake
10 Arrow Lakes
19 Revelstoke
20 Kootenay-Columbia
22 Vernon
23 Central Okanagan
27 Cariboo-Chilcotin
28 Quesnel
33 Chilliwack
34 Abbotsford
35 Langley
36 Surrey
37 Delta
38 Richmond
39 Vancouver
40 New Westminster
41 Burnaby
42 Maple Ridge-Pitt Meadows

Source: BC Statistics

see inset

43 Coquitlam
44 North Vancouver
45 West Vancouver
46 Sunshine Coast
47 Powell River
48 Howe Sound
49 Central Coast
50 Haida Gwaii/Queen Charlotte
51 Boundary
52 Prince Rupert
53 Okanagan Similkameen
54 Bulkley Valley
57 Prince George

58 Nicola-Similkameen
59 Peace River South
60 Peace River North
61 Greater Victoria
62 Sooke
63 Saanich
64 Gulf Islands
67 Okanagan Skaha
68 Nanaimo-Ladysmith
69 Qualicum
70 Alberni
71 Comox Valley
72 Campbell River

73 Kamloops/Thompson
74 Gold Trail
75 Mission
78 Fraser-Cascade
79 Cowichan Valley
81 Fort Nelson
82 Coast Mountains
83 North Okanagan-Shuswap
84 Vancouver Island West
85 Vancouver Island North
87 Stikine
91 Nechako Lakes
92 Nisga'a

Regional Districts

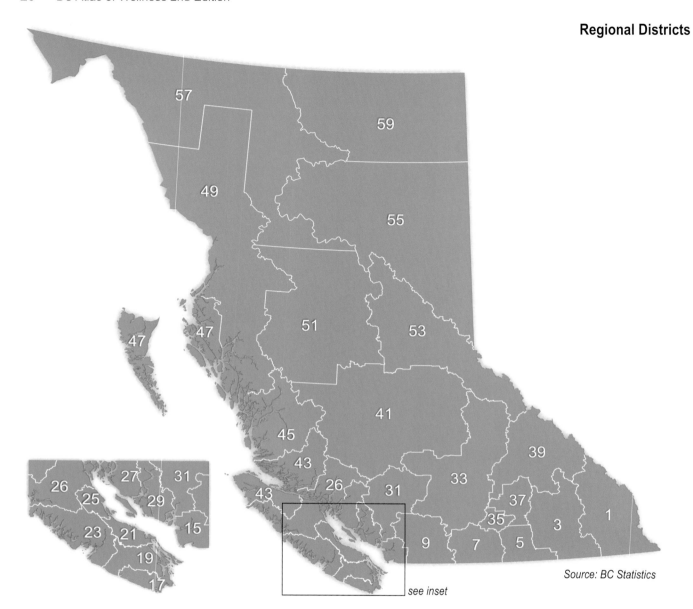

Source: BC Statistics

see inset

1	East Kootenay	25	Comox Valley	43	Mount Waddington
3	Central Kootenay	26	Strathcona	45	Central Coast
5	Kootenay Boundary	27	Powell River	47	Skeena-Queen Charlotte
7	Okanagan-Similkameen	29	Sunshine Coast	49	Kitimat-Stikine
9	Fraser Valley	31	Squamish-Lillooet	51	Bulkley-Nechako
15	Greater Vancouver	33	Thompson-Nicola	53	Fraser-Fort George
17	Capital	35	Central Okanagan	55	Peace River
19	Cowichan Valley	37	North Okanagan	57	Stikine
21	Nanaimo	39	Columbia-Shuswap	59	Northern Rockies
23	Alberni-Clayoquot	41	Cariboo		

Economic Development Regions

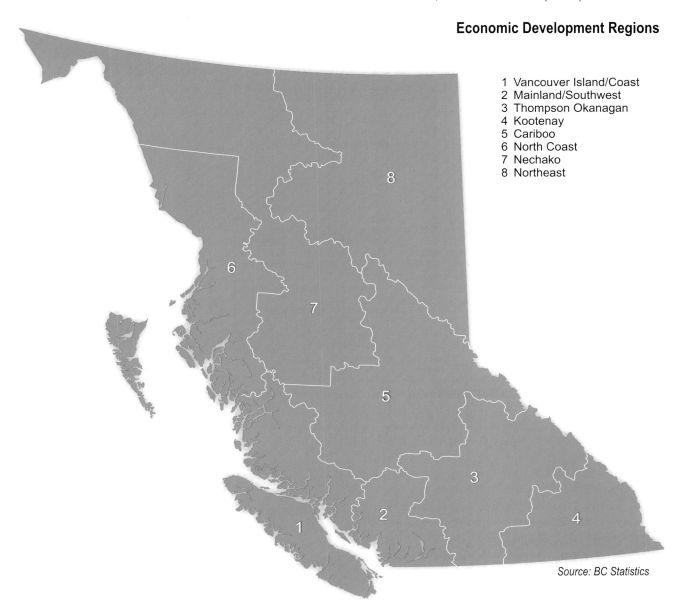

1 Vancouver Island/Coast
2 Mainland/Southwest
3 Thompson Okanagan
4 Kootenay
5 Cariboo
6 North Coast
7 Nechako
8 Northeast

Source: BC Statistics

Canadian Community Health Survey, sample data

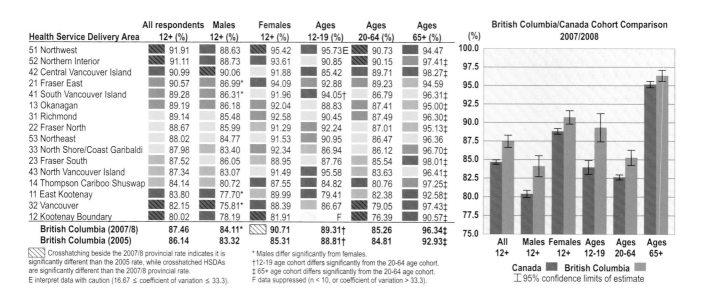

Health Service Delivery Area	All respondents 12+ (%)	Males 12+ (%)	Females 12+ (%)	Ages 12-19 (%)	Ages 20-64 (%)	Ages 65+ (%)
51 Northwest	91.91	88.63	95.42	95.73E	90.73	94.47
52 Northern Interior	91.11	88.73	93.61	90.85	90.15	97.41‡
42 Central Vancouver Island	90.99	90.06	91.88	85.42	89.71	98.27‡
21 Fraser East	90.57	86.99*	94.09	92.88	89.23	94.59
41 South Vancouver Island	89.28	86.31*	91.96	94.05†	86.79	96.31‡
13 Okanagan	89.19	86.18	92.04	88.83	87.41	95.00‡
31 Richmond	89.14	85.48	92.58	90.45	87.49	96.30‡
22 Fraser North	88.67	85.99	91.29	92.24	87.01	95.13‡
53 Northeast	88.02	84.77	91.53	90.95	86.47	96.36
33 North Shore/Coast Garibaldi	87.98	83.40	92.34	86.94	86.12	96.70‡
23 Fraser South	87.52	86.05	88.95	87.76	85.54	98.01‡
43 North Vancouver Island	87.34	83.07	91.49	95.58	83.63	96.41‡
14 Thompson Cariboo Shuswap	84.14	80.72	87.55	84.82	80.76	97.25‡
11 East Kootenay	83.80	77.70*	89.99	79.41	82.38	92.58‡
32 Vancouver	82.15	75.81*	88.39	86.67	79.05	97.43‡
12 Kootenay Boundary	80.02	78.19	81.91	F	76.39	90.57‡
British Columbia (2007/8)	**87.46**	**84.11***	**90.71**	**89.31†**	**85.26**	**96.34‡**
British Columbia (2005)	**86.14**	**83.32**	**85.31**	**88.81†**	**84.81**	**92.93‡**

Crosshatching beside the 2007/8 provincial rate indicates it is significantly different than the 2005 rate, while crosshatched HSDAs are significantly different than the 2007/8 provincial rate.
E interpret data with caution (16.67 ≤ coefficient of variation ≤ 33.3).

* Males differ significantly from females.
†12-19 age cohort differs significantly from the 20-64 age cohort.
‡ 65+ age cohort differs significantly from the 20-64 age cohort.
F data suppressed (n < 10, or coefficient of variation > 33.3).

The larger top map opposite shows data for the 12 years and over age cohort. The DARK GREEN group has a range of 90.99% - 91.91%, and includes the three HSDAs (Northwest, Northern Interior and Central Vancouver Island) with the highest values; the next highest group, in LIGHT GREEN, has a range of 89.19% - 90.57%, and includes the three HSDAs with the next highest values; the middle group contains the four HSDAs with the middle values which are coloured BEIGE; the next three HSDAs are coloured ORANGE and have lower values than the middle group; and finally, the three with the lowest values are RED and have a range of 80.02% - 83.80%. When HSDAs are GREY, data are not available for mapping, usually because the sample size is considered too small (<10) to report for that region. This is based on the Statistics Canada convention for CCHS data. CROSS HATCHED areas have values that are significantly different from the provincial average (see Northwest and Northern Interior, All respondents ages 12+ column above). The four smaller maps focus on different cohorts of respondents: all males, all females, age 12 to 19 years (youth), and age 65 years and over (seniors). CROSS HATCHING again denotes any areas that have statistically significantly higher or lower values than the BC average.

The table above supports the maps opposite. Using the same colour scheme and hatching symbols as the maps, the left hand column shows the values of the HSDAs from highest (best) to lowest (worst) for the 12+ age cohort. The other columns keep the order of the left hand column and provide the point estimate for each HSDA for males and females and for the other age cohorts. The two

bottom rows show results for BC for 2007/8 and 2005 respectively. A cross hatching symbol indicates there is a significant difference between the two results (e.g., Females 12+ column above).

F (e.g., Kootenay Boundary Ages 12 to 19) indicates the sample size was <10 or the coefficient of variation (CV) was greater than 33.33.

E following a value (e.g., 95.73E for Northwest Ages 12 to 19) indicates a coefficient of variation (16.67 ≤ CV ≤ 33.3) that yields a large confidence interval, rendering a caution in interpretation.

The * symbol indicates a significant difference between sexes within an HSDA, or at the provincial level (e.g., Males 12+ column above).

The † symbol indicates a significant difference between the youth cohort and the 20-64 age cohort within a particular HSDA, or at the provincial level.

The ‡ symbol similarly indicates a significant difference between the seniors cohort and the 20 to 64 age cohort.

The graph above provides the 95% confidence interval ranges (I) for key cohorts for BC and Canada so that comparisons can be made between the two jurisdictions, and between different age cohorts and between sexes.

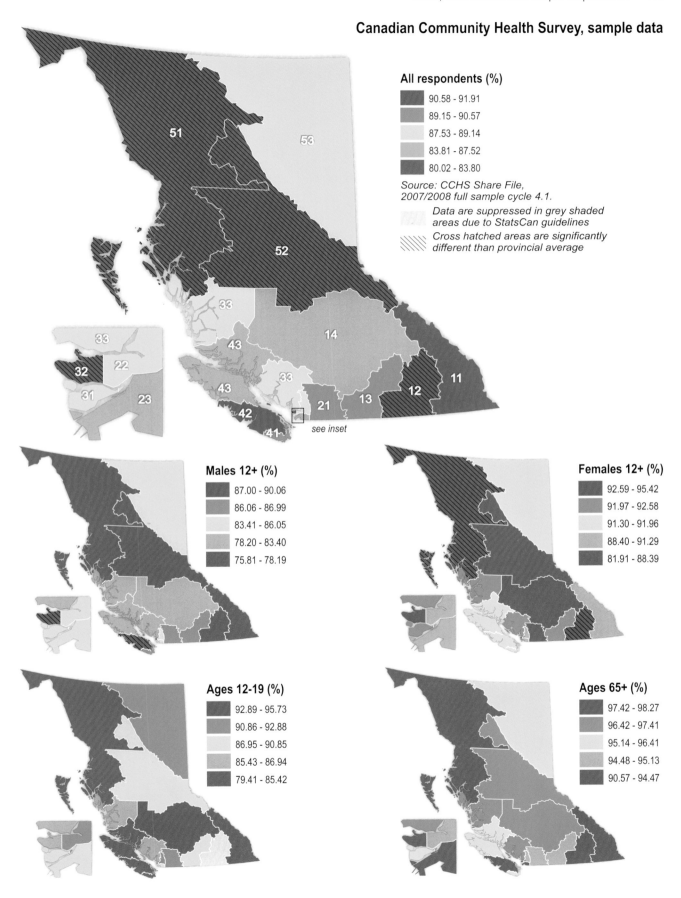

Canadian Community Health Survey, sample data

All respondents (%)

- 90.58 - 91.91
- 89.15 - 90.57
- 87.53 - 89.14
- 83.81 - 87.52
- 80.02 - 83.80

Source: CCHS Share File, 2007/2008 full sample cycle 4.1.

Data are suppressed in grey shaded areas due to StatsCan guidelines

Cross hatched areas are significantly different than provincial average

Males 12+ (%)

- 87.00 - 90.06
- 86.06 - 86.99
- 83.41 - 86.05
- 78.20 - 83.40
- 75.81 - 78.19

Females 12+ (%)

- 92.59 - 95.42
- 91.97 - 92.58
- 91.30 - 91.96
- 88.40 - 91.29
- 81.91 - 88.39

Ages 12-19 (%)

- 92.89 - 95.73
- 90.86 - 92.88
- 86.95 - 90.85
- 85.43 - 86.94
- 79.41 - 85.42

Ages 65+ (%)

- 97.42 - 98.27
- 96.42 - 97.41
- 95.14 - 96.41
- 94.48 - 95.13
- 90.57 - 94.47

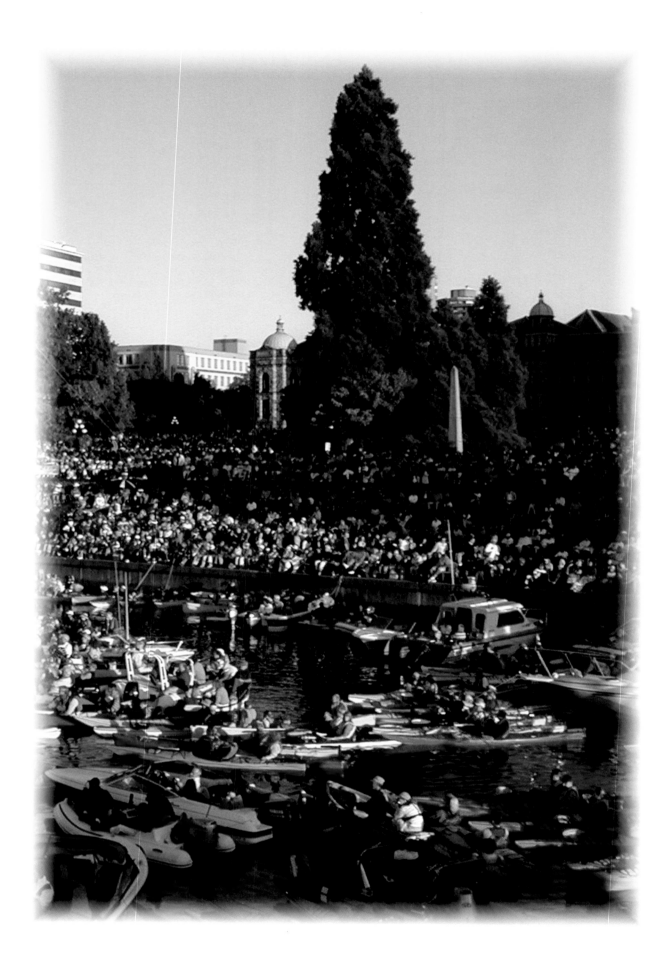

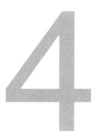

The British Columbia Demographic Context

This chapter provides background material on BC based on selective demographic characteristics. The original Atlas provided information on physical, climatic, and demographic characteristics, but because there have been no changes or updated data on the physical and climatic variables from those previously presented, we have not included them in this edition of the Atlas. Interested readers are referred to the original Atlas for these indicators and characteristics, which included physiography, precipitation-free days, hours of bright sunshine, seasonal trends in precipitation, and recent changes in maximum and minimum temperatures. The "wellness" of ecosystems and the physical environment (air, water, land, sea, biodiversity, toxic contaminants, climatic change, and sea) has been well researched. Interested readers can find the most recent documentation elsewhere (Ministry of Environment, 2007).

As a context for many of the data and maps that occur in the following chapters, the material presented here focuses on key demographic indicators that help describe the population of BC at the HSDA level, which is the primary administrative unit used for mapping purposes in this Atlas. The first three maps show total population, population density, and female population, and give a sense of where the population is in BC and also some idea of urbanicity and rurality. Research has shown that the rural population tends to be less well than those living in urban areas, and there are major differences in gender from a wellness perspective (Virtue et al., 2010). The next four maps show the proportion of the population in four key age categories: birth to 11 years; 12 to 19 years; 20 to 64 years; and 65 years and over. The last three categories are used extensively throughout the Atlas.

Next are six maps that focus on two key sub-populations in the province whose levels of wellness are known to be different from those of the average population in BC. The

first group is the Aboriginal population, and the relative importance of this group by location is provided, while the second group deals with characteristics of the immigrant population.

The next five maps provide a more detailed description of the population in each HSDA in the province. The HSDAs are organized in five groups based on the five geographical Health Authorities in BC: Interior; Fraser; Vancouver Coastal; Vancouver Island; and Northern.

A final map provides a sense of the overall distribution of the population in the province. The chapter concludes with a brief summary.

Population distribution within the province

The maps opposite provide important indicators of the geographical distribution of the population within BC, based on HSDA boundaries. The HSDA boundary set was chosen as it is the dominant administrative unit used in this *Atlas*. When viewed in conjunction with the nighttime map presented at the end of the chapter, a better perspective can be provided about the province's population and the majority of wellness maps that follow. Data are based on the P.E.O.P.L.E. 35 model population estimates (BC Stats, 2010b), when BC had an estimated population of 4,455,210 residents, with an annual 5 year growth rate of 1.4%.

Health Service Delivery Area	Total population (%)	Population density/ sq. km.	Female population (%)
23 Fraser South	15.62	802.29	50.21
32 Vancouver	14.44	4,809.81	50.33
22 Fraser North	13.39	200.66	50.29
41 South Vancouver Island	8.25	155.55	51.65
13 Okanagan	7.88	16.42	51.04
21 Fraser East	6.28	23.69	49.83
33 North Shore/Coast Garibaldi	6.24	5.23	50.88
42 Central Vancouver Island	5.87	20.66	50.64
14 Thompson Cariboo Shuswap	5.01	1.87	49.99
31 Richmond	4.34	1,245.71	51.17
52 Northern Interior	3.20	0.79	49.02
43 North Vancouver Island	2.70	2.92	50.10
11 East Kootenay	1.80	1.76	49.90
12 Kootenay Boundary	1.78	2.73	50.07
51 Northwest	1.68	0.29	48.70
53 Northeast	1.52	0.40	48.04
British Columbia	**100.00**	**4.66**	**50.39**

Percent of total population

There are three main population regions in BC. More than four in every ten (43.45%) people in the province are found in three HSDAs in the urban lower mainland in the southwest corner of the province. Fraser South (15.62%), with a 5 year annual growth rate of 2.0%, and Vancouver (14.44%) and Fraser North (13.39%), both with an annual 5 year growth rate of 1.5%, clearly dominate the population distribution within BC. Neighbouring HSDAs, such as North Shore/Coast Garibaldi, Richmond, and to a lesser extent Fraser East, also help to make up an ever-expanding lower mainland region, and when their populations are included, six in every ten people can be found in this region, which continues to grow and attract new residents.

The second major population region is also in the extreme southwest of the province on the southern tip of Vancouver Island, where 8.25% of the province's population resides, and which has been growing at an annual rate of 1.1% for the last 5 years. Okanagan, in the southern interior of the province, is the third major population region, with 7.88% of the province's population. It is the fastest growing HSDA in the province, with an annual growth rate of 2.2% since 2004.

Population density

Provincially, BC had an average population density of 4.66 per square kilometre. Vancouver dominates the province in terms of population density. As noted in the table, this HSDA had a population density of approximately 4,810 people per square kilometre. Next in importance was Richmond, with 1,246 people per square kilometre. Other lower mainland HSDAs were also prominent, particularly Fraser South and Fraser North. The only other HSDA with a relatively high population density was South Vancouver Island. Generally, population density was high in the

southwest of the province, while the whole of the northern half of BC and much of the interior had very low population densities. Most of the population in the north and interior are located in small towns and communities with one or two notable exceptions.

Female population

There are major differences in wellness between genders (McKee et al., 2010) and women live longer than men (see life expectancy in Chapter 13), so it is important to view the relative distribution of genders throughout the province. Overall, 50.39% of the province's population is female. The relative figures vary throughout the province, with a high of 51.65% females in South Vancouver Island and a low of 48.04% in Northeast. Higher relative concentrations of females are also found in Richmond and in Okanagan, while the northern HSDAs have the lowest concentrations.

Population distribution within the province

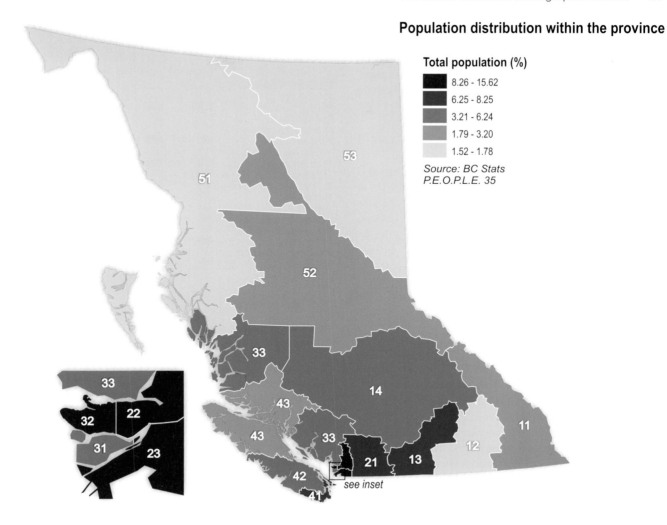

Total population (%)

- 8.26 - 15.62
- 6.25 - 8.25
- 3.21 - 6.24
- 1.79 - 3.20
- 1.52 - 1.78

Source: BC Stats
P.E.O.P.L.E. 35

see inset

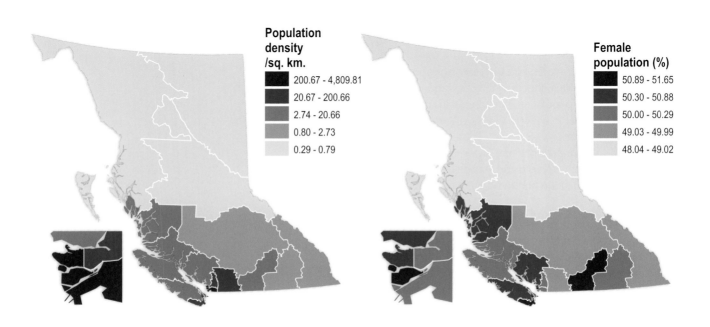

Population
density
/sq. km.

- 200.67 - 4,809.81
- 20.67 - 200.66
- 2.74 - 20.66
- 0.80 - 2.73
- 0.29 - 0.79

Female
population (%)

- 50.89 - 51.65
- 50.30 - 50.88
- 50.00 - 50.29
- 49.03 - 49.99
- 48.04 - 49.02

Population age patterns

Many of the wellness maps are based on population age cohorts, especially the wellness indicators derived from the CCHS 4.1, so this group of indicators provides a brief analysis of how key population cohorts are distributed throughout the province. Again, the population data are provided for 2009 and are derived from P.E.O.P.L.E. 35 from BC Stats. The data are provided at the HSDA level and show the percentage of population in any HSDA in four different age categories: under 12 years; 12 to 19 years; 20 to 64 years; and 65 years and over. The key age category for "ranking" HSDAs is the 20 to 64 age cohort, and this is shown in the top left corner on the page opposite. As can be seen from the table and maps opposite, there are fairly major geographical differences in the population of HSDAs based on these age categories.

Health Service Delivery Area	Ages < 12 (%)	Ages 12-19 (%)	Ages 20-64 (%)	Ages 65+ (%)
32 Vancouver	9.94	7.23	70.46	12.37
22 Fraser North	12.02	10.11	66.07	11.81
31 Richmond	11.17	10.04	65.76	13.02
41 South Vancouver Island	10.13	8.64	63.88	17.34
52 Northern Interior	13.99	11.42	63.03	11.57
33 North Shore/Coast Garibaldi	11.40	10.28	62.80	15.52
53 Northeast	17.05	11.61	62.78	8.56
11 East Kootenay	12.14	10.13	61.73	16.01
14 Thompson Cariboo Shuswap	11.72	10.33	61.32	16.63
51 Northwest	14.98	12.59	61.21	11.22
23 Fraser South	14.07	10.84	61.14	13.94
43 North Vancouver Island	11.89	10.41	61.10	16.59
12 Kootenay Boundary	10.94	10.13	60.90	18.03
21 Fraser East	14.55	11.08	60.02	14.36
42 Central Vancouver Island	10.73	9.90	59.49	19.87
13 Okanagan	10.93	9.80	59.26	20.01
British Columbia	**11.96**	**9.84**	**63.46**	**14.73**

Population 20 to 64 years old

More than six in every ten (63.46%) individuals provincially were in this mid-age population cohort in 2009, a marginal increase from 2005 (63.31%). This age cohort is broad in nature and includes young people still in post secondary education, but the dominant group is the post-war "baby boomers," which is a major demographic group in BC and elsewhere. This age cohort is mainly involved in the workforce and family formation and child rearing.

There were major differences in the relative importance of this age group throughout BC. More than seven in ten (70.46%) people in Vancouver were in this cohort, compared with 60% or less in Okanagan, Central Vancouver Island, and Fraser East. The highest HSDAs were found in the urban lower mainland, including Vancouver, Fraser North, and Richmond (all above 65%).

Population less than 12 years old

This youngest age cohort had a fairly large geographical spread in values. While the provincial average was 11.96% of the total population, this ranged from a high of 17.05% in Northeast to a low of 9.94% in Vancouver and 10.13% in South Vancouver Island. Generally, lower values were more prevalent in the lower mainland and the southern half of Vancouver Island, while the higher values were characteristic of the northern half of the province.

Population 12 to 19 years old

Individuals in this youth cohort are mainly in the school system. Nearly one in ten (9.84%) in the province were in this age cohort in 2009. Values ranged from 7.23% in Vancouver to 12.59% in Northwest. Generally, the highest values were found in the northern half of the province, while lower values were evident in South Vancouver Island and in the Okanagan.

Population 65 years and over

This seniors age cohort accounted for 14.73% of the province's population in 2009. The large majority in this cohort were retired. There were major geographical differences among the HSDAs, with Okanagan and Central Vancouver Island having the highest percentages (both with approximately 20%), while Northeast had only 8.56% of its population in this cohort. Geographically, the northern half of the province had the lowest percentages in this age cohort, while the highest were in the southern interior of the province, as well as Central Vancouver Island.

Population age patterns

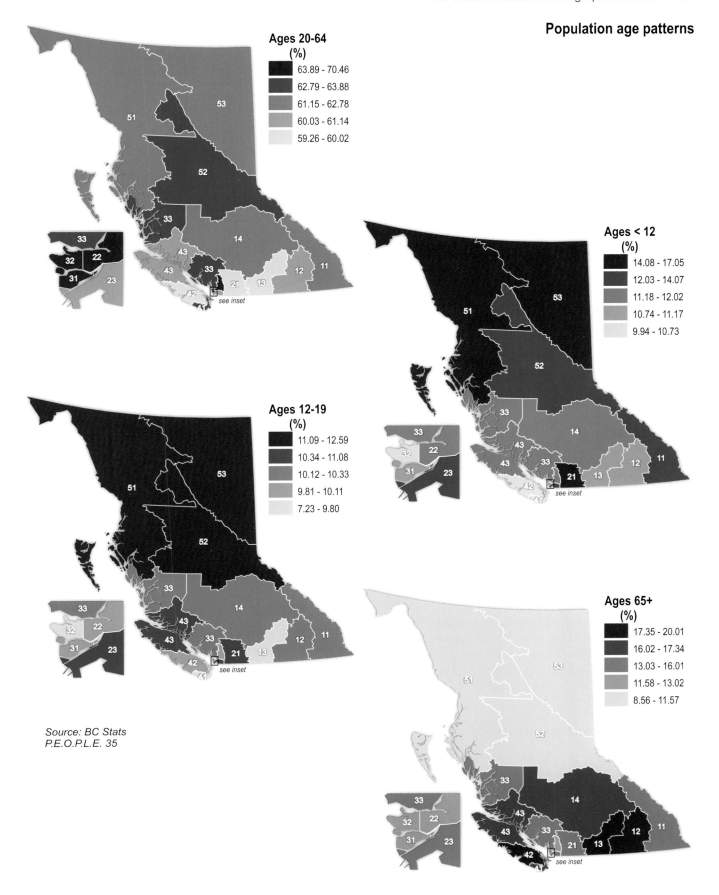

Ages 20-64 (%)
- 63.89 - 70.46
- 62.79 - 63.88
- 61.15 - 62.78
- 60.03 - 61.14
- 59.26 - 60.02

Ages < 12 (%)
- 14.08 - 17.05
- 12.03 - 14.07
- 11.18 - 12.02
- 10.74 - 11.17
- 9.94 - 10.73

Ages 12-19 (%)
- 11.09 - 12.59
- 10.34 - 11.08
- 10.12 - 10.33
- 9.81 - 10.11
- 7.23 - 9.80

Ages 65+ (%)
- 17.35 - 20.01
- 16.02 - 17.34
- 13.03 - 16.01
- 11.58 - 13.02
- 8.56 - 11.57

Source: BC Stats
P.E.O.P.L.E. 35

Aboriginal population distribution within the province

Although the proportion of the BC population who identified as Aboriginal was only 4.81% in the 2006 census (BC Stats, 2010b), up from 4.39% in 2001, they are an important sub-group of the BC population, especially from a health and wellness perspective. In a recent report on the health and well-being of BC's Aboriginal population, the Provincial Health Officer, Dr. Perry Kendall, noted that although there had been some improvements since an earlier report, significant gaps in health and wellness assets relative to the general BC population still remained (Kendall, 2009). Of the more than 196,000 individuals who self-identified as Aboriginal in 2006, approximately two-thirds were North American Indian (First Nations), with the other major group identifying as Metis (Norton, 2008).

Overall, the Aboriginal population is much younger than the general BC population, with 37% aged 19 or younger, compared to 22% for the BC population as a whole. The Aboriginal population has grown more rapidly than the non-Aboriginal population because of higher birth rates (Kendall, 2009).

Percent Aboriginal population

Although provincially the Aboriginal population represented only a small portion of the population, there are major differences geographically throughout the province. Nearly one-third (30.03%) of the population in Northwest was Aboriginal in 2006, an increase from one-quarter in 2001, while in Richmond, in the extreme southwest of the province, less than one percent self-identified as Aboriginal.

Generally, HSDAs in the northern half of the province, along with the central interior (Thompson Cariboo Shuswap), had the highest percentages of Aboriginal population (all above 11%). At the other extreme, the urban HSDAs of the lower mainland (Fraser South, Vancouver, Fraser North, and Richmond) had the lowest proportion (2% or less) of their population who were Aboriginal.

Distribution of Aboriginal population

Of the approximately 196,000 Aboriginal people in BC, nearly one-quarter were found in just two HSDAs in 2006: Thompson Cariboo Shuswap (11.89%) and Northwest (11.33%). Richmond had the lowest proportion, with less than one percent (0.65%). Small percentages also resided in the southeast of the province (Kootenay Boundary and East Kootenay), where only 4% of the Aboriginal population were found.

Health Service Delivery Area	Aboriginal population (%)	Distribution of Aboriginal population (%)	Female Aboriginal population (%)
51 Northwest	30.03	11.33	50.70
52 Northern Interior	13.14	9.18	49.99
53 Northeast	12.35	4.02	49.02
14 Thompson Cariboo Shuswap	11.27	11.89	52.20
43 North Vancouver Island	8.87	5.00	51.63
42 Central Vancouver Island	7.85	9.80	51.04
21 Fraser East	5.68	7.35	52.26
11 East Kootenay	5.66	2.12	53.61
13 Okanagan	4.57	7.36	52.91
33 North Shore/Coast Garibaldi	4.39	5.83	50.29
12 Kootenay Boundary	4.10	1.55	51.49
41 South Vancouver Island	3.34	5.80	53.10
23 Fraser South	2.14	6.83	53.61
32 Vancouver	2.02	6.03	50.55
22 Fraser North	1.92	5.27	53.32
31 Richmond	0.73	0.65	51.37
British Columbia	4.81	100.00	51.62

Although many of the lower mainland HSDAs had a small percentage of their population who were Aboriginal, collectively, approximately 30% of the Aboriginal population resided in that region in 2006.

Percent female Aboriginal population

Proportionately, there were more females (51.62%) in the Aboriginal population than in the BC population as a whole (50.39%). The lowest proportions were found in Northeast (49.02%) and Northern Interior (49.99%). With the exception of East Kootenay (53.61%), the highest proportion of females resided in the lower mainland HSDAs of Fraser North and Fraser South, and South Vancouver Island (all over 53%).

Aboriginal population distribution within the province

Aboriginal population (%)

- 11.28 - 30.03
- 5.69 - 11.27
- 4.11 - 5.68
- 2.03 - 4.10
- 0.73 - 2.02

Source: BC Stats, 2006 Census of Canada, Statistics Canada

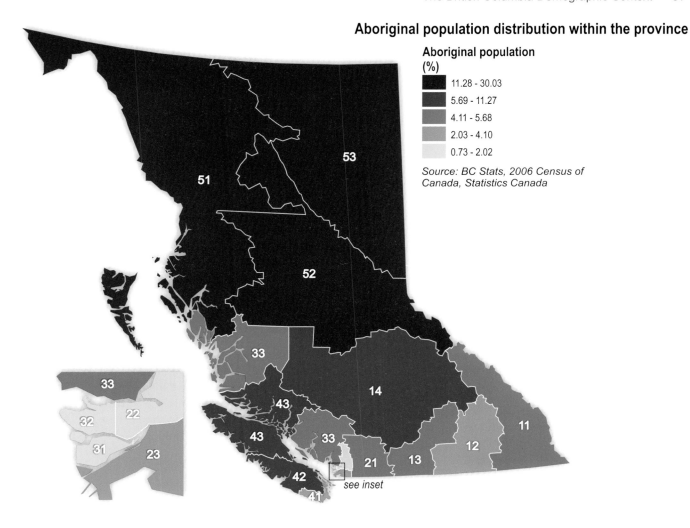

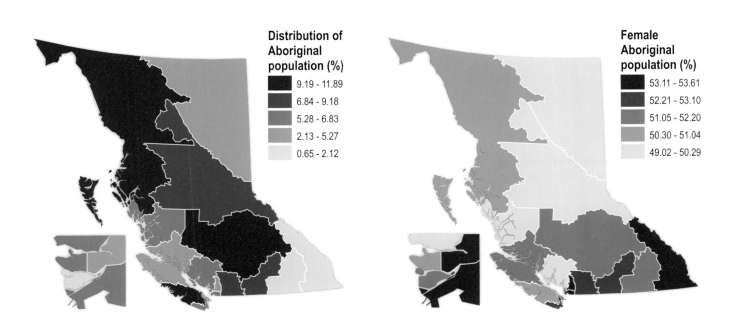

Distribution of Aboriginal population (%)

- 9.19 - 11.89
- 6.84 - 9.18
- 5.28 - 6.83
- 2.13 - 5.27
- 0.65 - 2.12

Female Aboriginal population (%)

- 53.11 - 53.61
- 52.21 - 53.10
- 51.05 - 52.20
- 50.30 - 51.04
- 49.02 - 50.29

Recent immigrants and language

Immigrant population refers to people who were foreign-born and have been granted citizenship, landed immigration or refugee status by Canadian authorities. According to the 2006 census, 27.5% of BC's population was foreign born, compared with 26.1% in 2001 (Ip, 2008a).

Within the BC population as a whole, foreign-born individuals are an important sub-group, and one that is increasing in importance. New arrivals, particularly new immigrants, tend to be healthier than native-born Canadians, partly because the population is younger, often better-educated (an important wellness asset), and have received medical screening prior to immigrating to Canada (McDonald & Kennedy, 2004). Further, there is often a degree of self-selection of potential immigrants which can affect the wellness of new immigrants (Ng et al., 2005). Over time, however, this health and wellness gap tends to fade as new immigrants take on some of the lifestyle characteristics of native-born Canadians (Guslulak, 2007).

Within Canada, BC was second only to Ontario in terms of the proportion of foreign-born people in the population. More than half (53.4%) of the foreign-born population came from Asia, primarily Mainland China, India, Hong Kong, the Philippines and the Middle East, while 31.2% were born in Europe. More than half had been living in Canada for more than 15 years. On balance, immigration has shifted in the past 15 to 20 years from European origin to Asian origin (Ip, 2008a).

From a gender perspective, 52% of the foreign-born population was female and the large majority was in the 25 to 54 age cohort. Nearly one quarter of the BC population indicated they were from a visible minority in 2006, and the populations of Richmond (65.1%) and Vancouver (51.1%) were more than half visible minorities, while Fraser North and Fraser South were about one third visible minorities.

Recent immigrants

Recent immigrants are those individuals who entered Canada between 2001 and 2006. They constituted 4.36% of BC's population in 2006. The geographical distribution was quite concentrated. More than 1 in 10 (10.82%) of Richmond's population were recent immigrants, followed by Vancouver and Fraser North (both over 7%). Other HSDAs in the urban lower mainland region of the province also had relatively large percentages (mostly over 5%) of recent immigrants in their populations, while the remainder of the province's HSDAs had less than 2%.

Health Service Delivery Area	Recent immigrants (%)	Change in recent immigrants since 2001 census (%)	Foreign language spoken at home (%)
31 Richmond	10.82	-3.76	43.35
32 Vancouver	7.82	-2.15	32.14
22 Fraser North	7.51	-1.92	23.85
23 Fraser South	5.84	0.48	21.14
33 North Shore/Coast Garibaldi	4.58	-0.67	10.63
21 Fraser East	2.70	0.13	11.44
41 South Vancouver Island	1.82	0.41	5.00
13 Okanagan	1.21	0.17	3.90
53 Northeast	1.01	0.00	4.39
42 Central Vancouver Island	1.00	0.19	2.89
12 Kootenay Boundary	0.74	0.10	2.54
51 Northwest	0.74	0.07	5.20
43 North Vancouver Island	0.72	0.14	2.01
14 Thompson Cariboo Shuswap	0.71	0.00	3.12
11 East Kootenay	0.63	-0.12	2.14
52 Northern Interior	0.56	0.06	3.18
British Columbia	**4.36**	**-0.58**	**15.69**

Change in recent immigrants since 2001

Richmond's recent immigrant population had fallen by 3.76 percentage points, while Vancouver and Fraser North saw reductions of approximately 2 percentage points. Elsewhere in the province, the majority of HSDAs witnessed a slight rise in the percentage of their populations who were new immigrants.

Foreign language spoken at home

Approximately 16% of the population spoke a language other than English or French in the home in 2006. The major foreign languages spoken were Chinese (nearly 240,000 over age 15 years) and Punjabi (nearly 96,000 over age 15 years) (Ip, 2008b). Again, this was most prevalent in the urban lower mainland HSDAs, with 43.35% in Richmond speaking a foreign language in the home. Nearly a third did so in Vancouver and over 20% did so in Fraser North and Fraser South. Outside of the lower mainland HSDAs, 5% or less spoke a foreign language at home. It is worth noting that 9% of foreign-born people in BC had no English language ability, while nearly 15% of those who arrived between 2001 and 2006 had no English (Ip, 2008a).

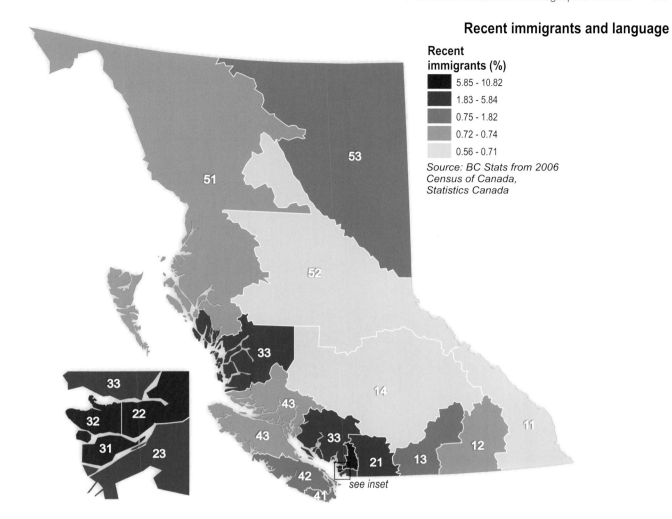

Recent immigrants and language

Recent immigrants (%)

- 5.85 - 10.82
- 1.83 - 5.84
- 0.75 - 1.82
- 0.72 - 0.74
- 0.56 - 0.71

Source: BC Stats from 2006 Census of Canada, Statistics Canada

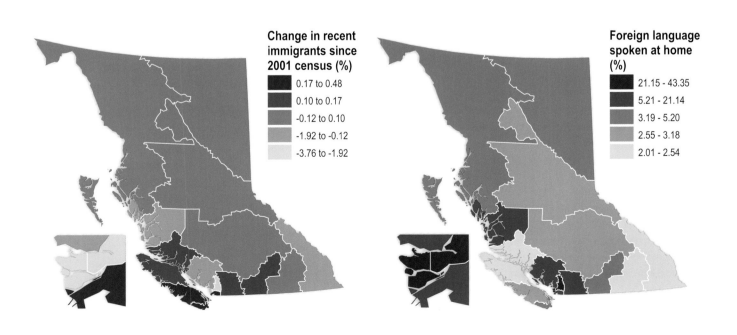

Change in recent immigrants since 2001 census (%)

- 0.17 to 0.48
- 0.10 to 0.17
- -0.12 to 0.10
- -1.92 to -0.12
- -3.76 to -1.92

Foreign language spoken at home (%)

- 21.15 - 43.35
- 5.21 - 21.14
- 3.19 - 5.20
- 2.55 - 3.18
- 2.01 - 2.54

Interior HSDAs

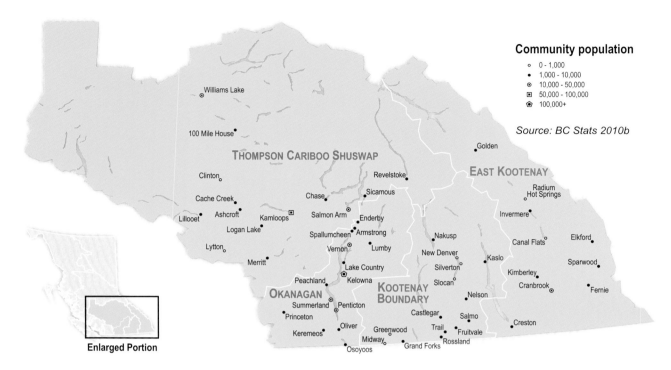

East Kootenay: HSDA 11

East Kootenay had one of the smallest populations of any HSDA in 2009 (less than 80,000). Half of the population was located in Cranbrook (population density more than 700 per square kilometre), followed by Kimberley (8% of the population), Creston and Fernie (both 6% of the population), and Golden and Sparwood (both 5% of the population). One third of the HSDA's population was scattered in rural areas. Most of the population was located in river valleys in this mountainous area. East Kootenay had the lowest proportion (2%) of visible minorities in its population, while nearly 6% of its population was Aboriginal.

Kootenay Boundary: HSDA 12

In 2009, close to half (47%) of the 79,000 population of this southeastern HSDA was scattered throughout the HSDA in rural areas. The remainder of the population was distributed in about a dozen small communities, the largest of which was Nelson with more than 12% of the population. Castlegar and Trail had about 10% each of the HSDA's population, followed by Grand Forks (5%) and Rossland (4%). Population tended to be in valley areas in what is quite a mountainous area. Population densities were highest in Warfield (more than 900 per square kilometre), Nelson (800 per square kilometre), and Fruitvale (over 700 per square kilometre). Only about 2.5% of the population was visible minorities, while nearly 5% was Aboriginal.

Okanagan: HSDA 13

There were over 350,000 people in this HSDA in 2009, with more than one-third in Kelowna (population density over 500 per square kilometre). Vernon and Penticton each had over 10% of the population, while Summerland, Lake Country, and Coldstream each had a little over 3%. Penticton's population density was approximately 760 per square kilometre. Spallumcheen, Peachland, Osoyoos, Oliver, Armstrong, and Enderby collectively had 8% of the population. These smaller communities were compact, with population densities of 300 to 800 per square kilometre. Many communities were located in the central part of the HSDA, running north south in the Okanagan Valley. Less than 5% of the population was visible minorities, and 4.6% self-identified as Aboriginal.

Thompson Cariboo Shuswap: HSDA 14

This HSDA had a population of almost 225,000 in 2009, and 38% resided in Kamloops, with a density of nearly 300 per square kilometre. Other notable communities were Salmon Arm (8%) and Williams Lake (5%), while Revelstoke and Merritt had over 7% of the population between them. About 35% was scattered throughout the HSDA in rural areas. Only about 4% of the population was visible minorities, while over 11% self-identified as Aboriginal.

Fraser HSDAs

Community population

- ○ 0 - 1,000
- • 1,000 - 10,000
- ⊙ 10,000 - 50,000
- ▣ 50,000 - 100,000
- ⬢ 100,000+

Source: BC Stats 2010b

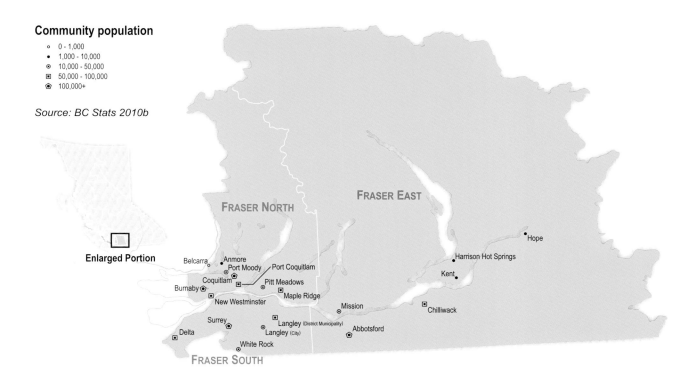

Fraser South: HSDA 23

Located to the south of the Fraser River, Fraser South had the largest population of any HSDA with an estimate of nearly 700,000 residents in 2009. The City of Surrey had approximately 63% of the total population, followed by Delta and Langley district municipalities with approximately 15% each. Population densities, however, were highest for the City of White Rock, with well over 3,500 people per square kilometre. It was the fastest growing HSDA in BC, and more than one third of its residents were visible minorities, particularly South Asian (20%) and Chinese (5%).

Fraser North: HSDA 22

Fraser North lies to the north of the Fraser River in the lower mainland of the province. With a population of nearly 600,000 in 2009, it was the third largest HSDA in BC. There were seven communities with populations of over 15,000, and two villages (Anmore and Belcarra) with a combined total population of about 2,500. Burnaby had almost 40% of the HSDA's population, followed by Coquitlam (over 20%) and Maple Ridge, New Westminster, and Port Coquitlam (all with more than 10%

each). New Westminster had the highest population density (over 3,300 per square kilometre), followed by Burnaby (over 2,300 per square kilometre). Port Coquitlam and Port Moody both had population densities well in excess of 1,000 per square kilometre. Close to 40% were visible minorities (the third highest HSDA in BC), primarily Chinese (more than 17%) and South Asian (more than 6%).

Fraser East: HSDA 21

Farther inland lies Fraser East, which straddles the Fraser River and is increasingly being viewed as part of the lower mainland region of the province. It had a population of 280,000 in 2009, and approximately half of the region's population resided in Abbotsford, with a population density of more than 360 per square kilometre. Chilliwack had half the population of Abbotsford and, in turn, Mission had half the population of Abbotsford. Hope, Kent, and Harrison Hot Springs, farther east up the Fraser Valley, while all were well-defined communities, had relatively small populations. Nearly 16% were visible minorities, dominated by South Asian (almost 11%), and close to 6% of the population were Aboriginal.

Vancouver Coastal HSDAs

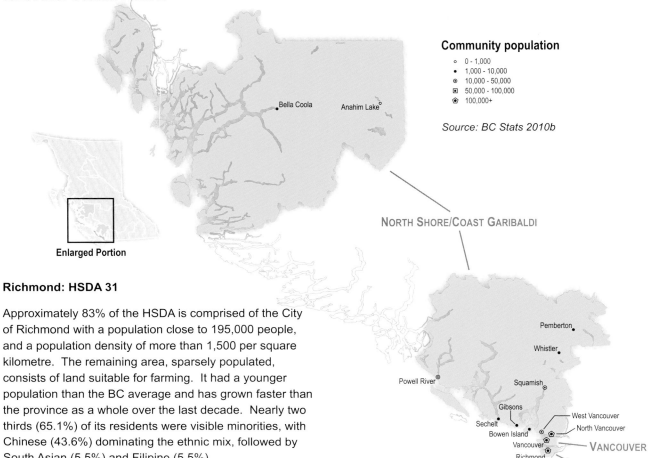

Community population

- o 0 - 1,000
- • 1,000 - 10,000
- ◉ 10,000 - 50,000
- ▣ 50,000 - 100,000
- ⬠ 100,000+

Source: BC Stats 2010b

Richmond: HSDA 31

Approximately 83% of the HSDA is comprised of the City of Richmond with a population close to 195,000 people, and a population density of more than 1,500 per square kilometre. The remaining area, sparsely populated, consists of land suitable for farming. It had a younger population than the BC average and has grown faster than the province as a whole over the last decade. Nearly two thirds (65.1%) of its residents were visible minorities, with Chinese (43.6%) dominating the ethnic mix, followed by South Asian (5.5%) and Filipino (5.5%).

Vancouver: HSDA 32

The City of Vancouver had a population of over 640,000 in 2009. With a population density of nearly 5,500 per square kilometre, it was by far the most densely populated part of BC. Proportionately more of its population was in the 25 to 64 age group than the rest of BC. More than half (51.1%) of its population was from a visible minority group, second only to Richmond, and the most prominent groups were Chinese (51.1%), followed by South Asian (5.6%) and Filipino (4.9%).

North Shore/Coast Garibaldi: HSDA 33

The North Shore/Coast Garibaldi HSDA consists of two large non-contiguous regions with a variety of urban, rural, mountain, and water body areas. The overall population of the HSDA was nearly 280,000 in 2009, but approximately one third of the population was located in the District Municipality of North Vancouver, in the lower mainland (southern) portion of the HSDA. The neighbouring City of North Vancouver and District Municipality of West Vancouver, which were about the same population size, comprised a second third of the

population. The City of North Vancouver was notable because of its compactness, with a population density of approximately 4,000 per square kilometre. Heading north from West Vancouver are several smaller but important settlements, including Squamish (more than 6% of the HSDA's population) and Whistler (4%) and Pemberton. Approximately 8% of the residents in this sub-area were Aboriginal.

The western part of the southern block of the HSDA consists of what is called the "Sunshine Coast," and is accessible only by ferry or sea plane. There are several smaller communities, but the key ones are Powell River in the extreme west, which had more than 5% of the HSDA's population, and Sechelt and Gibsons, which, combined, made up about 5% of the HSDA's population. Bowen Island, as its name suggests, is an island community with less than 3% of the HSDA's population.

The northern block of the HSDA is remote and had very few residents. The major population area was the Bella Coola Valley, which had a population of less than 3,000 in 2009, more than half of whom were Aboriginal.

Vancouver Island HSDAs

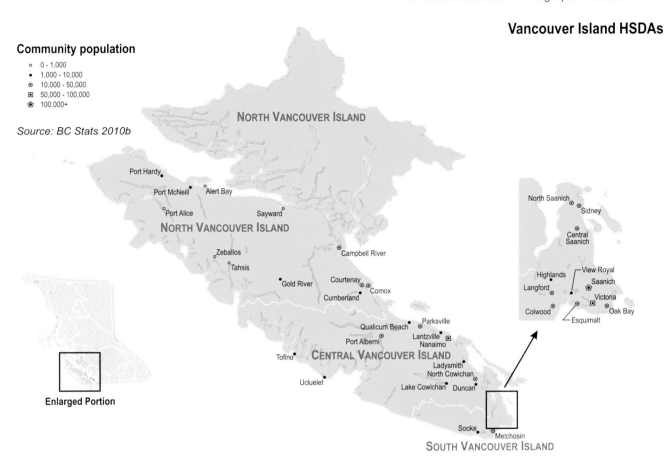

Community population

- ○ 0 - 1,000
- • 1,000 - 10,000
- ⊙ 10,000 - 50,000
- ▣ 50,000 - 100,000
- ◉ 100,000+

Source: BC Stats 2010b

NORTH VANCOUVER ISLAND

Port Hardy
Port McNeill   Alert Bay
Port Alice   Sayward
NORTH VANCOUVER ISLAND
Zeballos   Campbell River
Tahsis
Gold River   Courtenay
                  Comox
Cumberland
                  Parksville
Qualicum Beach
Port Alberni   Lantzville
                  Nanaimo
Tofino   CENTRAL VANCOUVER ISLAND
                  Ladysmith
                  North Cowichan
Ucluelet   Lake Cowichan Duncan

North Saanich
                  Sidney
Central
Saanich
Highlands   View Royal
Langford   Saanich
                  Victoria
Colwood   Oak Bay
          Esquimalt

Sooke
          Metchosin
SOUTH VANCOUVER ISLAND

Enlarged Portion

South Vancouver Island: HSDA 41

In 2009, the South Vancouver Island HSDA had a population of approximately 370,000, with most people residing in the east of the HSDA. It is comprised of many individual municipalities, but most of the population was concentrated in the four core municipalities of Saanich (31.4%), the provincial capital of Victoria (22.6%), Oak Bay (5.2%), and Esquimalt (4.9%). While Saanich had a population density of more than 1,000 per square kilometre, Victoria's density was more than 4,000 per square kilometre. Esquimalt had a density of over 2,400 people per square kilometre, while Oak Bay's population density was somewhat less than 1,800 per square kilometre. The dominant visible minority group was Chinese (3.6%), followed by South Asian (2.1%). Aboriginal people represented 3.3% of the HSDA's population.

Central Vancouver Island: HSDA 42

With a population of more than 260,000 in 2009, Central Vancouver Island had a variety of separate municipalities, most of which are on the east coast. Nanaimo had approximately one-third of the HSDA's population (more than 1,000 people per square kilometre), followed by

North Cowichan (over 11% of the population). A full third of the population, however, was found scattered through the region in rural areas. While Duncan had only about 2% of the HSDA's population, with a density of over 2,500 per square kilometre, it had the highest population density of any of the municipalities. Approximately 8% of the population was Aboriginal.

Northern Vancouver Island: HSDA 43

With a population of around 120,000 in 2009, North Vancouver Island was the least populated of the three HSDAs on Vancouver Island. Nearly 60% of the population was concentrated in three municipalities, Campbell River (26%), Courtenay (20%), and Comox (12%). Courtenay and Campbell River had population densities of over 800 per square kilometre. One third of the population was scattered in rural areas with a population density of less than 1 per square kilometre. A few small villages were located on the north part of the Island and the extreme west coast, all of which were quite remote. Fully 10% of the population was Aboriginal.

Northern HSDAs

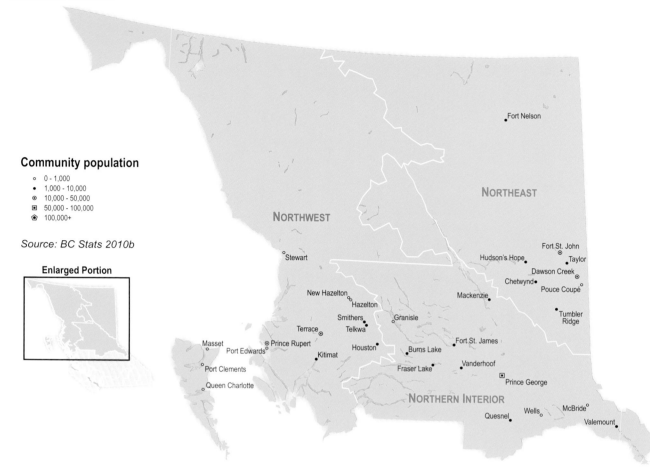

Community population

- ∘ 0 - 1,000
- • 1,000 - 10,000
- ⊚ 10,000 - 50,000
- ⊡ 50,000 - 100,000
- ⌖ 100,000+

Source: BC Stats 2010b

Enlarged Portion

Northwest: HSDA 51

With a population of only 75,000, this HSDA had the second smallest population in the province. It had also lost population over the past 10 years. Close to 50% of the population was scattered throughout the region in rural areas, while 45% was concentrated in four municipalities: Prince Rupert (over 17%), Terrace (over 15%), Kitimat (over 12%), and Houston (over 4%), all in the southern part of the HSDA. Much of the HSDA consists of mountainous areas dissected by river valleys where population density was very low, and even in the population centres, population density was only in the order of 300 per square kilometre. The HSDA also has an important offshore component, Haida Gwaii, consisting mainly of mountains and forests with a few small villages, including Masset, Queen Charlotte City, and Port Clements. One third of the population was Aboriginal.

Northern Interior: HSDA 52

More than half (nearly 52%) of the population of over 142,000 was concentrated in Prince George, while over 30% of the people were scattered around the HSDA in

rural, sometimes mountainous areas. Other important communities included Quesnel (nearly 7% of the population), Mackenzie, Vanderhoof, Burns Lake, and Fort St. James (collectively with about 9% of the HSDA's population), with Fraser Lake, Valemount, McBride, Granisle, and Wells providing the rest of the population. More than 13% of the HSDA's residents were Aboriginal.

Northeast: HSDA 53

The Northeast had only about 68,000 individuals. Approximately half of the population was found in Fort St. John (27%), Dawson Creek (17%), and Fort Nelson (7%), all with population densities of more than 400 per square kilometre. Approximately 36% of the population was scattered throughout the HSDA in rural areas, while the remaining population was located in Chetwynd, Taylor, Hudson's Hope, and Pouce Coupe. Over 13% of the population was Aboriginal.

Nighttime view of BC population distribution

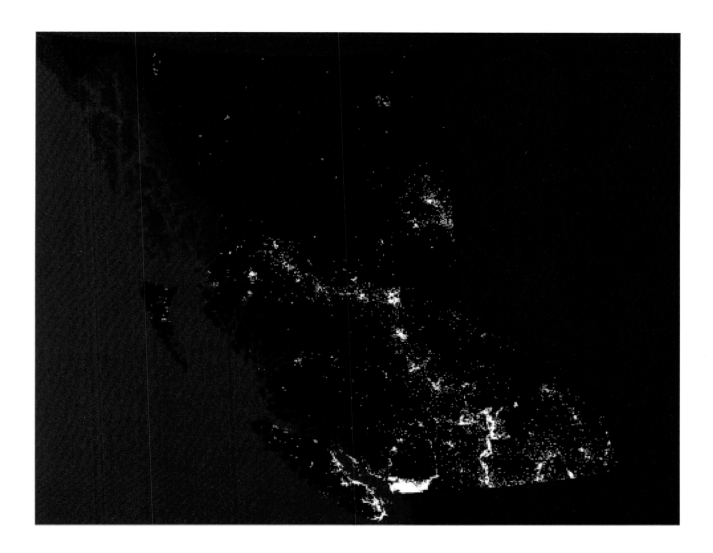

This map provides a visualization of how the population was distributed through the province in 2006, based on the census. One of the key points to note for those not familiar with BC is that much of the province is uninhabited, and where population does occur, it is clustered primarily in the southern most quarter.

Key population concentrations occur in the extreme southwestern part (lower mainland) of the province, and the southern tip and eastern part of Vancouver Island, which lies off the southwest coast of the mainland. In the southern central part of the mainland, population is concentrated in a north to south line in the Okanagan Valley. In the southeast of the province, population is centred on small communities, again often located in river valleys.

In the central interior part of the province, population is concentrated in several communities running in a general northwest to southeast direction, and settlements are usually in river valleys. Population in the northern half of the province is very sparse, with a concentration in small communities in the northeast.

Recent population growth has mostly been focused in the lower mainland, Okanagan Valley, and southern and eastern Vancouver Island. As such, the general geographical pattern will have changed very little since the 2006 census.

Summary

As noted already, the majority of the population in the province is far from equally distributed throughout the province and the most rapid population growth has taken place in those areas where there is already the greatest concentrations and densities of population: the lower mainland, especially Metropolitan Vancouver, along with South Vancouver Island, the Nanaimo area on the central part of Vancouver Island, and the Okanagan region.

While most of the province's population resided in these areas, the geography of the Aboriginal population was quite different from that of the BC population as a whole. Many lived in designated reserves, which are often very small and can be remote, some being accessible only by water. Approximately 26% of Aboriginal people lived on these reserves in 2006, down from 30% in 2001. North Shore/Coast Garibaldi, Northwest, and Thompson Cariboo Shuswap had the highest proportion of their Aboriginal population living on these designated reserves. Aboriginal males were more likely to live on reserve than Aboriginal females (Norton, 2008), although females outnumbered males overall. Aboriginal people were more likely to reside in the north and central regions of the province. Overall, the Aboriginal population was much younger than the province's population as a whole.

New immigrants to Canada who lived in BC were very much concentrated in the urban lower mainland, where there was an already large concentration of immigrants. Since 2001, however, there has been a small but noticeable trend of some new immigrants settling elsewhere in the province—a trend that has been noted in other provinces of Canada (Federation of Canadian Municipalities, 2009). A language other than English or French spoken in the home was quite common in the higher immigrant population regions, and there were many new immigrants who had very little command of English or French in 2006.

There has been little relative change in overall geographical patterns between the 2001 and 2006 censuses. The north continued to have a much higher proportion of its population in the younger age cohorts and was below average for the senior cohort. Parts of the lower mainland had proportionately more people in the mid-age cohort, while Central Vancouver Island, Okanagan and Kootenay Boundary had higher percentages of seniors, many of whom had moved from elsewhere to retire in those areas.

5

The Geography of Wellness Assets and Determinants

Introduction

Numerous factors can be viewed as wellness assets and health determinants, as discussed in Chapter 2. Research has shown that individuals, families, or communities that possess these wellness-related assets have greater prospects for better health and wellness status and outcomes than those who do not possess them. This chapter focuses on a variety of these assets.

Key indicators in this chapter are based on the 2006 Canada Census, the 2008 McCreary AHS IV, the 2007/8 CCHS 4.1 (share file), the 2008/9 Students Satisfaction Survey. A variety of other sources are also used, including the Ministry of Children and Family Development, Ministry of Public Safety and Solicitor General, Ministry of Education, Ministry of Community and Rural Development, as well as others. In total, there are six groupings of wellness asset indicators with a total of 112 maps, as described below.

Families, income, and housing

In total, 20 maps are included in this category of wellness assets and health determinants. The first three maps provide information on family structure. Children who live in the parental home do far better than those who live alone or are in the care of the state (Turpel-Lafond & Kendall, 2007; 2010; Turpel-Lafond, 2010). Further, children who live with two adults are generally happier and more likely to thrive than those who do not (Ermisch, Iacovou & Skew, 2011). Single parenthood is tough on both parent and child(ren), thus potentially compromising the wellness of both. Adults living together are able to provide support and companionship for each other throughout their lives together, thus increasing wellness for both individuals.

The next group of 10 maps covers a variety of income-related factors. As Mikkonen and Raphael (2010) have noted, "Level of income shapes overall living conditions, affects psychological functioning, and influences health-related behaviours such as quality of diet, extent of physical activity, tobacco use, and excessive alcohol use. In Canada, income determines the quality of other social determinants of health such as food security, housing, and other basic prerequisites of health" (p. 12). The ability of a population to support young and older people in the population, called dependency ratios, provides useful community wellness indicators. Individual and community wellness also generally increase with mean family income, while those living above the low income cut-off measure (LICO) spend a smaller percentage of their income on basic necessities such as shelter, food, and clothing than those below the cut-off level. The family group most likely to be below the cut-off level is the female-headed lone parent family (Sauve, 2010). Income equality within a geographical region has been shown to be important from a wellness perspective: the smaller the gradient between the highest and lowest income families, the more stable and secure the community tends to be. Within Canada as a whole, income inequality has been rising over the past 20 years (Sauve, 2010) – not a very encouraging wellness trend. The ratio of female income to male income is also a useful indicator of wellness, as it provides a measure of income equity between genders. Other important wellness indicators include income sources, such as income from employment or government transfers. The data we provide are based on the 2006 census and, being somewhat out-of-date, they do not include the impacts of the 2008/9 downturn in the global economy. However, relative patterns may not have changed markedly. Nevertheless, some caution in interpretation of the maps is required.

The next seven maps provide information on housing. Shelter is not only a fundamental human right, but housing provides a sense of security and stability and a place where families are nurtured and bond, and where friends and neighbours can play and socialize. It is an important wellness measure (Bryant, 2009). Poor housing or homelessness are associated with poorer health and insecurity. The maps presented here are based on the 2006 Canada Census, and look at differing components of housing. Adequate housing does not require any major repairs, according to residents. Housing is defined as affordable if it costs less than 30% of before-tax household income. For renters, shelter costs include rent and any payments for electricity, fuel, water, and other municipal services. For owners, costs include mortgage payments (principal and interest), property taxes, and any condominium fees, along with payments for electricity, fuel, water, and other municipal services. BC, especially in the lower mainland and southern part of Vancouver Island, has some of the highest cost housing in Canada, and in a recent international report on housing affordability in cities of over 1 million people, Metro Vancouver ranked the third most unaffordable housing city out of more than 80 cities worldwide (Cox & Pavletich, 2011). Suitable housing has enough bedrooms for the size and make-up of resident households, according to National Occupancy Standard requirements (Central Mortgage and Housing Corporation, 2011). The final three maps included in this group are based on data from the McCreary AHS IV and provide information on youth who have their own bedrooms.

Connections

Being connected to others is important from a wellness perspective. This group of 24 maps provides indicators that show different levels of connectedness. Youth and children who have generally higher levels of connectedness with their family are healthier, do better in school and engage in less risky behaviours, as do those who have regular meals with parents and those who have a strong connection to their school (Eisenberg et al., 2004; Franko et al., 2008; Saewyc et al., 2006; Smith et al., 2009; Fieldhouse, 2009). These three measures are mapped using survey data from the McCreary AHS IV. Three more indicators are mapped from CCHS 4.1 and also deal with issues of connectedness. A strong sense of connectedness to local community, positive social interactions, and emotional supports indicate a sense of inclusion, cohesion, trust in others and in the community, and promote health and longer life. Connectedness and social networks are also important in dealing with change and, as Keown (2009) has noted, more than one in four adult Canadians experienced a change in 2008 that had a significant impact on their lives. Connectedness is also a

measure of belongingness, which is an important wellness asset (Canadian Population Health Initiative, 2004).

Improving health

Actions that involve doing something to improve health and intentions to improve health are important from a wellness perspective. This group of 18 maps focuses on health improvements, as well as access to programs at or close to the work environment, and learning how to stay healthy at school. The first three indicators are based on CCHS 4.1, and the last one comes from the Student Satisfaction Survey for 2008/9. Given that many people spend a lot of time in the work environment, while younger individuals spend time at school, both these settings are important from the perspective of maintaining or improving and learning about health and wellness (Kendall, 2008a; Mikkonen & Raphael, 2010; Merrill et al., 2011).

Education, culture, arts and volunteerism

Overall, there are 30 maps in this grouping. The first 19 maps focus on educational and learning assets and achievements. Research has consistently shown the importance of a good education for health and wellness (Mikkonen & Raphael, 2010; Suhrcke & de Paz Nieves, 2011). The first map combines a couple of key pieces of information and looks at the distribution of Strong Start programs throughout BC relative to those areas that are likely to have the greatest proportion of youngsters who may be at risk of not being fully ready to learn when entering kindergarten. Early childhood development has been recognized as an important determinant of health (Mikkonen & Raphael, 2010), and therefore being ready to learn is an important wellness asset. Strong Start programs, although open to all youngsters and their caregivers, have been set up in BC primarily to help to level the playing field for those children that may be at a socioeconomic disadvantage. The next key indicators are based on the Early Development Instrument (EDI), which measures readiness to learn on entering kindergarten (Janus & Offord, 2007; Janus et al., 2007). These are followed by educational achievements at grades 4 and 7 in 2009/10, and high school graduation and post-secondary education completion in the adult population based on the 2006 census. While successful completion of key educational milestones is important, in today's world, lifelong learning is also a key wellness asset, and five maps are presented based on the Composite Learning Index (CLI) developed by the Canadian Council on Learning (2010a). The final two maps in this group show the availability of adult and child and youth programs within the public library system.

Many of the wellness and well-being frameworks discussed in Chapter 2 include cultural activities. Research shows that there are clear relationships between cultural activities and volunteering and donating, community and neighbourhood connections, sense of belonging, labour force participation, social activities, and overall quality of life. These are all very important wellness assets (Hill Strategies Research Inc, 2008). The next group of seven maps covers various components of culture and the arts. The first map looks at employment in the arts, while the next six maps provide information from the 2008/9 Student Satisfaction Survey related to students learning about arts and music. As Ewing (2010) notes, "immersion in the Arts can improve an individual's sense of enjoyment, purpose and identity, positively changing the direction of people's lives. The Arts, it is argued, by transforming learning in formal educational contexts, can ensure that the curriculum engages and has relevance for all children" (p.1). Further, involvement of students in the arts and music programs has been shown to increase academic achievement, IQ, attendance, performance on standardized reading and verbal tests, and literacy (Vaughan et al., 2011).

There are just four maps in the volunteerism group because there are few readily available geographical data related to volunteerism in BC. Volunteerism is an important individual and community wellness asset. A survey undertaken in 2010 suggested that volunteering made people happier, and improved both emotional and physical health (UnitedHealthcare, 2010). While geographical data for volunteerism in BC are hard to come by, there are data at the provincial level, although results are somewhat mixed. For BC as a whole, 46.6% of the population aged 15 and over indicated that they had volunteered during 2007, a slight increase over the 2004 results of 45%, similar results to those for Canada as a whole. But of those who did volunteer, the average number of hours volunteered in BC dropped significantly (14%) between the 2 years (Hall et al., 2009). Another measure looks at helping others. While BC had one of the lowest rates among provinces and territories of helping others directly, it had increased significantly between 2004 and 2007 from 78% to 83%. A third measure, which looks at charitable donations, shows that in 2008 BC also had one of the lowest donation rates of any province, based on the returns of tax filers (Gainer et al., 2010).

Information will become available with the release of the 2009/10 CCHS share file data, but this will only be available later in 2011. We have obtained data from the half sample (2009) for CCHS 5.1 on membership in

voluntary organizations. Samples are not large enough to usefully look at geographical variations, but provincially, 36.62% of all respondents indicated that they were members of voluntary organizations, and the youth (41.97%) and senior (44.54%) cohorts were significantly more likely to be members of voluntary organizations than the mid-age cohort (34.17%). Further, females (40.54%) were significantly more likely than males (29.94%) to be members of voluntary groups.

The first map looks at volunteerism in the BC library system, based on information from the Ministry of Education, while the next three maps use McCreary AHS IV data to examine volunteerism by students.

Safety

Feeling safe at home, at school, and in the community are important for wellness. This group of 14 maps provides a series of indicators related to students' perceptions of safety at school, and also crime rates within the community. Students spend a large part of their daily lives in a school setting, and feeling safe at school is important for learning and for a student's well-being (Kendall, 2008a). There is also "a recognition that a strong relationship exists between feelings of safety and belonging" (Ministry of Education, 2008, p. 3). The first six maps in this group deal with feelings of safety in the school environment. This is followed by three maps that describe issues related to bullying at school. Key dimensions of bullying include physical, psychological, or verbal actions that intend to and cause harm, and over time a victim may feel excluded, intimidated, and self-esteem becomes undermined (Baldrey & Farrington, 2007). These student-based maps use data from the 2008/9 Student Satisfaction Survey and McCreary AHS IV. The final five maps in this section provide information on crime. Crime rates, developed by BC Stats from data provided by the Ministry of Safety and Solicitor General for the period 2006 to 2008, while a "negative" indicator of community wellness, are an indicator of community cohesion and safety.

Community actions and capacities

The final six maps provide indicators related to actions by communities to improve capacity for improving the health and wellness of their populations. Several relate to specific programs that supported ActNow BC outcomes, especially with respect to sustainability. Such actions by communities tend to make them more cohesive, stronger, and healthier.

Family structure

Children not living in the family home

This indicator is reversed from that seen in the first edition of the Atlas: percentages were very low overall, and we felt it better to show the indicator in a manner that highlights geographical variations throughout BC. The proportion of children who are living in the care of the state or on a government-funded Youth Agreement is an important indicator of not only how we treat children as a society, but a useful measure of family and community social and economic wellness. It is also a measure of the effectiveness of community supports for families in need or at risk.

Children come into care because of a variety of protection concerns such as neglect, or physical, emotional, or sexual abuse. This measure provides an underestimate of children not being well cared for by their biological parents. Many are looked after by relatives through both formal and informal arrangements (MacKenzie et al., 2009). This is often associated with socioeconomic deprivation, which is connected to depression, low self-esteem, substance misuse, and other factors that undermine the ability of parents to look after their offspring. Key mediators are factors such as community support assets, social cohesiveness, inclusion, and social capital. Specific subgroups are at greater risk of having children taken into care, particularly Aboriginal groups because of a variety of economic, social, and historical issues (Foster & Wharf, 2007; Kendall, 2009). Youth Agreements allow older children to live independently, and cover those between the ages of 16 and 18 years, when there is no parent or other person willing to take responsibility, or a youth feels it is not safe to be in the home.

In BC, in 2009, 1.47% of all children between birth and 18 years, were in state care or on Youth Agreements. This ranged from a low of 0.47% in Richmond to 2.90% in Thompson Cariboo Shuswap. While this value for all children is very similar to the 1.48% in 2005, the range geographically has increased from 1.56 percentage points to 2.33 percentage points in 2009, indicating a greater geographical variation throughout the province. Overall, children were more likely to be in care or on Youth Agreements in the north and interior parts of BC, while lower values were more likely to be found in the lower mainland HSDAs.

Children living in 2 parent families

Generally, children living in two parent families do better developmentally than those living in care, on their own, or in lone parent families. Single parent families, especially those headed by females, which comprised about 80% of all lone parent families in 2006, experience greater challenges,

Health Service Delivery Area	Children not living at home (%)	Children in 2 parent families (%)	Couples living together (%)
31 Richmond	0.47	78.1	59.86
22 Fraser North	0.77	76.4	58.48
33 North Shore/Coast Garibaldi	0.92	75.4	59.67
23 Fraser South	1.03	78.2	62.11
32 Vancouver	1.30	73.4	50.59
53 Northeast	1.31	77.4	63.27
12 Kootenay Boundary	1.49	72.3	61.67
41 South Vancouver Island	1.66	70.3	56.73
13 Okanagan	1.74	71.3	62.14
43 North Vancouver Island	1.79	70.3	62.17
11 East Kootenay	1.80	74.0	64.18
21 Fraser East	2.00	75.0	61.93
42 Central Vancouver Island	2.41	69.7	62.08
52 Northern Interior	2.50	72.4	61.11
51 Northwest	2.70	70.5	59.96
14 Thompson Cariboo Shuswap	2.90	71.1	62.25
British Columbia	**1.47**	**74.3**	**59.17**

especially in child rearing. They are generally poorer, with only 50% of the average income of couple families, and have greater challenges balancing requirements around work and family. They tend to be more isolated, and often feel excluded from community happenings. The struggle to survive can be a tough one. Children raised in two parent families usually receive more attention and support, both in terms of time and finances, and have better opportunities to thrive.

In 2006, close to three in every four (74.3%) children were being raised in a two parent family. This was a reduction from 79.80% in 2001. Throughout the province, there was an 8.5 percentage point range, with Fraser South at 78.2% and Central Vancouver Island with only 69.7%. The reduction in children living in two parent families was found in every HSDA in the province, indicating a societal level change potentially putting more children at risk. Geographically, the lowest levels of two parent families were found throughout all of Vancouver Island, parts of the interior and Northwest, while higher levels were found in parts of the lower mainland (with the exception of Vancouver) and Northeast.

Couples living together

Couples living together (married or common law) are able to share living tasks, child rearing, and incomes. Emotional attachments provide supports at times of illness, and for males at least, marriage results in a longer life. In 2006, throughout BC, nearly six in every ten (59.17%) households on average had two adults living together, a marginal increase over 2001 (58.86%). Most HSDAs were between 58% and 64%, with Vancouver being the lowest at 50.59%, and an outlier from other HSDAs. South Vancouver Island (56.73%) also had a relatively low percentage. Those with the highest values were found in the extreme northeast and southeast of the province, as well as the central interior.

Family structure

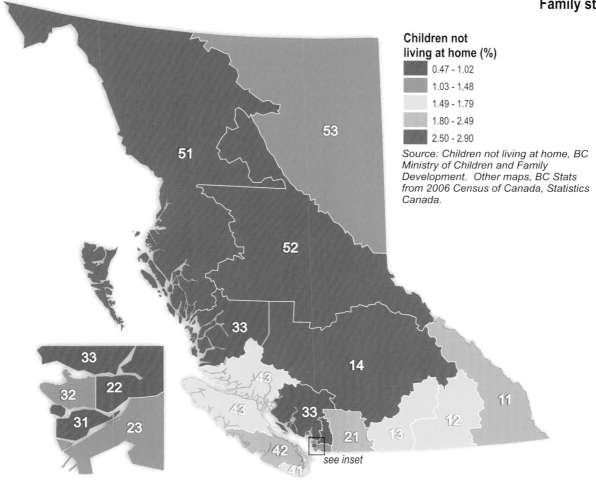

Children not living at home (%)

- 0.47 - 1.02
- 1.03 - 1.48
- 1.49 - 1.79
- 1.80 - 2.49
- 2.50 - 2.90

Source: Children not living at home, BC Ministry of Children and Family Development. Other maps, BC Stats from 2006 Census of Canada, Statistics Canada.

see inset

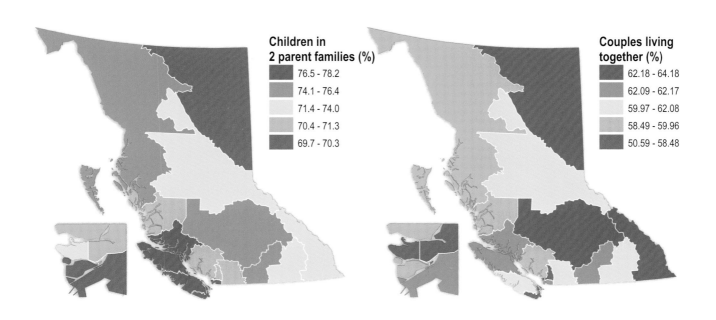

Children in 2 parent families (%)

- 76.5 - 78.2
- 74.1 - 76.4
- 71.4 - 74.0
- 70.4 - 71.3
- 69.7 - 70.3

Couples living together (%)

- 62.18 - 64.18
- 62.09 - 62.17
- 59.97 - 62.08
- 58.49 - 59.96
- 50.59 - 58.48

Demographic dependency rates

Dependency rates provide a measure of young and senior populations that can be supported by the proportion of the population that is often in the paid workforce. As such, it gives a measure of the "working age population" that can theoretically support those normally at either end of the age spectrum who are often retired or dependent upon parents.

Total dependency rate

The total dependency rate takes the combined number of children between birth and age 17 years and the number of seniors who are 65 years and older, and divides the total by the number of people in the population between the ages of 18 and 64 years, and multiplies that number by 100 to provide a percentage of those available to support the young and old in the population both economically and as potential caregivers and providers of other services. The lower the percentage, the greater the theoretical potential to support the young and old. For the province as a whole, the average dependency rate was 51.11% in 2009, a small, but not insignificant reduction since 2005 (50.78%). Values varied from a low of 37.93% in Vancouver, to a high of 61.42% in Okanagan, a range of 23 percentage points among HSDAs. Values were lowest in parts of the lower mainland (Vancouver, Richmond, Fraser North), while higher values were more characteristic of Fraser East, Okanagan, and Central Vancouver Island (all 59% or higher). Overall patterns were very similar to those observed in 2001.

Child dependency rate

This indicator, new to this edition of the Atlas, takes just the child population from birth to age 17 years and divides it by the population between the ages of 18 and 64 years, and multiplies that number by 100 to provide a percentage value. It provides a measure of the child population that is dependent on the general working age population. Again, the lower the value, the greater the potential of the community to support dependent children. It also gives a better sense of the component of the total dependency rate attributable to the child population. Values varied from a low of 20.87% for Vancouver to a high of 38.91% in Northeast, a range of 18 percentage points among HSDAs. Rates were also low in Richmond (26.54%) and South Vancouver Island (24.52%), while values were highest in parts of the north (Northeast and Northwest) and Fraser East (all above 36%).

Health Service Delivery Area	Total dependency (%)	Child dependency (%)	Senior dependency (%)
32 Vancouver	37.93	20.87	17.06
22 Fraser North	45.18	28.04	17.14
31 Richmond	45.49	26.54	18.95
41 South Vancouver Island	50.65	24.52	26.13
52 Northern Interior	51.14	33.66	17.48
53 Northeast	51.91	38.91	13.00
33 North Shore/Coast Garibaldi	52.52	28.84	23.67
51 Northwest	54.69	37.34	17.35
11 East Kootenay	54.74	29.97	24.77
14 Thompson Cariboo Shuswap	55.69	29.79	25.90
23 Fraser South	56.23	34.46	21.77
43 North Vancouver Island	56.34	30.40	25.94
12 Kootenay Boundary	56.93	28.63	28.29
21 Fraser East	58.94	36.12	22.82
42 Central Vancouver Island	60.54	28.63	31.91
13 Okanagan	61.42	29.13	32.30
British Columbia	**51.11**	**28.85**	**22.26**

Senior dependency rate

This is another indicator that is new to this edition of the Atlas. It takes the seniors population (age 65 and over) and divides it by the "normal" working age population (18 to 64 years) and multiplies by 100 to provide a percentage value. For the province as a whole, the average value is 22.26%, with a low of 13.00% in Northeast and a high of 32.30% in Okanagan, for a range of 19 percentage points among HSDAs. Geographically, the lowest rates are found in two general regions: the northern half of the province and parts of the lower mainland (Vancouver, Fraser North, and Richmond), all below 19%. High values are found in the southern interior and Central Vancouver Island (all above 28%).

Demographic dependency rates

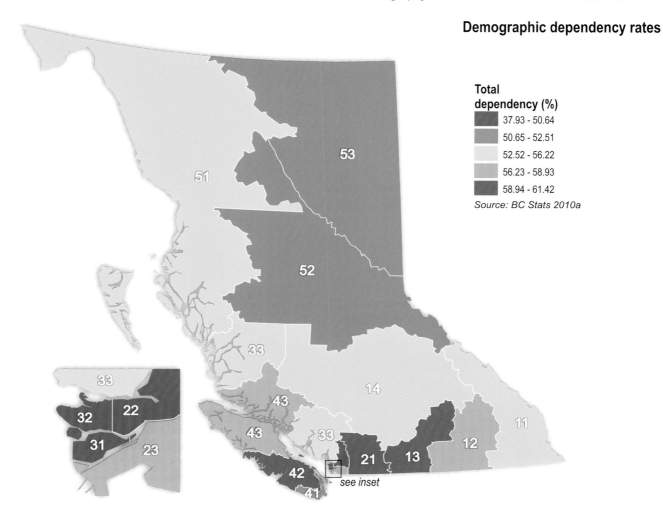

Total dependency (%)
- 37.93 - 50.64
- 50.65 - 52.51
- 52.52 - 56.22
- 56.23 - 58.93
- 58.94 - 61.42

Source: BC Stats 2010a

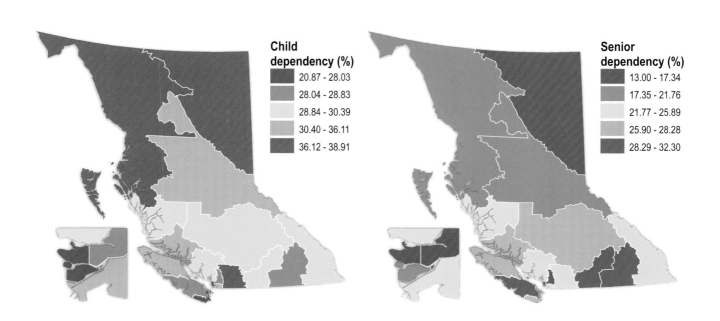

Child dependency (%)
- 20.87 - 28.03
- 28.04 - 28.83
- 28.84 - 30.39
- 30.40 - 36.11
- 36.12 - 38.91

Senior dependency (%)
- 13.00 - 17.34
- 17.35 - 21.76
- 21.77 - 25.89
- 25.90 - 28.28
- 28.29 - 32.30

Income distribution

Income and income equity are important for both families and communities, and are useful wellness indicators. Having a good income that is comparable to other community members, regardless of gender, allows more equity in opportunities and living. Four indicators are presented, two of which are new: income equality and female/male income comparisons.

Median family income

According to the 2006 census, the median annual family income in BC was $61,988, an increase from $46,802 in 2001. Geographically, the highest median family incomes were found in North Shore/ Coast Garibaldi and Northeast (both over $69,000), followed by Fraser South at nearly $68,000. At the other extreme, Kootenay Boundary had a median family income of only $53,803. There were some clear geographical patterns. Outside of the lower mainland, and South Vancouver Island, much of the southern half of the province, including Central and North Vancouver Island, had below the BC median family income.

Families above LICO

Canada has no official poverty measure, but there are several factors used to measure relative low incomes. A common one is the Low Income Cut-off (LICO). Using post-tax income, cut-offs are set at income levels where a family would spend a share of its post-tax income which is 20 percentage points higher than the average family would spend on three items: food, clothing and shelter. Cut-offs are calculated based on family size and type of community (Giles, 2004), but the measure is not without its critics (Shillington & Stapleton, 2010). In reality, the measure is an indicator of inequality, not poverty *per se* (Schrier, 2009). Over the last 10 years, BC has consistently ranked last among Canada's provinces on the LICO measure. The measure we use here, however, is the percentage of individuals who live above the LICO.

In BC in 2006, 86.7% were above the LICO, an improvement from 2001 (82.25%). The range was from 75.8% in Richmond to 93.9% in Northeast. South Vancouver Island also had a high percentage (91.7%). The lowest percentages were found in parts of the urban lower mainland of the province. Richmond was the only HSDA not to show an increase in the percentage above LICO between 2001 and 2006.

Health Service Delivery Area	Median income ($)	Above LICO (%)	Income equality (ratio)	Female/Male income (ratio)
33 North Shore/Coast Garibaldi	69,429	89.0	4.52	60.63
53 Northeast	69,394	93.9	3.39	56.74
23 Fraser South	67,974	86.9	3.41	71.71
52 Northern Interior	65,779	90.4	3.44	64.59
22 Fraser North	65,452	82.9	3.59	73.82
41 South Vancouver Island	65,384	91.7	3.59	76.97
32 Vancouver	61,503	78.8	4.92	74.62
51 Northwest	61,273	88.9	3.33	66.81
21 Fraser East	58,821	89.0	3.42	70.46
31 Richmond	58,511	75.8	3.83	76.83
11 East Kootenay	57,664	90.6	3.35	63.05
43 North Vancouver Island	56,890	88.8	3.42	65.47
14 Thompson Cariboo Shuswap	56,298	90.8	3.46	66.88
42 Central Vancouver Island	55,722	90.3	3.41	71.10
13 Okanagan	54,963	90.8	3.50	70.36
12 Kootenay Boundary	53,803	89.7	3.42	71.13
British Columbia	**61,988**	**86.7**	**3.83**	**71.09**

Family income equality

This new indicator measures the income share of the bottom half (poorest) households against the share of the top half. If there was complete equity in income, the value would be 1. Lower values indicate greater equity in income within HSDAs. For BC as a whole, the top half of households on average had 3.83 times the income that the bottom half had on average in 2005, based on the 2006 census. The greatest equity was found in Northwest, Northeast, and East Kootenay (all below 3.40), while the greatest inequities were found in the lower mainland HSDAs of Vancouver (4.92) and North Shore/Coast Garibaldi (4.52).

Female/male income comparisons

The equity in earnings of income between male and female employees is an important wellness indicator. There has been major concern about inequities based on gender, and females have had significant problems breaking the "glass ceiling" in terms of income equity. Based on data from the 2006 census, the income of females in full-time employment was 71.09% of that earned by males in full-time employment. Among HSDAs, this varied from a low of 56.74% in Northeast to a high of 76.97% in South Vancouver Island. Geographically, equity was higher in the urban lower mainland (with the exception of North Shore/Coast Garibaldi) and southern half of Vancouver Island, and lower throughout the northern half of the province and the extreme southeast.

Income distribution

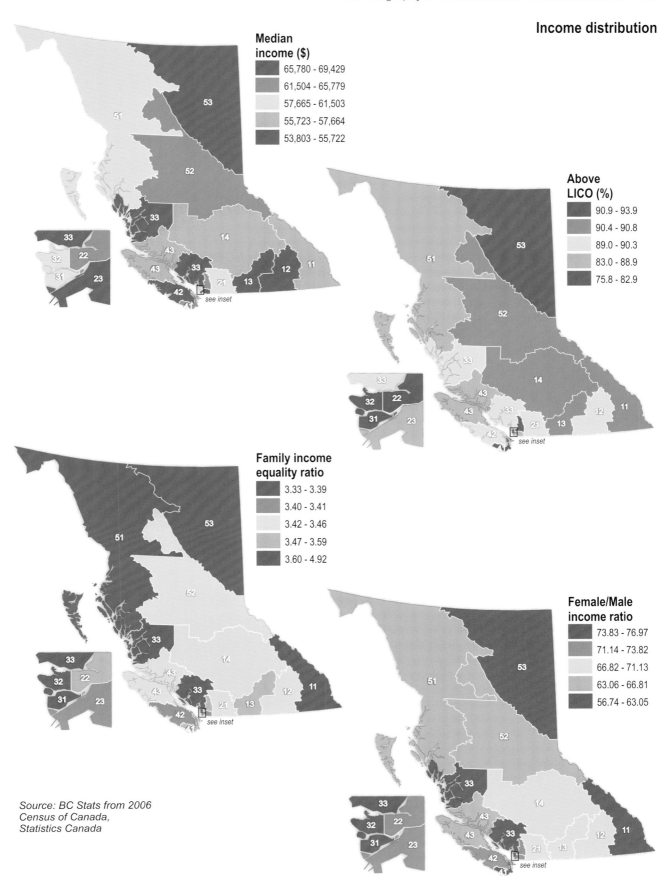

Median income ($)
- 65,780 - 69,429
- 61,504 - 65,779
- 57,665 - 61,503
- 55,723 - 57,664
- 53,803 - 55,722

Above LICO (%)
- 90.9 - 93.9
- 90.4 - 90.8
- 89.0 - 90.3
- 83.0 - 88.9
- 75.8 - 82.9

Family income equality ratio
- 3.33 - 3.39
- 3.40 - 3.41
- 3.42 - 3.46
- 3.47 - 3.59
- 3.60 - 4.92

Female/Male income ratio
- 73.83 - 76.97
- 71.14 - 73.82
- 66.82 - 71.13
- 63.06 - 66.81
- 56.74 - 63.05

Source: BC Stats from 2006 Census of Canada, Statistics Canada

Source of income

There are three main sources providing incomes to families. These are income from employment, income from government, and income from a variety of other sources. All are subject to variation over time. Each of these indicators is new to the Atlas.

Employment income

In BC as a whole in 2005, based on the 2006 Census, 77.1% of all income came from employment sources. Median employment income in BC in 2005 was $42,230, marginally higher than for Canada as a whole ($41,401). The largest employer in BC was trade (over 350,000), followed by health care and social assistance, manufacturing, construction, accommodation and food, professional, scientific and technical, and education, each with more than 150,000 employees. Average weekly wages were highest in forestry, fishing, mining, oil and gas, followed by utilities and public administration, all with weekly wages of over $1,000 in 2007 (Lu, 2010). Geographically, the importance of employment income varied by 20 percentage points between HSDAs. Northeast received 87.4% of its income from employment earnings, while at the other extreme, Central Vancouver Island received just over two-thirds (68.2%) of its income from this source. Geographically, employment income was relatively most important in the northern half of the province and parts of the lower mainland, and least important relatively speaking in the south and central interior of the province and on Vancouver Island.

Income from government transfers

This source of income provided close to one-tenth (9.6%) of all income to individuals and families in 2005. Income in this category consists of several sources, including a variety of income assistance payments, employment insurance for those who are unemployed, workers' compensation payments, and government pensions and supplements including tax credits. Government transfer income was relatively most important in Central Vancouver Island, which received 13.8% of all income from this source, while Northeast had half that amount (6.7%) in its income composition. Geographically, government transfer income was most important in the southern and central interior of the province as well as on Vancouver Island, except the extreme southern part, while it was least important in the southwest urban lower mainland region and the extreme northeast of the province.

Health Service Delivery Area	Income from employment (%)	Income from government transfers (%)	Income from other sources (%)
53 Northeast	87.4	6.7	5.9
52 Northern Interior	82.6	9.4	8.0
22 Fraser North	81.6	8.3	10.0
23 Fraser South	80.8	8.9	10.4
31 Richmond	79.7	8.8	11.5
51 Northwest	79.5	12.9	7.8
33 North Shore/Coast Garibaldi	77.3	7.2	15.4
32 Vancouver	77.2	7.6	15.2
21 Fraser East	76.9	12.1	11.0
11 East Kootenay	75.1	12.0	12.9
14 Thompson Cariboo Shuswap	74.0	12.8	13.2
41 South Vancouver Island	72.8	9.0	18.2
12 Kootenay Boundary	72.3	13.3	14.5
43 North Vancouver Island	71.9	12.9	15.2
13 Okanagan	69.8	13.4	16.8
42 Central Vancouver Island	68.2	13.8	18.0
British Columbia	**77.1**	**9.6**	**13.4**

Income from other sources

This source provided 13.4% of the total income of families in 2005. It consists primarily of private pension payments and investments. It was least important in Northeast, where it comprised only 5.9% of total income, and most important in South and Central Vancouver Island, where it made up three times that amount (both over 18%). Geographically, it was the least important source of income in the northern half of the province, while it was of much greater importance on Vancouver Island, Okanagan, and Vancouver and North Shore/Coast Garibaldi in the lower mainland.

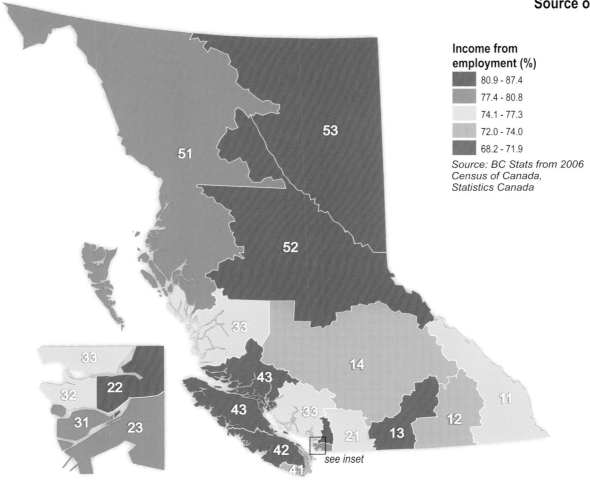

Source of income

Income from employment (%)

- 80.9 - 87.4
- 77.4 - 80.8
- 74.1 - 77.3
- 72.0 - 74.0
- 68.2 - 71.9

Source: BC Stats from 2006 Census of Canada, Statistics Canada

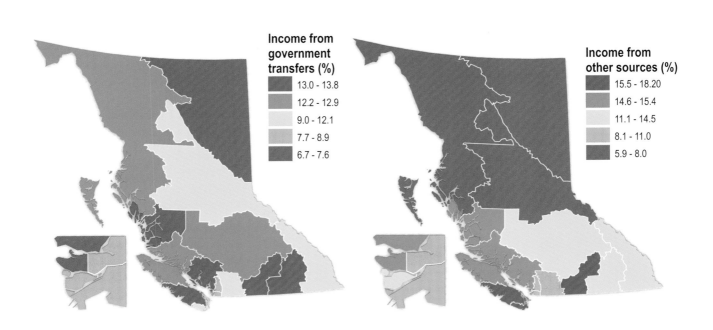

Income from government transfers (%)

- 13.0 - 13.8
- 12.2 - 12.9
- 9.0 - 12.1
- 7.7 - 8.9
- 6.7 - 7.6

Income from other sources (%)

- 15.5 - 18.20
- 14.6 - 15.4
- 11.1 - 14.5
- 8.1 - 11.0
- 5.9 - 8.0

Housing standards for all households

Shelter is a basic need. The table and maps opposite describe "acceptable" housing, based on three key dimensions defined by the Central Mortgage and Housing Corporation: adequacy, affordability, and suitability. Adequate housing does not require any major repairs. Housing is affordable if it costs less than 30% of before-tax household income. Suitable housing has enough bedrooms for the size and make-up of resident households. These data were based on residents' responses in the 2006 census.

Acceptable

Two out of every three households (66.03%) in BC reported having acceptable housing. This compared with 55.97% for Aboriginal households. Throughout BC, there was a 19 percentage point spread among regions. More than eight in every ten households in Stikine (80.85%), a very low population area in the extreme northwest of the province, indicated that they had acceptable housing, while at 61.68%, Greater Vancouver had the lowest levels of acceptable housing. Geographically, the most acceptable housing occurred *outside* of the urban lower mainland, Okanagan region, and southern and eastern parts of Vancouver Island. In addition to Greater Vancouver, Squamish-Lillooet was below the provincial average for housing acceptability.

Adequate

More than nine of every ten BC households (93.03%) indicated that they had adequate housing in 2006. This compares with only 86.82% for Aboriginal households. With a 12 percentage point spread, the geographical differences were not as great as for total acceptable standards. Central Okanagan (95.84%) households had the highest adequate housing, while only 83.31% of households in Central Coast indicated they had adequate housing. Geographically, the highest average adequate housing occurred in the southwestern quadrant of the province, and those with below provincial average adequate housing occurred in the north, central interior, and central and north coastal parts of the province, including parts of Vancouver Island. Overall, patterns tended to be reversed to those for the overall acceptability standard.

Affordable

Three of every four BC households (75.37%) indicated that they had affordable housing in 2006, compared with only 70.87% for Aboriginal households. Affordability of housing showed a great variation throughout the province: only

Regional District	Acceptable housing (%)	Adequate housing (%)	Affordable housing (%)	Suitable housing (%)
57 Stikine	80.85	91.49	93.62	95.74
51 Bulkley-Nechako	76.07	90.36	87.23	95.06
53 Fraser-Fort George	74.98	91.73	83.83	96.27
5 Kootenay Boundary	74.71	89.97	84.17	96.81
45 Central Coast	74.29	83.81	91.43	96.19
41 Cariboo	73.70	90.44	84.38	95.49
1 East Kootenay	73.50	91.93	82.78	96.24
55 Peace River	73.32	90.78	84.18	95.09
39 Columbia-Shuswap	73.27	91.11	81.56	96.75
49 Kitimat-Stikine	72.53	86.91	84.81	95.64
33 Thompson-Nicola	72.31	92.77	79.98	95.89
23 Alberni-Clayoquot	72.27	89.66	83.24	95.49
43 Mount Waddington	72.24	86.98	83.66	97.67
25 Comox Valley	72.02	92.23	80.06	96.07
26 Strathcona	72.02	92.23	80.06	96.07
27 Powell River	71.97	89.11	82.44	96.57
59 Northern Rockies	71.91	86.92	87.89	95.88
19 Cowichan Valley	71.60	92.42	79.15	96.35
7 Okanagan-Similkameen	70.52	93.70	76.85	96.65
35 Central Okanagan	70.22	95.84	75.16	96.42
37 North Okanagan	70.14	93.57	76.80	96.27
21 Nanaimo	70.13	93.40	76.67	96.56
29 Sunshine Coast	68.97	92.28	76.65	96.14
3 Central Kootenay	68.82	88.97	80.09	95.64
17 Capital	68.22	94.16	75.12	95.28
9 Fraser Valley	66.48	94.37	74.36	93.90
47 Skeena-Queen Charlotte	66.03	86.67	81.65	92.92
31 Squamish-Lillooet	63.01	93.23	72.93	92.53
15 Greater Vancouver	61.68	93.26	72.41	90.19
British Columbia	**66.03**	**93.03**	**75.37**	**92.93**

72.93% of Greater Vancouver households had affordable housing, compared with 93.62% of households in Stikine, a range of over 20 percentage points. The overall geographic pattern was quite similar to that for the overall acceptable housing indicator, showing the major impact of affordability on housing as a whole. The highest rates of affordable housing tended to be found in the northern two-thirds of the province, and the least affordable in the urban lower mainland, southern parts of Vancouver Island, and parts of the Okanagan region in the southern interior.

Suitable

Based on the number of bedrooms relative to the household composition, more than nine of every ten provincial households (92.93%) indicated they had suitable housing in 2006. This compared with 89.12% for Aboriginal households. The geographical spread, at about 5 percentage points, was quite small: Mt Waddington, at 97.67%, and Greater Vancouver, at 90.19%, had respectively the highest and lowest average regional values. Geographically, the lowest average values were found in the urban lower mainland, while those with higher average values were clustered in the southeast of the province (with the exception of Central Kootenay) and Powell River and Mt Waddington on the south central coast.

Housing standards for all households

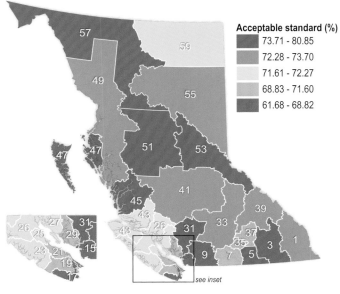

Acceptable standard (%)
- 73.71 - 80.85
- 72.28 - 73.70
- 71.61 - 72.27
- 68.83 - 71.60
- 61.68 - 68.82

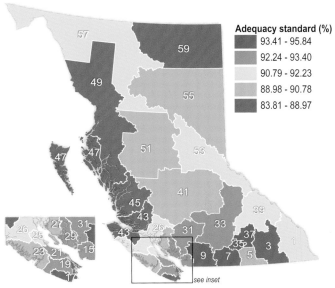

Adequacy standard (%)
- 93.41 - 95.84
- 92.24 - 93.40
- 90.79 - 92.23
- 88.98 - 90.78
- 83.81 - 88.97

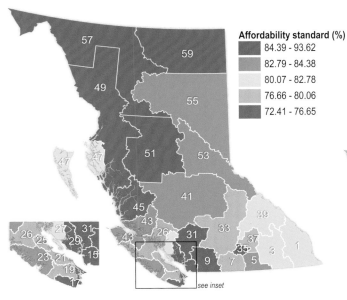

Affordability standard (%)
- 84.39 - 93.62
- 82.79 - 84.38
- 80.07 - 82.78
- 76.66 - 80.06
- 72.41 - 76.65

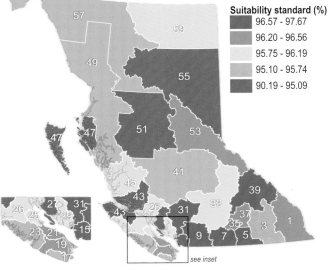

Suitability standard (%)
- 96.57 - 97.67
- 96.20 - 96.56
- 95.75 - 96.19
- 95.10 - 95.74
- 90.19 - 95.09

Source: CMHC (2006 census-based housing indicators and data).

Youth with their own bedroom

Suitable housing has enough bedrooms for the size and make-up of resident households, according to National Occupancy Standard (NOS) requirements. Enough bedrooms generally means one bedroom each for youth, especially in families with youth of different sexes (Canada Mortgage and Housing Corporation, 2011).

In 2008, the McCreary AHS IV asked students if they had their own bedroom. For the province as a whole, nearly nine in every ten (89.46%) students indicated that they had their own bedroom. The range between HSDAs was over 14 percentage points, indicating quite a geographical variation throughout the province, with Kootenay Boundary at 93.73% having the highest value, and Vancouver (79.07%) having the lowest. Many of the HSDAs were significantly different from the provincial average. Both Richmond and Vancouver were significantly lower than average, while all other HSDAs, with the exception of North Shore/Coast Garibaldi and Fraser South, were significantly higher than the provincial average.

There were no significant differences between genders at the provincial level, although in Vancouver, male students (83.77%) were significantly more likely to have their own bedroom when compared to female students (75.69%).

For male students, the range among HSDAs was just over 10 percentage points. Kootenay Boundary, Okanagan, South Vancouver Island, and Thompson Cariboo Shuswap (all greater than 92%) were significantly higher than the provincial average for male students, while Richmond and Vancouver (both below 86%) were significantly lower.

For female students, the range among HSDAs at 17 percentage points was much higher than that for males, showing a greater geographical variation throughout the province. Vancouver (75.67%) and Richmond (85.67%) were significantly lower than the provincial average, while all other HSDAs, with the exception of Fraser South/Fraser East and Fraser North, were significantly higher (all about 92%, or higher).

Geographically, there were clear geographical patterns. With the exception of North Shore/Coast Garibaldi, the percentage of students having their own bedroom was consistently lower than the provincial average in the lower mainland HSDAs, where housing costs were the highest in the province, while all other HSDAs were higher than the provincial average.

Health Service Delivery Area	All students (%)	Males (%)	Females (%)
12 Kootenay Boundary	93.73	94.47	93.07
13 Okanagan	93.55	94.13	93.18
41 South Vancouver Island	93.31	93.52	93.10
52 Northern Interior	93.01	91.98	94.34
51 Northwest	92.89	91.67	94.22
14 Thompson Cariboo Shuswap	92.81	92.65	92.98
11 East Kootenay	92.78	91.44	93.96
43 North Vancouver Island	92.47	92.26	92.60
42 Central Vancouver Island	92.29	91.03	93.57
33 North Shore/Coast Garibaldi	91.31	90.62	91.96
21 Fraser South/Fraser East	88.79	88.66	88.94
22 Fraser North	87.79	88.58	87.00
31 Richmond	85.73	85.86	85.67
32 Vancouver	79.07	83.77†	75.69
53 Northeast	N/A	N/A	N/A
British Columbia	**89.46**	**89.89**	**89.13**

† Male rate is significantly different than female rate.
Crosshatched HSDAs are significantly different than the provincial average.
N/A: No data available

Youth with their own bedroom

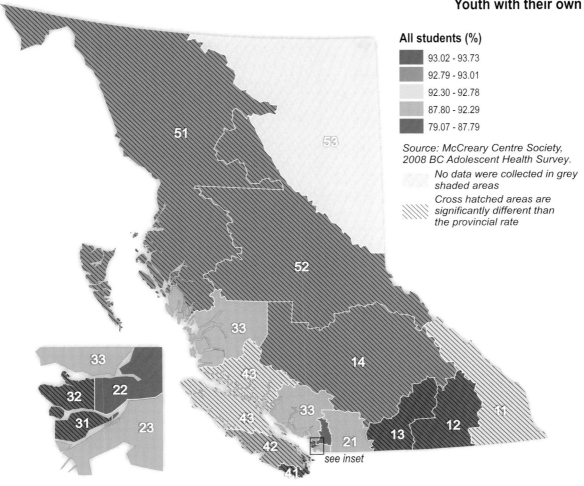

All students (%)

- 93.02 - 93.73
- 92.79 - 93.01
- 92.30 - 92.78
- 87.80 - 92.29
- 79.07 - 87.79

Source: McCreary Centre Society, 2008 BC Adolescent Health Survey.

No data were collected in grey shaded areas

Cross hatched areas are significantly different than the provincial rate

see inset

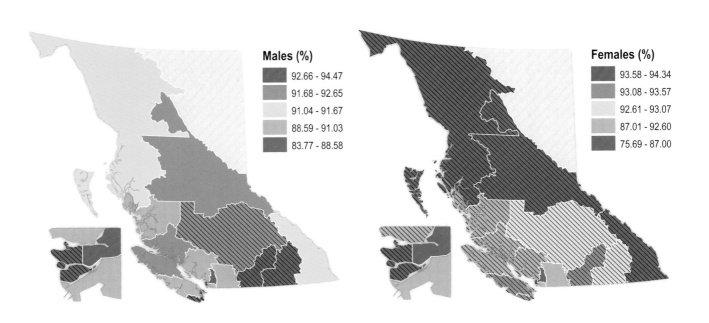

Males (%)

- 92.66 - 94.47
- 91.68 - 92.65
- 91.04 - 91.67
- 88.59 - 91.03
- 83.77 - 88.58

Females (%)

- 93.58 - 94.34
- 93.08 - 93.57
- 92.61 - 93.07
- 87.01 - 92.60
- 75.69 - 87.00

Youth with high family connectedness

Young people who feel strong connection to their family generally have higher emotional wellness values than those who do not. Family connection is therefore an important wellness asset indicator.

The McCreary AHS IV asked students questions related to their family relationships, including information about whether they felt close to their mothers and fathers (or the person considered to be the mother or father) and whether they felt their parents cared about them and were close to them. Questions also canvassed whether students felt their parents were warm and loving toward them most of the time, and whether they were satisfied with the relationship. Additional questions included whether respondents felt their family understood them, paid attention to them, and had fun together.

Results were used to create an index by averaging responses. Values ranged from 0 to 10; higher values denoted stronger levels of family connectedness. It should be noted that data were not collected in Northeast and the data for Fraser South and Fraser East have been combined because several school districts did not participate. Consequently, some caution in interpretation is required.

On average, students (grades 7 to 12) in BC had a family connectedness score of 7.86 (out of 10). This was significantly higher than in 2003 (7.80). The range among HSDA went from 8.11 to 7.65, and there were several HSDAs with significant differences from the provincial average. North Shore/Coast Garibaldi (8.11) had significantly stronger family connections than the provincial average, and at the other extreme, Northwest, North Vancouver Island, and Vancouver (all 7.69 or lower) had significantly less strong family connections.

There were some significant differences in scores by gender. Overall, male students had a significantly higher score (8.03) than female students (7.70), a result consistent with 2003. Furthermore, this stronger family connectedness for males was consistent in all HSDAs, and the difference was significant for nine individual HSDAs.

Among male students, scores ranged from 8.19 for North Shore/Coast Garibaldi to 7.79 for Vancouver. This latter score was significantly lower than the provincial average for male students. The majority of scores for female students ranged from 7.80 to 7.50, but North Shore/Coast Garibaldi scored 8.03, much higher than any other HSDA

Health Service Delivery Area		All students (Index)		Males (Index)		Females (Index)
33 North Shore/Coast Garibaldi	▨	8.11	■	8.19	▨	8.03
41 South Vancouver Island	■	7.93	■	8.14†	■	7.71
22 Fraser North	■	7.92	▨	8.04†	■	7.81
12 Kootenay Boundary	▨	7.91	▨	8.03	■	7.79
13 Okanagan	▨	7.91	▨	8.08†	■	7.76
21 Fraser South/Fraser East	▨	7.91	■	8.14†	■	7.70
14 Thompson Cariboo Shuswap	■	7.83	▨	8.00†	■	7.68
31 Richmond	▨	7.80	■	7.86	■	7.73
52 Northern Interior	▨	7.74	▨	7.97†	■	7.50
42 Central Vancouver Island	▨	7.72	▨	7.88†	■	7.57
11 East Kootenay	▨	7.71	▨	7.96†	■	7.48
32 Vancouver	▨	7.69	▨	7.79	■	7.63
43 North Vancouver Island	▨	7.69	▨	7.92†	▨	7.51
51 Northwest	▨	7.65	■	7.80	■	7.50
53 Northeast		N/A		N/A		N/A
British Columbia		**7.86**		**8.03†**		**7.70**

† Male rate is significantly different than female rate.
Crosshatched HSDAs are significantly different than the provincial average.
N/A: No data available

family connectedness score, and significantly higher than the provincial average for female students.

Geographically, family connectedness tended to be stronger than average in several urban lower mainland HSDAs (although Richmond and Vancouver were not consistent with this pattern) for all students and for male and female students separately. Parts of the southern interior also had higher than average scores, as did South Vancouver Island. Lower than average values were generally found in the north, central interior, and parts of Vancouver Island, as well as Vancouver and Richmond.

Youth with high family connectedness

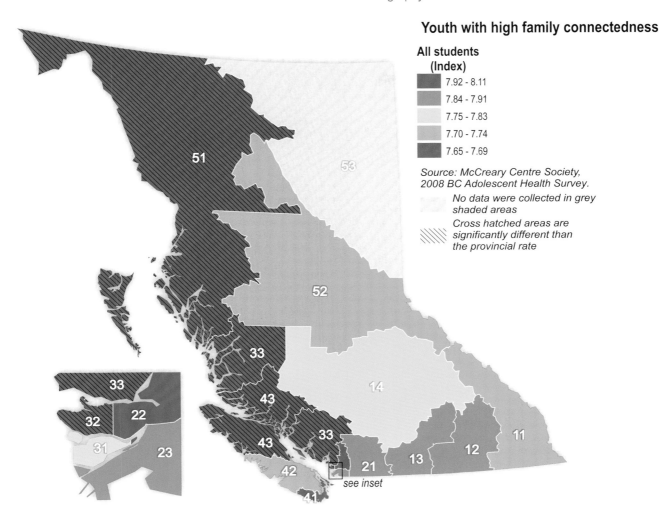

All students
(Index)

	7.92 - 8.11
	7.84 - 7.91
	7.75 - 7.83
	7.70 - 7.74
	7.65 - 7.69

Source: McCreary Centre Society, 2008 BC Adolescent Health Survey.

No data were collected in grey shaded areas

Cross hatched areas are significantly different than the provincial rate

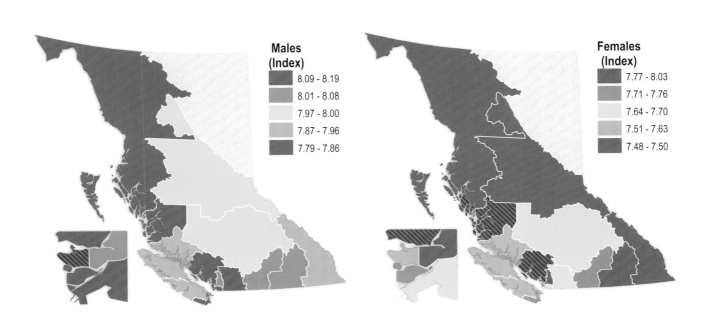

Males
(Index)

	8.09 - 8.19
	8.01 - 8.08
	7.97 - 8.00
	7.87 - 7.96
	7.79 - 7.86

Females
(Index)

	7.77 - 8.03
	7.71 - 7.76
	7.64 - 7.70
	7.51 - 7.63
	7.48 - 7.50

Youth eating their evening meal with at least one parent 4 or 5 times in the past five school days

The sharing of family meals has been shown increasingly to be an important wellness asset for both children and parents. The frequency of family dinners tends to decrease as children go through high school, and this is when the benefits of such meals might be most needed. Eating meals together keeps the doors open for communication at what is often a challenging time for adolescents. It also improves eating habits. Studies have shown that teens who eat dinner with their families are less likely to engage in risky behaviours such as illegal drug use, alcohol consumption, and tobacco smoking. Such teens also do better in school.

The McCreary AHS IV asked students *"On how many of the past five school days was at least one of your parents in the room with you while you ate your evening meal?"* Student respondents could answer anywhere from zero to five days.

In BC, nearly seven in every ten (68.37%) student respondents indicated that they ate evening meals with at least one parent present on four or more of the past five school days. There was a six percentage point range throughout the province. Students in Vancouver (71.66%) were most likely to have evening meals with one or more parents, while students in Central Vancouver Island were least likely at 65.19%, which was significantly lower than the provincial average for all students.

Comparing responses from male and female students, the provincial average for males (70.14%) was significantly higher than for females (66.74%). While this difference was evident for most HSDAs, only two (Northern Interior and Fraser South/Fraser East) registered this difference as being significant. Further, female students in Richmond (70.53%) were more likely than male students (67.81%) to have an evening meal four or more times a week with one or more parents, although this difference was not significant.

The response for male students among HSDAs ranged from a high of 72.36% for Vancouver to a low of 66.35% for Central Vancouver Island. None of the HSDAs, however, were significantly different from the provincial average for male students. Responses from female students ranged from a high of 71.15% for Vancouver, which was significantly higher than the provincial female average, to a low of 64.05% for Central Vancouver Island.

Overall, there was a relatively small variation among students who indicated eating evening meals with one or

Health Service Delivery Area	All students (%)	Males (%)	Females (%)
32 Vancouver	71.66	72.36	71.15
33 North Shore/Coast Garibaldi	69.70	71.20	68.32
22 Fraser North	69.59	70.75	68.55
31 Richmond	69.15	67.81	70.53
12 Kootenay Boundary	69.10	69.64	68.60
14 Thompson Cariboo Shuswap	68.49	71.74	65.47
13 Okanagan	68.46	69.27	67.69
51 Northwest	67.88	68.48	67.15
21 Fraser South/Fraser East	67.58	70.40†	65.02
41 South Vancouver Island	67.22	69.78	64.78
52 Northern Interior	66.99	70.46†	63.24
43 North Vancouver Island	66.62	70.38	63.44
11 East Kootenay	66.15	68.52	64.06
42 Central Vancouver Island	65.19	66.35	64.05
53 Northeast	N/A	N/A	N/A
British Columbia	**68.37**	**70.14†**	**66.74**

† Male rate is significantly different than female rate.
Crosshatched HSDAs are significantly different than the provincial average.
N/A: Data not available

more parent present. Nevertheless, there were clear geographical patterns: students in the urban lower mainland HSDAs had generally higher values than average, while those in Central Vancouver Island had consistently the lowest percentages for all students, and for males and females separately.

Youth eating their evening meal with at least one parent 4 or 5 times in the past five school days

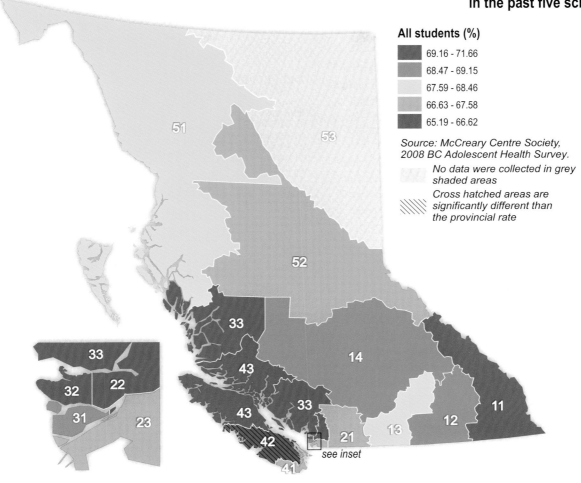

All students (%)

- 69.16 - 71.66
- 68.47 - 69.15
- 67.59 - 68.46
- 66.63 - 67.58
- 65.19 - 66.62

Source: McCreary Centre Society, 2008 BC Adolescent Health Survey.

No data were collected in grey shaded areas

Cross hatched areas are significantly different than the provincial rate

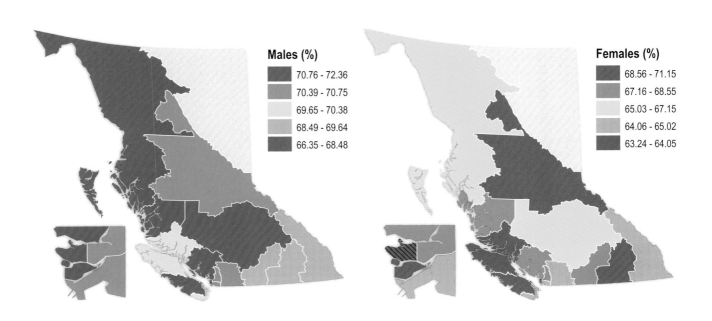

Males (%)

- 70.76 - 72.36
- 70.39 - 70.75
- 69.65 - 70.38
- 68.49 - 69.64
- 66.35 - 68.48

Females (%)

- 68.56 - 71.15
- 67.16 - 68.55
- 65.03 - 67.15
- 64.06 - 65.02
- 63.24 - 64.05

Youth with strong school connectedness

Students' strong connectedness to school is an important wellness asset. It represents a variety of factors, including security, and respect for school as a place for learning.

The McCreary AHS IV asked students questions related to their thoughts about school, and relationships with their teachers and other students. Questions included whether or not students liked and were happy at school, whether they felt part of their school, the degree to which they felt teachers cared about them and treated students fairly, whether they felt safe at school, and whether they got along with teachers and other students.

The school connectedness index combined the results, once they had been standardized on a scale of 0 to 1. The index ranged from 0 to 10, with higher values denoting stronger connections to school. It should be noted that data were not collected in Northeast, and data for Fraser South and Fraser East have been combined because several school districts did not participate. Consequently, some caution in interpretation is required.

Students (grades 7 to 12) as a whole in BC had an average school connectedness index of 6.83 (out of 10). This was significantly stronger than in 2003 (6.67). Scores among HSDAs for all students ranged from a high of 7.00 to a low of 6.39, with some significant differences geographically. South Vancouver Island, Fraser South/Fraser East, and North Shore/Coast Garibaldi were significantly higher (all 6.97 or higher) than the provincial average. On the other hand, Central Vancouver Island, Northeast, Northern Interior, and East Kootenay (all below 6.65) were significantly lower.

There were significant differences between genders for school connectedness. Provincially, female students on average were significantly more connected to school (6.94) than male students (6.72), a reversal of the family connectedness relationship. Furthermore, female students in six HSDAs had significantly stronger connections to their schools than did their male counterparts.

Index values among HSDAs for male students ranged from 6.87 to 6.33, and several HSDAs had values significantly different than the average for male students. Fraser South/Fraser East (6.89) had significantly stronger connections to school, while Northern Interior, Central and North Vancouver Island, East Kootenay, and Northwest (all under 6.50) had significantly less connection.

Health Service Delivery Area	All students (Index)		Males (Index)		Females (Index)
41 South Vancouver Island	7.00		6.87		7.12
21 Fraser South/Fraser East	6.98		6.89		7.05
33 North Shore/Coast Garibaldi	6.97		6.81†		7.13
22 Fraser North	6.87		6.76		6.97
31 Richmond	6.87		6.85		6.89
32 Vancouver	6.84		6.85		6.84
13 Okanagan	6.83		6.65†		6.98
12 Kootenay Boundary	6.72		6.52†		6.90
14 Thompson Cariboo Shuswap	6.67		6.52		6.83
43 North Vancouver Island	6.64		6.39†		6.85
42 Central Vancouver Island	6.62		6.46†		6.79
51 Northwest	6.53		6.30†		6.75
52 Northern Interior	6.52		6.49		6.57
11 East Kootenay	6.39		6.33		6.43
53 Northeast	N/A		N/A		N/A
British Columbia	**6.83**		**6.72†**		**6.94**

† Male rate is significantly different than female rate.
Crosshatched HSDAs are significantly different than the provincial average.
N/A: No data available

For female students, values among HSDAs ranged from 7.13 to 6.43. Female students in North Shore/Coast Garibaldi (7.13) and South Vancouver Island (7.12) had significantly stronger school connections than the average for female students, provincially. At the other extreme, Northern Interior (6.57) and East Kootenay (6.43) had significantly lower values than the provincial average.

Geographically, patterns for all students, and males and females separately, were similar. Stronger school connectedness was more prominent in parts of the lower mainland (except for Vancouver and Richmond), while lower levels were more characteristic of Central and North Vancouver Island, the northern part of the province, and East Kootenay.

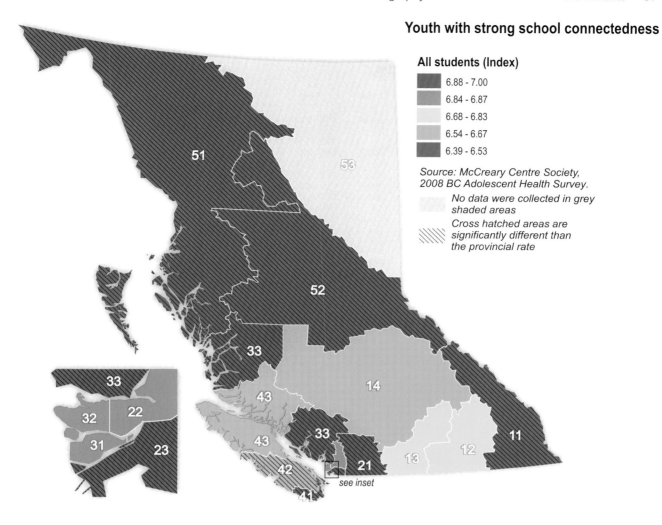

Youth with strong school connectedness

All students (Index)

- 6.88 - 7.00
- 6.84 - 6.87
- 6.68 - 6.83
- 6.54 - 6.67
- 6.39 - 6.53

Source: McCreary Centre Society, 2008 BC Adolescent Health Survey.

No data were collected in grey shaded areas

Cross hatched areas are significantly different than the provincial rate

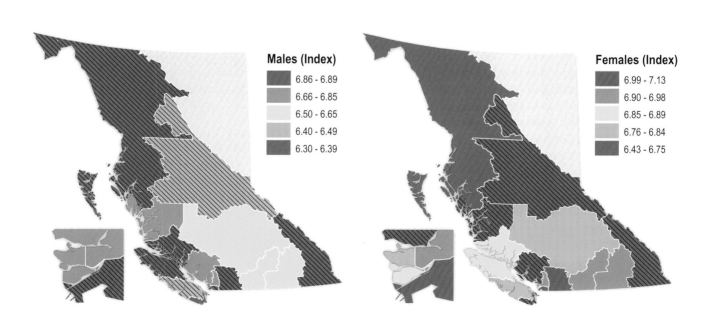

Males (Index)

- 6.86 - 6.89
- 6.66 - 6.85
- 6.50 - 6.65
- 6.40 - 6.49
- 6.30 - 6.39

Females (Index)

- 6.99 - 7.13
- 6.90 - 6.98
- 6.85 - 6.89
- 6.76 - 6.84
- 6.43 - 6.75

Strong sense of belonging to the local community

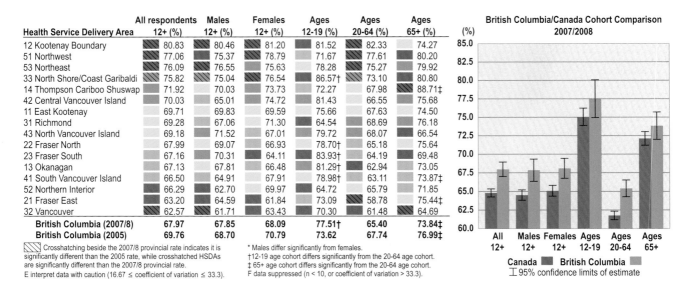

Health Service Delivery Area	All respondents 12+ (%)	Males 12+ (%)	Females 12+ (%)	Ages 12-19 (%)	Ages 20-64 (%)	Ages 65+ (%)
12 Kootenay Boundary	80.83	80.46	81.20	81.52	82.33	74.27
51 Northwest	77.06	75.37	78.79	71.67	77.61	80.20
53 Northeast	76.09	76.55	75.63	78.28	75.27	79.92
33 North Shore/Coast Garibaldi	75.82	75.04	76.54	86.57†	73.10	80.80
14 Thompson Cariboo Shuswap	71.92	70.03	73.73	72.27	67.98	88.71‡
42 Central Vancouver Island	70.03	65.01	74.72	81.43	66.55	75.68
11 East Kootenay	69.71	69.83	69.59	75.66	67.63	74.50
31 Richmond	69.28	67.06	71.30	64.54	68.69	76.18
43 North Vancouver Island	69.18	71.52	67.01	79.72	68.07	66.54
22 Fraser North	67.99	69.07	66.93	78.70†	65.18	75.64
23 Fraser South	67.16	70.31	64.11	83.93†	64.19	69.48
13 Okanagan	67.13	67.81	66.48	81.29†	62.94	73.05
41 South Vancouver Island	66.50	64.91	67.91	78.98†	63.11	73.87‡
52 Northern Interior	66.29	62.70	69.97	64.72	65.79	71.85
21 Fraser East	63.20	64.59	61.84	73.09	58.78	75.44‡
32 Vancouver	62.57	61.71	63.43	70.30	61.48	64.69
British Columbia (2007/8)	**67.97**	**67.85**	**68.09**	**77.51†**	**65.40**	**73.84‡**
British Columbia (2005)	**69.76**	**68.70**	**70.79**	**73.62**	**67.74**	**76.99‡**

▧ Crosshatching beside the 2007/8 provincial rate indicates it is significantly different than the 2005 rate, while crosshatched HSDAs are significantly different than the 2007/8 provincial rate.
E interpret data with caution (16.67 ≤ coefficient of variation ≤ 33.3).

* Males differ significantly from females.
† 12-19 age cohort differs significantly from the 20-64 age cohort.
‡ 65+ age cohort differs significantly from the 20-64 age cohort.
F data suppressed (n < 10, or coefficient of variation > 33.3).

British Columbia/Canada Cohort Comparison 2007/2008

Canada ■   British Columbia ▨
I 95% confidence limits of estimate

Individuals develop a sense of belonging to their local community through memberships in local organizations, or by helping neighbours and others when needed. Those with a strong sense of local belonging feel included in the "life" of their community. The CCHS asked respondents to describe their sense of belonging in their local community as either "*very strong, somewhat strong, somewhat weak, or very weak.*" Nearly seven out of every ten (67.97%) BC respondents indicated that they had a strong or somewhat strong sense of belonging to their local community. For all BC respondents, Kootenay Boundary, North Shore/Coast Garibaldi, Northwest, and Northeast (all over 75%) reported significantly higher values than the provincial average, while Vancouver had a significantly lower value.

While there were no significant differences between genders, either provincially or for individual HSDAs, for male respondents were significantly higher in Kootenay Boundary, North Shore/Coast Garibaldi, and the Northeast (all above 75%), and significantly lower in Vancouver (62.57%). For female respondents, Kootenay Boundary, North Shore/Coast Garibaldi, and Northwest (all above 75%) had significantly higher values than the provincial average for females.

There were no significant differences among individual HSDAs for youth respondents (age 12-19 years) when compared to the BC value for this cohort. Provincially, youth (77.51%) had a significantly higher level of belonging than the mid-age (20-64 years) cohort, as was the case in five HSDAs.

Senior respondents (age 65 years and over) had a

significantly higher value of community belonging (73.84%) than the mid-age cohort, provincially, and also for Thompson Cariboo Shuswap, Fraser East, and South Vancouver Island HSDAs. Compared to the provincial average for seniors, belonging was significantly higher in Thompson Cariboo Shuswap (88.71%), but significantly lower in Fraser East (64.69%).

Overall, there were major geographical variations, with a spread of approximately 20 percentage points for all cohorts, but geographical patterns were quite varied. North Shore/Coast Garibaldi in the lower mainland had consistently higher levels of belonging, as did Northwest, Northeast (except for youth), and Kootenay Boundary (except for seniors). Vancouver, and to a lesser extent Fraser East and Northern Interior, had relatively lower values of belonging. Values for youth were consistently low in the northern and central regions of the province, and higher on the south coast, except for Vancouver and Richmond.

Although values for all BC cohorts, with the exception of youth, declined, there were no statistical differences for any of the BC cohorts between the 2005 and 2007/8 samples. For 2007/8, all BC male, female, and mid-age respondents reported significantly higher values of community belonging than their peers nationally.

Strong sense of belonging to the local community

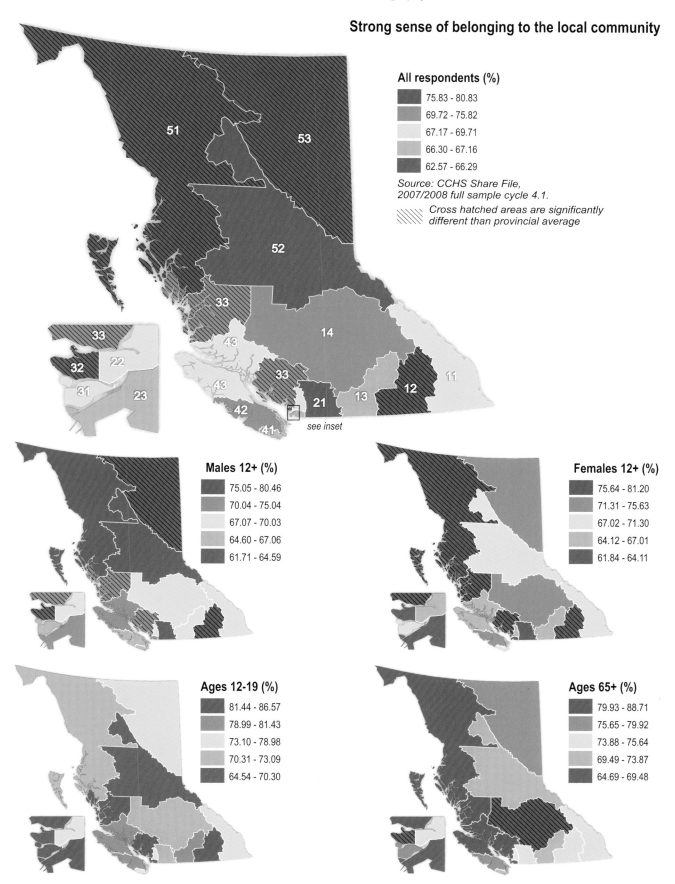

All respondents (%)

- 75.83 - 80.83
- 69.72 - 75.82
- 67.17 - 69.71
- 66.30 - 67.16
- 62.57 - 66.29

Source: CCHS Share File, 2007/2008 full sample cycle 4.1.

Cross hatched areas are significantly different than provincial average

see inset

Males 12+ (%)

- 75.05 - 80.46
- 70.04 - 75.04
- 67.07 - 70.03
- 64.60 - 67.06
- 61.71 - 64.59

Females 12+ (%)

- 75.64 - 81.20
- 71.31 - 75.63
- 67.02 - 71.30
- 64.12 - 67.01
- 61.84 - 64.11

Ages 12-19 (%)

- 81.44 - 86.57
- 78.99 - 81.43
- 73.10 - 78.98
- 70.31 - 73.09
- 64.54 - 70.30

Ages 65+ (%)

- 79.93 - 88.71
- 75.65 - 79.92
- 73.88 - 75.64
- 69.49 - 73.87
- 64.69 - 69.48

Strong positive social interaction

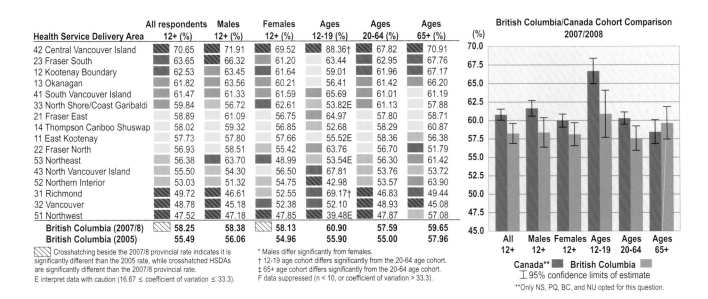

Health Service Delivery Area	All respondents 12+ (%)	Males 12+ (%)	Females 12+ (%)	Ages 12-19 (%)	Ages 20-64 (%)	Ages 65+ (%)
42 Central Vancouver Island	70.65	71.91	69.52	88.36†	67.82	70.91
23 Fraser South	63.65	66.32	61.20	63.44	62.95	67.76
12 Kootenay Boundary	62.53	63.45	61.64	59.01	61.96	67.17
13 Okanagan	61.82	63.56	60.21	56.41	61.42	66.20
41 South Vancouver Island	61.47	61.33	61.59	65.69	61.01	61.19
33 North Shore/Coast Garibaldi	59.84	56.72	62.61	53.82E	61.13	57.88
21 Fraser East	58.89	61.09	56.75	64.97	57.80	58.71
14 Thompson Cariboo Shuswap	58.02	59.32	56.85	52.68	58.29	60.87
11 East Kootenay	57.73	57.80	57.66	55.52E	58.36	56.38
22 Fraser North	56.93	58.51	55.42	63.76	56.70	51.79
53 Northeast	56.38	63.70	48.99	53.54E	56.30	61.42
43 North Vancouver Island	55.50	54.30	56.50	67.81	53.76	53.72
52 Northern Interior	53.03	51.32	54.75	42.98	53.57	63.90
31 Richmond	49.72	46.61	52.55	69.17†	46.83	49.44
32 Vancouver	48.78	45.18	52.38	52.10	48.93	45.08
51 Northwest	47.52	47.18	47.85	39.48E	47.87	57.08
British Columbia (2007/8)	**58.25**	**58.38**	**58.13**	**60.90**	**57.59**	**59.65**
British Columbia (2005)	**55.49**	**56.06**	**54.96**	**55.90**	**55.00**	**57.96**

Crosshatching beside the 2007/8 provincial rate indicates it is significantly different than the 2005 rate, while crosshatched HSDAs are significantly different than the 2007/8 provincial rate.
E interpret data with caution (16.67 ≤ coefficient of variation ≤ 33.3).

* Males differ significantly from females.
† 12-19 age cohort differs significantly from the 20-64 age cohort.
‡ 65+ age cohort differs significantly from the 20-64 age cohort.
F data suppressed (n < 10, or coefficient of variation > 33.3).

British Columbia/Canada Cohort Comparison 2007/2008

Canada** ■   British Columbia ▨
⊥ 95% confidence limits of estimate
**Only NS, PQ, BC, and NU opted for this question.

Spending time with others is important for wellness and feelings of inclusion. This index is based on the following CCHS questions: *"Do you have someone to: have a good time with; get together with for relaxation; do things to get mind off things; and do something enjoyable with?"*. The index (0 to 16), measures the social interaction available to an individual (Statistics Canada, nd). This indicator is based on the percentage of respondents who scored 15 or 16, indicating a high level of positive social interaction.

Well over half (58.25%) of BC respondents had a high level of positive social interaction, with Central Vancouver Island (70.65%) significantly higher than the BC average value, and Richmond, Vancouver, and Northwest (all less than 50%) significantly lower than the BC average value.

There were no significant gender differences at the provincial level or for individual HSDAs. For males, Fraser South (66.32%) and Central Vancouver Island (71.91%) had significantly more respondents reporting a high level of positive social interaction than the provincial average, while Richmond, Vancouver, and the Northwest (all below 48%) had significantly fewer. For females, Central Vancouver Island (69.52%) had significantly more, while Northwest (47.85%) had significantly fewer respondents with positive social interaction compared to the female average.

Provincially, there were no significant differences between youth and the mid-age cohort, although youth in Richmond and Central Vancouver had significantly higher values of positive social interaction than the mid-age cohorts in those HSDAs. Within BC, Central Vancouver Island youth had by far the highest significant value (88.36%) when compared

with the provincial youth value (60.09%). Northwest and Northern Interior youth, both under 43%, had significantly lower values than the BC average.

There were no significant differences between the senior and mid-age cohorts for BC or for any HSDA. Central Vancouver Island (70.91%) had significantly higher values, while Vancouver (45.08%) had significantly lower values of positive social interaction than seniors provincially.

Geographically, cohort ranges among HSDAs were between 20 and 25 percentage points, except for youth, which had a range in excess of 50 percentage points. High values occurred consistently in the southernmost interior regions (Kootenay Boundary and the Okanagan) and on the southwest coast (South and Central Vancouver Island and Fraser South); however, Vancouver and the Northwest had consistently low values for this variable.

Each BC cohort increased in value between 2005 and 2007/8, and this was significant for all respondents and for females. In comparison to Canadian averages, BC had significantly lower values for all respondents, males, youth, and mid-age cohorts. Not all provinces/territories opted for this question, therefore caution is advised in interpreting comparisons to the Canada averages.

Strong positive social interaction

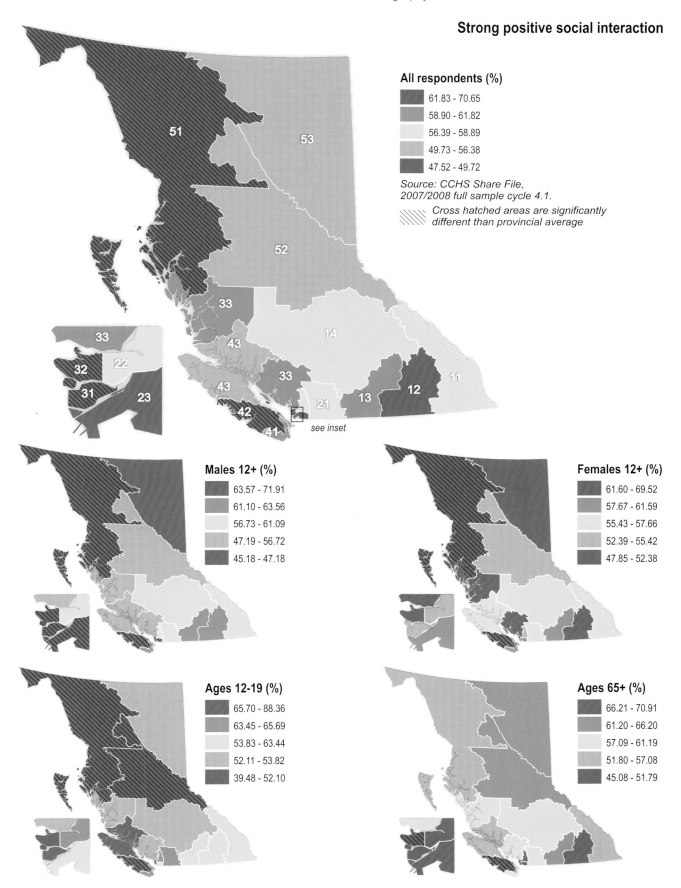

All respondents (%)

- 61.83 - 70.65
- 58.90 - 61.82
- 56.39 - 58.89
- 49.73 - 56.38
- 47.52 - 49.72

Source: CCHS Share File, 2007/2008 full sample cycle 4.1.

Cross hatched areas are significantly different than provincial average

see inset

Males 12+ (%)

- 63.57 - 71.91
- 61.10 - 63.56
- 56.73 - 61.09
- 47.19 - 56.72
- 45.18 - 47.18

Females 12+ (%)

- 61.60 - 69.52
- 57.67 - 61.59
- 55.43 - 57.66
- 52.39 - 55.42
- 47.85 - 52.38

Ages 12-19 (%)

- 65.70 - 88.36
- 63.45 - 65.69
- 53.83 - 63.44
- 52.11 - 53.82
- 39.48 - 52.10

Ages 65+ (%)

- 66.21 - 70.91
- 61.20 - 66.20
- 57.09 - 61.19
- 51.80 - 57.08
- 45.08 - 51.79

Strong emotional/informational support

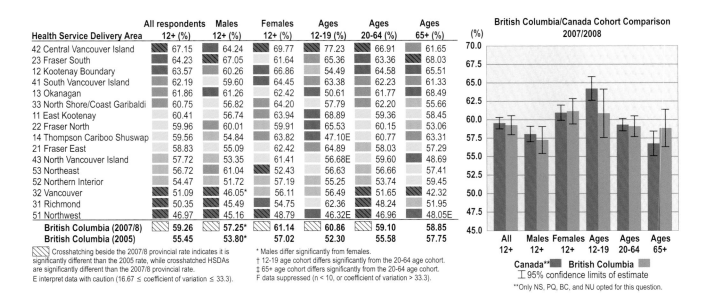

Health Service Delivery Area	All respondents 12+ (%)	Males 12+ (%)	Females 12+ (%)	Ages 12-19 (%)	Ages 20-64 (%)	Ages 65+ (%)
42 Central Vancouver Island	67.15	64.24	69.77	77.23	66.91	61.65
23 Fraser South	64.23	67.05	61.64	65.36	63.36	68.03
12 Kootenay Boundary	63.57	60.26	66.86	54.49	64.58	65.51
41 South Vancouver Island	62.19	59.60	64.45	63.38	62.23	61.33
13 Okanagan	61.86	61.26	62.42	50.61	61.77	68.49
33 North Shore/Coast Garibaldi	60.75	56.82	64.20	57.79	62.20	55.66
11 East Kootenay	60.41	56.74	63.94	68.89	59.36	58.45
22 Fraser North	59.96	60.01	59.91	65.53	60.15	53.06
14 Thompson Cariboo Shuswap	59.56	54.84	63.82	47.10E	60.77	63.31
21 Fraser East	58.83	55.09	62.42	64.89	58.03	57.29
43 North Vancouver Island	57.72	53.35	61.41	56.68E	59.60	48.69
53 Northeast	56.72	61.04	52.43	56.63	56.66	57.41
52 Northern Interior	54.47	51.72	57.19	55.25	53.74	59.45
32 Vancouver	51.09	46.05*	56.11	56.49	51.65	42.32
31 Richmond	50.35	45.49	54.75	62.36	48.24	51.95
51 Northwest	46.97	45.16	48.79	46.32E	46.96	48.05E
British Columbia (2007/8)	**59.26**	**57.25***	**61.14**	**60.86**	**59.10**	**58.85**
British Columbia (2005)	**55.45**	**53.80***	**57.02**	**52.30**	**55.58**	**57.75**

Crosshatching beside the 2007/8 provincial rate indicates it is significantly different than the 2005 rate, while crosshatched HSDAs are significantly different than the 2007/8 provincial rate.
E interpret data with caution (16.67 ≤ coefficient of variation ≤ 33.3).

* Males differ significantly from females.
† 12-19 age cohort differs significantly from the 20-64 age cohort.
‡ 65+ age cohort differs significantly from the 20-64 age cohort.
F data suppressed (n < 10, or coefficient of variation > 33.3).

British Columbia/Canada Cohort Comparison 2007/2008

Canada** ▮   British Columbia ▮
⊥ 95% confidence limits of estimate
**Only NS, PQ, BC, and NU opted for this question.

This index was derived from the following CCHS questions: *"Do you have someone to: listen; receive advice about a crisis; help understand a problem; confide in; give advice; share most private worries and fears; turn to for suggestions for personal problems; and who understands problems?"* Results were amalgamated to create the index with a score from 0 to 32 (Statistics Canada, nd). Data were based on the percentage of respondents who scored 29 to 32, indicating a high level of support.

Six in every ten (59.26%) BC respondents reported a high level of emotional or informational support. Within BC, Central Vancouver Island (67.15%) had significantly more, while Richmond, Vancouver, and the Northwest (all 51% or less) had significantly fewer respondents than average with high levels of emotional or informational support.

Provincially, females (61.14%) fared significantly better than males (57.25%) for emotional or informational support. Vancouver had a significant difference of 10 percentage points between genders. Males in Fraser South (67.05%) had a significantly higher level of support than males provincially, while males in Richmond, Vancouver, and the Northwest had significantly lower values, with 46% or less reporting a high level of support. For females, Central Vancouver Island (69.77%) had significantly more respondents reporting a high level of support, while Northeast (52.43%) and Northwest (48.79%) were significantly lower.

For BC youth respondents, Central Vancouver Island (77.23%) had significantly higher levels of strong support

than the provincial youth average (60.86%). Fraser South (68.03%) had significantly more seniors with high levels of support in comparison to the BC seniors' average (58.85%), while Vancouver had significantly fewer seniors (42.32%) with high levels of support.

Overall, there were major geographical variations, with a spread of approximately 20 percentage points for all cohorts, although the spread for youth was over 30 percentage points. Consistently higher values occurred in Fraser South and Central Vancouver Island. Northwest and Vancouver had consistently lower values. For youth, high values occurred mostly in the southernmost coastal areas, with relatively lower values throughout the rest of the province. Lower values for seniors were clustered along the coastal areas, while higher values occurred in Fraser South, South Vancouver Island, and the south central HSDAs.

All BC cohorts had significantly higher support values in 2007/8 than in 2005, except for seniors. There were no significant differences between BC and Canadian respondents for any cohorts, although Canadian youth and seniors had significantly higher and lower values, respectively, than the Canadian mid-age cohort. Not all provinces/territories opted for this question, therefore caution is advised in interpreting comparisons to the Canada averages.

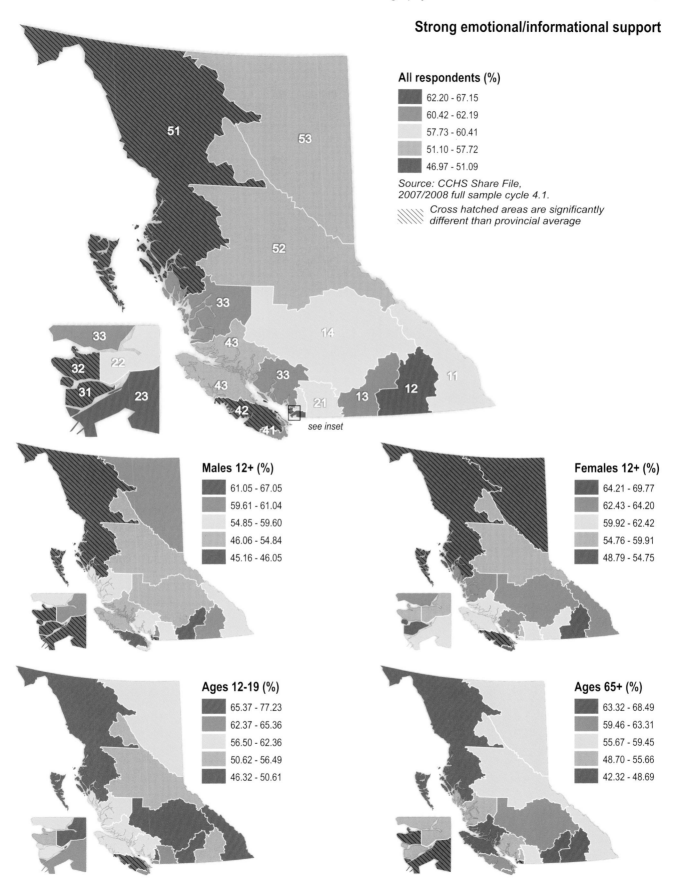

Strong emotional/informational support

All respondents (%)

- 62.20 - 67.15
- 60.42 - 62.19
- 57.73 - 60.41
- 51.10 - 57.72
- 46.97 - 51.09

Source: CCHS Share File, 2007/2008 full sample cycle 4.1.

Cross hatched areas are significantly different than provincial average

Males 12+ (%)

- 61.05 - 67.05
- 59.61 - 61.04
- 54.85 - 59.60
- 46.06 - 54.84
- 45.16 - 46.05

Females 12+ (%)

- 64.21 - 69.77
- 62.43 - 64.20
- 59.92 - 62.42
- 54.76 - 59.91
- 48.79 - 54.75

Ages 12-19 (%)

- 65.37 - 77.23
- 62.37 - 65.36
- 56.50 - 62.36
- 50.62 - 56.49
- 46.32 - 50.61

Ages 65+ (%)

- 63.32 - 68.49
- 59.46 - 63.31
- 55.67 - 59.45
- 48.70 - 55.66
- 42.32 - 48.69

see inset

Did something to improve health in the past 12 months

Health Service Delivery Area	All respondents 12+ (%)	Males 12+ (%)	Females 12+ (%)	Ages 12-19 (%)	Ages 20-64 (%)	Ages 65+ (%)
32 Vancouver	63.30	62.60	63.98	63.41	65.82	47.10‡
42 Central Vancouver Island	63.22	64.92	61.63	80.17	65.38	45.71‡
12 Kootenay Boundary	63.12	60.36	65.94	74.50	66.44	42.92‡
41 South Vancouver Island	61.22	56.13*	65.78	68.08	65.91	37.75‡
52 Northern Interior	60.57	58.26	62.90	71.83	61.29	41.70‡
43 North Vancouver Island	59.91	54.77	64.69	68.78	61.91	45.42
13 Okanagan	59.78	55.78	63.55	65.37	60.37	54.93
31 Richmond	58.66	57.81	59.44	63.28	60.10	47.40
21 Fraser East	57.47	52.15	62.68	63.47	59.80	42.24‡
11 East Kootenay	56.89	48.51*	65.01	46.78E	61.28	45.20‡
14 Thompson Cariboo Shuswap	56.61	49.66*	63.24	63.64	57.88	46.40
33 North Shore/Coast Garibaldi	56.15	57.75	54.65	69.91	56.25	46.42
23 Fraser South	55.60	53.30	57.84	60.07	55.28	53.44
51 Northwest	54.86	44.93*	65.20	55.00	56.07	46.86
53 Northeast	54.84	50.10	59.69	63.03	55.23	38.88E
22 Fraser North	54.29	54.13	54.45	65.45	54.85	40.99‡
British Columbia (2007/8)	**58.58**	**56.22***	**60.84**	**65.34†**	**60.07**	**46.35‡**

No comparable 2005 data available

⬚ Crosshatching beside the 2007/8 provincial rate indicates it is significantly different than the 2005 rate, while crosshatched HSDAs are significantly different than the 2007/8 provincial rate.
E interpret data with caution (16.67 ≤ coefficient of variation ≤ 33.3).

* Males differ significantly from females.
† 12-19 age cohort differs significantly from the 20-64 age cohort.
‡ 65+ age cohort differs significantly from the 20-64 age cohort.
F data suppressed (n < 10, or coefficient of variation > 33.3).

British Columbia/Canada Cohort Comparison 2007/2008

Canada ■ British Columbia ▨
⊥ 95% confidence limits of estimate

Individuals can adopt certain lifestyle habits and behaviours to help attain and maintain an optimum state of health and wellness. A willingness to take steps to improve health when there is room for improvement is an essential component of a healthy lifestyle leading to improved wellness. This indicator presents the percentage of individuals who responded positively to the CCHS question: *"In the past 12 months, did you do anything to improve your health (for example, lost weight, quit smoking, increased exercise)?"*. In BC, 58.58% of all respondents had done something in the past year to improve their health, and Vancouver (63.3%) was significantly higher than the provincial average.

Across BC, females as a whole fared significantly better than males for this indicator: only 56.22% of males had taken action to improve health, compared to 60.84% for female respondents. There were four individual HSDAs (East Kootenay, Thompson Cariboo Shuswap, South Vancouver Island, and Northwest) in which this same trend was apparent.

Males in Vancouver (62.60%) were significantly more proactive about health improvement than males provincially, while those in the Northwest (44.93%) were significantly less proactive. For females, respondents in Fraser North (54.45%) were significantly less likely than females provincially to have taken action to improve their health in the past year.

For youth, the percent of individuals reporting having done something to improve health in the past year (65.34%) was significantly higher than for the mid-age cohort at the provincial level, and youth in Central Vancouver Island (80.17%) were significantly higher than the provincial average.

Provincially, the older age cohort (46.35%) was significantly lower than the mid-age cohort, and this trend also occurred in half of the HSDAs. In comparison to their peers provincially, older respondents in the Okanagan (54.93%) were significantly more likely to have taken action to improve their health in the past year, while in South Vancouver Island, only 37.85% of older respondents had done something to improve health, significantly lower than the provincial average for this cohort.

Generally, the geographic variation among HSDAs was modest, with approximately a 10 percentage point range in values. The range for youth, however, at over 30 percentage points, was considerably higher. There was little regional consistency among the different cohorts, except for Northeast and Fraser North, which both consistently had relatively low values.

Data were not available to compare results for BC between 2005 and 2007/8, and British Columbians for all age and gender cohorts had comparable values to the Canadian averages for taking action to improve health in the past 12 months.

Did something to improve health in the past 12 months

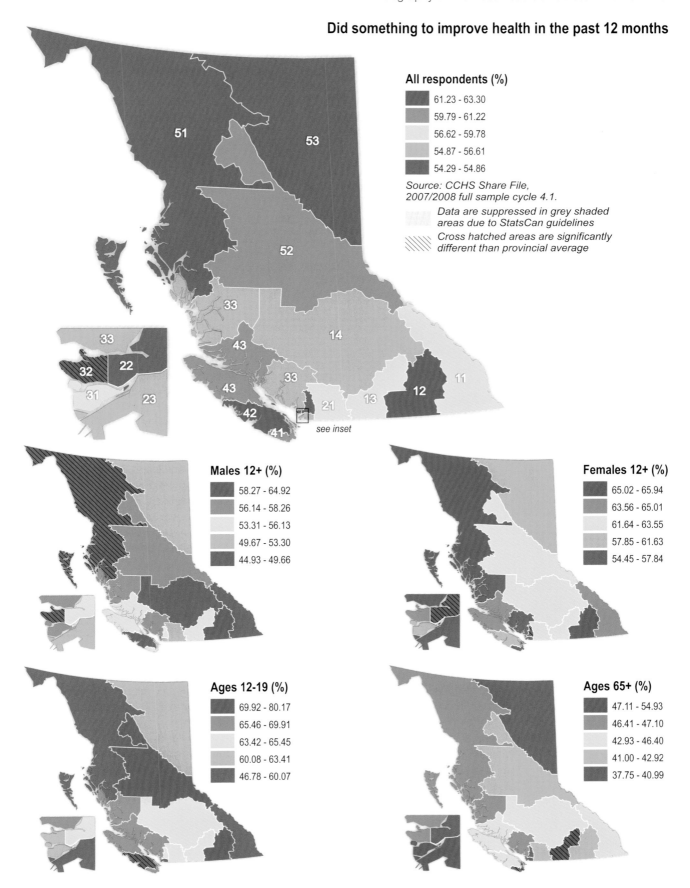

All respondents (%)

- 61.23 - 63.30
- 59.79 - 61.22
- 56.62 - 59.78
- 54.87 - 56.61
- 54.29 - 54.86

Source: CCHS Share File, 2007/2008 full sample cycle 4.1.

Data are suppressed in grey shaded areas due to StatsCan guidelines

Cross hatched areas are significantly different than provincial average

Males 12+ (%)

- 58.27 - 64.92
- 56.14 - 58.26
- 53.31 - 56.13
- 49.67 - 53.30
- 44.93 - 49.66

Females 12+ (%)

- 65.02 - 65.94
- 63.56 - 65.01
- 61.64 - 63.55
- 57.85 - 61.63
- 54.45 - 57.84

Ages 12-19 (%)

- 69.92 - 80.17
- 65.46 - 69.91
- 63.42 - 65.45
- 60.08 - 63.41
- 46.78 - 60.07

Ages 65+ (%)

- 47.11 - 54.93
- 46.41 - 47.10
- 42.93 - 46.40
- 41.00 - 42.92
- 37.75 - 40.99

Intends to improve health over the next year

Health Service Delivery Area	All respondents 12+ (%)	Males 12+ (%)	Females 12+ (%)	Ages 12-19 (%)	Ages 20-64 (%)	Ages 65+ (%)
41 South Vancouver Island	58.65	57.92	59.32	45.28†	65.96	35.33‡
52 Northern Interior	57.27	53.60	60.98	64.78	58.08	42.15‡
14 Thompson Cariboo Shuswap	56.66	51.95	61.04	59.99	61.48	33.87‡
12 Kootenay Boundary	54.69	50.71	58.67	36.82E†	64.07	28.80E‡
42 Central Vancouver Island	51.46	49.10	53.65	48.22E	58.30	29.49‡
51 Northwest	51.44	50.25	52.70	30.71E†	57.45	36.74E‡
11 East Kootenay	49.33	44.79	53.66	45.73E	54.16	31.07‡
53 Northeast	48.19	41.75	54.73	36.66E	51.05	41.66
13 Okanagan	47.78	44.23	51.12	26.40E†	57.16	28.56‡
32 Vancouver	45.94	48.49	43.49	50.43	49.68	19.41‡
33 North Shore/Coast Garibaldi	45.39	46.08	44.76	37.16E	48.77	35.83
31 Richmond	45.08	42.68	47.27	41.72	50.49	19.50E‡
22 Fraser North	44.99	40.85	48.97	41.85	48.71	25.06E‡
43 North Vancouver Island	43.79	39.93	47.38	54.89E	46.71	24.02E‡
21 Fraser East	43.04	41.44	44.60	43.01	47.46	22.88‡
23 Fraser South	41.47	35.85*	46.98	40.26	45.17	21.91‡
British Columbia (2007/8)	**47.63**	**45.18***	**49.96**	**43.52†**	**52.34**	**27.37‡**
No comparable 2005 data available						

Crosshatching beside the 2007/8 provincial rate indicates it is significantly different than the 2005 rate, while crosshatched HSDAs are significantly different than the 2007/8 provincial rate.
E interpret data with caution (16.67 ≤ coefficient of variation ≤ 33.3).

* Males differ significantly from females.
† 12-19 age cohort differs significantly from the 20-64 age cohort.
‡ 65+ age cohort differs significantly from the 20-64 age cohort.
F data suppressed (n < 10, or coefficient of variation > 33.3).

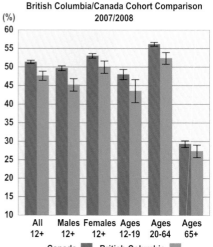

British Columbia/Canada Cohort Comparison 2007/2008

Canada ■   British Columbia ▨
⊥ 95% confidence limits of estimate

This indicator presents the percentage of individuals who responded positively to the CCHS question: *"Is there anything you intend to do to improve your physical health in the next year?".* Nearly half of BC respondents (47.63%) indicated some intention to improve their health within the next year. Thompson Cariboo Shuswap, South Vancouver Island, and Northern Interior (all over 56%) had significantly greater intentions, while Fraser South (41.47%) had significantly lower intentions than BC respondents as a whole.

Across BC, females (49.96%) had significantly higher intentions than males (45.18%) to improve their health in the next year, although within HSDAs, only female respondents in Fraser South (46.98%) were significantly higher than males (35.85%).

Males in South Vancouver Island (57.92%) and Northern Interior (53.6%) had significantly greater intentions to improve their health than males provincially, while those in Fraser South (35.85%) were significantly less likely to do so. For females, Thompson Cariboo Shuswap, South Vancouver Island, and Northern Interior (all over 59%) had significantly greater intentions to improve their health than females provincially, while females in Vancouver (43.49%) had significantly lower intentions.Youth respondents provincially had significantly lower intentions (43.52%) than the mid-age cohort (52.34%), and youth in Okanagan, South Vancouver Island, and Northwest had significantly lower intentions than their mid-age counterparts. Compared to the provincial average for youth, Thompson Cariboo Shuswap and Northern Interior

(both over 59%) had significantly higher intentions, while Okanagan (26.40%) had significantly lower intentions.

For the older age cohort provincially, respondents reporting intentions to improve health (27.37%) were significantly lower than the mid-age cohort. There were only two HSDAs, Northeast and North Shore/Coast Garibaldi, in which older respondents did not have a significantly lower intention than the mid-age group. Older respondents in South Vancouver Island, Northern Interior, and Northeast (all over 35%) had significantly greater intentions than their peers provincially to improve health in the next year, while older respondents in the Okanagan (19.41%) had significantly lower intentions. Caution interpreting the results for the youth and older age cohorts at the HSDA level is required because several had relatively high coefficients of variation.

Geographical patterns for this indicator were quite varied. Consistently higher values across all cohorts were seen in Northern Interior and Thompson Cariboo Shuswap, and lower values occurred in parts of the southwest of BC.

Data were unavailable to make BC comparisons between 2005 and 2007/8. British Columbians overall had significantly lower intentions to improve health in the next year when compared to Canadians as a whole, and BC males, females, youth, and mid-age cohorts all were significantly lower than the Canadian cohort averages.

Intends to improve health over the next year

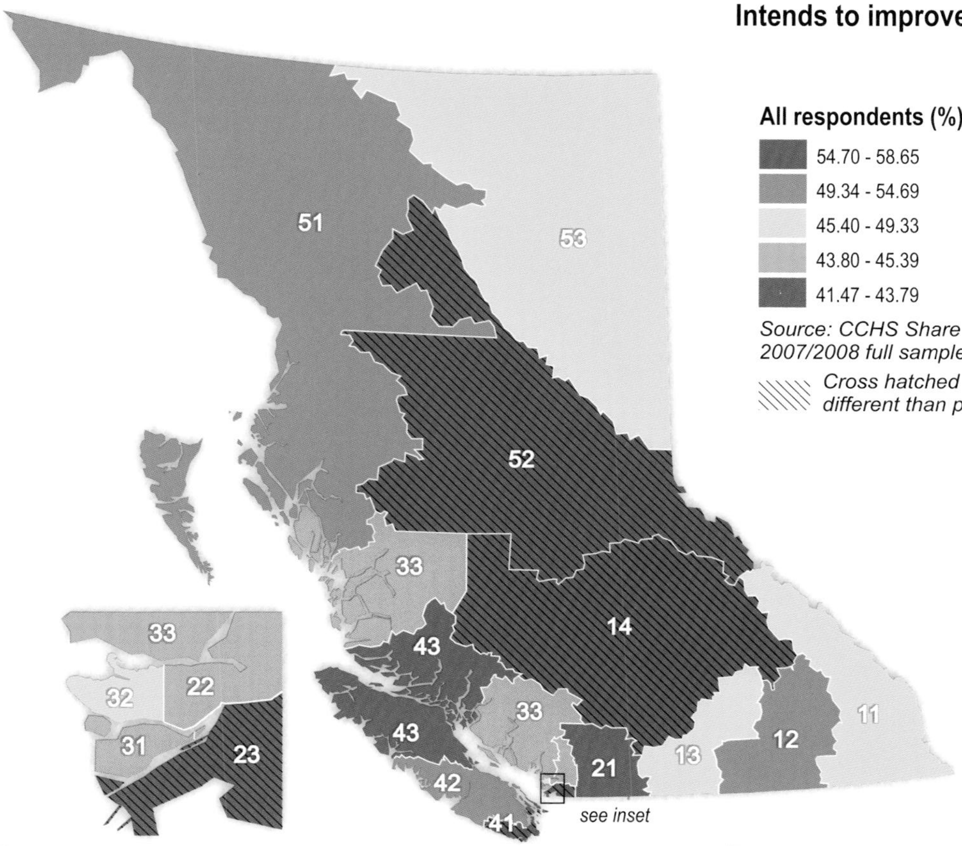
All respondents (%)
54.70 - 58.65
49.34 - 54.69
45.40 - 49.33
43.80 - 45.39
41.47 - 43.79
Source: CCHS Share File, 2007/2008 full sample cycle 4.1.
Cross hatched areas are significantly different than provincial average
51
53
52
33
14
43
43
33
11
12
13
21
42
41
33
32
22
31
23
see inset

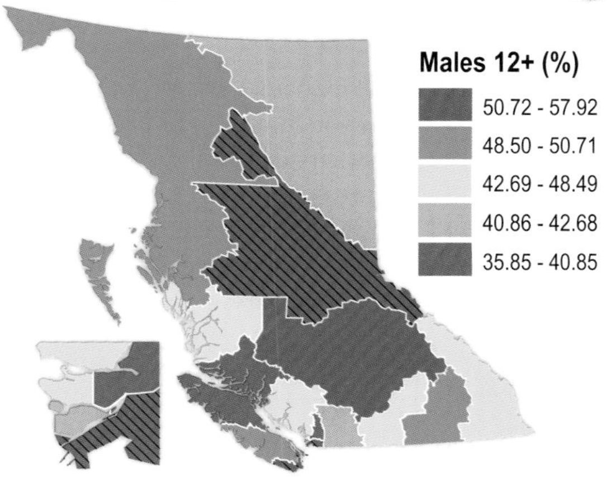
Males 12+ (%)
50.72 - 57.92
48.50 - 50.71
42.69 - 48.49
40.86 - 42.68
35.85 - 40.85

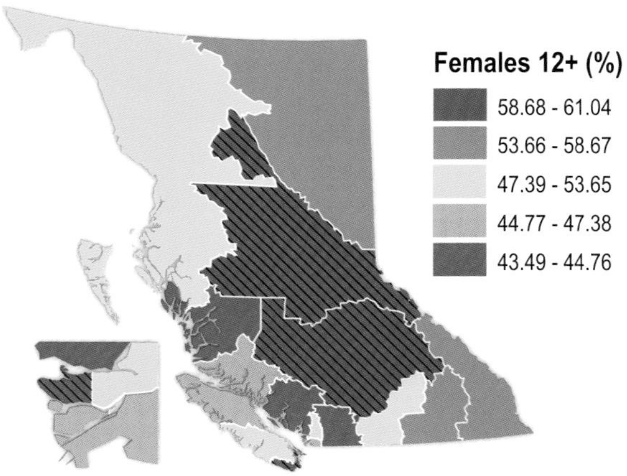
Females 12+ (%)
58.68 - 61.04
53.66 - 58.67
47.39 - 53.65
44.77 - 47.38
43.49 - 44.76

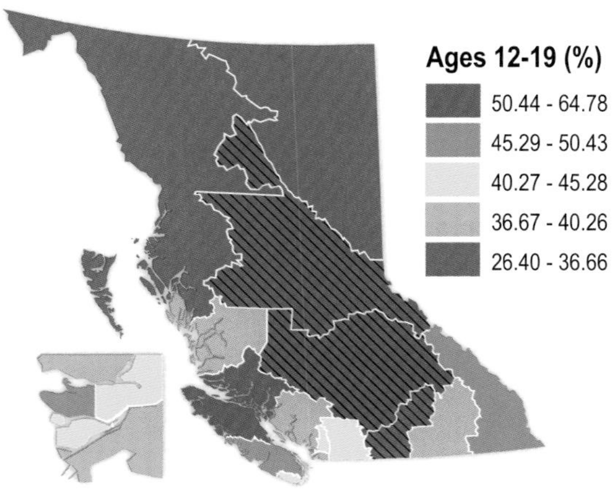
Ages 12-19 (%)
50.44 - 64.78
45.29 - 50.43
40.27 - 45.28
36.67 - 40.26
26.40 - 36.66

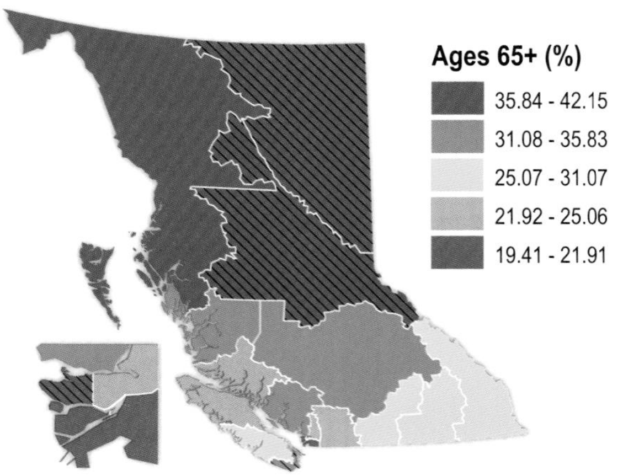
Ages 65+ (%)
35.84 - 42.15
31.08 - 35.83
25.07 - 31.07
21.92 - 25.06
19.41 - 21.91

Has access to programs at or near work to improve health

Health Service Delivery Area	All respondents 15-75 (%)	Males 15-75 (%)	Females 15-75 (%)	Ages 15-24 (%)	Ages 25-44 (%)	Ages 45-75 (%)
13 Okanagan	54.52	51.65	57.99	50.26E	54.95	56.14
12 Kootenay Boundary	53.83	50.37	58.26	F	63.31	44.81
41 South Vancouver Island	52.57	50.53	55.12	51.31	51.67	54.26
33 North Shore/Coast Garibaldi	48.05	41.89	57.10	48.36	46.91	48.99
14 Thompson Cariboo Shuswap	46.15	39.92	53.57	40.57	48.33	46.57
32 Vancouver	45.28	44.02	46.84	41.33	47.38	43.05
42 Central Vancouver Island	41.03	36.89	46.35	28.86E	41.28	45.44
11 East Kootenay	40.84	34.15E	49.02	F	46.48	39.44
51 Northwest	39.73	37.62E	42.42	35.61E	43.23	37.05E
53 Northeast	36.16	35.32E	37.37E	43.94E	30.55E	40.57E
43 North Vancouver Island	33.76	36.11	30.16E	F	37.87	32.85E
52 Northern Interior	33.23	36.52	28.79	F	45.03	29.69
22 Fraser North	33.15	27.33	40.32	35.75E	30.16	35.96
23 Fraser South	32.36	25.71*	40.78	43.36	28.43	32.96
31 Richmond	31.07	29.02E	33.51	F	29.64	32.93E
21 Fraser East	24.39	20.08E	30.37	F	28.15	27.49
British Columbia (2007/8)	**40.09**	**36.27***	**44.96**	**38.10**	**40.01**	**41.00**
No comparable 2005 data available						

Crosshatching beside the 2007/8 provincial rate indicates it is significantly different than the 2005 rate, while crosshatched HSDAs are significantly different than the 2007/8 provincial rate.
E interpret data with caution (16.67 ≤ coefficient of variation ≤ 33.3).

* Males differ significantly from females.
†15-24 age cohort differs significantly from the 25-44 age cohort.
‡ 45-75 age cohort differs significantly from the 25-44 age cohort.
F data suppressed (n < 10, or coefficient of variation > 33.3).

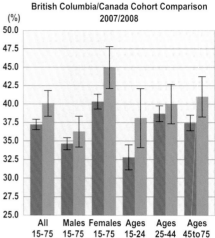

British Columbia/Canada Cohort Comparison 2007/2008

Canada ■   British Columbia ■
⊥ 95% confidence limits of estimate

In response to the CCHS question *"At or near your place of work, do you have access to programs to improve health, physical fitness or nutrition?"* four out of ten (40.09%) respondents in BC aged 15 - 75 years who worked outside the home answered positively. Kootenay Boundary, Okanagan, and South Vancouver Island (all above 52%) were significantly more likely than the provincial average to have access to such programs, while Fraser East, Fraser North, Fraser South, and Richmond (all below 34%) were significantly less likely.

Female respondents (44.96%) were significantly more likely than males (36.27%) to have access to programs at or near work to improve their health. Within HSDAs, Fraser South was the only area in which the value for males was significantly different than that of females.

Male respondents in Okanagan (51.65%) and South Vancouver Island (50.53%) were significantly more likely than males provincially to have access to health improvement programs at or near work, while males in Fraser East, Fraser North, and Fraser South (all below 28%) were significantly lower than the provincial average for male respondents.

Female respondents in Okanagan (57.99%) and South Vancouver Island (55.12%) were significantly more likely, and females in Fraser East, Richmond, North Vancouver Island, and Northern Interior (all below 34%) were significantly less likely than their peers provincially to have access to health improvement programs at or near work.

At the provincial level, there were no significant differences

between the younger (15 - 24 years) and mid-age (25 - 44 years) cohorts overall. The sample size was too small to report values for six of the HSDAs for the younger cohort, and for another five HSDAs, samples had high coefficients of variation, or small sample sizes, so interpretation should be made with caution.

There were no significant differences between older respondents (45 - 75 years) and the mid-age cohort. Older respondents in Okanagan and South Vancouver Island (both above 54%) were significantly more likely, while those in Fraser East and the Northern Interior (both below 30%) were significantly less likely than their peers provincially to have access to health improvement programs at or near work.

There was approximately a 30 percentage point spread for all cohorts (except the younger cohort), indicating large geographic variations. Higher values occurred in the south central part of the province, and North Shore/Coast Garibaldi. The lower mainland and Fraser regions had lower values.

There were no comparative CCHS data for 2005. The 2007/8 sample respondents in BC were more likely to have access to programs to improve health at or near work than their Canadian counterparts for all cohorts. These differences were significant for all respondents and for females.

Has access to programs at or near work to improve health

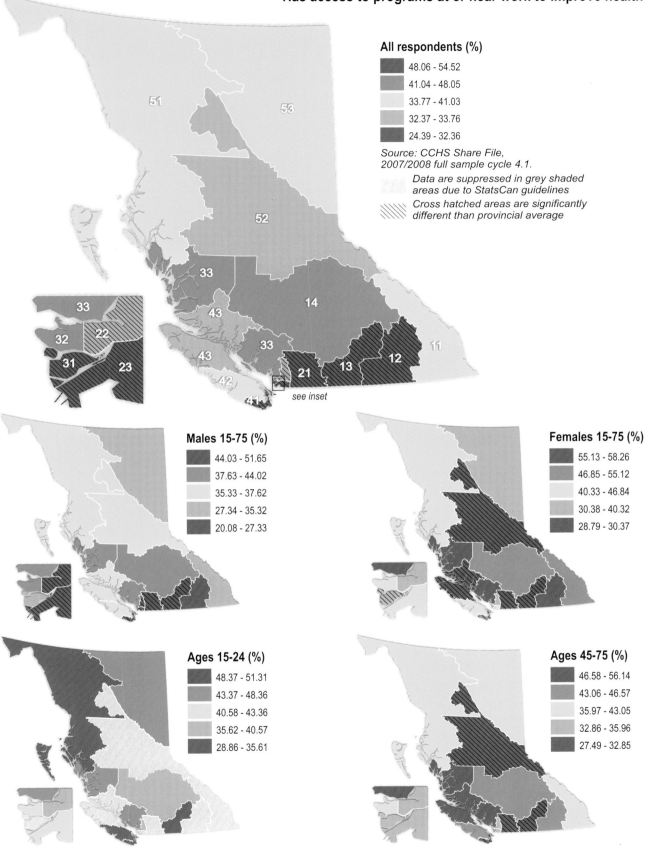

All respondents (%)

- 48.06 - 54.52
- 41.04 - 48.05
- 33.77 - 41.03
- 32.37 - 33.76
- 24.39 - 32.36

Source: CCHS Share File, 2007/2008 full sample cycle 4.1.

Data are suppressed in grey shaded areas due to StatsCan guidelines

Cross hatched areas are significantly different than provincial average

see inset

Males 15-75 (%)

- 44.03 - 51.65
- 37.63 - 44.02
- 35.33 - 37.62
- 27.34 - 35.32
- 20.08 - 27.33

Females 15-75 (%)

- 55.13 - 58.26
- 46.85 - 55.12
- 40.33 - 46.84
- 30.38 - 40.32
- 28.79 - 30.37

Ages 15-24 (%)

- 48.37 - 51.31
- 43.37 - 48.36
- 40.58 - 43.36
- 35.62 - 40.57
- 28.86 - 35.61

Ages 45-75 (%)

- 46.58 - 56.14
- 43.06 - 46.57
- 35.97 - 43.05
- 32.86 - 35.96
- 27.49 - 32.85

Students learning about how to stay healthy at school

The school is an important setting for learning about how to be healthy and to promote health and wellness among students (Kendall, 2008). The Student Satisfaction Survey asked students *"At school, are you learning how to stay healthy?"* and those students who answered "all of the time" or "many times" in 2008/9 are analysed in the table and maps opposite. This is a new indicator for the Atlas.

Grades 3/4

Nearly two-thirds (63.07%) of students in these grades responded positively to this question by indicating *"all of the time"* or *"many times."* There was a large differential among school districts: 74.16% of students in Rocky Mountain responded positively, while less than half did so in Gulf Islands, Alberni and Vancouver Island West. There were few clear clusters regionally, although a group in the southern central interior had relatively high values, with positive outliers in Fort Nelson (71.91%), North Vancouver Island (68.89%), Saanich (70.42%), and Delta (68.42%). Areas with lower values occurred on Vancouver Island, parts of the southeast and northwest and Peace River region, the central interior, and coastal parts of the province.

Grade 7

Just six in ten respondents indicated that they had learned how to stay healthy in grade 7. Abbotsford and Gold Trail (both above 71%) had the highest percentage of students with positive response, while Central Coast again had the lowest percentage of students with a positive response (25.00%). Geographically, there were no distinct patterns, except for higher positive values in the lower mainland, Coast Mountains (63.47%), and several school districts in the southern interior (Gold Trail, Kamloops/Thompson), Rocky Mountain in the southeast, and Qualicum on Vancouver Island. Low values occurred throughout parts of the north, central coastal areas, northern parts of Vancouver Island, and the extreme southern interior and southeastern parts of the province.

Grade 10

Less than half (49.24%) of grade 10 respondents indicated that they learned how to stay healthy at school *"all of the time"* or *"many times."* Arrow Lakes (74.58%) had by far the highest positive value, followed by 61.90% in Vancouver Island West. At the other extreme, only 26.67% of students in Central Coast responded positively. Again, there were very few clear regional clusters, except for a group of school districts in the lower mainland area that had higher than average positive values, along with parts of the northeast and interior. Most of the northwest and north coast had lower than average values, although Haida Gwaii (57.50%) was a positive outlier.

School District	All students grades 3/4 (%)	All students grade 7 (%)	All students grade 10 (%)
6 Rocky Mountain	74.16	69.75	55.15
78 Fraser-Cascade	73.44	49.23	48.62
22 Vernon	71.22	54.61	52.20
81 Fort Nelson	71.19	34.85	57.41
63 Saanich	70.42	53.45	55.07
74 Gold Trail	70.37	71.26	43.75
58 Nicola-Similkameen	68.93	57.38	53.42
85 Vancouver Island North	68.89	50.96	50.00
37 Delta	68.42	59.29	46.75
67 Okanagan Skaha	67.29	51.41	34.59
79 Cowichan Valley	67.28	57.64	51.89
75 Mission	67.21	57.81	44.60
42 Maple Ridge-Pitt Meadows	67.06	57.86	41.47
83 North Okanagan-Shuswap	66.42	44.86	35.38
73 Kamloops/Thompson	66.07	63.78	46.01
23 Central Okanagan	66.01	62.53	35.14
69 Qualicum	65.43	63.61	42.37
36 Surrey	65.21	66.88	55.66
57 Prince George	64.95	56.00	47.20
91 Nechako Lakes	64.93	52.55	55.31
50 Haida Gwaii/Queen Charlotte	64.86	52.73	57.50
72 Campbell River	64.04	40.92	48.68
41 Burnaby	63.86	65.52	54.74
20 Kootenay-Columbia	63.32	50.67	48.78
38 Richmond	63.16	68.82	47.25
28 Quesnel	62.96	54.75	41.10
5 Southeast Kootenay	62.65	47.48	47.08
39 Vancouver	62.54	63.86	53.78
51 Boundary	62.50	48.39	43.75
35 Langley	62.46	59.19	43.75
44 North Vancouver	62.32	60.51	54.33
52 Prince Rupert	62.28	47.66	42.02
34 Abbotsford	61.75	71.42	54.01
19 Revelstoke	61.67	61.54	46.38
43 Coquitlam	61.10	68.50	60.31
47 Powell River	60.58	61.70	46.25
87 Stikine	60.00	54.55	42.86
48 Howe Sound	59.62	42.37	48.96
46 Sunshine Coast	59.60	46.33	45.65
40 New Westminster	59.13	57.60	35.52
82 Coast Mountains	59.06	63.47	45.38
59 Peace River South	59.03	59.89	50.41
53 Okanagan Similkameen	58.54	56.35	38.06
45 West Vancouver	58.54	61.12	54.82
33 Chilliwack	58.25	51.07	52.55
68 Nanaimo-Ladysmith	58.23	61.95	55.97
61 Greater Victoria	57.47	44.48	42.03
10 Arrow Lakes	57.45	54.76	74.58
8 Kootenay Lake	57.25	53.05	41.67
62 Sooke	56.57	59.89	21.53
27 Cariboo-Chilcotin	56.48	56.40	50.99
60 Peace River North	56.48	53.99	51.69
71 Comox Valley	52.55	48.91	46.09
54 Bulkley Valley	51.35	57.87	55.87
64 Gulf Islands	49.30	29.67	33.10
70 Alberni	45.49	60.63	28.77
84 Vancouver Island West	42.31	40.00	61.90
49 Central Coast	Msk	25.00	26.67
92 Nisga'a	Msk	61.54	23.08
British Columbia	**63.07**	**60.04**	**49.24**

Msk: Data masked for privacy

Students learning about how to stay healthy at school

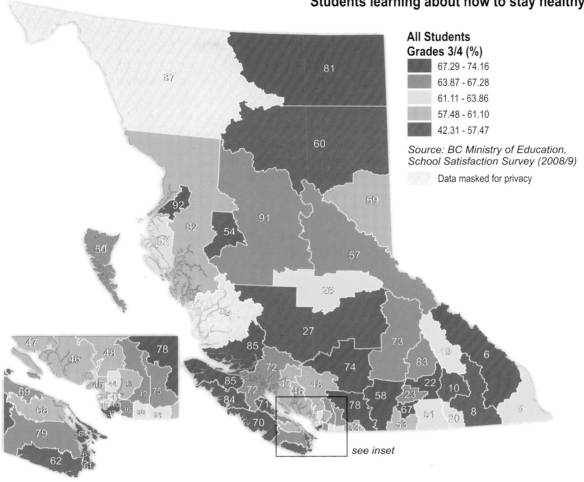

**All Students
Grades 3/4 (%)**

- 67.29 - 74.16
- 63.87 - 67.28
- 61.11 - 63.86
- 57.48 - 61.10
- 42.31 - 57.47

*Source: BC Ministry of Education,
School Satisfaction Survey (2008/9)*

Data masked for privacy

see inset

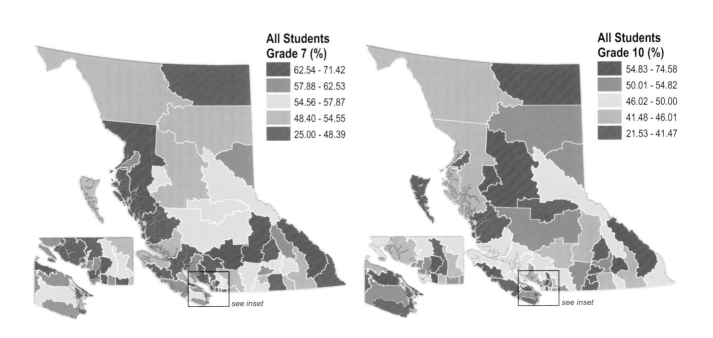

**All Students
Grade 7 (%)**

- 62.54 - 71.42
- 57.88 - 62.53
- 54.56 - 57.87
- 48.40 - 54.55
- 25.00 - 48.39

see inset

**All Students
Grade 10 (%)**

- 54.83 - 74.58
- 50.01 - 54.82
- 46.02 - 50.00
- 41.48 - 46.01
- 21.53 - 41.47

see inset

Strong start programs

Children who are exposed to language-rich environments and play-based early learning experiences are more likely to be ready to learn once they enter kindergarten. StrongStart BC centres provide free school-based early learning services for adults and their young children, from birth to 5 years. They are operated by school districts in available school space, preferably in a school offering kindergarten, and young children have access to learning environments and benefit from social interactions. Adults also learn ways to support learning, both at the centre and at home. Activities are led by certified early childhood educators and healthy snacks are provided (Ministry of Education, 2010a).

Two types of early learning programs have been made available: centres and learning outreach programs. Centres are located in school facilities and operate 5 days per week, for a minimum of 3 hours per day. Outreach programs operate in rural and remote communities on a reduced schedule to accommodate a variety of remote locations. The major intent of these initiatives is to help level the "playing field" and improve readiness to learn, especially for low socio-economic and hard-to-reach children and families.

Programs were introduced over several phases starting in the fall of 2006. By 2010, there were 315 programs in place, including 284 centres and 31 outreach programs in 24 school districts covering more than 85 communities (Powell, 2010). In addition, a virtual program has been established online to help reach those who cannot connect with either a centre or outreach program (Wormley, 2010).

The table and map opposite provide a perspective of these programs by school district. The indicator developed includes three key components. First is the number of programs (centres and outreach programs) by school district. Second, the proportion of "at-risk" children in any school district is used, based on the percentage of children entering kindergarten between 2007/8 to 2008/9 who were vulnerable on one or more of the components of the Early Development Instrument (EDI) (see readiness to learn indicator on the next page). This percentage is then applied to the total number of children between birth and 5 years old using the population based on BC Stats P.E.O.P.L.E. 35 model (BC Stats, 2010a), the target group for the StrongStart initiatives. The final indicator provides the number of strong start programs per 1,000 at-risk children between birth and 5 years old. These indicators are new to the Atlas.

The BC average was 4.15 programs per 1,000 at-risk young children. At one extreme, Arrow Lakes had nearly 135 programs per 1,000 young children at-risk, while Vancouver had only 1.49 programs per 1,000 at-risk children. Arrow Lakes was an outlier, and had only a small number of young children overall, with very few at-risk based on the EDI, so caution is required in interpreting this number. Those with the highest numbers of programs per 1,000 at-risk children are clustered in southern interior and Kootenay Boundary areas of the province. Relatively high numbers are also found in rural school districts such as Haida Gwaii, Fort Nelson, Vancouver Island North, and Gulf Islands (all above 10 programs per 1,000 at-risk children). Those with the smallest numbers were concentrated in the urban lower mainland (Vancouver, Surrey, Richmond, Burnaby) and Greater Victoria. Outliers were also evident in Peace River North, Kamloops/Thompson, and Central Okanagan.

School District	Strong start programs per 1,000 at-risk children	
10 Arrow Lakes		134.53
50 Haida Gwaii/Queen Charlotte		35.11
19 Revelstoke		33.39
64 Gulf Islands		28.99
51 Boundary		25.37
47 Powell River		15.93
20 Kootenay-Columbia		15.28
81 Fort Nelson		14.10
53 Okanagan Similkameen		11.21
58 Nicola-Similkameen		10.18
85 Vancouver Island North		10.06
8 Kootenay Lake		9.72
91 Nechako Lakes		9.72
74 Gold Trail		9.49
27 Cariboo-Chilcotin		9.27
46 Sunshine Coast		9.16
59 Peace River South		9.10
28 Quesnel		8.31
54 Bulkley Valley		8.28
6 Rocky Mountain		8.10
78 Fraser-Cascade		7.97
69 Qualicum		7.87
70 Alberni		7.86
83 North Okanagan-Shuswap		7.54
67 Okanagan Skaha		6.74
79 Cowichan Valley		6.39
57 Prince George		6.35
72 Campbell River		6.02
5 Southeast Kootenay		5.86
62 Sooke		5.73
52 Prince Rupert		5.68
63 Saanich		5.53
37 Delta		5.51
22 Vernon		5.31
68 Nanaimo-Ladysmith		4.98
42 Maple Ridge-Pitt Meadows		4.95
75 Mission		4.89
45 West Vancouver		4.71
35 Langley		4.30
44 North Vancouver		4.07
43 Coquitlam		3.97
34 Abbotsford		3.85
48 Howe Sound		3.79
82 Coast Mountains		3.56
71 Comox Valley		3.56
40 New Westminster		3.49
23 Central Okanagan		3.45
33 Chilliwack		3.45
73 Kamloops/Thompson		3.29
60 Peace River North		3.13
41 Burnaby		2.94
61 Greater Victoria		2.24
38 Richmond		2.21
36 Surrey		2.18
39 Vancouver		1.49
49 Central Coast		N/A
92 Nisga'a		N/A
87 Stikine		N/A
84 Vancouver Island West		N/A
British Columbia		**4.15**

N/A: No data

Strong start programs

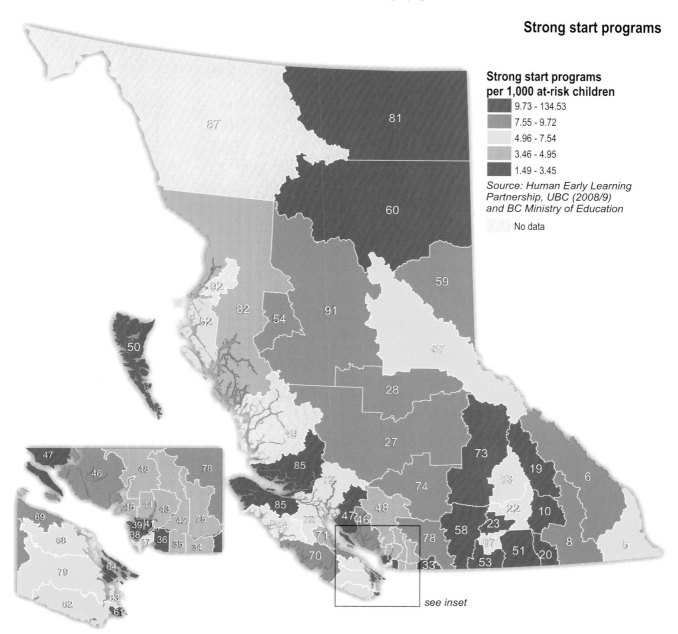

**Strong start programs
per 1,000 at-risk children**

- 9.73 - 134.53
- 7.55 - 9.72
- 4.96 - 7.54
- 3.46 - 4.95
- 1.49 - 3.45

*Source: Human Early Learning
Partnership, UBC (2008/9)
and BC Ministry of Education*

No data

see inset

Readiness to learn

Getting a good start in life is important for later health and wellness (Mikkonen & Raphael, 2010). Students who enter kindergarten "ready to learn" do much better educationally than those who have some "vulnerabilities," and there is a clear relationship between education and health and wellness outcomes. The Early Development Instrument (EDI) has been designed to evaluate a child's development as they enter kindergarten.

The EDI has approximately 130 questions that kindergarten teachers answer for each child after they have been in kindergarten for several months. There are five components to the EDI: physical health and well-being; social competence; emotional maturity; language and cognitive development; and communication skills and general knowledge. On average, a little over 10% of kindergarten students who are evaluated are rated as being vulnerable on each of the five components noted above (Human Early Learning Partnership, 2010). Because the communication and general knowledge factor is often overwhelmed by high numbers of new immigrant youngsters, we have chosen to not include this factor in our analyses of readiness to learn.

Overall ready

Approximately three out of every four (75.1%) kindergarten students were ready to learn for the 2 year period 2007/8 to 2008/9. Readiness to learn showed major geographical variation, and ranged from a high of 93.3% in Revelstoke to a low of 50.3% in Prince Rupert. The highest performing kindergarten students were found in the southeastern part of the province, parts of the lower mainland, and the southern part of Vancouver Island. Those least ready to learn were found in much of the interior and coastal areas outside of the lower mainland.

Socially ready

The pattern for this indicator was fairly similar to overall ready to learn. Values ranged from a high of 97.3% in Revelstoke to a low of 71.3% in Prince Rupert.

Emotionally ready

Again, the pattern for this indicator was fairly similar to the other two, although there were a couple of outliers worthy of note: Vancouver Island North and Quesnel (both above 91%) performed relatively higher, given their values for overall readiness to learn. Overall values ranged from 96.7% in Revelstoke to a low of 80.1% in both Nicola-Similkameen and Okanagan-Similkameen.

School District	Ready to learn (%)	Socially ready (%)	Emotionally ready (%)
19 Revelstoke	93.3	97.3	96.7
10 Arrow Lakes	90.0	95.0	92.5
20 Kootenay-Columbia	85.6	93.3	92.9
45 West Vancouver	82.4	89.7	90.0
23 Central Okanagan	82.2	92.5	90.1
22 Vernon	81.3	93.7	91.9
40 New Westminster	80.5	91.7	92.8
63 Saanich	80.3	88.6	87.3
44 North Vancouver	79.8	89.1	88.4
79 Cowichan Valley	79.2	89.6	91.3
83 North Okanagan-Shuswap	79.2	89.5	87.9
35 Langley	79.0	89.2	89.2
62 Sooke	78.2	90.6	90.4
69 Qualicum	77.9	89.1	88.3
34 Abbotsford	77.7	88.3	89.7
61 Greater Victoria	77.7	88.9	89.4
6 Rocky Mountain	77.6	88.9	86.2
43 Coquitlam	77.5	87.5	89.0
81 Fort Nelson	77.2	87.0	91.1
38 Richmond	77.1	84.8	87.6
42 Maple Ridge-Pitt Meadows	77.0	85.5	90.4
8 Kootenay Lake	76.4	90.3	83.4
51 Boundary	76.2	91.0	88.9
37 Delta	76.0	87.3	87.4
57 Prince George	75.9	88.1	88.5
36 Surrey	75.9	87.9	88.7
64 Gulf Islands	75.6	94.9	87.2
70 Alberni	75.2	88.6	87.1
73 Kamloops/Thompson	74.8	88.0	88.3
68 Nanaimo-Ladysmith	74.7	85.7	89.8
41 Burnaby	74.5	87.4	88.8
50 Haida Gwaii/Queen Charlotte	74.5	84.5	85.5
72 Campbell River	73.7	87.8	85.9
5 Southeast Kootenay	73.5	86.4	83.4
54 Bulkley Valley	73.4	85.1	85.0
48 Howe Sound	73.4	87.5	87.2
67 Okanagan Skaha	73.4	86.5	85.0
85 Vancouver Island North	72.6	88.2	91.2
47 Powell River	72.3	83.2	81.4
53 Okanagan Similkameen	72.0	85.3	80.1
27 Cariboo-Chilcotin	71.0	87.5	87.0
33 Chilliwack	70.2	84.8	83.1
39 Vancouver	70.0	83.6	84.3
82 Coast Mountains	69.9	86.5	87.9
59 Peace River South	69.9	85.6	86.3
75 Mission	69.1	83.7	81.6
28 Quesnel	69.0	85.0	91.1
71 Comox Valley	67.8	83.4	81.9
91 Nechako Lakes	67.4	85.0	84.2
78 Fraser-Cascade	67.3	78.5	85.6
60 Peace River North	64.8	84.9	87.6
58 Nicola-Similkameen	62.4	85.1	80.1
46 Sunshine Coast	60.7	85.7	86.3
74 Gold Trail	59.5	81.4	86.0
52 Prince Rupert	50.3	71.3	81.0
49 Central Coast	N/A	N/A	N/A
92 Nisga'a	N/A	N/A	N/A
87 Stikine	N/A	N/A	N/A
84 Vancouver Island West	N/A	N/A	N/A
British Columbia	**75.1**	**87.3**	**87.6**

N/A: Data masked (small cell sizes)

Readiness to learn

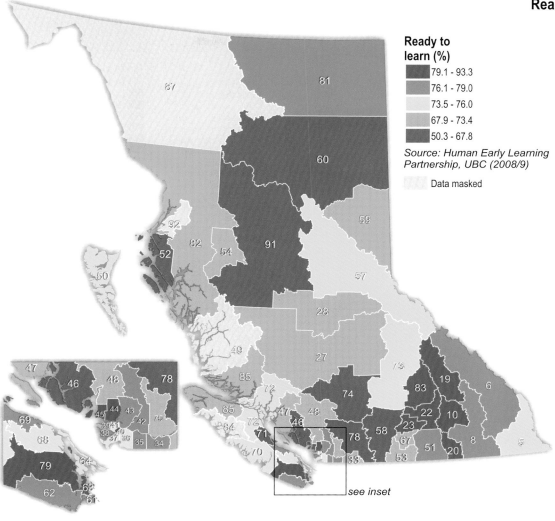

Ready to learn (%)

- 79.1 - 93.3
- 76.1 - 79.0
- 73.5 - 76.0
- 67.9 - 73.4
- 50.3 - 67.8

Source: Human Early Learning Partnership, UBC (2008/9)

Data masked

see inset

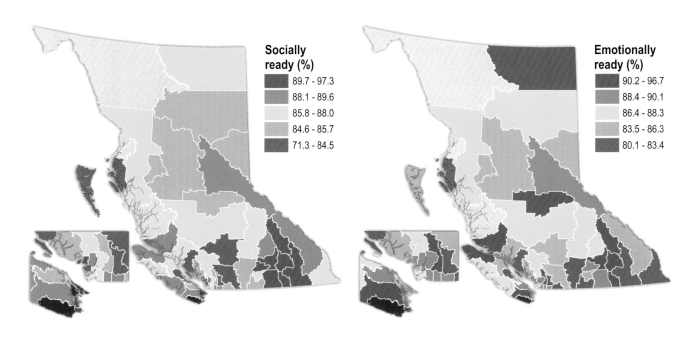

Socially ready (%)

- 89.7 - 97.3
- 88.1 - 89.6
- 85.8 - 88.0
- 84.6 - 85.7
- 71.3 - 84.5

Emotionally ready (%)

- 90.2 - 96.7
- 88.4 - 90.1
- 86.4 - 88.3
- 83.5 - 86.3
- 80.1 - 83.4

Foundation skills assessment, grade 4

Grade 4 students in public and independent schools are assessed annually on their ability to meet expectations related to reading, writing, and numeracy. Students are assessed in terms of 'not yet meeting,' 'meeting,' or 'exceeding' expectations. Approximately 7,000 to 8,000 (16%) of the more than 43,000 students were not assessed for a variety of reasons. The table and maps opposite provide the results, by school district, from the BC Ministry of Education and this is a new indicator for this Atlas.

Reading

Over two-thirds (67.12%) of the 43,000 grade 4 students provincially met or exceeded reading expectations. Female students (71%) were more likely to meet or exceed requirements than male students (64%), while only 51% of Aboriginal students did so. Fort Nelson had the highest value (91.53%), while Nisga'a (9.68%) and Stikine (26.09%) did poorly. Geographically, there were three general regions where students out-performed the average: the northeast (especially Fort Nelson), parts of the southeast quadrant of the province (Revelstoke, Okanagan Similkameen, Central Okanagan, Kamloops Thompson) and parts of the lower mainland (West Vancouver, Howe Sound, Abbotsford). Many of the school districts in the northwest quadrant did not do well, apart from Haida Gwaii and Bulkley Valley, and poorer results occurred on parts of Vancouver Island.

Writing

Nearly seven in every ten students (68.93%) met or exceeded the grade 4 writing assessment. Again, female students had a higher percentage (74%) that met or exceeded expectations than male students (64%), and Aboriginal students did not do as well (54%). The geographical patterns were quite similar to those described for reading assessments, although the spread among school districts was not as dramatic as it was for reading. Revelstoke had the highest positive assessments, with 86.30% of students meeting or exceeding expectations, compared with only 22% in Nisga'a. Revelstoke and Comox Valley did relatively poorly when compared to their results for reading.

Numeracy

Less than two-thirds (63.71%) of students met or exceeded grade 4 numeracy requirements, with 65% of female and 53% of male students meeting or exceeding expectations. Less than half (47%) of Aboriginal students did so. Fort Nelson scored best overall, while Stikine had no students who met or exceeded requirements. Extreme caution is required in interpreting this number. Nisga'a had only a quarter (25.81%) of their students meet or exceed requirements. Geographically, the patterns were very similar to those for reading and writing.

School District	Reading (%)	Writing (%)	Numeracy (%)
81 Fort Nelson	91.53	83.05	91.53
45 West Vancouver	86.82	85.45	86.82
19 Revelstoke	80.82	86.30	80.82
53 Okanagan Similkameen	79.58	72.77	79.58
48 Howe Sound	77.52	73.29	66.45
73 Kamloops/Thompson	77.41	84.52	73.59
34 Abbotsford	77.02	77.75	76.51
23 Central Okanagan	76.57	72.53	71.67
54 Bulkley Valley	76.22	76.92	72.73
64 Gulf Islands	74.53	74.53	75.47
50 Haida Gwaii/Queen Charlotte	74.47	85.11	65.96
35 Langley	73.52	76.36	66.79
10 Arrow Lakes	72.97	83.78	70.27
38 Richmond	71.51	76.99	71.71
22 Vernon	70.90	66.85	60.96
67 Okanagan Skaha	70.83	68.98	66.90
44 North Vancouver	70.49	66.96	65.28
70 Alberni	69.88	67.95	58.69
69 Qualicum	69.59	62.84	63.18
20 Kootenay-Columbia	69.17	62.78	59.40
33 Chilliwack	68.80	72.48	65.48
6 Rocky Mountain	68.12	70.74	70.74
60 Peace River North	68.05	80.74	66.08
75 Mission	68.01	67.34	63.98
63 Saanich	67.65	76.53	69.56
40 New Westminster	67.36	65.28	66.32
49 Central Coast	66.67	60.00	60.00
59 Peace River South	66.54	59.85	53.53
27 Cariboo-Chilcotin	66.31	70.56	60.48
71 Comox Valley	66.31	57.71	58.96
61 Greater Victoria	66.19	62.77	60.96
47 Powell River	66.00	64.00	64.67
8 Kootenay Lake	65.63	64.79	61.69
42 Maple Ridge-Pitt Meadows	65.17	72.16	57.98
5 Southeast Kootenay	64.55	60.52	63.11
37 Delta	64.36	68.14	59.21
57 Prince George	64.36	73.03	57.46
36 Surrey	64.15	71.52	58.66
58 Nicola-Similkameen	63.89	68.75	57.64
41 Burnaby	63.66	63.37	65.92
43 Coquitlam	63.39	66.46	62.16
79 Cowichan Valley	63.07	66.67	54.25
85 Vancouver Island North	62.38	72.28	61.39
74 Gold Trail	61.73	62.96	49.38
68 Nanaimo-Ladysmith	60.20	64.21	57.48
83 North Okanagan-Shuswap	58.58	60.64	56.06
46 Sunshine Coast	58.04	58.93	54.02
51 Boundary	57.14	64.76	60.95
62 Sooke	56.75	56.27	52.57
82 Coast Mountains	53.43	54.03	42.99
84 Vancouver Island West	53.33	60.00	50.00
28 Quesnel	52.28	32.99	40.61
52 Prince Rupert	50.65	66.23	40.91
39 Vancouver	49.20	50.21	48.86
72 Campbell River	47.41	55.70	47.93
91 Nechako Lakes	46.69	53.97	40.40
78 Fraser-Cascade	41.82	31.82	35.45
87 Stikine	26.09	34.78	0.00
92 Nisga'a	9.68	22.58	25.81
British Columbia	**67.12**	**68.93**	**63.71**

Foundation skills assessment, grade 4

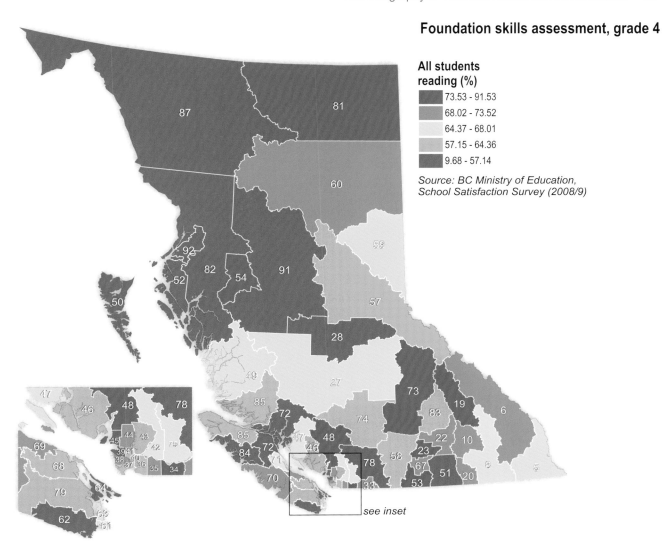

All students reading (%)

- 73.53 - 91.53
- 68.02 - 73.52
- 64.37 - 68.01
- 57.15 - 64.36
- 9.68 - 57.14

Source: BC Ministry of Education, School Satisfaction Survey (2008/9)

see inset

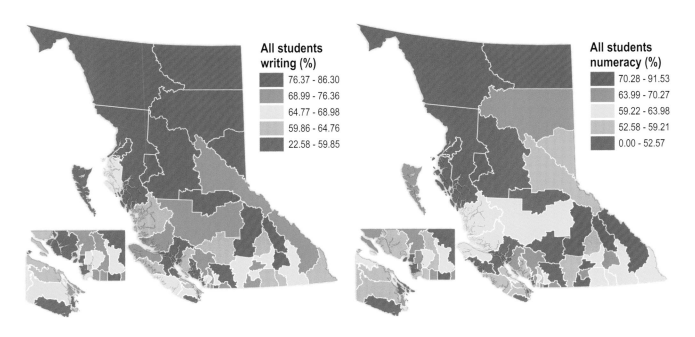

All students writing (%)

- 76.37 - 86.30
- 68.99 - 76.36
- 64.77 - 68.98
- 59.86 - 64.76
- 22.58 - 59.85

All students numeracy (%)

- 70.28 - 91.53
- 63.99 - 70.27
- 59.22 - 63.98
- 52.58 - 59.21
- 0.00 - 52.57

Foundation skills assessment, grade 7

As with grade 4 students, grade 7 students in public and independent schools were assessed on reading, writing, and numeracy. Again, results are reported in terms of 'not yet meeting,' 'meeting,' or 'exceeding' expectations. Of the more than 47,000 grade 7 students in 2009/10, between 8,000 and 9,000 had an unknown performance level, according to the data from the BC Ministry of Education. The results of those students who met or exceeded expected performance are given in the table and maps on the opposite page. This is a new indicator for this Atlas.

Reading

Less than two-thirds (64.81%) of all grade 7 students met or exceeded expected performance for reading skills. As was the case for grade 4 students, females (68%) out-performed males (62%), while Aboriginal students again did not do as well (46%). The values among school districts ranged from 87.65% for Revelstoke to 30.00% for Nisga'a. Geographically, there was a cluster of school districts in the central eastern interior (Revelstoke, Arrow Lakes, and Kamloops Thompson), as well as a group in the lower mainland area (West Vancouver, Howe Sound, Abbotsford, and Richmond) that were well above the provincial average. Fort Nelson, Gulf Islands, and Okanagan Similkameen were all positive outliers. Several parts of Vancouver Island, and school districts on the central coast and parts of the north and northern interior did not perform as well. Vancouver also did not do as well as neighbouring school districts.

Writing

Assessments for writing were higher than those for reading, with 67.93% of all BC students meeting or exceeding performance expectations. Females (74%) did substantially better than males (62%), and Aboriginal students (49%) were below the average for grade 7 students. Among school districts, there was a range of 94.29% in Arrow Lakes to just 20.83% in Central Coast and 37.50% in Quesnel. Geographical patterns were quite similar to those observed for reading, although Vancouver Island West was substantially lower when compared to the reading assessment results.

Numeracy

Just over six in every ten (62.21%) students in BC met or exceeded expected performance for numeracy, and females (63%) and males (62%) had quite similar overall assessments, compared with an average of only 39% for Aboriginal students. There was a range among school districts of 88.48% for West Vancouver to only 16.67% for Nisga'a and 32.14% for Quesnel. Patterns were quite similar to those of the other two indicators.

School District	Reading (%)	Writing (%)	Numeracy (%)
19 Revelstoke	87.65	88.89	85.19
45 West Vancouver	85.87	81.74	88.48
10 Arrow Lakes	80.00	94.29	85.71
48 Howe Sound	77.56	83.33	68.91
81 Fort Nelson	75.64	83.33	79.49
73 Kamloops/Thompson	74.24	84.02	66.97
34 Abbotsford	72.82	81.34	73.64
53 Okanagan Similkameen	72.82	71.84	66.02
38 Richmond	72.41	79.54	76.46
64 Gulf Islands	71.93	74.56	64.04
6 Rocky Mountain	71.03	69.05	69.05
47 Powell River	70.65	65.22	64.13
27 Cariboo-Chilcotin	70.55	73.87	64.13
35 Langley	70.47	71.73	68.25
36 Surrey	69.39	74.09	68.02
44 North Vancouver	69.01	64.72	68.77
22 Vernon	68.38	61.53	59.03
70 Alberni	67.07	58.08	50.60
54 Bulkley Valley	66.84	76.84	66.84
41 Burnaby	66.61	68.14	70.68
40 New Westminster	66.53	77.89	67.36
46 Sunshine Coast	66.43	73.93	63.21
75 Mission	65.52	65.92	59.03
43 Coquitlam	65.42	72.38	63.33
83 North Okanagan-Shuswap	65.12	67.25	58.72
60 Peace River North	64.91	77.52	55.96
37 Delta	62.23	63.91	58.94
51 Boundary	61.80	65.17	62.92
20 Kootenay-Columbia	61.74	63.76	54.70
67 Okanagan Skaha	61.30	60.71	51.28
84 Vancouver Island West	60.61	36.36	36.36
82 Coast Mountains	60.42	50.92	47.76
57 Prince George	60.32	59.18	52.14
23 Central Okanagan	60.21	62.90	57.13
71 Comox Valley	60.16	64.96	57.44
63 Saanich	60.13	64.09	53.71
79 Cowichan Valley	59.84	63.17	48.41
8 Kootenay Lake	59.79	59.01	52.22
68 Nanaimo-Ladysmith	56.83	59.19	50.95
61 Greater Victoria	56.76	54.68	49.64
59 Peace River South	56.75	61.96	50.00
50 Haida Gwaii/Queen Charlotte	56.00	62.00	52.00
74 Gold Trail	55.28	64.23	56.10
52 Prince Rupert	54.49	64.61	43.82
58 Nicola-Similkameen	54.36	54.36	43.08
42 Maple Ridge-Pitt Meadows	53.96	69.51	52.09
69 Qualicum	53.37	44.94	48.88
33 Chilliwack	53.00	55.27	45.87
5 Southeast Kootenay	51.75	61.77	45.92
91 Nechako Lakes	50.82	56.56	46.72
39 Vancouver	46.85	50.82	49.99
85 Vancouver Island North	46.85	59.46	36.94
62 Sooke	45.16	43.34	39.83
87 Stikine	42.86	50.00	42.86
28 Quesnel	42.50	37.50	32.14
49 Central Coast	41.67	20.83	45.83
72 Campbell River	40.96	44.82	40.48
78 Fraser-Cascade	35.29	41.18	33.82
92 Nisga'a	30.00	56.67	16.67
British Columbia	**64.81**	**67.93**	**62.21**

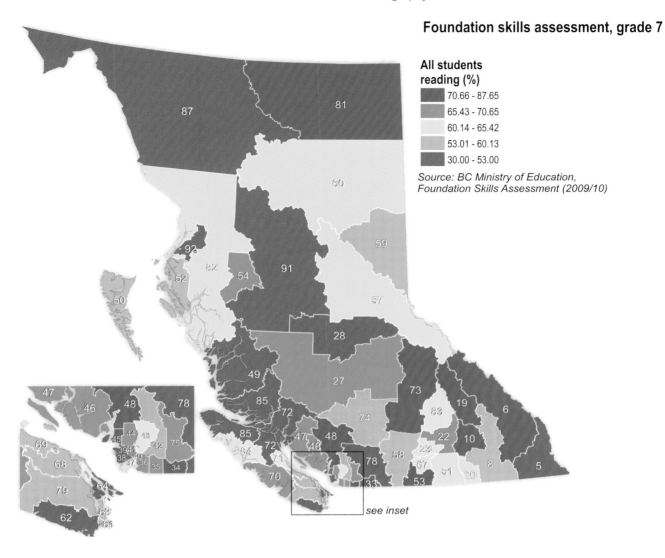

Foundation skills assessment, grade 7

All students reading (%)

- 70.66 - 87.65
- 65.43 - 70.65
- 60.14 - 65.42
- 53.01 - 60.13
- 30.00 - 53.00

Source: BC Ministry of Education, Foundation Skills Assessment (2009/10)

see inset

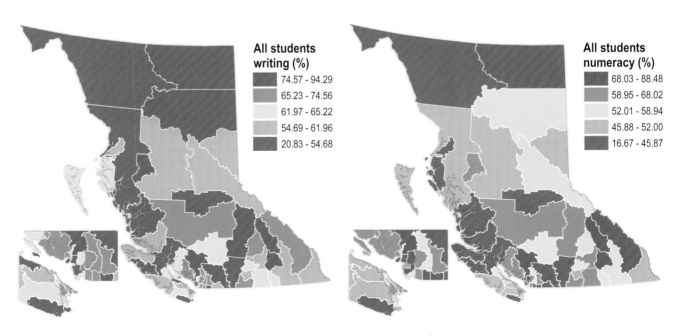

All students writing (%)

- 74.57 - 94.29
- 65.23 - 74.56
- 61.97 - 65.22
- 54.69 - 61.96
- 20.83 - 54.68

All students numeracy (%)

- 68.03 - 88.48
- 58.95 - 68.02
- 52.01 - 58.94
- 45.88 - 52.00
- 16.67 - 45.87

Adult education completion

Education is a key wellness asset. Those with higher levels of education are able to have greater job choices and better overall job opportunities. With this improved employment potential comes the ability to generate better incomes, greater wealth, and higher retirement incomes, which can result in improved housing, better nutrition, and more opportunities for contributing to positive family development, all important wellness assets which generally result in longer healthy life expectancies (Mikkonen & Raphael, 2010; McIntosh, et al., 2009; Canadian Population Health Initiative, 2008a; May, 2007).

Better education is closely associated with healthier lifestyles and healthy living. For example, higher education appears to be associated with a lower likelihood of obesity, especially among women. The positive effect of education on obesity is probably related to greater access to health-related information and improved ability to use such information (health literacy), clearer perception and understanding of the risks associated with lifestyle choices, and improved self-control and consistency of preferences over time (Sassi, 2009).

Higher levels of education are also related to greater social, cultural, and civic engagement (Campbell, 2006), again important wellness assets. In short, level of education is one of the most important overall wellness assets because of its relationship with so many other positive wellness factors.

The data presented in the table and two maps opposite are based on the 2006 census, and look at the proportion of population with a high school diploma, and with completed post-secondary education (BC Stats, 2010a).

High school graduates

In BC as a whole, nearly nine out of every ten (88.9%) residents between the ages of 25 and 54 had successfully graduated from high school in 2006. This was quite an improvement over the 5 years from 2001 (82.8%). North Shore/Coast Garibaldi (93.8%) had the highest proportion of graduates, while Northwest, at 79.2%, had the lowest proportion of their population with high school graduation, giving a range of almost 15 percentage points among HSDAs. Within the province, there were very clear geographic patterns. Most of the lower mainland (with the exception of Fraser South and Fraser East) and South Vancouver Island had above provincial averages of high school graduates, while the remainder of the province was below average. The lowest levels were found in the three

Health Service Delivery Area	High school graduation (%)		Post-secondary education (%)	
33 North Shore/Coast Garibaldi		93.8		71.6
31 Richmond		92.3		68.5
22 Fraser North		91.8		67.6
41 South Vancouver Island		91.7		66.5
32 Vancouver		91.4		71.9
23 Fraser South		88.5		59.5
12 Kootenay Boundary		87.9		59.2
13 Okanagan		87.9		58.2
11 East Kootenay		86.5		55.4
42 Central Vancouver Island		85.7		57.3
43 North Vancouver Island		85.1		55.8
21 Fraser East		84.1		52.7
14 Thompson Cariboo Shuswap		84.0		53.7
52 Northern Interior		81.8		50.4
53 Northeast		79.3		50.0
51 Northwest		79.2		49.9
British Columbia		**88.9**		**62.8**

northern HSDAs: Northwest and Northeast were both just above 79%, while Northern Interior was higher, but still below 82%.

Post-secondary graduates

In 2006, more than six in every ten (62.8%) residents in BC between the ages of 25 and 54 had completed some kind of post-secondary education. This was an increase from 57.7% recorded in the 2001 census. There was a 22 percentage point difference in values between the highest and lowest HSDAs. Vancouver and North Shore/Coast Garibaldi both had approximately 72% of residents between the ages of 25 and 54 with post-secondary education, compared with just less than half (49.9%) of the residents in Northwest. Geographically, patterns were quite similar to those for high school completion. The lower mainland HSDAs (with the exception of Fraser South and Fraser East) and South Vancouver Island had above provincial averages (all above 66%), while the three northern HSDAs all had only about one-half of their residents between the ages of 25 and 54 with post secondary education. The remainder of the HSDAs were also below the provincial average.

Adult education completion

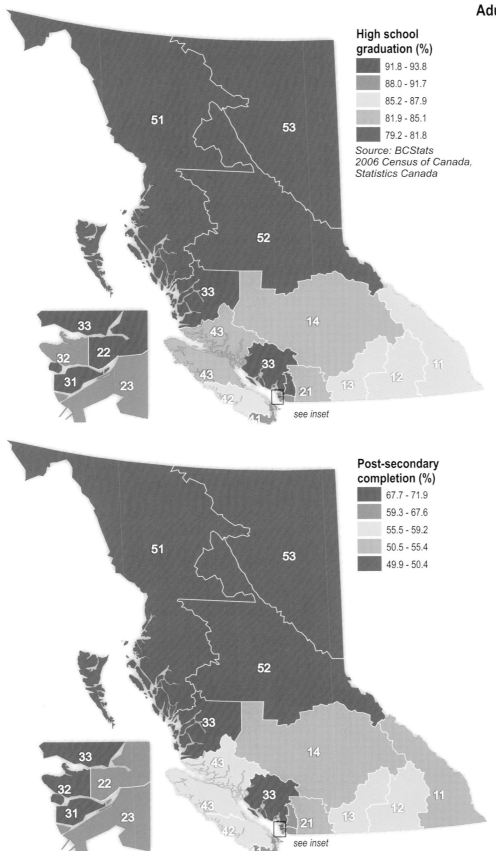

High school graduation (%)

- 91.8 - 93.8
- 88.0 - 91.7
- 85.2 - 87.9
- 81.9 - 85.1
- 79.2 - 81.8

Source: BCStats
2006 Census of Canada,
Statistics Canada

Post-secondary completion (%)

- 67.7 - 71.9
- 59.3 - 67.6
- 55.5 - 59.2
- 50.5 - 55.4
- 49.9 - 50.4

Composite learning index: lifelong learning

The Composite Learning Index (CLI) measures lifelong learning. It is based on a combination of indicators that reflect how Canadians learn. Lifelong learning results in higher wages, better job prospects, improved health, and more fulfilling lives, which result in a more resilient economy and stronger connections both within and between communities (Canadian Council on Learning (CCL), 2010a). The CLI combines 17 indicators covering four domains. A high value not only represents the state of learning and means that a region or community has the learning conditions needed to succeed economically and socially. Only three divisions (terciles rather than quintiles) are used here because there are only eight Economic Development Regions mapped, but data for more than 4,500 cities, towns, and rural communities in Canada are available (CCL, 2010b).

Economic Development Region	Overall CLI value	Learning to know	Learning to do	Learning to live together	Learning to be
1 Vancouver Island and Coast	82	5.6	6.2	5.1	6.3
5 Cariboo	79	4.8	6.4	5.1	5.6
3 Thompson-Okanagan	78	5.2	5.9	5.1	5.6
2 Lower Mainland-Southwest	76	6.3	6.1	4.6	5.1
4 Kootenay	75	5.0	6.3	3.2	5.4
7 Nechako	70	4.7	4.6	4.0	5.0
6 North Coast	70	4.8	4.4	3.9	5.1
8 Northeast	70	4.7	4.4	4.9	5.0
British Columbia	**77**	**5.9**	**6.1**	**4.7**	**5.4**

Overall CLI value

For BC as a whole, the CLI value was 77 (out of a possible 100) for 2009. This compares with a value of 68 for Canada as a whole, and BC was second only to Alberta among provinces. Values ranged from a high of 82 for Vancouver Island and Coast, to a low of 70 for each of the three northern regions. All regions showed a reduction from values recorded for 2007 and 2008, although all but the three northern regions had higher values than recorded in 2006. Among regions across Canada, Calgary had the highest value (88), while Notre Dame - Central Bonavista Bay in Newfoundland and Labrador had the lowest (51).

Learning to know

Five indicators make up this domain: access to learning institutions; university attainment; post-secondary participation; high school drop out rate; and youth literacy skills. BC had a value of 5.9 in 2009, and has remained close to this value since 2006. It has consistently had the highest value of any province, and compared with a value of 5 for Canada in 2009. Within BC, for 2009, the Lower Mainland-Southwest region had the highest value (6.3, which was also the highest value of any region within Canada), while Nechako and Northeast had the lowest value (both 4.7). Across Canada, the Northern region in Saskatchewan had the lowest value (2.4).

Learning to do

Three indicators make up this domain: availability of workplace training; participation in job-related training; and access to vocational training. BC had a value of 6.1 in 2009, one of only three provinces with a lower value than in 2006. Canada's value for 2009 was 5.9, while Alberta (6.8) had the highest value of all provinces. Within BC, the Cariboo region had the highest value (6.4), while North Coast and Northeast had the lowest (both 4.4). Kootenay was the only region to show an increase in value between 2006 (6.0) and 2009 (6.3). Across Canada, Lethbridge - Medicine Hat in Alberta had the highest value (7.4), and Gaspesie - Iles de la Madeleine in Quebec had the lowest (2.2).

Learning to live together

This domain has four indicators: access to community institutions; volunteering; participation in social clubs and organizations; and learning from other cultures. BC had a value of 4.7 in 2009, the same value as for Canada as a whole. While BC's value was lower than the other three western provinces and Ontario, it was one of only two provinces with a higher value in 2009 than in 2006. Within BC, Vancouver Island and Coast, Thompson-Okanagan, and Cariboo all had the highest value (5.1), while Kootenay had the lowest value (3.2). Across Canada, Regina - Moose Mountain in Saskatchewan had the highest value (6.3), while Nord du Quebec and Gaspesie - Iles de la Madeleine in Quebec had the lowest (both 2.2).

Learning to be

Five indicators make up this domain: exposure to media; learning through culture; learning through sports; broadband internet access; and access to cultural resources. BC, with a value of 5.4, was second only to Alberta (6.0) among provinces in 2009. Canada as a whole had a value of 5.0. BC was one of four provinces that had a higher value in 2009 than in 2006. Within BC, Vancouver Island and Coast had the highest value (6.3) in 2009, while Nechako and Northeast had the lowest (both 5.0). All regions in BC had a higher value in 2009 than in 2006. Across Canada, Calgary (7.3) had the highest value in 2009, and Notre Dame - Central Bonavista Bay (1.5) in Newfoundland and Labrador had the lowest.

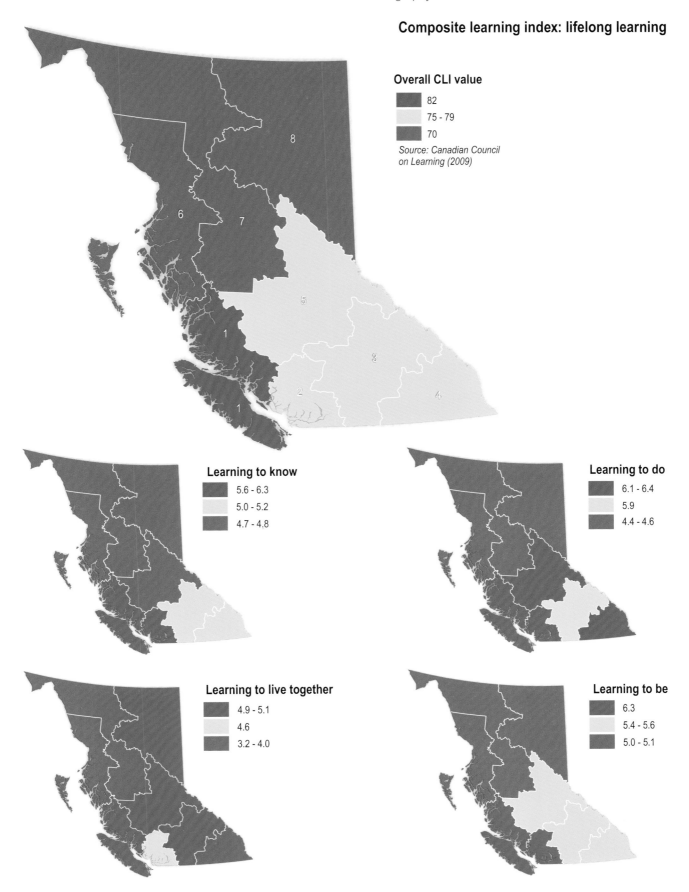

Composite learning index: lifelong learning

Overall CLI value

- 82
- 75 - 79
- 70

Source: Canadian Council on Learning (2009)

Learning to know

- 5.6 - 6.3
- 5.0 - 5.2
- 4.7 - 4.8

Learning to do

- 6.1 - 6.4
- 5.9
- 4.4 - 4.6

Learning to live together

- 4.9 - 5.1
- 4.6
- 3.2 - 4.0

Learning to be

- 6.3
- 5.4 - 5.6
- 5.0 - 5.1

Adult library programs

Public libraries offer information services and provide users with the support to find, evaluate, and use the information needed to pursue interests and achieve goals (Ministry of Community, Aboriginal and Women's Services, 2004).

They provide functions which:

- promote literacy and an enjoyment of reading;

- encourage a love of lifelong learning;

- support democratic values through free access to information for everyone;

- provide resources and programs that enhance the lives of children and families;

- support the local and provincial economy by providing information on jobs, skills, and markets;

- support local culture and leisure by partnering with arts and recreation organizations;

- reflect the personalities of their communities through local culture and heritage collections;

- serve as community meeting places; and

- offer an array of services including those for children and seniors, job-seekers and retirees, new Canadians, and individuals with special needs (Ministry of Community, Aboriginal and Women's Services, 2004, Ministry of Education, 2010d).

BC had over 240 separate public library service outlets in 2008 (Ministry of Education, 2010d). There were 71 locally appointed library boards consisting of 31 public library systems, each of which had a number of outlets (branches), and 40 small libraries run by library associations. In addition, there were six library federations that coordinated three regionally focused library services (Vancouver Island, Fraser Valley, and Okanagan) and two integrated systems (Cariboo and Thompson Nicola). These are shown in the table and map opposite.

Community	Programs/1000 pop. ages 19+	Community	Programs/1000 pop. ages 19+
1 Whistler (M)	82.44	37 Kaslo & District (A)	2.04
2 Houston (A)	30.98	38 Taylor (M)	2.00
3 Fernie (A)	19.57	39 Vanderhoof (A)	1.72
4 Hazelton District (A)	19.17	40 Pemberton & District (A)	1.71
5 Castlegar & District (A)	16.48	41 Prince Rupert (M)	1.54
6 West Vancouver (M)	12.68	42 North Vancouver City (M)	1.47
7 Tumbler Ridge (A)	11.13	43 Salmo (A)	1.46
8 Squamish (M)	10.72	44 North Vancouver District (M)	1.45
9 Hudson's Hope (A)	8.94	45 Burnaby (M)	1.36
10 Smithers (M)	8.50	46 Cranbrook (M)	1.35
11 Kitimat (A)	8.44	47 Fort St. John (A)	1.22
12 Nakusp (A)	7.41	48 Sechelt (A)	1.17
13 Pouce Coupe (M)	6.92	49 Beaver Valley (A)	1.04
14 Powell River (M)	6.63	50 Nelson (M)	0.92
15 Prince George (M)	5.89	51 Lillooet Area (A)	0.91
16 Greenwood (A)	5.83	52 Fort St. James (A)	0.71
17 Grand Forks & District (A)	5.06	53 Fort Nelson (A)	0.70
18 Surrey (M)	4.64	54 Kimberley (M)	0.62
19 Richmond (M)	4.45	55 Sparwood (A)	0.56
20 Port Moody (M)	4.29	56 Penticton (M)	0.55
21 Burns Lake (A)	3.96	57 Cariboo (I)	0.49
22 Midway (A)	3.66	58 Okanagan (R)	0.48
23 Chetwynd (A)	3.45	59 Vancouver Island (R)	0.48
24 Fraser Lake (A)	3.36	60 Pender Island (A)	0.42
25 Gibsons & District (A)	3.35	61 Salt Spring Island (A)	0.38
26 Fraser Valley (R)	3.22	62 Rossland (A)	0.35
27 Dawson Creek (M)	3.13	63 Creston (A)	0.30
28 McBride (A)	3.02	64 Mackenzie (M)	0.29
29 Coquitlam (M)	2.88	65 Greater Victoria (M)	0.11
30 Trail & District (M)	2.88	66 Alert Bay (A)	0.00
31 Vancouver (M)	2.70	67 Bowen Island (A)	0.00
32 Stewart (A)	2.50	68 Elkford (A)	0.00
33 Thompson-Nicola (I)	2.32	69 Granisle (A)	0.00
34 New Westminster (M)	2.17	70 Radium Hot Springs (M)	0.00
35 Terrace (A)	2.05	71 Valemount (A)	0.00
36 Invermere (M)	2.04	**British Columbia**	**2.77**

(A) Library Association (M) Municipal Library (R) Regional Library (I) Integrated Public Library System

In BC, there was a total of 9,128 adult programs provided in 2008 with an average of 2.77 programs per 1,000 adult residents (19 years of age and older). Programs ranged from literacy programs to cultural discussions to basic computer skills training, job searching sessions, and information on starting a business. These programs are important wellness assets, particularly for populations such as low-income or new immigrant residents, who may not have the resources to access these programs outside of the public library system.

Geographically, adult programming ranged from a high of more than 82 programs per 1,000 adult residents in Whistler to a low of only 0.11 programs per 1,000 residents in Greater Victoria. There were six communities that had no adult programming in 2008. Generally, there were more adult programs per capita outside of the lower mainland and southern part of Vancouver Island.

Adult library programs

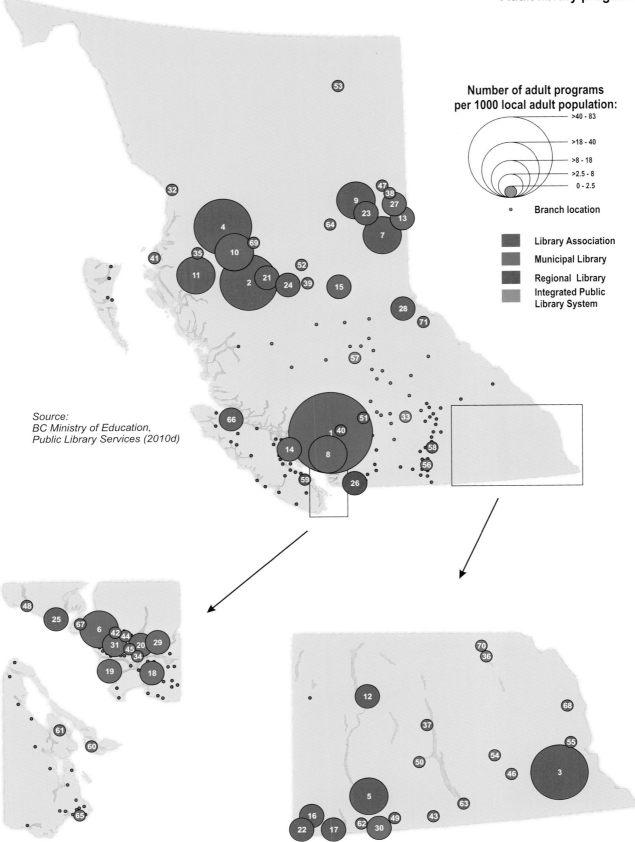

Number of adult programs
per 1000 local adult population:

>40 - 83
>18 - 40
>8 - 18
>2.5 - 8
0 - 2.5

○ Branch location

Library Association
Municipal Library
Regional Library
Integrated Public
Library System

Source:
BC Ministry of Education,
Public Library Services (2010d)

Child and youth library programs

As noted previously, public libraries are important public institutions because they offer information services that the public trust. While they offer important services for adults, they are just as important for the successful development of young children and youth.

In BC, there was a total of 31,104 child and youth programs provided throughout 2008, with an average of 31.10 programs per 1,000 child residents (aged 0-18 years). This average is much higher than that for adult programs, indicating the importance of libraries for children and youth. Child and youth programming ranged from a high of 284.63 programs per 1,000 children and youth in Greenwood to a low of 2.67 programs per 1,000 in Fort Nelson. Elkford was the only community in BC that recorded no child and youth programming in 2008.

Child and youth programming in public libraries can vary from literacy programs, such as reading clubs, to cultural programming, such as singing and arts and crafts. Such programming in public libraries is an important wellness asset. Early childhood education establishes a foundation that will impact a child's school readiness and high school completion because libraries become important resources for students in higher grades for information related to homework assignments. Successful development and high school graduation will ultimately contribute to future employment, income security, and health (BC Healthy Living Alliance, 2009).

Community	Programs/ 1,000 pop. age 0 to 18	Community	Programs/ 1,000 pop. age 0 to 18
1 Greenwood (A)	284.63	37 Cariboo (I)	31.24
2 Fernie (A)	244.59	38 Coquitlam (M)	30.00
3 Hudson's Hope (A)	218.92	39 Prince George (M)	28.15
4 Houston (A)	205.38	40 Salt Spring Island (A)	25.75
5 Whistler (M)	187.27	41 Fraser Lake (A)	25.68
6 Salmo (A)	141.94	42 Port Moody (M)	23.99
7 Rossland (A)	127.45	43 Tumbler Ridge (A)	21.54
8 Castlegar & District (A)	114.78	44 Fraser Valley (R)	19.68
9 Nelson (M)	88.89	45 Prince Rupert (M)	19.09
10 Nakusp (A)	71.41	46 Vanderhoof (A)	18.92
11 Vancouver (M)	71.34	47 Powell River (M)	18.22
12 Bowen Island (A)	67.36	48 Burnaby (M)	18.10
13 Beaver Valley (A)	66.07	49 Surrey (M)	16.14
14 Grand Forks & District (A)	62.66	50 Thompson-Nicola (I)	15.91
15 Squamish (M)	61.73	51 New Westminster (M)	15.91
16 Kitimat (A)	61.34	52 Pender Island (A)	15.50
17 Mackenzie (M)	54.76	53 Granisle (A)	15.48
18 North Vancouver City (M)	52.43	54 Pouce Coupe (M)	14.50
19 Alert Bay (A)	51.38	55 Vancouver Island (R)	14.36
20 West Vancouver (M)	50.93	56 Greater Victoria (M)	12.56
21 Dawson Creek (M)	50.10	57 Lillooet Area (A)	12.34
22 Fort St. James (A)	49.77	58 Kaslo & District (A)	10.96
23 Richmond (M)	48.17	59 McBride (A)	10.07
24 Burns Lake (A)	46.63	60 Taylor (M)	6.54
25 Penticton (M)	46.56	61 Pemberton & District (A)	6.48
26 Smithers (M)	45.72	62 Radium Hot Springs (M)	5.67
27 Fort St. John (A)	45.60	63 Sechelt (A)	5.56
28 Gibsons & District (A)	45.00	64 Sparwood (A)	5.56
29 Trail & District (M)	44.69	65 Creston (A)	4.98
30 Hazelton District (A)	42.25	66 Invermere (M)	4.51
31 Okanagan (R)	38.98	67 Valemount (A)	4.37
32 Midway (A)	38.52	68 Chetwynd (A)	3.79
33 Cranbrook (M)	37.05	69 Kimberley (M)	3.04
34 North Vancouver District (M)	36.25	70 Fort Nelson (A)	2.67
35 Terrace (A)	33.84	71 Elkford (A)	0.00
36 Stewart (A)	31.25	**British Columbia**	**31.10**

(A) Library Association (M) Municipal Library (R) Regional Library (I) Integrated Public Library System

Child and youth library programs

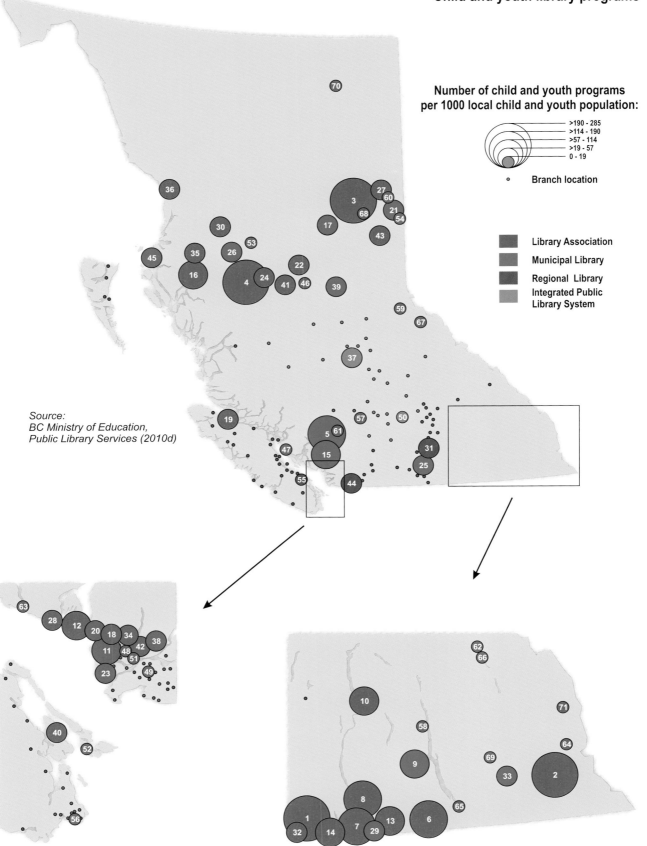

Number of child and youth programs
per 1000 local child and youth population:

>190 - 285
>114 - 190
>57 - 114
>19 - 57
0 - 19

• Branch location

Library Association
Municipal Library
Regional Library
Integrated Public Library System

Source:
BC Ministry of Education,
Public Library Services (2010d)

Employed in culture, arts or recreation

There has been an increasing recognition of the importance of culture and the arts to health and wellbeing (Ministry of Culture and Heritage, 2009). For example, the Gross National Happiness Index has cultural components as one of its indicators (The Centre for Bhutan Studies, 2008), as does the Canadian Index of Wellbeing (Institute of Wellbeing, 2009). Among Aboriginal peoples, culture is very important for wellness (National Collaborating Centre for Aboriginal Health, 2009; Kendall, 2009; Dockery, 2009; Ewing, 2010).

Arts, culture, and other creative industries have been major generators of economic activity over the past 15 years or so. They contribute in terms of job growth and wealth creation, through the creation, distribution, and retail of goods and services, as well as providing inputs to other parts of the economy. They form part of a package of attractions encouraging tourism, and create part of the necessary infrastructure of a modern region, helping to attract and retain investors, skilled workers, other creative people, and students. They also play an important role in innovation (Florida, 2003; Coish, 2004; Propris et al., 2009).

Within BC, a cultural mapping tool kit has been developed to help communities identify their strengths and resources (2010 LegaciesNow, nd). Obtaining good data on arts and culture within BC is difficult, other than at the provincial level.

The indicator presented in the table and map opposite analyses employment in the arts and culture based on the 2006 census and is a new indicator for the Atlas. A couple of cautions are required in looking at these data. First, with cutbacks in financial support for the arts and cultural groups by the BC government in 2009, employment figures and distribution may have changed. Second, we are using readily accessible geographical data from BC Stats (2010a) which combines professional occupations in arts and culture with technical, trades, and other highly skilled occupations in arts, culture, and recreation.

A report based on data from the 2006 census showed that BC had the largest percentage of employment in the arts of any province, and had the largest growth rate (58%) between 1991 and 2006 of any province. Among artists, 23% were musicians and singers, 17% were authors and writers, and 15% were visual artists. The broader cultural sector had more than 87,000 workers in the labour force in 2006 (Hill Strategies Research Inc, 2009).

Health Service Delivery Area	Employed in culture, arts and recreation (%)
32 Vancouver	6.5
33 North Shore/Coast Garibaldi	5.5
41 South Vancouver Island	4.2
12 Kootenay Boundary	3.7
31 Richmond	3.2
42 Central Vancouver Island	3.2
22 Fraser North	3.1
43 North Vancouver Island	2.6
13 Okanagan	2.5
11 East Kootenay	2.3
23 Fraser South	2.3
51 Northwest	2.3
14 Thompson Cariboo Shuswap	2.1
21 Fraser East	2.1
53 Northeast	1.5
52 Northern Interior	1.4
British Columbia	**3.3**

The table shows that 3.3% of the labour force was in arts and culture. There were major differences throughout the province. Vancouver had 6.5% of its labour force in arts and culture, followed by North Shore/Coast Garibaldi (5.5%). This compared with only 1.4% in Northern Interior and 1.5% in Northeast.

Geographically, higher numbers in arts and culture occupations were found in parts of the lower mainland and the southern half of Vancouver Island. In addition, Kootenay Boundary (3.7%) in the southeast interior was a geographical positive outlier. Lower levels of arts and culture employment were found throughout much of the north and central interior (Thompson Shuswap Cariboo) and Fraser East. Based on the 2001 census, an analysis of employment in culture-related occupations in Canada's metropolitan areas showed that Victoria and Vancouver were the two highest ranked in the country (Coish, 2004).

Employed in culture, arts or recreation

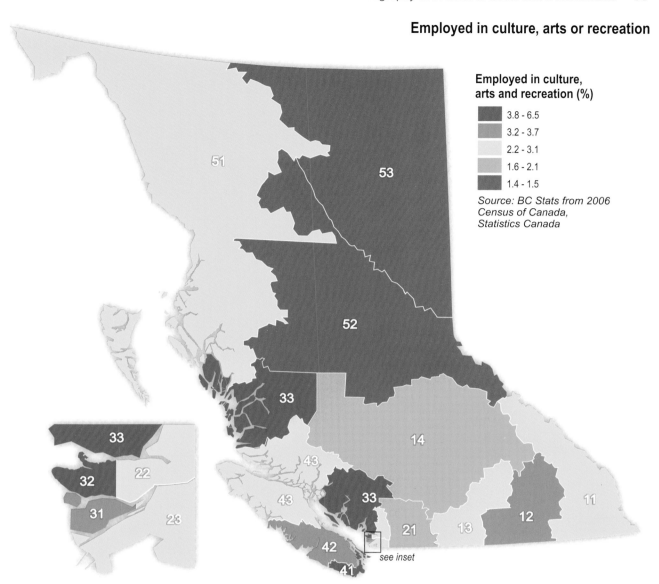

Employed in culture,
arts and recreation (%)

- 3.8 - 6.5
- 3.2 - 3.7
- 2.2 - 3.1
- 1.6 - 2.1
- 1.4 - 1.5

*Source: BC Stats from 2006
Census of Canada,
Statistics Canada*

see inset

Students learning about art at school

As noted earlier, art and culture are important wellness assets. While schools focus on academic subjects, learning about the arts is also important and can help improve learning in all subjects (Dunleavy & Dunning, 2009). For the 2005/6 Student Satisfaction Survey, the Ministry of Education introduced the question: *"At school, are you learning about art?"* This is a new indicator for the *Atlas*, and the table and maps presented here analyse responses from students for 2008/9 who answered positively by indicating *"all of the time"* or *"many times."*

Grades 3/4

An average of 61.72% of students indicated that they were learning about art in school in 2008/9. There were major geographical difference: 82.98% of students in Arrow Lakes, but only 38.96% of students in Gulf Islands felt they were learning about art *"all of the time"* or *"many times."* Geographical clusters worthy of note include higher positive responses evident in the southern and central interior (with the exception of Central Okanagan), while much of the southern half of Vancouver Island and the lower mainland had lower than average positive responses.

Grade 7

Fewer than half (49.65%) of all grade 7 students in BC answered positively to learning about art in school. As with grades 3/4 students, there was a wide variation between school districts, with 64.71% in Kootenay-Columbia but only 20.43% in Gulf Islands answering positively. Most of Vancouver Island, the extreme north, and areas surrounding the core of the lower mainland, along with outliers such as Rocky Mountain, and parts of the Okanagan had low values. Higher values were found in the lower mainland and much of the interior part of the province.

Grade 10

Only about one-fifth (22.22%) of grade 10 students indicated that they were learning about art at school. This ranged from 43.01% in Sunshine Coast to 6.67% in the tiny northwestern Stikine school district. Lower values occurred in parts of the central interior, and in much of Vancouver Island and the eastern lower mainland school districts. Higher values tended to be clustered in the northeast and central southeastern parts of the province.

School District	All students grades 3/4 (%)	All students grade 7 (%)	All students grade 10 (%)
10 Arrow Lakes	82.98	48.84	34.43
51 Boundary	79.82	53.40	31.72
84 Vancouver Island West	77.78	45.83	25.00
52 Prince Rupert	76.07	58.02	31.05
6 Rocky Mountain	73.45	39.16	22.16
27 Cariboo-Chilcotin	71.56	53.64	24.16
73 Kamloops/Thompson	71.10	57.95	15.59
20 Kootenay-Columbia	70.94	64.71	26.96
22 Vernon	69.98	52.68	20.67
67 Okanagan Skaha	69.69	48.64	23.92
58 Nicola-Similkameen	69.23	57.14	23.75
60 Peace River North	68.03	59.63	28.43
83 North Okanagan-Shuswap	67.81	23.03	24.08
50 Haida Gwaii/Queen Charlotte	66.67	55.36	41.03
37 Delta	66.63	55.44	24.69
53 Okanagan Similkameen	66.47	37.84	26.45
78 Fraser-Cascade	66.18	43.70	28.83
41 Burnaby	66.10	61.66	22.92
40 New Westminster	65.10	34.19	15.22
28 Quesnel	64.71	52.04	16.44
87 Stikine	64.71	30.00	6.67
79 Cowichan Valley	64.33	37.97	21.97
45 West Vancouver	63.35	60.71	25.87
57 Prince George	63.29	46.50	19.05
85 Vancouver Island North	63.16	54.46	19.47
8 Kootenay Lake	63.14	49.37	31.74
91 Nechako Lakes	63.07	61.38	21.03
42 Maple Ridge-Pitt Meadows	62.53	49.66	16.65
19 Revelstoke	62.30	54.35	30.43
36 Surrey	61.79	53.20	19.45
35 Langley	61.69	41.59	22.42
44 North Vancouver	61.41	50.19	22.91
5 Southeast Kootenay	61.22	58.60	23.29
72 Campbell River	61.05	29.18	17.54
59 Peace River South	60.81	56.02	31.20
47 Powell River	60.71	47.22	18.87
54 Bulkley Valley	60.67	45.60	26.82
39 Vancouver	60.36	62.46	24.70
71 Comox Valley	60.04	46.87	25.21
46 Sunshine Coast	59.80	38.40	43.01
68 Nanaimo-Ladysmith	59.79	46.50	19.82
43 Coquitlam	59.57	45.49	20.93
69 Qualicum	59.57	35.37	14.57
74 Gold Trail	59.34	48.94	31.00
75 Mission	59.01	49.66	20.77
48 Howe Sound	58.30	41.28	19.01
23 Central Okanagan	57.95	40.68	20.84
38 Richmond	57.18	54.06	28.40
33 Chilliwack	56.58	39.72	21.73
82 Coast Mountains	56.55	51.65	23.21
70 Alberni	56.42	50.87	15.35
62 Sooke	55.77	44.15	19.67
34 Abbotsford	55.68	49.21	20.30
61 Greater Victoria	54.75	42.82	22.25
81 Fort Nelson	54.10	38.89	36.54
63 Saanich	52.96	24.23	15.82
49 Central Coast	43.75	53.85	33.33
64 Gulf Islands	38.96	20.43	25.00
92 Nisga'a	Msk	46.15	23.08
British Columbia	**61.72**	**49.65**	**22.22**

Msk: Data masked for privacy

Students learning about art at school

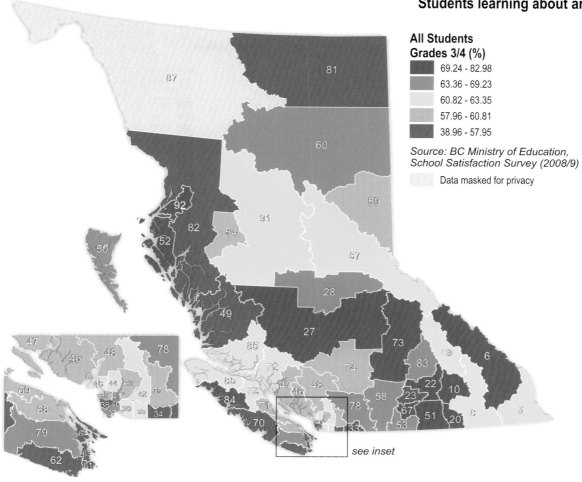

**All Students
Grades 3/4 (%)**

- 69.24 - 82.98
- 63.36 - 69.23
- 60.82 - 63.35
- 57.96 - 60.81
- 38.96 - 57.95

*Source: BC Ministry of Education,
School Satisfaction Survey (2008/9)*

Data masked for privacy

see inset

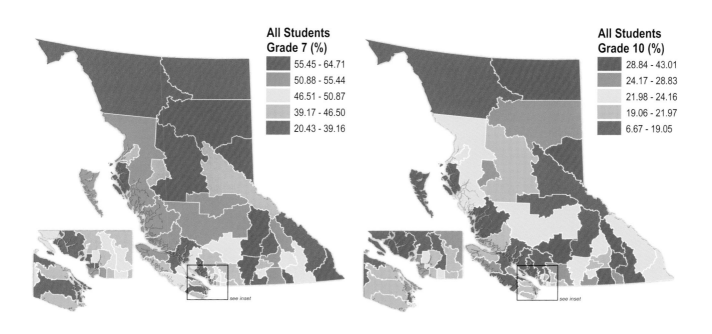

**All Students
Grade 7 (%)**

- 55.45 - 64.71
- 50.88 - 55.44
- 46.51 - 50.87
- 39.17 - 46.50
- 20.43 - 39.16

see inset

**All Students
Grade 10 (%)**

- 28.84 - 43.01
- 24.17 - 28.83
- 21.98 - 24.16
- 19.06 - 21.97
- 6.67 - 19.05

see inset

Students learning about music at school

There is evidence that listening to music enhances spatial skills. The arts can help students learn more effectively and students benefit by becoming more motivated and engaged and develop stronger skills in reading, writing and mathematics (Canadian Council on Learning, 2010c). The Student Satisfaction Survey asked, *"At school, are you learning about music?"* This is a new wellness indicator for the Atlas and the table and maps analyse responses from students for 2008/9 who answered positively by indicating *"all of the time"* or *"many times."*

Grades 3/4

More than six in every ten (62.86%) grades 3/4 students indicated that they were learning about music *"all of the time"* or *"many times."* There was a 70 percentage point difference among school districts, including major geographical variations throughout the province. Cowichan Valley (84.12%) and Stikine (12.50%) had the highest and lowest values, respectively. Geographically, much of the northern two-thirds of the province (with a few exceptions) had lower than average values, along with the northern part of Vancouver Island, and Revelstoke and Arrow Lakes which were outliers in the southeast. Much of the southeastern part of the province was above average, along with the central part of Vancouver Island and a couple of school districts in the lower mainland.

Grade 7

Only 47.26% of students in grade 7 responded positively to the music question. Responses ranged from 79.35% in Revelstoke and 70.36% in Burnaby, to zero in the tiny Stikine school district, and 7.69% in both Haida Gwaii and Central Coast. Again, with a couple of exceptions, much of the northern two-thirds of the province had lower than average values, along with most of Vancouver Island and eastern parts of the lower mainland. Higher than average values were clustered in the southeast of the province and parts of the lower mainland, with outliers in Comox Valley on Vancouver Island and Bulkley Valley in the north.

Grade 10

Less than one-fifth (18.13%) of grade 10 students answered positively. The highest value occurred in Nisga'a (30.77%), compared with zero in Central Coast and 5.56% in Quesnel. Lower values were again found in much of the northern two-thirds of the province, with the exception of a cluster in the north coastal region, and with one or two exceptions on much of Vancouver Island. While there were several school districts in the southeast

School District	All students grades 3/4 (%)	All students grade 7 (%)	All students grade 10 (%)
79 Cowichan Valley	84.12	38.43	10.49
70 Alberni	81.08	48.79	15.02
41 Burnaby	80.53	70.36	18.95
72 Campbell River	79.83	31.27	15.12
83 North Okanagan-Shuswap	79.26	49.58	27.98
69 Qualicum	78.29	23.39	19.06
22 Vernon	78.25	61.74	13.18
44 North Vancouver	77.89	48.79	23.20
6 Rocky Mountain	76.79	62.05	19.49
53 Okanagan Similkameen	75.76	48.62	11.84
71 Comox Valley	75.45	67.38	17.53
47 Powell River	74.11	57.75	18.87
68 Nanaimo-Ladysmith	73.94	53.16	18.14
36 Surrey	73.76	48.17	17.79
28 Quesnel	72.43	58.23	5.56
45 West Vancouver	72.37	59.51	15.76
35 Langley	71.37	53.31	19.60
40 New Westminster	70.57	59.54	22.28
8 Kootenay Lake	69.82	51.42	12.29
20 Kootenay-Columbia	69.81	67.33	12.07
54 Bulkley Valley	68.00	66.30	26.52
5 Southeast Kootenay	67.84	54.09	19.45
51 Boundary	66.67	59.41	23.97
61 Greater Victoria	66.64	44.84	21.05
33 Chilliwack	64.89	38.43	28.37
23 Central Okanagan	61.53	42.92	20.02
82 Coast Mountains	61.29	41.26	19.42
48 Howe Sound	60.89	48.99	19.59
43 Coquitlam	60.65	48.92	20.39
73 Kamloops/Thompson	60.00	53.27	13.97
75 Mission	59.55	37.13	18.13
67 Okanagan Skaha	59.38	40.42	18.95
46 Sunshine Coast	58.54	46.01	9.24
39 Vancouver	57.86	53.96	23.33
78 Fraser-Cascade	57.04	50.75	27.68
57 Prince George	55.43	28.67	13.72
58 Nicola-Similkameen	54.44	48.68	9.49
38 Richmond	52.59	64.42	20.26
81 Fort Nelson	52.46	18.57	15.38
91 Nechako Lakes	52.16	29.47	7.46
64 Gulf Islands	50.65	46.24	12.93
62 Sooke	46.81	38.65	12.80
27 Cariboo-Chilcotin	44.85	29.38	17.11
42 Maple Ridge-Pitt Meadows	42.87	23.69	16.53
74 Gold Trail	42.86	30.43	7.07
37 Delta	41.39	36.18	17.55
63 Saanich	39.57	23.68	16.26
19 Revelstoke	38.71	79.35	29.41
84 Vancouver Island West	38.46	36.00	18.18
85 Vancouver Island North	37.89	29.46	8.04
52 Prince Rupert	35.96	24.81	17.37
34 Abbotsford	35.30	38.92	14.29
49 Central Coast	31.25	7.69	0.00
59 Peace River South	30.36	44.15	10.12
60 Peace River North	22.47	13.60	7.77
10 Arrow Lakes	21.28	60.47	25.42
50 Haida Gwaii/Queen Charlotte	19.44	7.69	20.00
87 Stikine	12.50	0.00	13.33
92 Nisga'a	Msk	46.15	30.77
British Columbia	**62.86**	**47.26**	**18.13**

Msk: Data masked for privacy

with relatively high values (e.g., Arrow Lakes), there were also several with low values (e.g., Kootenay-Columbia). Vancouver and North Vancouver in the lower mainland also had relatively high values.

Students learning about music at school

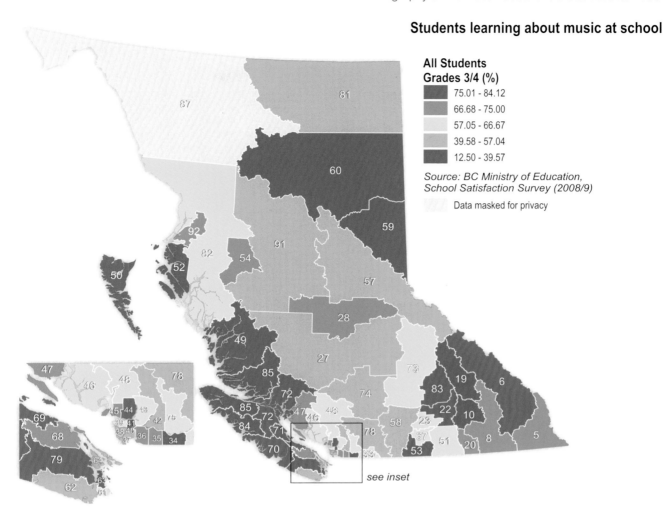

**All Students
Grades 3/4 (%)**

- 75.01 - 84.12
- 66.68 - 75.00
- 57.05 - 66.67
- 39.58 - 57.04
- 12.50 - 39.57

*Source: BC Ministry of Education,
School Satisfaction Survey (2008/9)*

Data masked for privacy

see inset

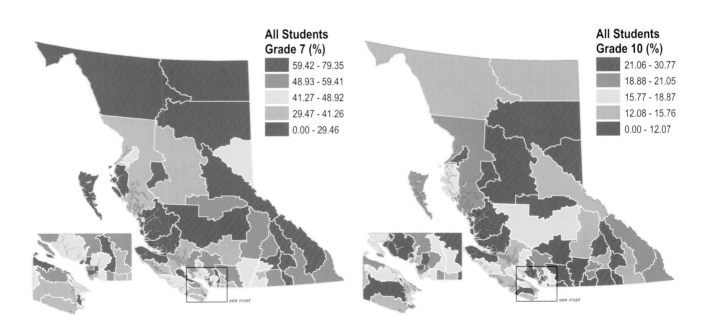

**All Students
Grade 7 (%)**

- 59.42 - 79.35
- 48.93 - 59.41
- 41.27 - 48.92
- 29.47 - 41.26
- 0.00 - 29.46

see inset

**All Students
Grade 10 (%)**

- 21.06 - 30.77
- 18.88 - 21.05
- 15.77 - 18.87
- 12.08 - 15.76
- 0.00 - 12.07

see inset

Library volunteers

Volunteering is an important indicator of civic engagement and caring about community. It is increasingly viewed as an important wellness asset, not only for the individuals involved, but also for their communities.

A report from the Corporation for National and Community Service indicated that "research has established a strong relationship between volunteering and health: those who volunteer have lower mortality rates, greater functional ability, and lower rates of depression later in life than those who do not volunteer" (Grimm et al., p. 1). Volunteering can also increase social cohesion and employment opportunities (Wilson & Musick, 1999).

There are very limited data at this time on the geography of volunteerism in BC, but one source where data are routinely collected and reported is for library services. Volunteers can be integral to the operation of public libraries, particularly in smaller communities where funding for libraries may be more stretched or limited. Furthermore, recent funding cutbacks to libraries by the provincial government have increased the need for volunteerism if services are to be maintained.

Community	Volunteers/ 1000 pop. ages 19+	Community	Volunteers/ 1000 pop. ages 19+
1 Pender Island (A)	29.43	37 Tumbler Ridge (A)	0.80
2 Midway (A)	22.19	38 Kitimat (A)	0.75
3 Salt Spring Island (A)	14.52	39 Invermere (M)	0.74
4 Radium Hot Springs (M)	9.94	40 Coquitlam (M)	0.69
5 Burns Lake (A)	9.90	41 Vanderhoof (A)	0.66
6 Greenwood (A)	9.89	42 New Westminster (M)	0.64
7 Bowen Island (A)	9.57	43 Cranbrook (M)	0.63
8 Fraser Lake (A)	8.12	44 Powell River (M)	0.59
9 Houston (A)	7.50	45 McBride (A)	0.55
10 Prince George (M)	7.03	46 Fort St. James (A)	0.49
11 Taylor (M)	6.85	47 Cariboo (I)	0.43
12 Kaslo & District (A)	6.60	48 Surrey (M)	0.25
13 Nakusp (A)	5.15	49 Fort St. John (A)	0.19
14 Hazelton District (A)	5.05	50 Penticton (M)	0.15
15 Lillooet Area (A)	4.84	51 North Vancouver District (M)	0.12
16 Salmo (A)	4.46	52 Greater Victoria (M)	0.10
17 Creston (A)	3.46	53 Terrace (A)	0.05
18 Castlegar & District (A)	3.00	54 Burnaby (M)	0.00
19 Gibsons & District (A)	2.97	55 Dawson Creek (M)	0.00
20 Rossland (A)	2.64	56 Elkford (A)	0.00
21 Fernie (A)	2.61	57 Fort Nelson (A)	0.00
22 Granisle (A)	2.54	58 Fraser Valley (R)	0.00
23 Smithers (M)	2.19	59 Hudson's Hope (A)	0.00
24 Pemberton & District (A)	2.13	60 Mackenzie (M)	0.00
25 Sechelt (A)	1.99	61 Port Moody (M)	0.00
26 Chetwynd (A)	1.98	62 Pouce Coupe (M)	0.00
27 Beaver Valley (A)	1.94	63 Prince Rupert (M)	0.00
28 Stewart (A)	1.89	64 Richmond (M)	0.00
29 Grand Forks & District (A)	1.68	65 Trail & District (M)	0.00
30 Kimberley (M)	1.44	66 Valemount (A)	0.00
31 Nelson (A)	1.21	67 Vancouver (M)	0.00
32 Squamish (M)	1.06	68 North Vancouver City (M)	N/A
33 Whistler (M)	0.98	69 Okanagan (R)	N/A
34 West Vancouver (M)	0.97	70 Thompson-Nicola (I)	N/A
35 Alert Bay (A)	0.96	71 Vancouver Island (R)	N/A
36 Sparwood (A)	0.83	**British Columbia**	**0.57***

N/A: No Data
* Excludes communities reporting no data.

(A) Library Association (M) Municipal Library (R) Regional Library (I) Integrated Public Library System

libraries by the provincial government have increased the need for volunteerism if services are to be maintained.

In BC, a total of 1,928 volunteers were working in public libraries throughout 2008, with an average of 0.57 volunteers per 1,000 residents. Volunteering in public libraries varied from a high of 29.43 volunteers per 1,000 residents on Pender Island to a low of 0.05 volunteers per 1,000 residents in Terrace. There were 14 communities that had no volunteers in 2008, and four that had no data on volunteerism in their service area. Generally, volunteering in libraries was more common in the less densely populated parts of the province, and less common in the lower mainland and southern part of Vancouver Island.

Library volunteers

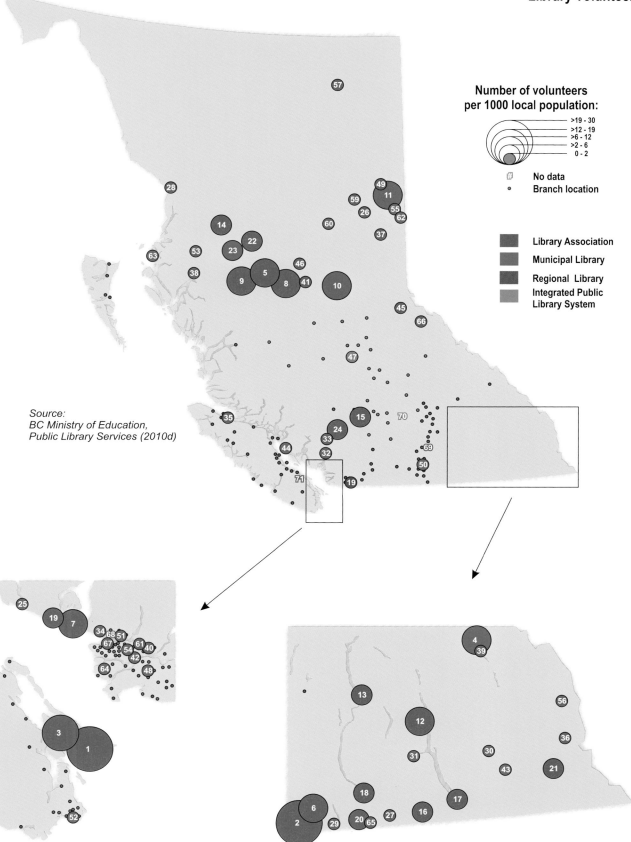

Number of volunteers
per 1000 local population:

>19 - 30
>12 - 19
>6 - 12
>2 - 6
0 - 2

No data
• Branch location

Library Association
Municipal Library
Regional Library
Integrated Public
Library System

Source:
BC Ministry of Education,
Public Library Services (2010d)

Youth who have volunteered in the past 12 months

As noted earlier, volunteering is an important wellness asset for both the individual and for the community at large. Those who volunteer receive non-financial rewards in knowing that they have helped to make a difference and contributed to something of value. It is also a useful measure of civic engagement.

The McCreary AHS IV asked students how often they had volunteered (helping others without pay) in the past 12 months. Examples given of volunteering included helping a charity, and unpaid babysitting or yard work. The table and maps opposite are based on the percentage of students who responded in the affirmative to this question.

Six out of every ten student respondents (61.92%) indicated that they had done some kind of volunteer work in the past 12 months, and at six percentage points, the difference among HSDAs across the province was quite small. Vancouver (66.78%) had the greatest percentage, while Fraser South/Fraser East (60.39%) had the lowest percentage who responded that they had volunteered in the past 12 months. Both Vancouver and Northwest (66.40%) were significantly higher than the provincial average, and no HSDA had significantly lower values than the average for all students.

There was a dramatic and significant difference between genders. Nearly seven in every ten (69.96%) female students responded that they had volunteered in the past 12 months, compared to only about half (53.08%) of male students, and this difference was consistent and significant for every individual HSDA. Furthermore, the lowest level of female student volunteer response among HSDAs, which occurred in Thompson Cariboo Shuswap (66.36%), was substantially higher than the highest volunteer response for male students, which was recorded for Northwest (58.59%).

Among HSDAs, the range between the highest and lowest HSDAs for male students was eight percentage points. While Northwest had the highest percentage who responded they had volunteered in the past 12 months, only Vancouver was significantly higher than the provincial average for male students. At the other extreme, Fraser North (49.87%), an adjoining neighbour of Vancouver, had the lowest percentage of male students who indicated that they had volunteered.

For female students, no HSDA was significantly different from the provincial overall average for females who indicated that they had volunteered in the past 12 months.

Health Service Delivery Area	All students (%)	Males (%)	Females (%)
32 Vancouver	66.78	58.30†	73.20
51 Northwest	66.40	58.59†	73.46
12 Kootenay Boundary	65.17	57.09†	72.36
33 North Shore/Coast Garibaldi	63.27	55.82†	70.41
13 Okanagan	63.11	53.57†	71.57
31 Richmond	61.73	52.46†	70.93
11 East Kootenay	61.63	52.95†	69.29
14 Thompson Cariboo Shuswap	61.00	55.12†	66.36
41 South Vancouver Island	60.95	52.80†	68.78
43 North Vancouver Island	60.93	52.76†	67.87
52 Northern Interior	60.79	53.45†	67.96
22 Fraser North	60.75	49.87†	71.29
42 Central Vancouver Island	60.41	50.64†	70.07
21 Fraser South/Fraser East	60.39	51.53†	68.19
53 Northeast	N/A	N/A	N/A
British Columbia	**61.92**	**53.08†**	**69.96**

† Male rate is significantly different than female rate.
Crosshatched HSDAs are significantly different than the provincial average.
N/A: No data

Geographically, the range between the highest and lowest HSDAs was seven percentage points: Northwest (73.46%) had the highest and Thompson Cariboo Shuswap (66.36%) the lowest percentage, respectively, of female students who responded they had volunteered.

Geographically, there were no clear regional patterns evident, and the major result for this indicator was the large difference between genders, which raises the question why male students are so different from female students when it comes to volunteer participation.

Youth who have volunteered in the past 12 months

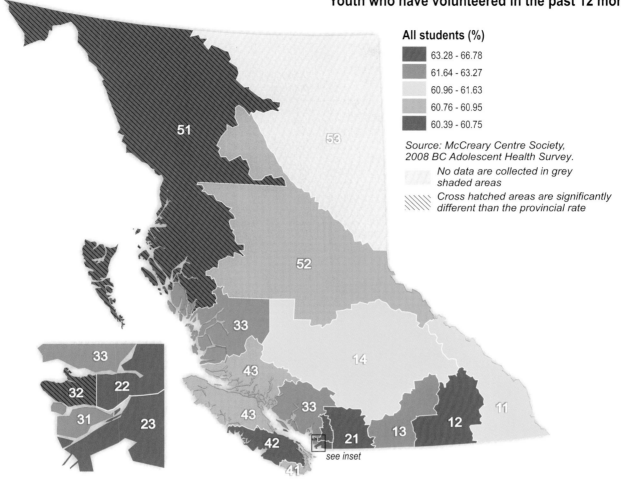

All students (%)

- 63.28 - 66.78
- 61.64 - 63.27
- 60.96 - 61.63
- 60.76 - 60.95
- 60.39 - 60.75

Source: McCreary Centre Society,
2008 BC Adolescent Health Survey.

No data are collected in grey
shaded areas

Cross hatched areas are significantly
different than the provincial rate

see inset

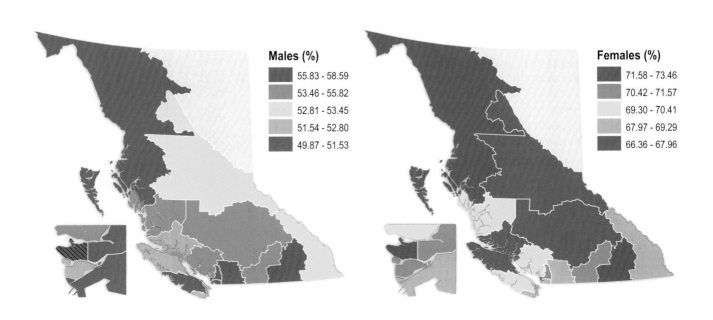

Males (%)

- 55.83 - 58.59
- 53.46 - 55.82
- 52.81 - 53.45
- 51.54 - 52.80
- 49.87 - 51.53

Females (%)

- 71.58 - 73.46
- 70.42 - 71.57
- 69.30 - 70.41
- 67.97 - 69.29
- 66.36 - 67.96

Students feeling safe at school

Safe schools are "ones in which members of the school community are free of the fear of harm, including potential threats from inside or outside the school" (Ministry of Education, 2008, p.11). A positive and welcoming school environment is one that also promotes learning (Kendall, 2008), and students who feel safe are more likely to learn and socialize than those who do not.

The Student Satisfaction Survey has asked about whether students feel safe and we provide analysis here for the youngest students. The older students are discussed on the next pages, based on the Adolescent Health Survey. Those grades 3/4 students (total, and males and females separately) who indicated that they felt safe "all the time" or "many times" in 2008/9 are analysed in the table and maps opposite.

All grades 3/4 students

On average, 83.69% of grades 3/4 students responded positively to feeling safe at school. Among school districts, responses ranged from a high of 92.86% in Central Coast to a low of 64.86% in Haida Gwaii, indicating important geographic differences. Higher than average values were clustered in the lower mainland, parts of the north coast (except Prince Rupert), and parts of the southern interior (Okanagan Skaha, Central Okanagan, and Rocky Mountain – all greater than 86%). Lower than average values of feeling safe were scattered around the province, and were mainly in rural school districts. A cluster of school districts with low values was found in the north and west part of Vancouver Island.

Male grades 3/4 students

At 81.78%, the average for male students was less than that for students as a whole. The school districts with the highest values were Arrow Lakes and Fraser Cascade (both above 89%), while at the other extreme, fewer than four in every ten male students (38.46%) felt safe in Haida Gwaii, followed by 61.54% in Vancouver Island North. Patterns were generally similar to those for total students, although males in Fort Nelson (70.00%) did comparatively more poorly than the student body as a whole.

Female grades 3/4 students

Provincially, female students on average (85.78%) were more likely to feel safe in school than male students. This result was also the case for all but eight of the individual school districts. While the average difference between male and female students was four percentage points, in some school districts the difference was much greater (40 percentage points for Haida Gwaii and 26 percentage points for Fort Nelson). While patterns were fairly similar

School District	All students grades 3/4 (%)	Males grades 3/4 (%)	Females grades 3/4 (%)
49 Central Coast	92.86	85.71	100.00
45 West Vancouver	87.59	84.74	90.41
67 Okanagan Skaha	86.68	85.87	87.63
38 Richmond	86.58	83.14	90.10
37 Delta	86.55	85.96	87.21
23 Central Okanagan	86.47	82.74	90.18
6 Rocky Mountain	86.39	82.93	89.53
78 Fraser-Cascade	86.03	89.39	84.06
39 Vancouver	85.92	85.46	86.65
34 Abbotsford	85.42	82.40	88.50
63 Saanich	85.37	80.68	90.38
36 Surrey	85.36	84.18	86.65
83 North Okanagan-Shuswap	85.15	84.83	86.10
41 Burnaby	85.00	83.22	86.79
44 North Vancouver	84.90	82.50	87.87
72 Campbell River	84.68	85.33	83.82
35 Langley	84.52	83.48	85.62
43 Coquitlam	84.49	83.48	85.89
51 Boundary	84.26	83.33	86.79
82 Coast Mountains	84.21	84.28	83.80
10 Arrow Lakes	84.09	89.47	80.00
61 Greater Victoria	83.76	82.78	85.17
69 Qualicum	83.75	79.86	88.55
42 Maple Ridge-Pitt Meadows	83.26	79.67	86.70
73 Kamloops/Thompson	83.24	79.72	86.94
53 Okanagan Similkameen	83.23	80.00	85.90
81 Fort Nelson	83.05	70.00	96.43
33 Chilliwack	82.52	79.11	85.75
62 Sooke	82.00	80.81	83.40
57 Prince George	81.99	Msk	Msk
79 Cowichan Valley	81.96	79.55	84.58
59 Peace River South	81.86	76.92	87.04
22 Vernon	81.59	78.35	85.33
40 New Westminster	81.44	81.68	81.19
54 Bulkley Valley	80.67	84.15	76.47
75 Mission	80.54	79.91	81.28
8 Kootenay Lake	80.51	76.81	83.94
27 Cariboo-Chilcotin	80.42	80.37	80.86
68 Nanaimo-Ladysmith	80.41	78.96	81.76
58 Nicola-Similkameen	80.23	75.79	85.19
20 Kootenay-Columbia	79.92	73.61	87.39
46 Sunshine Coast	79.90	78.76	80.90
91 Nechako Lakes	79.67	74.58	87.20
71 Comox Valley	79.24	78.66	80.42
48 Howe Sound	78.89	76.67	82.05
28 Quesnel	77.94	74.48	81.45
70 Alberni	77.38	73.33	80.56
74 Gold Trail	77.27	72.09	81.40
84 Vancouver Island West	76.92	76.92	76.92
47 Powell River	76.58	75.00	77.97
5 Southeast Kootenay	76.04	Msk	Msk
87 Stikine	75.00	66.67	80.00
60 Peace River North	74.06	75.00	72.60
64 Gulf Islands	73.33	69.05	78.13
52 Prince Rupert	73.33	66.67	77.03
19 Revelstoke	70.49	75.00	67.57
85 Vancouver Island North	70.21	Msk	Msk
50 Haida Gwaii/Queen Charlotte	64.86	38.46	79.17
92 Nisga'a	Msk	Msk	Msk
British Columbia	**83.69**	**81.78**	**85.78**

Msk: Data masked for privacy

to the other two cohorts, Arrow Lakes and Bulkley Valley had relatively lower percentages of female students who felt safe in school, while percentages in Fort Nelson, Kootenay-Columbia, and Nechako Lakes were relatively higher.

Students feeling safe at school

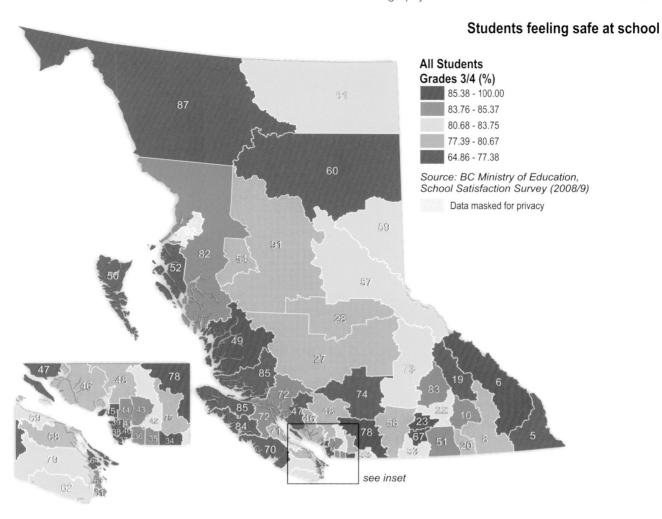

**All Students
Grades 3/4 (%)**

- 85.38 - 100.00
- 83.76 - 85.37
- 80.68 - 83.75
- 77.39 - 80.67
- 64.86 - 77.38

*Source: BC Ministry of Education,
School Satisfaction Survey (2008/9)*

Data masked for privacy

see inset

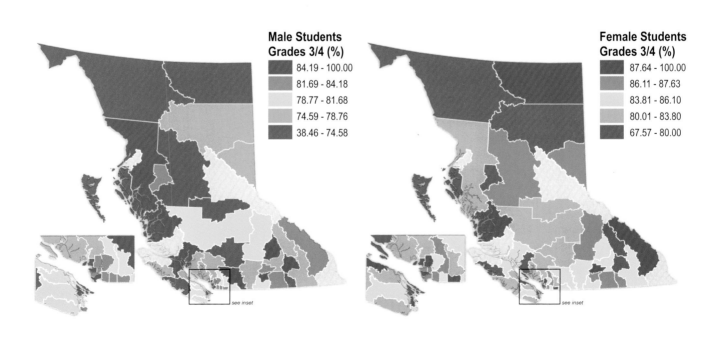

**Male Students
Grades 3/4 (%)**

- 84.19 - 100.00
- 81.69 - 84.18
- 78.77 - 81.68
- 74.59 - 78.76
- 38.46 - 74.58

see inset

**Female Students
Grades 3/4 (%)**

- 87.64 - 100.00
- 86.11 - 87.63
- 83.81 - 86.10
- 80.01 - 83.80
- 67.57 - 80.00

see inset

Youth who always feel safe at school

Students spend many hours a day at school. A school environment needs to be a safe environment if students are to flourish academically and socially. Students who are bullied or otherwise do not feel safe at school are less likely to want to go to school, may find it difficult to concentrate, and may skip school, thus undermining their ability to receive the best education they can. This, in turn, can create emotional problems, and hinder their future education, as well as employment prospects. As such, feeling safe at school is an important wellness asset for students.

The McCreary AHS IV asked students: *"How often do you feel safe at school. Always, often, sometimes, rarely, never?"* The results reported here include those students who responded "always" or "often."

Among BC student respondents, eight in every ten (81.43%) indicated that they always or often felt safe at school. The range among HSDAs went from a high of 87.39% for North Shore/Coast Garibaldi to 76.83% for East Kootenay, a spread of just over 10 percentage points. North Shore Coast Garibaldi and South Vancouver Island (84.41%) were both significantly higher than the provincial average, and East Kootenay was significantly lower than average.

Higher values occurred along the southernmost parts of the province (except for East Kootenay) and the southern half of Vancouver Island, while the lowest levels of those who had always or often felt safe at school occurred in the Northern HSDAs and adjoining central interior area, along with East Kootenay in the extreme south east of the province. In addition, students in both Vancouver and Richmond in the lower mainland had relatively low values in terms of having felt safe at school.

There were no significant differences between genders, either at the provincial level or for individual HSDAs. For male students, the range in values went from 85.92% for North Shore/Coast Garibaldi (significantly higher than the provincial average for males) to a low of 78.17% for Northwest, a range of 8 percentage points.

The range in values among HSDAs for female students who always or often felt safe was much higher than that for males, at 14 percentage points. Again, North Shore/Coast Garibaldi (88.77%) was significantly higher than the provincial average as was South Vancouver Island (85.20%), and East Kootenay, at 74.17%, was

Health Service Delivery Area	All students (%)	Males (%)	Females (%)
33 North Shore/Coast Garibaldi	87.39	85.92	88.77
41 South Vancouver Island	84.41	83.58	85.20
12 Kootenay Boundary	83.92	84.04	83.80
13 Okanagan	83.07	82.76	83.34
21 Fraser South/Fraser East	81.74	81.62	81.88
42 Central Vancouver Island	81.12	80.16	82.05
22 Fraser North	80.71	80.09	81.34
43 North Vancouver Island	79.84	79.63	80.05
31 Richmond	79.82	80.03	79.68
52 Northern Interior	79.69	81.94	77.51
32 Vancouver	79.31	81.12	78.19
51 Northwest	78.73	78.17	79.28
14 Thompson Cariboo Shuswap	78.69	78.19	79.35
11 East Kootenay	76.83	79.83	74.17
53 Northeast	N/A	N/A	N/A
British Columbia	**81.43**	**81.39**	**81.51**

† Male rate is significantly different than female rate.
Crosshatched HSDAs are significantly different than the provincial average.
N/A: No data.

significantly lower than the provincial average for female student respondents.

Geographically, patterns for male and female students separately were quite similar to those observed for the total student population.

Youth who always feel safe at school

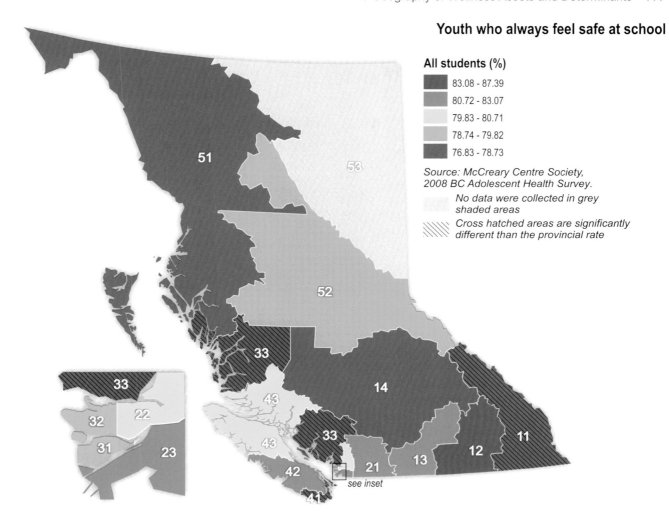

All students (%)

- 83.08 - 87.39
- 80.72 - 83.07
- 79.83 - 80.71
- 78.74 - 79.82
- 76.83 - 78.73

Source: McCreary Centre Society, 2008 BC Adolescent Health Survey.

No data were collected in grey shaded areas

Cross hatched areas are significantly different than the provincial rate

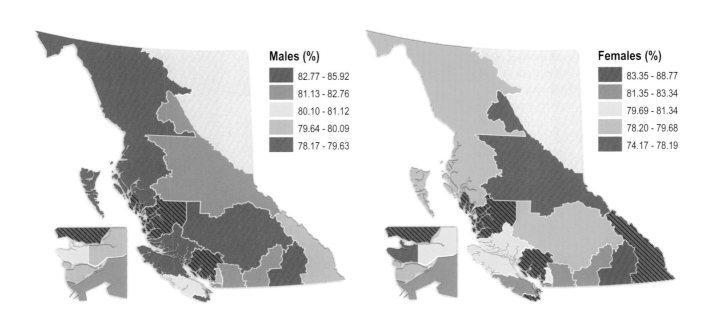

Males (%)

- 82.77 - 85.92
- 81.13 - 82.76
- 80.10 - 81.12
- 79.64 - 80.09
- 78.17 - 79.63

Females (%)

- 83.35 - 88.77
- 81.35 - 83.34
- 79.69 - 81.34
- 78.20 - 79.68
- 74.17 - 78.19

Students not bullied, teased, or picked on at school

An important component of a healthy school is one where students do not feel that they are bullied, teased, or otherwise harassed. Such bully-free environments support both positive academic learning, as well as positive social development among students (Kendall, 2008), both important wellness assets. The Student Satisfaction Survey asked whether students were bullied, teased, or picked on at school, and the results of those who answered that they were not bullied, teased, or picked on at school are shown in the table and maps opposite for 2008/9. This is a new indicator for the Atlas.

All students grade 7

Provincially, 77.92% of students responded negatively to the "bullying" question. There was a 40 percentage point difference among school districts: both Vancouver Island West and Revelstoke had values above 86%, while Central Coast had only 46.15%, and Fort Nelson had 57.97% of their grade 7 student respondents indicating that they were free of bullying or harassment at school. Geographically, the lowest values were clustered in the northeast and southeast of the province, with outliers along parts of coastal BC. Much of the lower mainland school districts had better than average values, as did parts of Vancouver Island, the northwest, and parts of the central eastern portion of the province.

All students grade 10

For BC as a whole, 81.75% were not bullied or picked on at school. There was a 20 percentage point difference among school districts. Nine in every ten students (90.54%) in Gulf Islands, compared with 69.23% in Central Coast, answered that they had not been bullied in 2008/9. Many of the lower mainland school districts had above average values, along with a cluster in the southern and eastern part of the province and parts of Vancouver Island. Otherwise, much of the remainder of the province had below average values for being bully-free, except for Quesnel in the central interior, Fort Nelson in the northeast, and Nisga'a in the northwest.

All students grade 12

The BC average for being bully-free among grade 12 students was 84.78%. Values ranged from a low of 70.00% in Fort Nelson in the northeast, to a high of 93.75% in Revelstoke. Geographically, there were two distinct clusters with above average values: the southeast of the province, except for Southeast Kootenay, and the

School District	All students grade 7 (%)	All students grade 10 (%)	All students grade 12 (%)
84 Vancouver Island West	86.96	81.82	82.35
19 Revelstoke	86.36	79.71	93.75
6 Rocky Mountain	83.44	75.77	90.73
78 Fraser-Cascade	82.44	78.76	85.57
41 Burnaby	81.90	82.98	84.84
38 Richmond	81.45	82.15	85.75
43 Coquitlam	80.72	82.97	85.54
45 West Vancouver	80.72	87.68	85.93
36 Surrey	80.59	83.46	83.42
63 Saanich	80.18	84.99	86.48
82 Coast Mountains	79.78	79.83	91.67
62 Sooke	79.42	76.63	80.88
37 Delta	79.38	83.88	86.18
72 Campbell River	79.35	80.41	86.27
46 Sunshine Coast	79.15	78.80	89.83
39 Vancouver	79.12	83.41	86.04
44 North Vancouver	78.84	82.70	86.69
42 Maple Ridge-Pitt Meadows	78.15	81.16	81.45
61 Greater Victoria	78.05	80.51	86.78
85 Vancouver Island North	77.98	75.89	78.48
48 Howe Sound	77.70	75.62	79.78
23 Central Okanagan	77.68	81.90	83.89
68 Nanaimo-Ladysmith	77.67	80.08	83.83
34 Abbotsford	77.12	81.20	81.96
20 Kootenay-Columbia	77.10	79.58	84.72
92 Nisga'a	76.92	88.46	Msk
52 Prince Rupert	76.92	75.81	77.64
73 Kamloops/Thompson	76.49	77.41	82.87
35 Langley	76.44	83.13	83.49
53 Okanagan Similkameen	76.37	77.07	85.48
57 Prince George	76.24	79.08	83.11
71 Comox Valley	76.04	81.61	86.59
27 Cariboo-Chilcotin	75.61	73.15	78.50
58 Nicola-Similkameen	75.54	77.36	84.96
69 Qualicum	75.35	81.33	85.65
67 Okanagan Skaha	75.26	80.75	86.82
64 Gulf Islands	75.00	90.54	87.21
79 Cowichan Valley	74.95	83.47	86.03
33 Chilliwack	74.70	83.87	79.74
83 North Okanagan-Shuswap	74.62	82.38	75.40
54 Bulkley Valley	74.30	81.56	84.87
75 Mission	74.25	84.10	91.73
70 Alberni	74.22	78.14	79.62
40 New Westminster	74.00	81.01	88.35
22 Vernon	73.33	79.90	89.66
28 Quesnel	73.23	84.14	87.23
87 Stikine	72.73	66.67	Msk
91 Nechako Lakes	72.03	78.51	87.31
50 Haida Gwaii/Queen Charlotte	71.70	75.00	78.95
8 Kootenay Lake	71.38	82.47	88.07
60 Peace River North	71.12	81.10	83.09
51 Boundary	71.00	83.10	77.22
47 Powell River	70.63	77.02	77.57
5 Southeast Kootenay	70.54	79.24	80.73
59 Peace River South	70.27	79.92	84.93
10 Arrow Lakes	69.77	85.25	88.89
74 Gold Trail	65.56	78.00	86.30
81 Fort Nelson	57.97	84.62	70.00
49 Central Coast	46.15	69.23	90.00
British Columbia	**77.92**	**81.75**	**84.78**

Msk: Data masked for privacy

north and central coastal area, except for Prince Rupert and Haida Gwaii. The lowest values were scattered around the province, including Vancouver Island.

Students not bullied, teased, or picked on at school

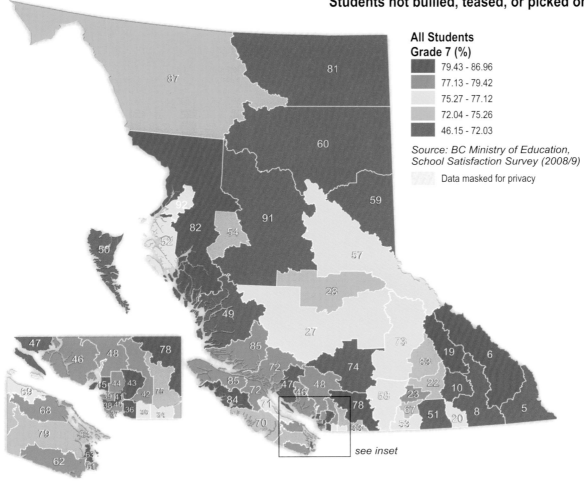

**All Students
Grade 7 (%)**

- 79.43 - 86.96
- 77.13 - 79.42
- 75.27 - 77.12
- 72.04 - 75.26
- 46.15 - 72.03

*Source: BC Ministry of Education,
School Satisfaction Survey (2008/9)*

Data masked for privacy

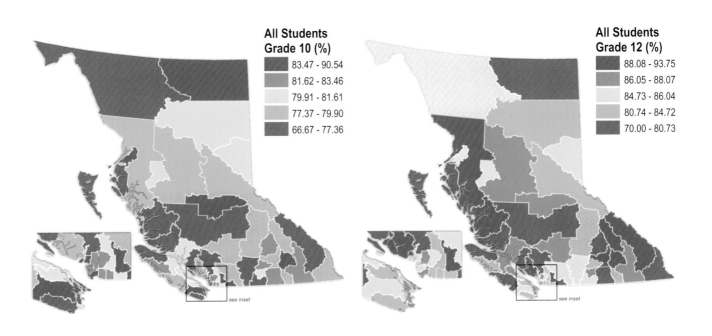

**All Students
Grade 10 (%)**

- 83.47 - 90.54
- 81.62 - 83.46
- 79.91 - 81.61
- 77.37 - 79.90
- 66.67 - 77.36

**All Students
Grade 12 (%)**

- 88.08 - 93.75
- 86.05 - 88.07
- 84.73 - 86.04
- 80.74 - 84.72
- 70.00 - 80.73

Crime rates

A measure of community safety includes crime rates. Communities with lower crime rates are often viewed as being healthy communities and citizens generally feel safer, an important community wellness indicator. Five key indicators of community safety are provided here, two of which are new to this edition of the Atlas: non-cannabis drug crime and motor vehicle theft. The three indicators included in the first Atlas have been updated to include more recent data. Each of the five indicators is based on averages of 3 years of statistics for the period 2006 to 2008, collected by the Ministry of Public Safety and Solicitor General (BC Stats, 2010a).

Health Service Delivery Area	Serious violent crime/ 1,000 pop.	Serious property crime/ 1,000 pop.	Change in total serious crime (%)	Non-cannabis crime/ 1,000 pop.	Motor vehicle theft/ 1,000 pop.
12 Kootenay Boundary	1.5	5.6	-25.44	1.6	2.5
11 East Kootenay	1.8	7.3	-23.77	1.7	3.3
31 Richmond	2.0	7.4	-27.65	2.4	3.5
33 North Shore/Coast Garibaldi	2.0	6.9	-23.00	1.7	2.5
41 South Vancouver Island	2.4	7.9	-0.64	1.8	3.3
42 Central Vancouver Island	2.4	10.7	-2.31	2.2	5.5
13 Okanagan	2.6	9.1	-19.34	2.7	7.2
21 Fraser East	3.5	13.6	-2.83	1.7	10.2
22 Fraser North	3.5	10.0	-18.17	1.4	6.7
43 North Vancouver Island	3.5	12.8	-26.28	3.1	4.0
23 Fraser South	4.1	10.1	-9.23	2.4	8.9
53 Northeast	4.1	9.7	-21.82	5.5	9.2
52 Northern Interior	5.4	11.2	-12.23	2.6	8.2
51 Northwest	5.8	15.2	-15.91	3.0	3.7
32 Vancouver	5.9	12.3	-16.13	4.8	5.1
14 Thompson Cariboo Shuswap	7.9	31.3	-10.79	6.8	26.8
British Columbia	**3.5**	**10.0**	**-13.63**	**2.5**	**6.1**

Serious violent crime

This indicator provides the 3 year average (2006 to 2008) rate of violent crime per 1,000 population. Serious violent crime includes: homicide, attempted murder, sexual and non-sexual assault resulting in bodily harm, robbery, and abduction. The rate in BC as a whole was 3.5 per 1,000 population, an increase of 12.0% from the 2003 to 2005 average. The highest rate (7.9 per 1,000 population) was found in Thompson Cariboo Shuswap, while the lowest rate (1.5 per 1,000 population) was recorded in Kootenay Boundary. Above average rates were found in the northern part of the province, the central interior, and parts of the lower mainland (Vancouver and Fraser South), while the lowest rates were found in the southeast of the province, the southern half of Vancouver Island, and North Shore/Coast Garibaldi. All but three HSDAs (Northeast, Richmond, and North Vancouver Island) had increases when compared to the 2003 to 2005 rate.

Serious property crime

The 3 year average for this indicator was 10.0 per 1,000 population for the province, a reduction of 20.1% from the average rate for 2003 to 2005. Rates varied from a low of 5.6 per 1,000 in Kootenay Boundary to a high of 31.3 per 1,000 for Thompson Cariboo Shuswap. Below average rates were found in the southeast quadrant of the province, as well as Richmond and North Shore/Coast Garibaldi in the lower mainland, and South Vancouver Island. Higher rates occurred in the north (other than Northeast), central interior, and Fraser East and Vancouver in the lower mainland. All HSDAs recorded decreases from the 2003 to 2005 average rate, with Richmond, Kootenay Boundary, Vancouver Island North,

and East Kootenay all recording rate reductions in excess of 30%.

Change in total serious crime

BC saw a reduction in total serious crime of 13.63% between 2003 to 2005 and 2006 to 2008. While every HSDA saw a rate reduction, the greatest reductions (in excess of 20%) were found in parts of the lower mainland (Richmond, North Shore/Coast Garibaldi), the southeast (East Kootenay, Kootenay Boundary), and Northeast and North Vancouver Island.

Non-cannabis drug crime

The rate for this category for the 2006 to 2008 period was 2.5 per 1,000 population. The highest rates (in excess of 5 per 1,000 population) occurred in Thompson Cariboo Shuswap and Northeast. The lowest rates were focused in the lower mainland (Fraser North, Fraser East, and North Shore/Coast Garibaldi), the southeast, and South Vancouver Island (all 1.8 per 1,000 or lower).

Motor vehicle theft

For the province as a whole, motor vehicle theft averaged 6.1 per 1,000 population for the period 2006 to 2008. By far the highest rate occurred in Thompson Cariboo Shuswap (26.8 per 1,000 population). Rates were also higher than average throughout much of the north (except Northwest) and the central and southern interior of the province. Much lower rates occurred in the south east, parts of the lower mainland, and South Vancouver Island, all 3.5 per 1,000 population or lower.

Crime rates

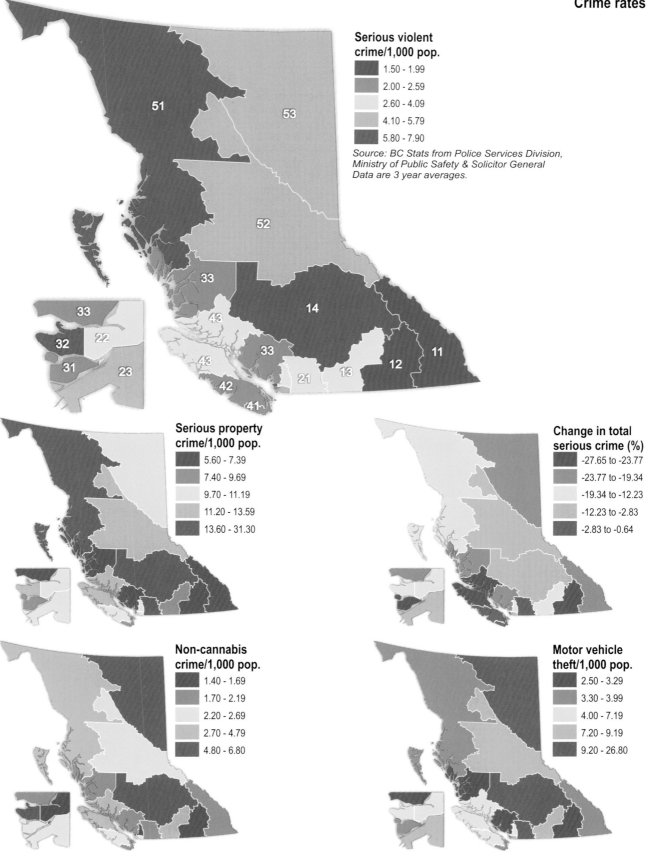

Serious violent crime/1,000 pop.

- 1.50 - 1.99
- 2.00 - 2.59
- 2.60 - 4.09
- 4.10 - 5.79
- 5.80 - 7.90

Source: BC Stats from Police Services Division, Ministry of Public Safety & Solicitor General Data are 3 year averages.

Serious property crime/1,000 pop.

- 5.60 - 7.39
- 7.40 - 9.69
- 9.70 - 11.19
- 11.20 - 13.59
- 13.60 - 31.30

Change in total serious crime (%)

- -27.65 to -23.77
- -23.77 to -19.34
- -19.34 to -12.23
- -12.23 to -2.83
- -2.83 to -0.64

Non-cannabis crime/1,000 pop.

- 1.40 - 1.69
- 1.70 - 2.19
- 2.20 - 2.69
- 2.70 - 4.79
- 4.80 - 6.80

Motor vehicle theft/1,000 pop.

- 2.50 - 3.29
- 3.30 - 3.99
- 4.00 - 7.19
- 7.20 - 9.19
- 9.20 - 26.80

Spirit squares

In 2006, the spirit squares initiative was one of three new programs announced to encourage British Columbians to live healthier lives by being more physically active, and to support the original goals of ActNow BC. The creation of the squares, while supporting ActNow BC initiatives, were also part of the celebrations related to the 150th anniversary of the founding of the Crown Colony of British Columbia. Key partners in this program included the Ministry of Community and Rural Development and the Ministry of Tourism, Culture and the Arts.

Funding was made available so that communities across the province could create or enhance existing outdoor public spaces to allow local community residents to gather, socialize, and share community pride and spirit. The concept was to help communities remain vibrant, connected, and sustainable, and ensure communities had a public space similar to traditional town squares or community commons. These spaces could host public celebrations and festivals to recognize a community's past, celebrate its future, and to provide a lasting legacy to celebrate a community's unique characteristics and culture. Such squares could help give towns and cities their identity and be recognized as *the* place to go to for community activities and gathering points. These squares would be an important community asset for socializing and meeting other citizens (Ministry of Community and Rural Development, 2008).

In total, up to $20 million was made available to undertake these projects, and costs were shared equally between the province and municipalities and regional districts, with a maximum provincial contribution of $500,000.

As the table and map opposite indicate, a total of 64 spirit squares were created: 29 in 2007, and 35 in 2008. The scope of projects varied substantially, and provincial grants ranged from $500,000 (18 communities) to $25,000 for Okanagan-Similkameen Regional District. Ten other communities received grants of less than $100,000.

Community	Community
1 Abbotsford	34 New Hazelton
2 Armstrong	35 New Westminster
3 Burnaby	36 North Vancouver (City)
4 Burns Lake	37 Okanagan-Similkameen
5 Campbell River	Regional District (Hedley)
6 Castlegar	38 Peachland
7 Chase	39 Penticton
8 Chetwynd	40 Pitt Meadows
9 Coquitlam	41 Port Alberni
10 Cranbrook	42 Powell River
11 Creston	43 Prince George
12 Cumberland	44 Prince Rupert
13 Delta	45 Princeton
14 Fort St. James	46 Qualicum Beach
15 Golden	47 Queen Charlotte
16 Harrison Hot Springs	48 Quesnel
17 Hope	49 Revelstoke
18 Houston	50 Richmond
19 Invermere	51 Salmon Arm
20 Kamloops	52 Sechelt
21 Kelowna	53 Sidney
22 Keremeos	54 Sooke
23 Ladysmith	55 Stewart
24 Lake Country	56 Summerland
25 Langley (City)	57 Surrey
26 Langley (District)	58 Terrace
27 Logan Lake	59 Trail
28 Lytton	60 Vernon
29 Mackenzie	61 Victoria
30 Maple Ridge	62 West Vancouver
31 Merritt	63 Westside
32 Mission	64 Williams Lake
33 Nanaimo (City)	

Spirit squares

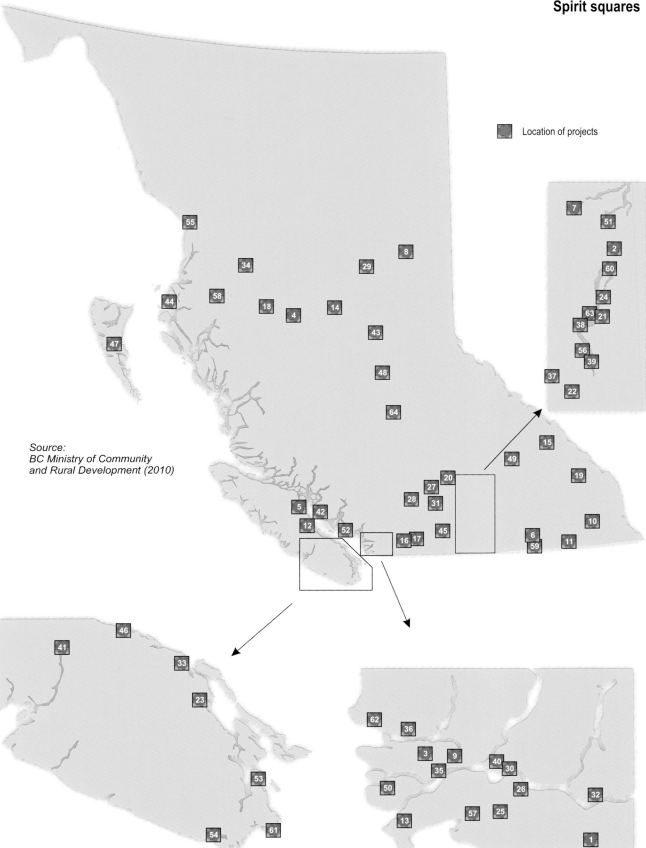

Location of projects

Source:
BC Ministry of Community
and Rural Development (2010)

Green cities awards

In 2006, the *LiveSmart BC Green Cities Award* was initiated. It recognized innovation and provided awards to local governments to help them achieve integrated community design and management, and increase urban densities that improved physical activity, energy conservation, and environmental benefits. The awards were to challenge local governments to create environmental and health and wellness improvements, and enable them to invest further in initiatives that resulted in greener and healthier communities.

The awards were administered by the Ministry of Community and Rural Development, with the support of several other provincial ministries, as well as ActNow BC.

The *Green Cities Awards* were distributed in 2007 and 2008 to local governments that were actively and effectively initiating change in the years preceding the awards. In all, there were 16 communities that received a *LiveSmart BC Green Cities Award* and 19 other finalists, as noted in the table and map opposite. Criteria for the winners included:

- Contribution toward community greenhouse gas emission reductions;

- Urban forests and new urban design to increase density and reduce urban sprawl;

- Reducing water use;

- Building seniors-friendly and disability-friendly communities; and

- Extent to which the community is advancing the ActNow BC principle of being more physically active.

Award winners included projects related to sustainable

community development, drinking water improvements and conservation, rainwater (storm water) management, wastewater treatment improvements, energy, and green buildings. Awards were provided in eight categories based on type of local government (Regional Districts) and population size.

2007	Category	Community
1	Regional District (Regional)	Nanaimo Regional District
2		Greater Vancouver Regional District
3	Regional District (Electoral Areas)	Capital Regional District - Area F - Saltspring Island
4		Regional District of Central Kootenay - Area D
5	Population of 1,500 - 5,000	Town of Oliver
6		Town of Gibsons
7		District of Houston
8	Population of 5,000 - 10,000	Resort Municipality of Whistler
9		Town of Ladysmith
10	Population of 10,000 - 25,000	City of Dawson Creek
11		District of Squamish
12		City of Fort St. John
13	Population of 25,000 - 100,000	City of North Vancouver
14		City of Kamloops
15		City of Maple Ridge
16	Population of 100,000+	City of Vancouver
17		City of Kelowna
2008		
18	Regional District (Regional)	Capital Regional District
19	Population less than 1,500	District of Taylor
20		Village of Pouce Coupe
21	Population of 1,500 - 5,000	City of Grand Forks
22		District of Chetwynd
23	Population of 5,000 - 10,000	Town of Smithers
24		District of Sechelt
25	Population of 10,000 - 25,000	City of Dawson Creek
26		City of White Rock
27		City of Langford
28	Population of 25,000 - 100,000	City of Prince George
29		City of Kamloops
30		City of North Vancouver
31	Population of 100,000+	City of Surrey
32		City of Kelowna
33	Partnership Award	City of Victoria and Dockside Green Ltd
34		District of Sechelt and the Sunshine Coast Association for Community Living

Green cities awards

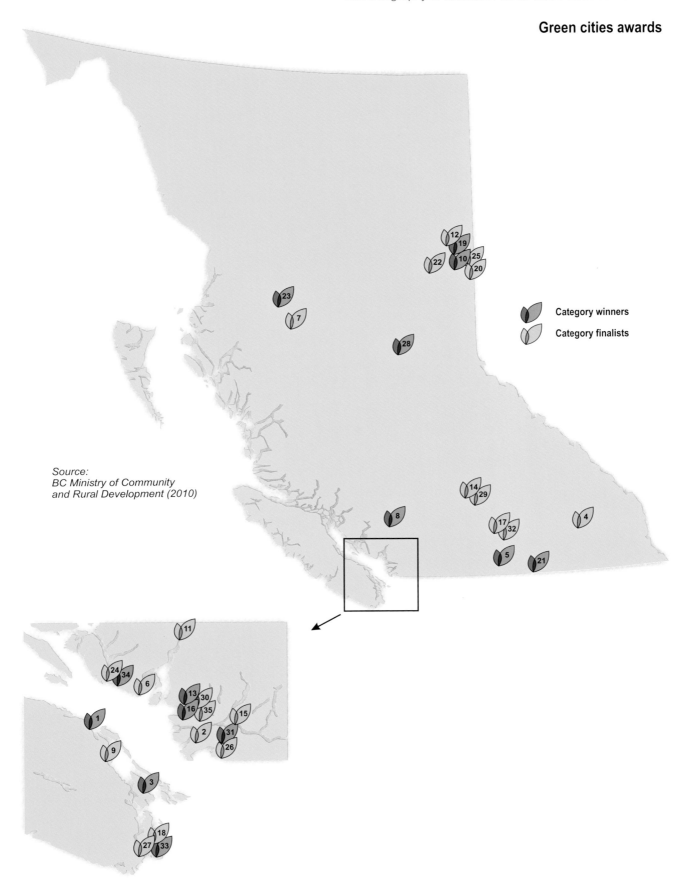

Category winners

Category finalists

Source:
BC Ministry of Community
and Rural Development (2010)

Towns for tomorrow

Part of the original ActNow BC program was to help maintain the sustainability of communities with populations of 15,000 or less. Towns for Tomorrow was announced in late 2006, in part to address these challenges. The program provided funding for infrastructure projects that address climate change and contribute to the overall health, sustainability, and livability of communities (Ministry of Community and Rural Development, 2010a).

Communities with populations under 5,000 had to cost-share with the Province on an 80/20 basis, with a maximum provincial contribution of $400,000, while those with populations between 5,000 and 15,000 shared on a 75/25 basis, with a maximum provincial contribution of $375,000.

Eligible proposals included projects related to water, wastewater, public transit, environmental energy improvement, local roads, recreation and culture, tourism, protective and emergency services, and community development.

Small communities were also encouraged to invest in training and other professional development initiatives that had a 'capacity building' component, and up to 10% of eligible costs could be spent to develop capacity in sustainable approaches to infrastructure planning and management.

Project selection criteria included advancing ActNow BC's principle of being more physically active, contribution towards community greenhouse gas emissions reduction, improved public and environmental health, and building seniors-friendly and disability-friendly communities.

In 2007, 24 projects were initiated, with a further 20 commencing in 2008. Finally, in 2009, 110 projects were funded. A total of 154 projects had been approved for 125 local governments, including 24 regional districts (Ministry of Community and Rural Development, 2010b), as indicated in the table and map opposite. These are new to the Atlas.

Community		Community		Community	
1	100 Mile House	44	Houston	86	Pouce Coupe
2	Alberni-Clayoquot RD	45	Hudson's Hope	87	Powell River
3	Armstrong	46	Invermere	88	Powell River RD
4	Barriere	47	Kaslo	89	Prince Rupert
5	Bowen Island	48	Kent	90	Princeton
6	Bulkley Nechako RD	49	Keremeos	91	Qualicum Beach
7	Burns Lake	50	Kimberley	92	Queen Charlotte
8	Cache Creek	51	Kitimat	93	Quesnel
9	Canal Flats	52	Kitimat Stikine RD	94	Radium Hot Springs
10	Capital RD	53	Kootenay Boundary RD	95	Revelstoke
11	Cariboo RD	54	Ladysmith	96	Rossland
12	Castlegar	55	Lake Country	97	Salmo
13	Central Coast RD	56	Lake Cowichan	98	Sayward
14	Central Kootenay RD	57	Lantzville	99	Sechelt
15	Central Okanagan RD	58	Lillooet	100	Sechelt Indian Government District
16	Chase	59	Lions Bay	101	Sicamous
17	Chetwynd	60	Logan Lake	102	Silverton
18	Clearwater	61	Lumby	103	Skeena Queen Charlotte RD
19	Clinton	62	Mackenzie	104	Smithers
20	Coldstream	63	Masset	105	Sooke
21	Columbia Shuswap RD	64	McBride	106	Spallumcheen
22	Comox	65	Merritt	107	Sparwood
23	Comox Valley RD	66	Metchosin	108	Squamish
24	Cowichan Valley RD	67	Mount Waddington RD	109	Stewart
25	Cumberland	68	Nakusp	110	Summerland
26	Dawson Creek	69	Nanaimo RD	111	Sunshine Coast RD
27	Duncan	70	Nelson	112	Tahsis
28	East Kootenay RD	71	New Denver	113	Taylor
29	Elkford	72	North Okanagan RD	114	Telkwa
30	Enderby	73	Northern Rockies RM	115	Terrace
31	Fort Nelson	74	Okanagan Similkameen RD	116	Thompson Nicola RD
32	Fort St. James	75	Oliver	117	Tofino
33	Fraser Fort George RD	76	Osoyoos	118	Trail
34	Fraser Lake	77	Parksville	119	Tumbler Ridge
35	Fraser Valley RD	78	Peace River RD	120	Ucluelet
36	Gibsons	79	Peachland	121	Valemount
37	Gold River	80	Pemberton	122	Vanderhoof
38	Golden	81	Port Alice	123	Wells
39	Grand Forks	82	Port Clements	124	Whistler
40	Harrison Hot Springs	83	Port Edward	125	Williams Lake
41	Hazelton	84	Port Hardy		
42	Highlands	85	Port McNeill		
43	Hope				

Towns for tomorrow

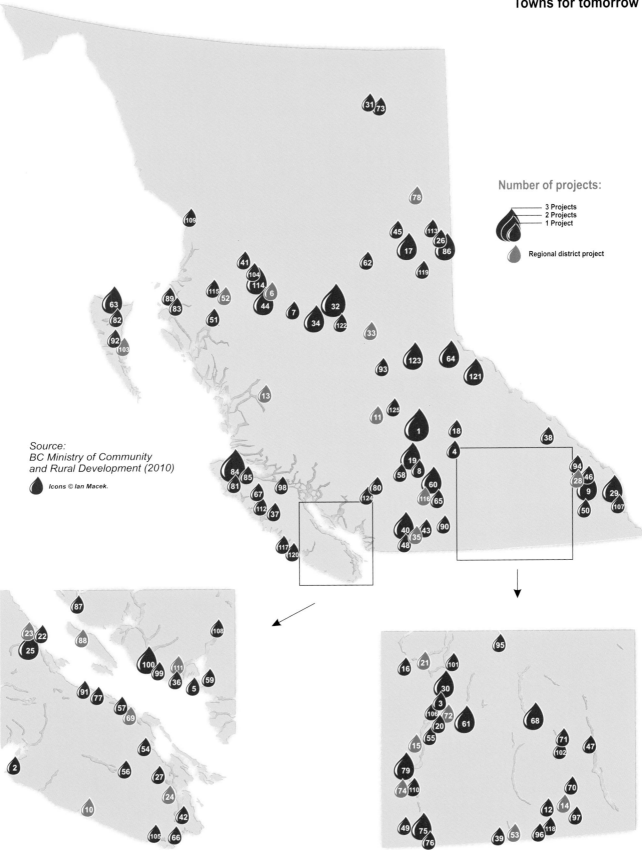

Number of projects:

3 Projects
2 Projects
1 Project

Regional district project

Source:
BC Ministry of Community
and Rural Development (2010)

Icons © Ian Macek.

Trees for tomorrow

The Trees for Tomorrow program, a $13 million cost-sharing venture to plant millions of trees in the public areas of cities, towns, villages, and regional districts throughout BC was announced in September 2008. The news release noted: "Planting trees in urban areas will help lock away greenhouse gases that would otherwise contribute to climate change. This is a great opportunity for communities to come together to improve air quality and beautify their communities" (Ministry of Community Development, 2010c).

By April 2009, approximately 130 projects in almost 100 communities throughout BC were funded as part of the plan aimed at planting four million trees in schoolyards, hospital grounds, civic parks, and other public spaces in BC over 5 years. These communities, in partnership with the Province, engaged volunteers to not only plant shrubs and seedlings, but also to educate residents about the benefits of urban afforestation in the hope that they would recognize the importance of becoming stewards of their own communities.

Community	Community	Community
1 108 Mile Ranch	34 Fruitvale	65 Oliver
2 Abbotsford	35 Gibsons	66 Pemberton
3 Ashcroft	36 Gitanmaax Reserve	67 Penticton
4 Barriere	37 Grand Forks	68 Pitt Meadows
5 Brentwood Bay	38 Hagensborg	69 Port Alberni
6 Burnaby	39 Houston	70 Port Clements
7 Burns Lake	40 Invermere	71 Port Coquitlam
8 Cache Creek	41 Kamloops	72 Port Hardy
9 Campbell River	42 Kelowna	73 Port Moody
10 Capital RD	43 Keremeos	74 Powell River
11 Castlegar	44 Kimberley	75 Prince George
12 Cawston	45 Kitimat	76 Prince Rupert
13 Central Saanich	46 Kitimat-Stikinie RD	77 Princeton
14 Chase	47 Kitselas First Nation/	78 Qualicum Beach
15 Chase and	Terrace	79 Quesnel
Salmon Arm	48 Kootenay/Columbia	80 Richmond
16 Chemainus	49 Kootenay-	81 Saanich
17 Chetwynd	Boundary RD	82 Salmon Arm
18 Coldstream	50 Lake Country	83 Sechelt
19 Colwood	51 Lake Cowichan	84 Shawnigan Lake
20 Comox	52 Langford	85 Sparwood
21 Comox Valley RD	53 Langley District	86 Surrey
22 Coquitlam	54 Lillooet	87 Taylor
23 Courtney	55 Lions Bay	88 Terrace
24 Cowichan Valley RD	56 Lytton	89 Tumbler Ridge
25 Cranbrook	57 Mayne Island (NLG)	90 Ucluelet
26 Creston	58 Merritt	91 Valemount
27 Dawson Creek	59 Mission	92 Vancouver
28 Delta	60 Nanaimo	93 Vernon
29 Duncan	61 Nelson	94 Victoria
30 Edgewood	62 Nelson/Castlegar	95 West Kelowna
31 Esquimalt	63 North Vancouver	96 West Vancouver
32 Fernie	64 Okanagan-	97 White Rock
33 Fraser Valley RD	Similkameen RD	98 Xaxli'p

There were several program streams:

- The CommuniTree Program was an application-based program for matching funding by local governments, First Nations, and community organizations to have trees planted in community and regional parks, hospital grounds, boulevards, and parking lots, as well as on school grounds and post secondary campuses.

- The Urban Mountain Pine Beetle Affected Area Renewal Program provided seedlings for urban areas affected by the pine beetle epidemic.

- Local governments could create groves of trees to commemorate the 150th anniversary of BC and to raise awareness about the importance of achieving climate change milestones in participating communities.

The table and map opposite, which are new to this Atlas, provide the location of projects throughout the province as of April 2009, which was when the last projects were announced. By late 2010, only $3 million of the proposed $13 million had been allocated. Of the approximately 100 communities benefitting from this initiative, 10 were Indian communities, while a further 7 were Regional Districts. While most communities had single projects, Okanagan-Similkameen Regional District had five separate projects, while Burnaby, Kelowna, and Vancouver each had four funded projects.

Trees for tomorrow

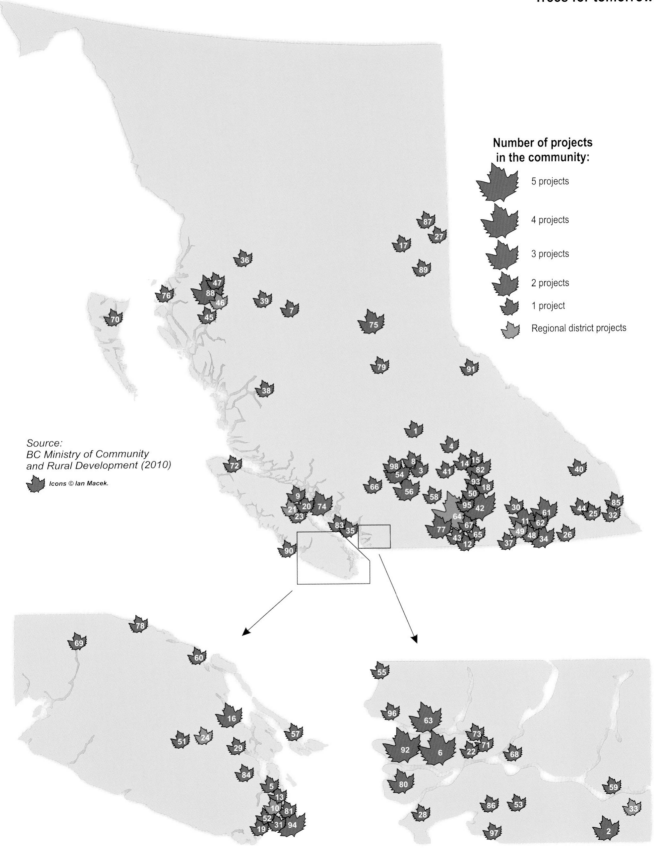

Number of projects in the community:

5 projects

4 projects

3 projects

2 projects

1 project

Regional district projects

Source:
BC Ministry of Community
and Rural Development (2010)

Icons © Ian Macek.

Pesticide-free communities

Pesticides kill weeds (herbicides), rodents (rodenticides), insects (insecticides), and fungi and bacteria (fungicides). Cosmetic pesticides are synthetic, chemical compounds that are generally used to improve the appearance of lawns, gardens, golf courses, playing fields, parks, school yards, and playgrounds. There have been many concerns about the health impacts of pesticides, starting perhaps half a century ago with *Silent Spring* (Carson, 1961), warning of the cumulative dangers of the use of DDT (Irwin, 1991).

Federal and provincial governments have the key responsibilities to protect against health and environmental risks of cosmetic pesticide exposure. Nevertheless, by 2010 there were nearly 170 communities across Canada that had instituted municipal by-laws banning or limiting the use of cosmetic pesticides in their municipalities. More than 30 were in BC and are shown in the map opposite. This is a new indicator of healthy public policy for this Atlas.

Within BC, municipalities can pass local by-laws that restrict cosmetic pesticide use only on private residential and municipal lands (Pesticide Free BC, 2010). Municipalities cannot, however, stop pesticide use on non-residential private property, or stop the sale of pesticides. Restricting cosmetic pesticide use on commercial, industrial, and multi-residential properties is voluntary, and this includes lands related to daycare centres, schools, colleges and universities, hospital grounds, golf courses, and other sports fields.

The Union of BC Municipalities, which represents the municipalities in BC, has passed resolutions at annual meetings asking the provincial government to bring in legislation to ban the sale and use of cosmetic pesticides. Further, a group of eight medical and health organizations have supported the Canadian Cancer Society, BC and Yukon Division's request for the BC Government to legislate a ban on the use of cosmetic pesticides to protect citizens from unnecessary cancer risks (Canadian Cancer Society, BC and Yukon Division, 2010).

More than half (57.76%) of residents in BC live in a community that has some type of restriction on the use of cosmetic pesticides. This compares with about 63% in Canada as a whole (Pesticide Free BC, 2010). Port Moody was the first BC municipality to pass a by-law restricting cosmetic pesticide use, starting in 2003 with municipal properties, and expanding to private residences in 2006. Many by-laws have been phased in this

manner so that residents and businesses can become educated about the initiative (Kassirer et al., 2004). In BC, all but 4 of the 34 communities had an educational program in place.

By April 2011, 33 communities will have some type of by-law in place, and eight others were considering draft by-laws (Abbotsford, Castlegar, Oak Bay, Penticton, Port Coquitlam, Revelstoke, Rossland, and Ucluelet).

Health Service Delivery Area	Protected by a pesticide by-law (%)
31 Richmond	100.00
32 Vancouver	97.93
23 Fraser South	81.12
33 North Shore/Coast Garibaldi	73.32
22 Fraser North	65.84
41 South Vancouver Island	58.86
14 Thompson Cariboo Shuswap	46.20
42 Central Vancouver Island	39.70
13 Okanagan	33.44
43 North Vancouver Island	32.53
11 East Kootenay	17.99
12 Kootenay Boundary	12.36
21 Fraser East	0.00
53 Northeast	0.00
52 Northern Interior	0.00
51 Northwest	0.00
British Columbia	**57.76**

There are large variations among HSDAs in terms of the percentage of population covered by a by-law. The three northern HSDAs and Fraser East have no communities with a cosmetic pesticide by-law, while at the other extreme, Vancouver and Richmond have complete population coverage (100%) on municipal and private residential lands. Generally, coverage is more complete in the southwest part of the province, including the lower mainland and South Vancouver Island.

Only 14 communities, with approximately one-quarter (24%) of the province's population, had by-laws that have banned pesticide use on both residential and municipal lands. These are: Comox, Courtenay, Delta, Esquimalt, Harrison Hot Springs, Invermere, Kimberley, Nanaimo, Qualicum Beach, Richmond, Tofino, Vancouver (City), Whistler, and White Rock (Pesticide Free BC, 2010).

The other 20 communities, with 33% of BC's population, have only limited restrictions on the cosmetic use of pesticides, and they can be used by permit or exemption. Integrated Pest Management Practices applicators can apply cosmetic pesticides on municipal lands like sports fields and playgrounds in Kamloops, Kelowna, North Vancouver (City and District), Port Alberni, Saanich, Salmon Arm, Sechelt, Surrey, and Victoria. Pesticides are allowed on "hardened surfaces" such as patios, driveways, and sidewalks in Burnaby, Cumberland, Delta, Golden, Kamloops, Maple Ridge, Port Moody, Salmon Arm, Surrey, Victoria, and West Vancouver (District). Turf facilities are exempted in Cumberland, Esquimalt, Kimberley, Maple Ridge, Nelson, Port Alberni, Qualicum Beach, Salmon Arm, and Whistler (Pesticide Free BC, 2010).

Pesticide-free communities

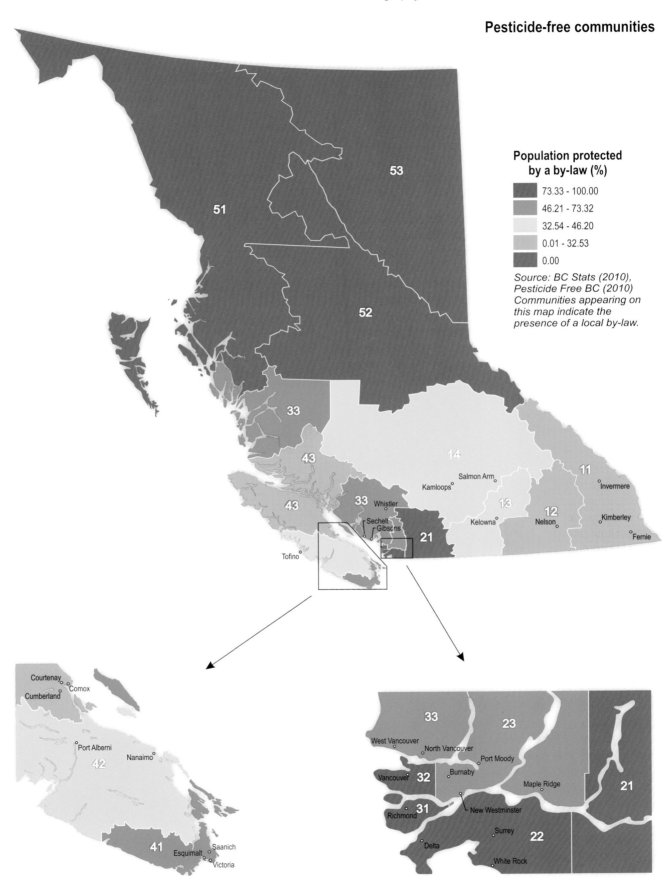

**Population protected
by a by-law (%)**

- 73.33 - 100.00
- 46.21 - 73.32
- 32.54 - 46.20
- 0.01 - 32.53
- 0.00

*Source: BC Stats (2010),
Pesticide Free BC (2010)
Communities appearing on
this map indicate the
presence of a local by-law.*

BC Healthy Living Alliance building community capacity initiatives

As noted earlier, in 2005, the BC Healthy Living Alliance (BCHLA) received a one-time grant of $25.2 million from the BC Ministry of Health to implement healthy living initiatives throughout the province. From the outset, the BCHLA initiatives were focused on reaching those areas and individuals in the province that had been under-served by healthy living programs in the past (BCHLA, 2010).

As part of this work, BCHLA developed and produced the *Community Capacity Building Strategy* (BCHLA, 2007a) in order to help guide the community capacity building initiative. "Capacity building is an effective health promotion tool that can lead to improvements in the health of communities, but also in their capability to develop locally directed, sustainable positive change" (BCHLA, 2007a, p15). The community capacity building initiative used individuals from the community to help implement projects and programs, thus ensuring a certain level of trust among community participants and gaining greater engagement from members of the community.

The community capacity building objectives were to support the implementation of BCHLA-approved initiatives under the three pillars – physical activity, healthy eating and tobacco cessation; to identify and align BCHLA-approved initiatives with regional network partners; to provide a central point of contact and information on BCHLA initiatives; and to seek opportunities to expand initiatives under the three pillars into identified at-risk communities.

Community capacity building was led by the Canadian Cancer Society, BC and Yukon Division, and not only set out to meet the above objectives, but also to ensure that communities gained the skills and resources necessary to sustain the healthy eating, physical activity, and tobacco reduction initiatives.

The adjacent map, which is new to this Atlas, represents the reach throughout the province of the community capacity building initiative, which took place from 2007 until 2010, when funding for the initiative ran out. In total, nearly 70 grants were provided to support 50 communities, most of which had small populations, were often somewhat remote, had minimal infrastructure, and included several Indian bands. In this initiative, nearly 1,500 individuals were trained to strengthen community capacity building, and partnerships were developed with over 400 regional and provincial organizations to support the work.

Community	Community
1 100 Mile House and Area	25 Lytton
2 Abbotsford	26 Maple Ridge
3 Alert Bay	27 McBride
4 Bamfield	28 Mission
5 Beecher Bay (Sooke)	29 Moricetown
6 Bella Bella	30 Mount Waddington
7 Bella Coola	31 Namgis First Nation
8 Burnaby	32 New Westminster
9 Castlegar	33 North Island
10 Chase	34 Okanagan
11 Chemainus/ Kuper Island	35 Pitt Meadows
12 Chetwynd	36 Port Alberni
13 Delta	37 Port Hardy
14 Fort Fraser	38 Port McNeill
15 Fort St. James	39 Port Renfrew
16 Fort St. John	40 Powell River
17 Granisle	41 Princeton
18 Greenville	42 Salmo
19 Haida Gwaiss	43 Sea to Sky Corridor
20 Hazeltons	44 Sliammon/ Powell River
21 Kingcome	45 Sunshine Coast
22 Kitamaat	46 Telegraph Creek
23 Langleys	47 Tofino
24 Lantzville	48 Trail
	49 Tumbler Ridge
	50 Ucluelet

BC Healthy Living Alliance building community capacity initiatives

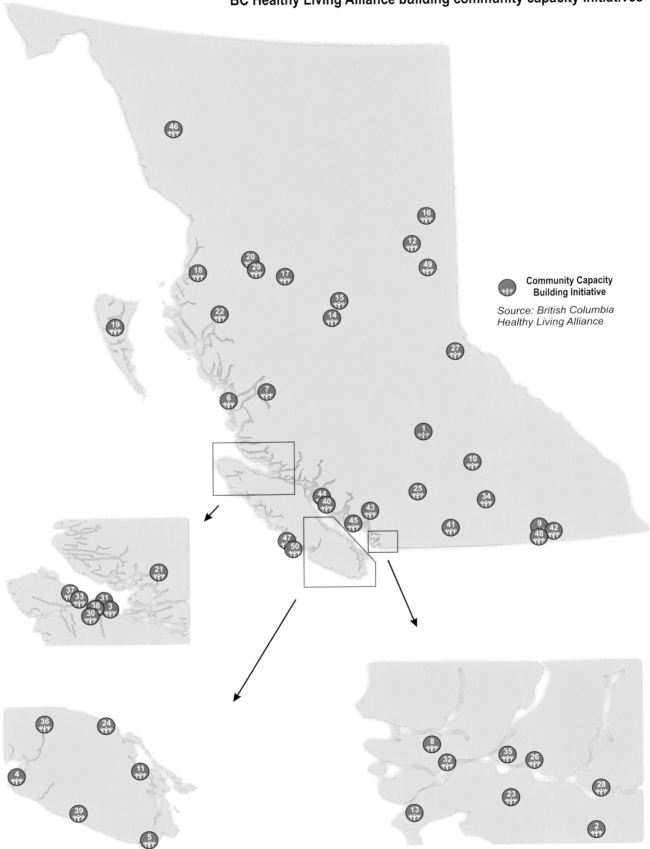

Community Capacity
Building Initiative

*Source: British Columbia
Healthy Living Alliance*

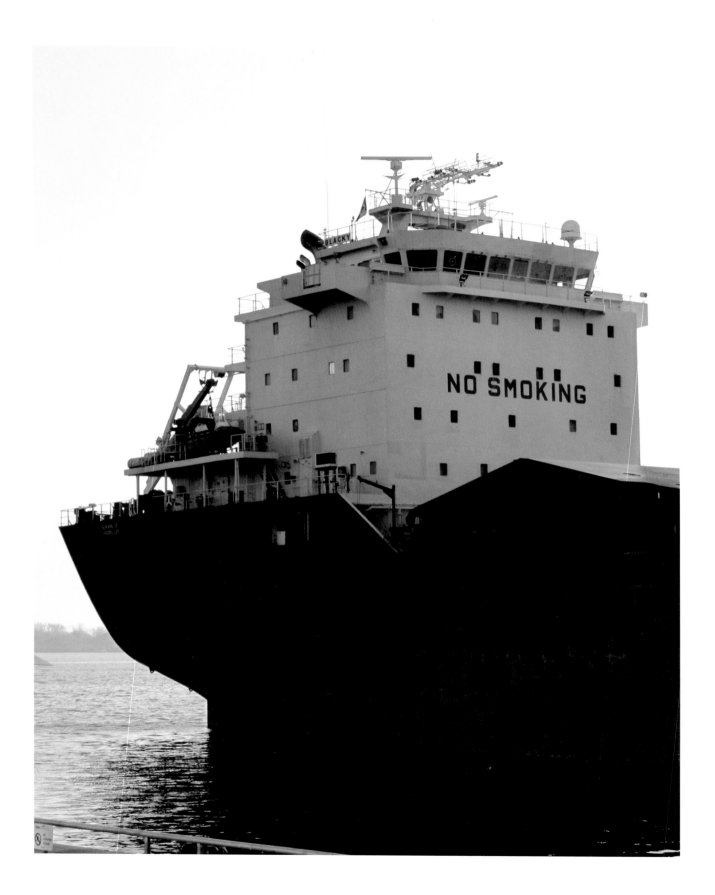

The Geography of Smoke-free Environments and Behaviours

British Columbia is acknowledged as having the lowest tobacco smoking rates in Canada (Shields, 2007; Health Canada, 2011), with only 12% of those 15 years and over indicating that they smoked in the first half of 2010. BC also has low rates of smoking when compared internationally (Studlar, 2007). However, smoking and frequenting areas where others are smoking or have smoked, which results in second-hand or environmental tobacco smoke, as well as third-hand tobacco smoke (the invisible remains of cigarette smoke that deposits on carpeting, clothing, furniture, and other surfaces), are still causes and contributors to many key chronic diseases and illnesses in the province, many of which are responsible for mortality. As a consequence, smoking reduction was one of the key pillars of ActNow BC.

Tobacco is still the greatest preventable cause of death and illness in Canada (Patra et al., 2007; Baliunas et al., 2007). Annually, the Vital Statistics Agency publishes an estimate of the Smoking Attributable Mortality based on a variety of diagnoses related to smoking. These include:

- Circulatory system diseases, such as hypertension, ischemic heart diseases, cerebrovascular diseases, other forms of heart diseases, and others;

- Cancers, such as cancers of the trachea, lung, pancreas, esophagus, and bladder, among others;

- Respiratory system diseases, such as chronic obstructive pulmonary disease, pneumonia and influenza, and bronchitis and emphysema.

The average annual number of deaths attributable to smoking and its effects in BC was more than 6,100, or approximately 20% of all deaths, for the 5 year period 2005 to 2009 based on the BC Vital Statistics Agency Annual Reports for those years. On average, it has been

estimated that smokers who quit can realize a reversal of the effects fairly quickly after quitting and could gain back up to 4.2 years of life that would otherwise have been lost through the impacts of continued smoking (Bridge & Turpin, 2004).

Of particular concern is the number of young people who smoke. While the prevalence of smoking among young people has been declining in recent years, there are still many young people who first experiment and then continue to smoke into adulthood. Research has shown that more than one-quarter of young people in BC are susceptible to smoking based on family and peer factors (Chen et. al., 2007; Hutchinson et al., 2008).

Not only are current smokers at risk of chronic health problems and premature mortality, but so are non-smokers who inhale other people's exhaled smoke, known as "mainstream" smoke, and/or substances from cigarettes, known as "sidestream" smoke. The latter is likely the more dangerous of the two. Effects can be felt not only by those in the immediate vicinity of a smoker, but also those who may be in neighbouring apartments or housing units in multi-unit buildings. Smoke from one unit can enter a neighbouring unit through a variety of mechanisms, such as neighbouring patios, common ventilation systems, electrical outlets, and cracks and gaps around sinks and countertops. A report by the US Office of the Surgeon General (2006) reviewed the health effects of second-hand smoke and concluded that there is no risk-free level of exposure. Children in particular are vulnerable, because their bodies are still developing. Recent concern has also been expressed about the effects of third-hand smoke, especially for babies who may be crawling on carpets and surfaces that have absorbed toxins from tobacco smoke. Nicotine from third-hand smoke can react with ozone in indoor air, and surfaces such as clothing and furniture, to form other pollutants. Exposure can occur not only for babies, but to individuals napping on a sofa in a smoking environment (Petrick et al., 2011).

While BC was often viewed as a leader in tobacco reduction legislation and other initiatives to reduce tobacco use, it has fallen behind other jurisdictions. Nevertheless, the Province has taken a series of initiatives within the past few years to reduce tobacco use. In 2007, tobacco use in schools and on school grounds was banned, and also smoking in foster homes was prohibited by the Ministry of Children and Family Development. In 2008, the Province introduced a series of new regulations under the Tobacco Control Act that banned:

- Smoking in all indoor public spaces and workplaces, with exemptions made for the ceremonial use of tobacco by Aboriginal people;

- Smoking within 3 metres of public and workplace doorways, open windows, or air intakes;

- Tobacco sales in public buildings, including hospitals and health facilities, universities and colleges, athletic and recreational facilities, and provincial government buildings; and

- Display and promotion of tobacco products in all places where tobacco is sold that are accessible to youth under 19 years.

And in 2009, BC implemented a ban on smoking in a vehicle if a child under the age of 16 years was riding in the vehicle, following the lead of Nova Scotia which implemented legislation in 2008, and the adoption of local by-laws by Surrey, White Rock, and Richmond (Saltman et al., 2010).

More than 20 municipalities throughout the province have adopted smoke-free local by-laws that exceed provincial requirements. These include: smoke-free patios in bars and restaurants, beaches, playgrounds, parks, and other outdoor spaces; buffer zones around patios, doorways, windows, air intakes, and transit shelters; smoke-free vehicles with children present; and a broad definition of smoking, not exclusive to tobacco and/or including hookahs (Non-Smokers' Rights Association, 2011).

This chapter includes 37 separate maps related to smoke-free activities and environments. Most of the maps are based on the five map CCHS model described in Chapter 3, and provide data at the HSDA level for all respondents, males, females, and for different age cohorts, while maps from McCreary AHS IV and the Student Satisfaction Survey are also provided. The first five indicators and 25 maps look at smoke-free or smoking restricted environments in public places, and other environments:

work, vehicles, and homes. This is followed by three maps that look at smoke-free environments specific to youth. The next five maps show non-smoking behaviours for the BC population as a whole, and these are followed by three maps that focus on non-smoking behaviours of students in grades 7, 10 and 12. The final map is based on the activities undertaken by BCHLA as part of its tobacco reduction strategy in support of ActNow BC (BCHLA, 2007d).

A couple of cautions are required in examining the data. First, data were not available for the Northeast for the McCreary AHS IV indicator set, and second, the indicator for smoke-free workplace has different age cohorts than the other CCHS indicators.

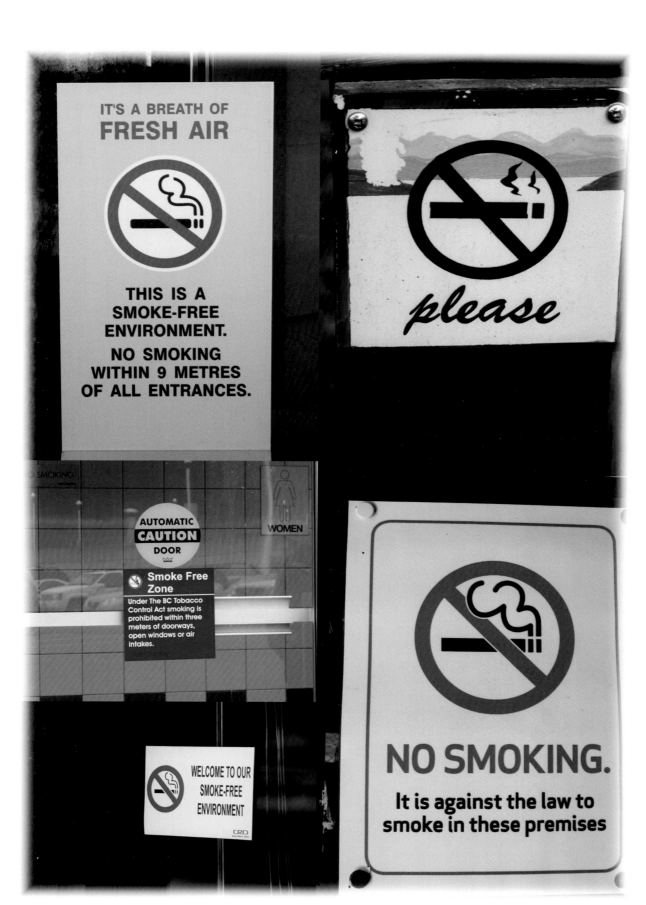

Smoke-free environment in frequented public places in the past month

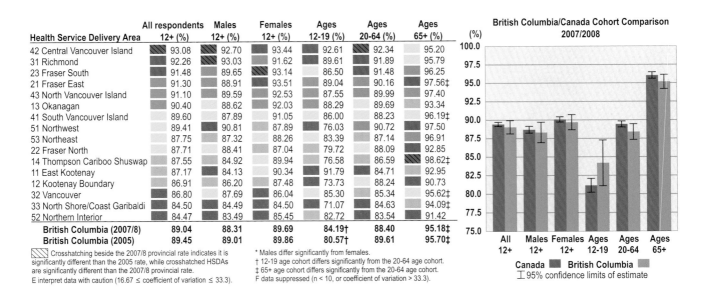

Health Service Delivery Area	All respondents 12+ (%)	Males 12+ (%)	Females 12+ (%)	Ages 12-19 (%)	Ages 20-64 (%)	Ages 65+ (%)
42 Central Vancouver Island	93.08	92.70	93.44	92.61	92.34	95.20
31 Richmond	92.26	93.03	91.62	89.61	91.89	95.79
23 Fraser South	91.48	89.65	93.14	86.50	91.48	96.25
21 Fraser East	91.30	88.91	93.51	89.04	90.16	97.56‡
43 North Vancouver Island	91.10	89.59	92.53	87.55	89.99	97.40
13 Okanagan	90.40	88.62	92.03	88.29	89.69	93.34
41 South Vancouver Island	89.60	87.89	91.05	86.00	88.23	96.19‡
51 Northwest	89.41	90.81	87.89	76.03	90.72	97.50
53 Northeast	87.75	87.32	88.26	83.39	87.14	96.91
22 Fraser North	87.71	88.41	87.04	79.72	88.09	92.85
14 Thompson Cariboo Shuswap	87.55	84.92	89.94	76.58	86.59	98.62‡
11 East Kootenay	87.17	84.13	90.34	91.79	84.71	92.95
12 Kootenay Boundary	86.91	86.20	87.48	73.73	88.24	90.73
32 Vancouver	86.80	87.69	86.04	85.30	85.34	95.62‡
33 North Shore/Coast Garibaldi	84.50	84.49	84.50	71.07	84.63	94.09‡
52 Northern Interior	84.47	83.49	85.45	82.72	83.54	91.42
British Columbia (2007/8)	89.04	88.31	89.69	84.19†	88.40	95.18‡
British Columbia (2005)	89.45	89.01	89.86	80.57†	89.61	95.70‡

Crosshatching beside the 2007/8 provincial rate indicates it is significantly different than the 2005 rate, while crosshatched HSDAs are significantly different than the 2007/8 provincial rate.
E interpret data with caution (16.67 ≤ coefficient of variation ≤ 33.3).

* Males differ significantly from females.
† 12-19 age cohort differs significantly from the 20-64 age cohort.
‡ 65+ age cohort differs significantly from the 20-64 age cohort.
F data suppressed (n < 10, or coefficient of variation > 33.3).

Places where people gather can be smoke-free, establishing an environmental asset for wellness. The CCHS asked if, in the past month, they were *"exposed to second-hand smoke every day or almost everyday in public places such as bars, restaurants, shopping malls, arenas, bingo halls, bowling alleys."* These maps represent the number of respondents who answered in the negative (i.e., had not been exposed to smoke regularly in those places). In BC, nearly nine out of ten respondents (89.04%) were not frequently exposed to second-hand smoke in public spaces. Central Vancouver Island was the only HSDA with a significantly higher value (93.08%) than the provincial average.

There were no significant differences between the genders at the provincial level or for any individual HSDA. For males, Richmond (93.03%) and Central Vancouver Island (92.70%) each had significantly more respondents reporting smoke-free experiences of public spaces compared to the male average in BC. For females, respondents in Fraser South (93.14%) were significantly more likely to experience smoke-free public places. No HSDA had significantly low values for either gender.

Provincially, 84.19% of youth reported smoke-free experiences of public places, making them significantly less likely to experience smoke-free public places than the mid-age cohort. While not significant, youth in North Shore/Coast Garibaldi and Kootenay Boundary had low averages (less than 74%) when compared to the provincial average for youth.

Older respondents in BC (95.18%) were significantly more

likely to report experiencing smoke-free public places at the provincial level than the mid-age cohort, and this pattern was reflected in five individual HSDAs. Thompson Cariboo Shuswap stood out, with a significantly higher percentage of older respondents reporting smoke-free experiences in frequented public places in the last month, at 98.62%.

While the spread in values among HSDAs was approximately 10 percentage points or less, youth had a spread of 20 percentage points, showing greater geographical variation within the province. Overall, consistently higher values were clustered around the southern regions of the province, while lower averages occurred in the northern and south eastern regions. However, there were some variations in that trend, including North Shore/Coast Garibaldi, Fraser North, and Vancouver, all of which had lower averages for all cohorts.

There were no significant differences for any BC cohorts between 2005 and 2007/8. Looking at BC in comparison to the Canadian picture, rates for frequenting smoke-free public places were quite similar to Canadian rates for all age and gender cohorts.

Smoke-free environment in frequented public places in the past month

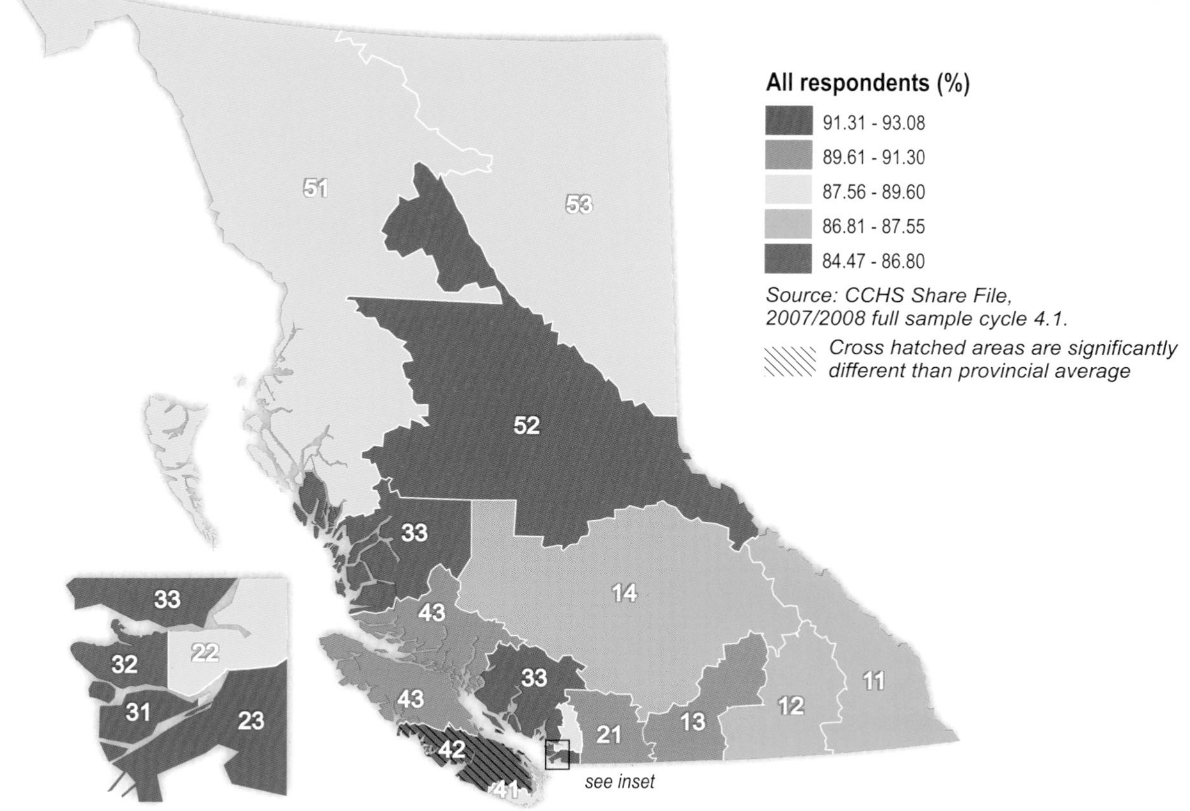

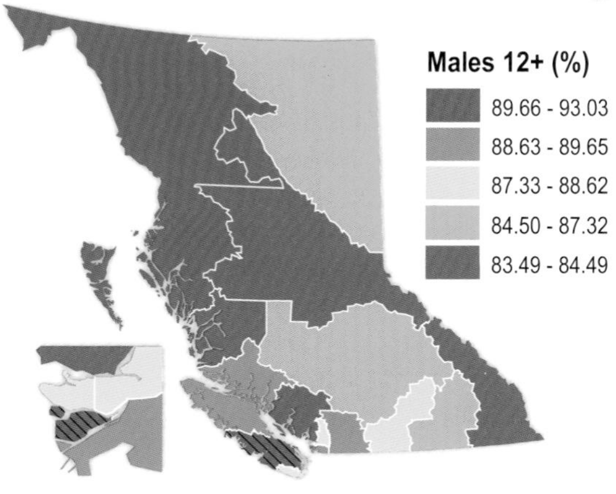

All respondents (%)

- 91.31 - 93.08
- 89.61 - 91.30
- 87.56 - 89.60
- 86.81 - 87.55
- 84.47 - 86.80

Source: CCHS Share File, 2007/2008 full sample cycle 4.1.

Cross hatched areas are significantly different than provincial average

51   53   52   33   43   14   11   33   43   13   12   21   42   41

33   32   22   31   23

see inset

Males 12+ (%)

- 89.66 - 93.03
- 88.63 - 89.65
- 87.33 - 88.62
- 84.50 - 87.32
- 83.49 - 84.49

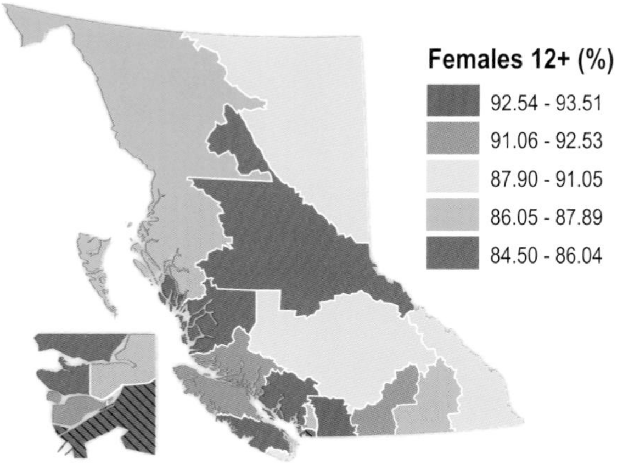

Females 12+ (%)

- 92.54 - 93.51
- 91.06 - 92.53
- 87.90 - 91.05
- 86.05 - 87.89
- 84.50 - 86.04

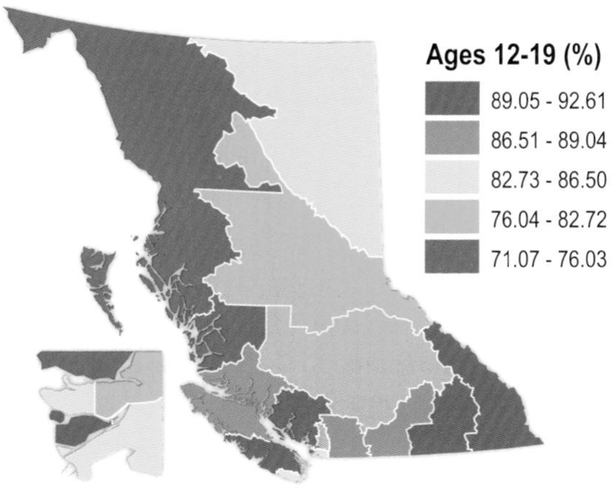

Ages 12-19 (%)

- 89.05 - 92.61
- 86.51 - 89.04
- 82.73 - 86.50
- 76.04 - 82.72
- 71.07 - 76.03

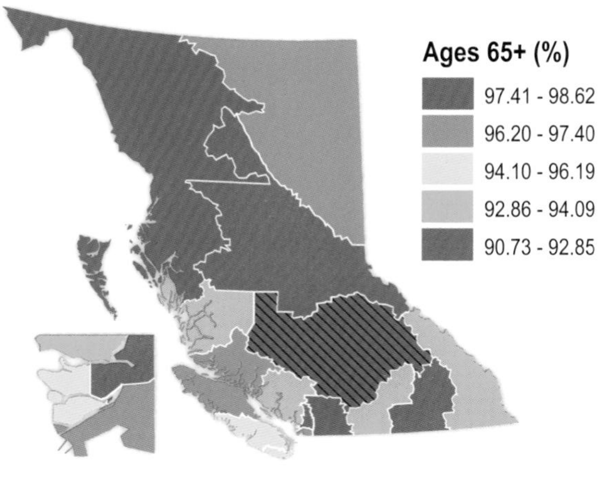

Ages 65+ (%)

- 97.41 - 98.62
- 96.20 - 97.40
- 94.10 - 96.19
- 92.86 - 94.09
- 90.73 - 92.85

Smoke-free work environment

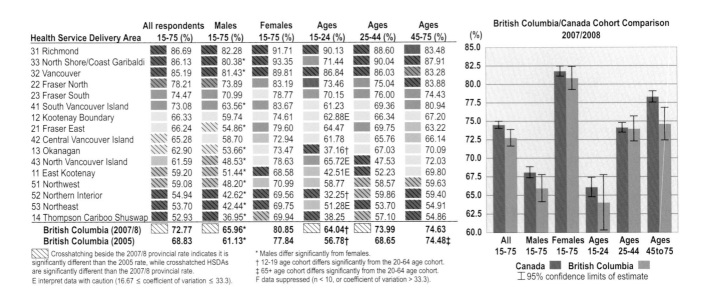

Health Service Delivery Area	All respondents 15-75 (%)	Males 15-75 (%)	Females 15-75 (%)	Ages 15-24 (%)	Ages 25-44 (%)	Ages 45-75 (%)
31 Richmond	86.69	82.28	91.71	90.13	88.60	83.48
33 North Shore/Coast Garibaldi	86.13	80.38*	93.35	71.44	90.04	87.91
32 Vancouver	85.19	81.43*	89.81	86.84	86.03	83.28
22 Fraser North	78.21	73.89	83.19	73.46	75.04	83.88
23 Fraser South	74.47	70.99	78.77	70.15	76.00	74.43
41 South Vancouver Island	73.08	63.56*	83.67	61.23	69.36	80.94
12 Kootenay Boundary	66.33	59.74	74.61	62.88E	66.34	67.20
21 Fraser East	66.24	54.86*	79.60	64.47	69.75	63.22
42 Central Vancouver Island	65.28	58.70	72.94	61.78	65.76	66.14
13 Okanagan	62.90	53.66*	73.47	37.16†	67.03	70.09
43 North Vancouver Island	61.59	48.53*	78.63	65.72E	47.53	72.03
11 East Kootenay	59.20	51.44*	68.58	42.51E	52.23	69.80
51 Northwest	59.08	48.20*	70.99	58.77	58.57	59.63
52 Northern Interior	54.94	42.62*	69.56	32.25†	59.86	59.40
53 Northeast	53.70	42.44*	69.75	51.28E	53.70	54.91
14 Thompson Cariboo Shuswap	52.93	36.95*	69.94	38.25	57.10	54.86
British Columbia (2007/8)	**72.77**	**65.96***	**80.85**	**64.04†**	**73.99**	**74.63**
British Columbia (2005)	**68.83**	**61.13***	**77.84**	**56.78†**	**68.65**	**74.48‡**

Crosshatching beside the 2007/8 provincial rate indicates it is significantly different than the 2005 rate, while crosshatched HSDAs are significantly different than the 2007/8 provincial rate.
E interpret data with caution (16.67 ≤ coefficient of variation ≤ 33.3).

* Males differ significantly from females.
† 12-19 age cohort differs significantly from the 20-64 age cohort.
‡ 65+ age cohort differs significantly from the 20-64 age cohort.
F data suppressed (n < 10, or coefficient of variation > 33.3).

British Columbia/Canada Cohort Comparison 2007/2008

Canada ■   British Columbia ▨
⊥ 95% confidence limits of estimate

The work place can be a significant venue for exposure to environmental tobacco smoke, especially for those in full time employment. Having a work place completely free of smoke is an important wellness asset. The CCHS asked respondents "*At your place of work, what are the restrictions on smoking?*" Among all respondents (age 15 to 75 years) who had paid work, 72.77% indicated that smoking was completely restricted in their work place. Fraser North, Richmond, Vancouver, and North Shore/Coast Garibaldi (all above 78%) were significantly more likely, while workers in seven HSDAs in the north and interior areas of BC (all below 66%) were significantly less likely to have smoke-free work environments.

Males (65.96%) were significantly less likely than females (80.85%) to have smoke-free work environments. This significant difference occurred in all but five HSDAs. Males in Fraser North, Richmond, Vancouver, and North Shore/Coast Garibaldi (all above 73%) had significantly higher values, whereas males in eight HSDAs, mostly in rural regions of the province, had significantly lower values for smoke-free work environments. Female respondents in Richmond, Vancouver, and North Shore/Coast Garibaldi (all above 89%) had significantly higher values of smoke-free work environments, whereas females in East Kootenay, Thompson Cariboo Shuswap, Northern Interior, and Northeast (all below 70%) had significantly lower values than females provincially.

The younger age cohort (15 to 24 years) was significantly less likely than the mid-age cohort (25 to 44 years) to have smoke-free work environments. This significant difference

also occurred in Okanagan and Northern Interior. Compared to the provincial average, younger respondents in Vancouver (86.84%) and Richmond (90.13%) had significantly higher values, while those in Okanagan, Thompson Cariboo Shuswap and Northern Interior (all below 39%) were significantly lower than the provincial average for the younger age cohort.

For the 45-75 year cohort, 74.63% respondents provincially reported having smoke-free work environments. There were no significant differences between this cohort and the mid-age cohort. Fraser North, Vancouver, and North Shore/Coast Garibaldi (all above 83%) had significantly higher values of smoke-free work environments, while Thompson Cariboo Shuswap, Northwest, Northern Interior, and Northeast (all below 60%) had significantly lower values than the older age BC average.

Geographically there were major variations across the province for all cohorts. Younger age respondents had almost a 60 percentage point spread among HSDAs, while all other cohorts had at least a 20 percentage point spread. Generally, the urban lower mainland had higher values, while the north and central interior HSDAs were lower.

For BC respondents, the 2007/8 cohorts had significantly higher values than in 2005, except for female and older respondents. When compared to Canadian averages for 2007/8, BC respondents were less likely to have smoke-free environments, and this difference was significant for the all respondents and older age cohorts.

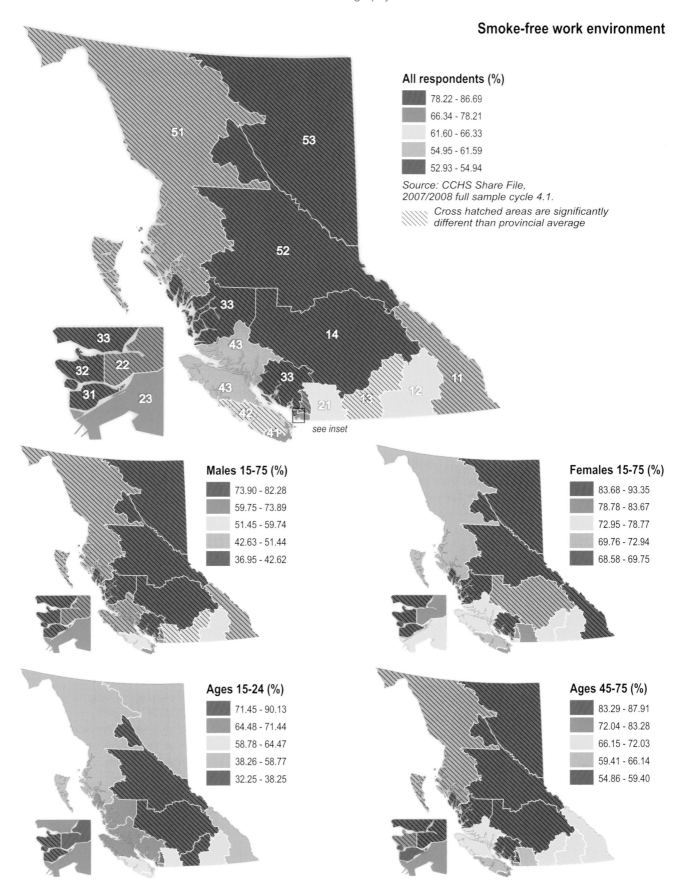

Smoke-free work environment

All respondents (%)

- 78.22 - 86.69
- 66.34 - 78.21
- 61.60 - 66.33
- 54.95 - 61.59
- 52.93 - 54.94

Source: CCHS Share File, 2007/2008 full sample cycle 4.1.

Cross hatched areas are significantly different than provincial average

Males 15-75 (%)

- 73.90 - 82.28
- 59.75 - 73.89
- 51.45 - 59.74
- 42.63 - 51.44
- 36.95 - 42.62

Females 15-75 (%)

- 83.68 - 93.35
- 78.78 - 83.67
- 72.95 - 78.77
- 69.76 - 72.94
- 68.58 - 69.75

Ages 15-24 (%)

- 71.45 - 90.13
- 64.48 - 71.44
- 58.78 - 64.47
- 38.26 - 58.77
- 32.25 - 38.25

Ages 45-75 (%)

- 83.29 - 87.91
- 72.04 - 83.28
- 66.15 - 72.03
- 59.41 - 66.14
- 54.86 - 59.40

Smoke-free vehicle environment in the past month

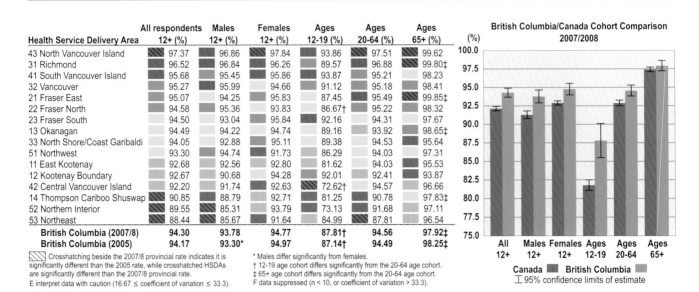

Health Service Delivery Area	All respondents 12+ (%)	Males 12+ (%)	Females 12+ (%)	Ages 12-19 (%)	Ages 20-64 (%)	Ages 65+ (%)
43 North Vancouver Island	97.37	96.86	97.84	93.86	97.51	99.62
31 Richmond	96.52	96.84	96.26	89.57	96.88	99.80‡
41 South Vancouver Island	95.68	95.45	95.86	93.87	95.21	98.23
32 Vancouver	95.27	95.99	94.66	91.12	95.18	98.41
21 Fraser East	95.07	94.25	95.83	87.45	95.49	99.85‡
22 Fraser North	94.58	95.36	93.83	86.67†	95.22	98.32
23 Fraser South	94.50	93.04	95.84	92.16	94.31	97.67
13 Okanagan	94.49	94.22	94.74	89.16	93.92	98.65‡
33 North Shore/Coast Garibaldi	94.05	92.88	95.11	89.38	94.53	95.64
51 Northwest	93.30	94.74	91.73	86.29	94.03	97.31
11 East Kootenay	92.68	92.56	92.80	81.62	94.03	95.53
12 Kootenay Boundary	92.67	90.68	94.28	92.01	92.41	93.87
42 Central Vancouver Island	92.20	91.74	92.63	72.62†	94.57	96.66
14 Thompson Cariboo Shuswap	90.85	88.79	92.71	81.25	90.78	97.83‡
52 Northern Interior	89.55	85.31	93.79	73.13	91.68	97.11
53 Northeast	88.44	85.67	91.64	84.99	87.81	96.54
British Columbia (2007/8)	**94.30**	**93.78**	**94.77**	**87.81†**	**94.56**	**97.92‡**
British Columbia (2005)	**94.17**	**93.30***	**94.97**	**87.14†**	**94.49**	**98.25‡**

⊠ Crosshatching beside the 2007/8 provincial rate indicates it is significantly different than the 2005 rate, while crosshatched HSDAs are significantly different than the 2007/8 provincial rate.
E interpret data with caution (16.67 ≤ coefficient of variation ≤ 33.3).

* Males differ significantly from females.
† 12-19 age cohort differs significantly from the 20-64 age cohort.
‡ 65+ age cohort differs significantly from the 20-64 age cohort.
F data suppressed (n < 10, or coefficient of variation > 33.3).

Many Canadians commute by car and use a vehicle to undertake other activities, particularly in the suburbs or smaller communities. The environment of a vehicle is confined and so a smoke-free vehicle environment is an asset that can maintain present and future wellness.

The CCHS asked respondents if, in the past month, they were *"exposed to second-hand smoke everyday or almost every day in a car or private vehicle."* Nearly 95% of respondents answered in the negative, indicating that most British Columbians are able to enjoy mainly smoke-free vehicle environments. For all respondents, North Vancouver Island (97.37%) had a significantly higher percentage of respondents reporting smoke-free vehicle environments than the provincial average, while Thompson Cariboo Shuswap, Northern Interior, and Northeast (all below 91%) had significantly lower levels.

There were no significant differences between genders for this variable at either the provincial or HSDA level. For males, Northern Interior (85.31%) and Northeast (85.67%) were significantly less likely to have reported experiencing mainly smoke-free vehicle environments when compared to males provincially (93.78%). For females, North Vancouver Island (97.84%) had significantly more respondents reporting smoke-free vehicles compared to the female provincial average (94.77%).

For youth in BC, 87.81% reported travelling in primarily smoke-free vehicle environments. Provincially, youth as a whole and those in Fraser North and Central Vancouver Island were significantly less likely to experience mainly smoke-free vehicle environments than the mid-age cohort.

Compared to the provincial average for youth, those in Central Vancouver Island (72.62%) were significantly less likely to report smoke-free vehicle environments.

Older respondents in BC (97.92%) were significantly more likely to experience smoke-free vehicle environments than the mid-age cohort. At the HSDA level, older respondents in Okanagan, Thompson Cariboo Shuswap, Fraser East, and Richmond were significantly more likely to experience smoke-free vehicle environments than their mid-age counterparts. Seniors in Fraser East, Richmond, and North Vancouver Island (99% and above) all had significantly higher values than the BC rate.

Geographically, there was a modest 10 percentage point spread for most cohorts, although the spread among HSDAs for youth was 30 percentage points. The highest values for this variable occurred on Vancouver Island, with the exception of Central Vancouver Island, and in the urban lower mainland region of the province.

There were no significant differences for any of the BC cohorts between 2005 and 2007/8. In comparison to the national average, all BC age and gender cohorts, with the exception of older respondents, were significantly more likely to experience smoke-free vehicle environments.

Smoke-free vehicle environment in the past month

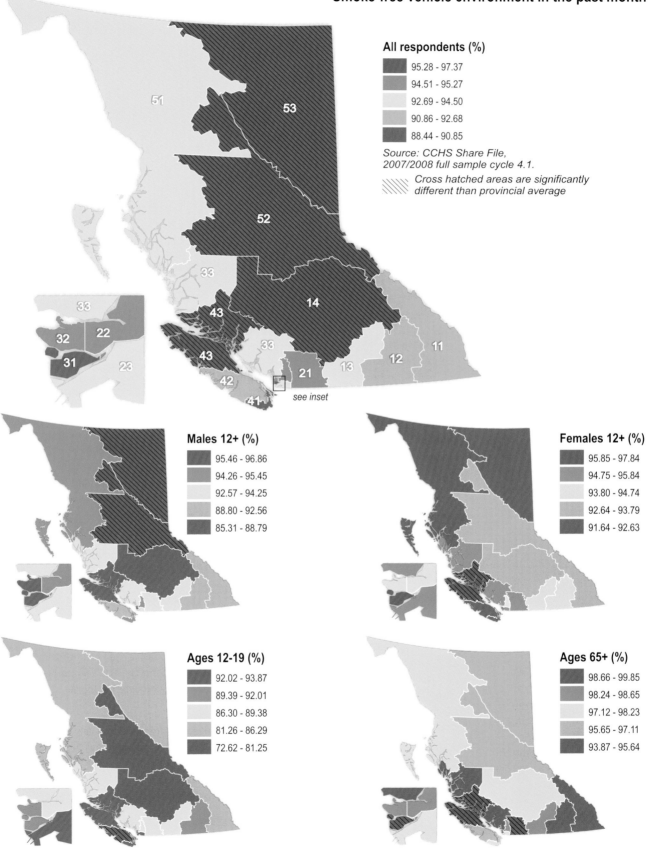

All respondents (%)

- 95.28 - 97.37
- 94.51 - 95.27
- 92.69 - 94.50
- 90.86 - 92.68
- 88.44 - 90.85

Source: CCHS Share File, 2007/2008 full sample cycle 4.1.

Cross hatched areas are significantly different than provincial average

see inset

Males 12+ (%)

- 95.46 - 96.86
- 94.26 - 95.45
- 92.57 - 94.25
- 88.80 - 92.56
- 85.31 - 88.79

Females 12+ (%)

- 95.85 - 97.84
- 94.75 - 95.84
- 93.80 - 94.74
- 92.64 - 93.79
- 91.64 - 92.63

Ages 12-19 (%)

- 92.02 - 93.87
- 89.39 - 92.01
- 86.30 - 89.38
- 81.26 - 86.29
- 72.62 - 81.25

Ages 65+ (%)

- 98.66 - 99.85
- 98.24 - 98.65
- 97.12 - 98.23
- 95.65 - 97.11
- 93.87 - 95.64

Smoke-free home environment

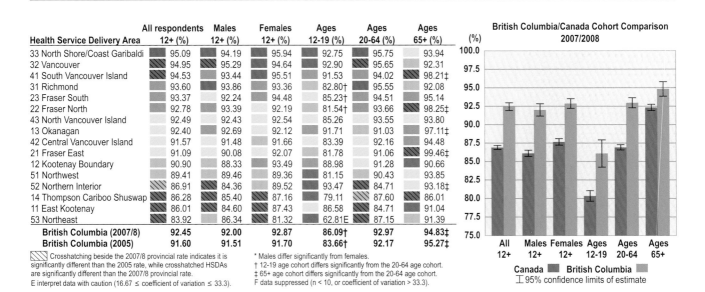

Health Service Delivery Area	All respondents 12+ (%)	Males 12+ (%)	Females 12+ (%)	Ages 12-19 (%)	Ages 20-64 (%)	Ages 65+ (%)
33 North Shore/Coast Garibaldi	95.09	94.19	95.94	92.75	95.75	93.94
32 Vancouver	94.95	95.29	94.64	92.90	95.65	92.31
41 South Vancouver Island	94.53	93.44	95.51	91.53	94.02	98.21‡
31 Richmond	93.60	93.86	93.36	82.80†	95.55	92.08
23 Fraser South	93.37	92.24	94.48	85.23†	94.51	95.14
22 Fraser North	92.78	93.39	92.19	81.54†	93.66	98.25‡
43 North Vancouver Island	92.49	92.43	92.54	85.26	93.55	93.80
13 Okanagan	92.40	92.69	92.12	91.71	91.03	97.11‡
42 Central Vancouver Island	91.57	91.48	91.66	83.39	92.16	94.48
21 Fraser East	91.09	90.08	92.07	81.78	91.06	99.46‡
12 Kootenay Boundary	90.90	88.33	93.49	88.98	91.28	90.66
51 Northwest	89.41	89.46	89.36	81.15	90.43	93.85
52 Northern Interior	86.91	84.36	89.52	93.47	84.71	93.18‡
14 Thompson Cariboo Shuswap	86.28	85.40	87.16	79.11	87.60	86.01
11 East Kootenay	86.01	84.60	87.43	86.58	84.71	91.04
53 Northeast	83.92	86.34	81.32	62.81E	87.15	91.39
British Columbia (2007/8)	**92.45**	**92.00**	**92.87**	**86.09†**	**92.97**	**94.83‡**
British Columbia (2005)	**91.60**	**91.51**	**91.70**	**83.66†**	**92.17**	**95.27‡**

Crosshatching beside the 2007/8 provincial rate indicates it is significantly different than the 2005 rate, while crosshatched HSDAs are significantly different than the 2007/8 provincial rate.
E interpret data with caution (16.67 ≤ coefficient of variation ≤ 33.3).

* Males differ significantly from females.
† 12-19 age cohort differs significantly from the 20-64 age cohort.
‡ 65+ age cohort differs significantly from the 20-64 age cohort.
F data suppressed (n < 10, or coefficient of variation > 33.3).

Individuals and families generally spend more than one-third of their time in their homes. Home environments can either foster good health or create challenges for health, depending on behaviours within the home. Because of relatively small spaces within the home, from a wellness perspective, creating a home environment that is free of tobacco smoke is important for all inhabitants. As noted earlier, there is no risk-free level of smoke exposure, and babies and younger children are particularly at-risk to the ill-effects of second-hand smoke in the home.

In BC, 92.45% of respondents indicated that their homes were smoke-free. Vancouver (94.95%) and South Vancouver Island (94.53%) had significantly more respondents reporting smoke-free homes than the provincial average, while East Kootenay, Thompson Cariboo Shuswap, Northern Interior, and the Northeast (all below 87%) had significantly fewer.

Provincially, 92% of males and 92.87% of females reported having a smoke-free home. There were no significant differences between genders at the provincial or individual HSDA level. For males, Vancouver had significantly more respondents, while East Kootenay, Thompson Cariboo Shuswap, and Northern Interior (all below 86%) had significantly fewer respondents reporting smoke-free homes compared to all males in BC. For females, East Kootenay, Thompson Cariboo Shuswap, and the Northeast (all below 88%) had significantly fewer respondents reporting smoke-free homes compared to all females in BC.

Youth in BC (86.09%) were significantly less likely to

report a smoke-free home environment when compared to the mid-age cohort, and particularly in Fraser North, Fraser South, and Richmond. No HSDA was significantly different than the provincial average for youth.

For older respondents, 94.83% reported living in a smoke-free home, which was significantly higher than the mid-age cohort. This difference was also seen in five individual HSDAs: Okanagan, Fraser East, Fraser North, South Vancouver Island, and Northern Interior. Older respondents in Fraser East, Fraser North, and South Vancouver Island (all above 97%) were significantly more likely than their provincial peers as a whole to live in a smoke-free home, while those in Thompson Cariboo Shuswap (86.01%) were significantly less likely.

Although there was a modest 10 percentage point spread among HSDAs for all cohorts geographically, except youth (30 percentage points), the northern and interior regions of the province had lower levels of smoke-free homes, whereas the southern and coastal areas of the province had higher levels for most cohorts. The Okanagan was the lone interior HSDA with consistently higher values of smoke-free homes.

There were no significant differences for any BC cohorts between 2005 and 2007/8. In comparison to the Canadian averages for smoke-free homes, British Columbians in all age and gender cohorts had significantly higher values of smoke-free homes.

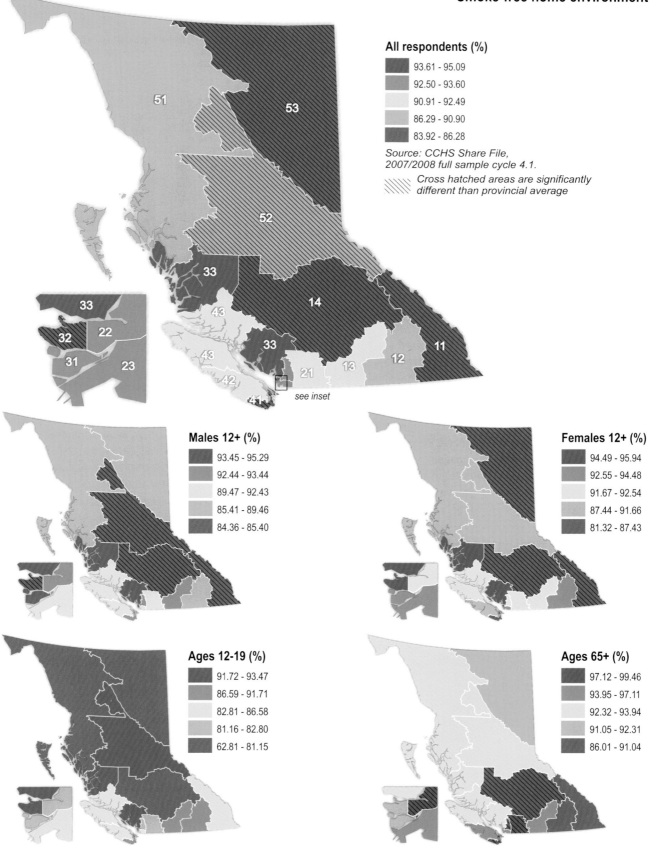

Smoke-free home environment

All respondents (%)
- 93.61 - 95.09
- 92.50 - 93.60
- 90.91 - 92.49
- 86.29 - 90.90
- 83.92 - 86.28

Source: CCHS Share File, 2007/2008 full sample cycle 4.1.

Cross hatched areas are significantly different than provincial average

Males 12+ (%)
- 93.45 - 95.29
- 92.44 - 93.44
- 89.47 - 92.43
- 85.41 - 89.46
- 84.36 - 85.40

Females 12+ (%)
- 94.49 - 95.94
- 92.55 - 94.48
- 91.67 - 92.54
- 87.44 - 91.66
- 81.32 - 87.43

Ages 12-19 (%)
- 91.72 - 93.47
- 86.59 - 91.71
- 82.81 - 86.58
- 81.16 - 82.80
- 62.81 - 81.15

Ages 65+ (%)
- 97.12 - 99.46
- 93.95 - 97.11
- 92.32 - 93.94
- 91.05 - 92.31
- 86.01 - 91.04

Some restriction against smoking cigarettes at home

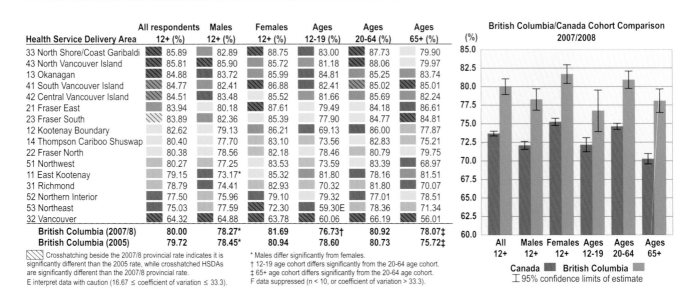

Health Service Delivery Area	All respondents 12+ (%)	Males 12+ (%)	Females 12+ (%)	Ages 12-19 (%)	Ages 20-64 (%)	Ages 65+ (%)
33 North Shore/Coast Garibaldi	85.89	82.89	88.75	83.00	87.73	79.90
43 North Vancouver Island	85.81	85.90	85.72	81.18	88.06	79.97
13 Okanagan	84.88	83.72	85.99	84.81	85.25	83.74
41 South Vancouver Island	84.77	82.41	86.88	82.41	85.02	85.01
42 Central Vancouver Island	84.51	83.48	85.52	81.66	85.69	82.24
21 Fraser East	83.94	80.18	87.61	79.49	84.18	86.61
23 Fraser South	83.89	82.36	85.39	77.90	84.77	84.81
12 Kootenay Boundary	82.62	79.13	86.21	69.13	86.00	77.87
14 Thompson Cariboo Shuswap	80.40	77.70	83.10	73.56	82.83	75.21
22 Fraser North	80.38	78.56	82.18	78.46	80.79	79.75
51 Northwest	80.27	77.25	83.53	73.59	83.39	68.97
11 East Kootenay	79.15	73.17*	85.32	81.80	78.16	81.51
31 Richmond	78.79	74.41	82.93	70.32	81.80	70.07
52 Northern Interior	77.50	75.96	79.10	79.32	77.01	78.51
53 Northeast	75.03	77.59	72.30	59.30E	78.36	71.34
32 Vancouver	64.32	64.88	63.78	60.06	66.19	56.01
British Columbia (2007/8)	**80.00**	**78.27***	**81.69**	**76.73†**	**80.92**	**78.07‡**
British Columbia (2005)	**79.72**	**78.45***	**80.94**	**78.60**	**80.73**	**75.72‡**

Crosshatching beside the 2007/8 provincial rate indicates it is significantly different than the 2005 rate, while crosshatched HSDAs are significantly different than the 2007/8 provincial rate.
E interpret data with caution (16.67 ≤ coefficient of variation ≤ 33.3).

* Males differ significantly from females.
† 12-19 age cohort differs significantly from the 20-64 age cohort.
‡ 65+ age cohort differs significantly from the 20-64 age cohort.
F data suppressed (n < 10, or coefficient of variation > 33.3).

Exposure to second-hand smoke is recognized as a major risk factor for lung cancer, respiratory diseases, and many other health problems. Individuals and families spend much of their time at home, and having some restrictions against smoking in the home is an important step toward creating healthy smoke-free home environments. This indicator presents the percentage of CCHS participants who responded positively to the question *"Are there any restrictions against smoking cigarettes in your home?"*. Among all respondents in BC, eight out of ten (80%) had some restrictions against smoking at home. There were six HSDAs (all with values over 83%) that were significantly higher than the provincial average. Vancouver (64.32%) was the only HSDA that reported significantly lower than average values for this indicator.

Among BC respondents, males (78.27%) were significantly less likely than females (81.69%) to have some restrictions against smoking at home. East Kootenay was the only HSDA with a significant difference between genders, and males were significantly lower than females.

For North Vancouver Island (85.90%), there were significantly more males with smoking restrictions at home than in the rest of the province, whereas males in Vancouver (64.88%) were significantly less likely to have smoking restrictions. Females in Fraser East, North Shore/Coast Garibaldi, and South Vancouver Island (all above 86%) were significantly more likely to have smoking restrictions at home than females provincially, while females in Vancouver (63.78%) and Northeast (72.30%)

were significantly less likely than females provincially to have smoking restrictions at home.

Both younger and older respondents were significantly less likely than the mid-age cohort to have restrictions on smoking at home; however, there were no significant differences at the individual HSDA level. Compared to the provincial average for youth, respondents in Vancouver (60.06%) were significantly less likely to have restrictions against smoking at home. For older respondents, Fraser South (84.81%) and South Vancouver Island (85.01%) had significantly higher values than the provincial average, and Vancouver (56.01%) had a significantly lower value.

Geographically, there were major variations between HSDAs with a spread of over 20 percentage points for all cohorts, and a more than 30 percent spread in the oldest cohort. Most of the south coastal area of the province had consistently high values for this variable with the exception of Vancouver, Richmond, and Fraser North, all of which had consistently lower values. Once again, the northern and central areas of the province had consistently lower values.

There were no significant differences for BC respondents between 2005 and 2007/8 for any of the cohorts. In comparison to the 2007/8 national averages, British Columbians in every cohort had significantly higher values than their Canadian peers for restrictions on smoking at home.

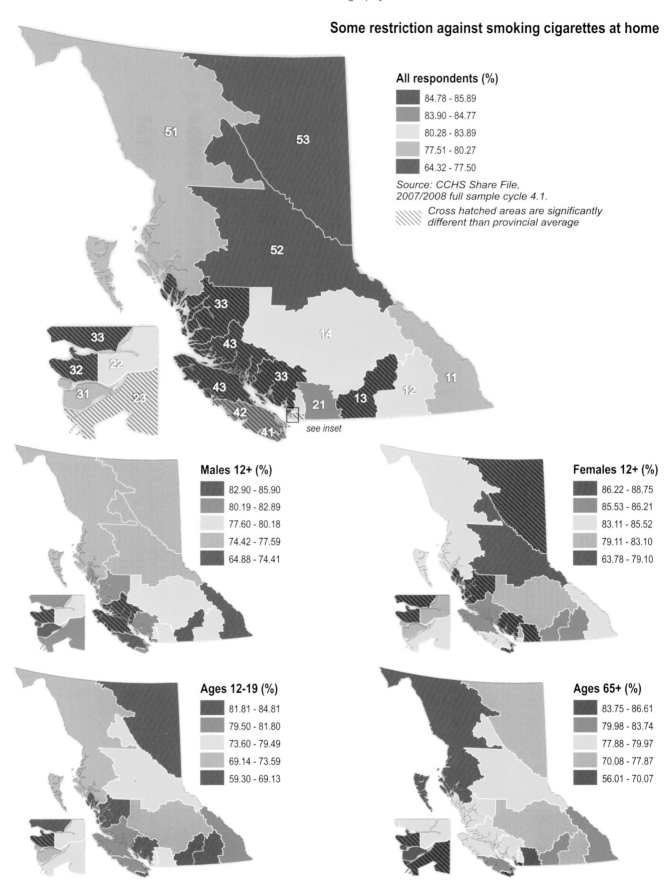

Some restriction against smoking cigarettes at home

All respondents (%)

- 84.78 - 85.89
- 83.90 - 84.77
- 80.28 - 83.89
- 77.51 - 80.27
- 64.32 - 77.50

Source: CCHS Share File, 2007/2008 full sample cycle 4.1.

Cross hatched areas are significantly different than provincial average

Males 12+ (%)

- 82.90 - 85.90
- 80.19 - 82.89
- 77.60 - 80.18
- 74.42 - 77.59
- 64.88 - 74.41

Females 12+ (%)

- 86.22 - 88.75
- 85.53 - 86.21
- 83.11 - 85.52
- 79.11 - 83.10
- 63.78 - 79.10

Ages 12-19 (%)

- 81.81 - 84.81
- 79.50 - 81.80
- 73.60 - 79.49
- 69.14 - 73.59
- 59.30 - 69.13

Ages 65+ (%)

- 83.75 - 86.61
- 79.98 - 83.74
- 77.88 - 79.97
- 70.08 - 77.87
- 56.01 - 70.07

Youth who are never exposed to tobacco smoke in their home or family vehicle

As indicated earlier, exposure to environmental tobacco smoke can be very damaging to a person's health. Young people, in particular, are vulnerable to problems created by such exposure. Being free from exposure to environmental tobacco smoke, especially in more confined spaces such as rooms in the home and vehicles, can be an important wellness asset.

The McCreary AHS IV asked students the following question: *"How often are you usually exposed to tobacco smoke inside your home or your family vehicle. Never, sometimes, almost every day or every day? (Note: if you are a smoker include your own smoke as well as other people's smoke)"* Responses in the table and maps opposite provide the percentage of students who answered that they were never exposed to tobacco smoke in their home or family vehicle.

More than seven in every ten (72.33%) student respondents in BC indicated that they were never exposed to tobacco smoke in their home or family vehicle. However, there was a large variation among HSDAs, with more than 20 percentage points between the highest and lowest value HSDAs. Richmond (80.29%) had the highest percentage, and East Kootenay (59.32%) the lowest percentage of students who responded that they were never exposed to tobacco smoke.

Geographically, there were major regional differences, with HSDAs in the urban lower mainland and South Vancouver Island all higher than the provincial average, while all other HSDAs were lower than the provincial average. Richmond, North Shore/Coast Garibaldi, Vancouver, and Fraser North (all above 75%) were significantly higher than the provincial average. All other HSDAs, with the exception of South Vancouver Island, Fraser South/Fraser East, and Okanagan, were significantly lower than the provincial student average.

There were no significant differences between male students and female students, either at the provincial level or for any individual HSDA, although provincially, males were marginally more likely to indicate that they were not exposed to tobacco smoke. The difference between the highest and lowest value HSDAs for males was 17 percentage points, while there was a 24 percentage point range for female students, considerably higher than that for males.

For male students, Richmond (80.76%) had the highest percentage, while Northern Interior (61.83%) had the

Health Service Delivery Area	All students (%)	Males (%)	Females (%)
31 Richmond	80.29	80.76	79.86
33 North Shore/Coast Garibaldi	79.54	78.91	80.11
32 Vancouver	78.93	79.92	78.25
22 Fraser North	75.65	76.00	75.34
41 South Vancouver Island	74.70	75.64	73.85
21 Fraser South/Fraser East	73.77	74.41	73.19
13 Okanagan	69.83	71.60	68.29
42 Central Vancouver Island	67.94	66.38	69.47
12 Kootenay Boundary	66.54	64.14	68.63
43 North Vancouver Island	63.77	66.06	62.00
51 Northwest	62.57	62.28	62.92
14 Thompson Cariboo Shuswap	62.38	62.57	62.30
52 Northern Interior	62.02	61.83	62.12
11 East Kootenay	59.32	63.06	55.98
53 Northeast	N/A	N/A	N/A
British Columbia	**72.33**	**72.73**	**71.98**

† Male rate is significantly different than female rate.
Crosshatched HSDAs are significantly different than the provincial average.
N/A: No data

lowest percentage of students who responded that they were never exposed to tobacco smoke in the home or family vehicle. For female students, North Shore/Coast Garibaldi (80.11%) and East Kootenay (55.98%) had the highest and lowest percentages, respectively. The geographical patterns for both male and female students were the same as those for all students combined, with the urban southwest having significantly higher values than the rest of the province.

Youth who are never exposed to tobacco smoke in their home or family vehicle

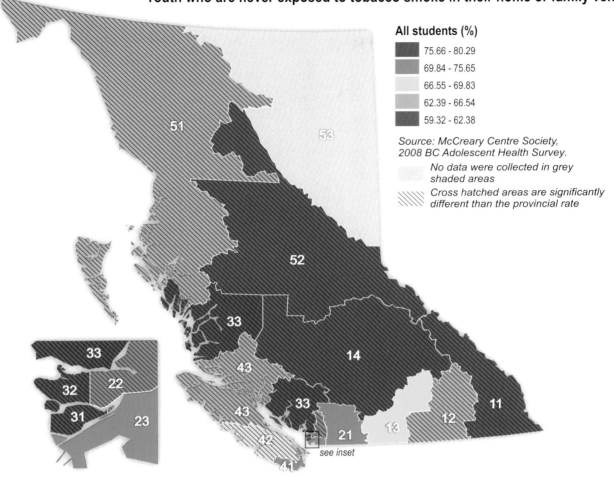

All students (%)

- 75.66 - 80.29
- 69.84 - 75.65
- 66.55 - 69.83
- 62.39 - 66.54
- 59.32 - 62.38

Source: McCreary Centre Society, 2008 BC Adolescent Health Survey.

No data were collected in grey shaded areas

Cross hatched areas are significantly different than the provincial rate

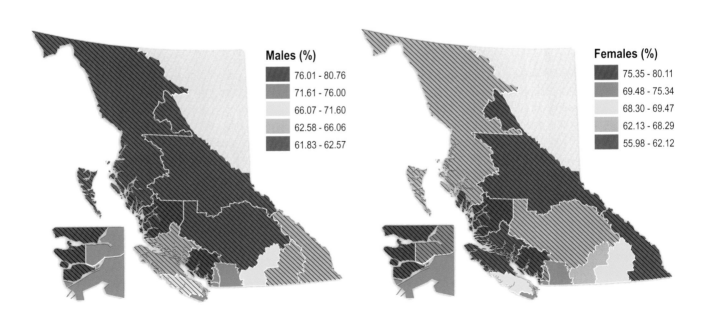

Males (%)

- 76.01 - 80.76
- 71.61 - 76.00
- 66.07 - 71.60
- 62.58 - 66.06
- 61.83 - 62.57

Females (%)

- 75.35 - 80.11
- 69.48 - 75.34
- 68.30 - 69.47
- 62.13 - 68.29
- 55.98 - 62.12

Presently a non-smoker

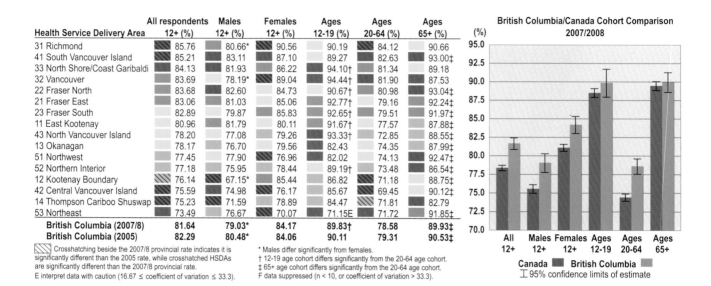

Health Service Delivery Area	All respondents 12+ (%)	Males 12+ (%)	Females 12+ (%)	Ages 12-19 (%)	Ages 20-64 (%)	Ages 65+ (%)
31 Richmond	85.76	80.66*	90.56	90.19	84.12	90.66
41 South Vancouver Island	85.21	83.11	87.10	89.27	82.63	93.00‡
33 North Shore/Coast Garibaldi	84.13	81.93	86.22	94.10†	81.34	89.18
32 Vancouver	83.69	78.19*	89.04	94.44†	81.90	87.53
22 Fraser North	83.68	82.60	84.73	90.67†	80.98	93.04‡
21 Fraser East	83.06	81.03	85.06	92.77†	79.16	92.24‡
23 Fraser South	82.89	79.87	85.83	92.65†	79.51	91.97‡
11 East Kootenay	80.96	81.79	80.11	91.67†	77.57	87.88‡
43 North Vancouver Island	78.20	77.08	79.26	93.33†	72.85	88.55‡
13 Okanagan	78.17	76.70	79.56	82.43	74.35	87.99‡
51 Northwest	77.45	77.90	76.96	82.02	74.13	92.47‡
52 Northern Interior	77.18	75.95	78.44	89.19†	73.48	86.54‡
12 Kootenay Boundary	76.14	67.15*	85.44	86.82	71.18	88.75‡
42 Central Vancouver Island	75.59	74.98	76.17	85.67	69.45	90.12‡
14 Thompson Cariboo Shuswap	75.23	71.59	78.89	84.47	71.81	82.79
53 Northeast	73.49	76.67	70.07	71.15E	71.72	91.85‡
British Columbia (2007/8)	**81.64**	**79.03***	**84.17**	**89.83†**	**78.58**	**89.93‡**
British Columbia (2005)	**82.29**	**80.48***	**84.06**	**90.11**	**79.31**	**90.53‡**

⧅ Crosshatching beside the 2007/8 provincial rate indicates it is significantly different than the 2005 rate, while crosshatched HSDAs are significantly different than the 2007/8 provincial rate.
E interpret data with caution (16.67 ≤ coefficient of variation ≤ 33.3).

* Males differ significantly from females.
† 12-19 age cohort differs significantly from the 20-64 age cohort.
‡ 65+ age cohort differs significantly from the 20-64 age cohort.
F data suppressed (n < 10, or coefficient of variation > 33.3).

Tobacco smoke is related to many major diseases, and smoking is still the single largest cause of preventable death in BC. Being a non-smoker is an important asset for wellness. The CCHS asked participants *"At the present time, do you smoke cigarettes daily, occasionally or not at all?"* More than eight out of ten (81.64%) respondents in BC were presently non-smokers. Richmond (85.76%) and South Vancouver Island (85.21%) had significantly more non-smokers than the provincial average, while Kootenay Boundary, Thompson Cariboo Shuswap, and Central Vancouver Island (all bellow 77%) had significantly fewer non-smokers.

Provincially, there were significantly fewer non-smoking males (79.03%) than females (84.17%). The same trend of significantly fewer non-smoking males was also seen in Kootenay Boundary, Richmond, and Vancouver.

Within the male cohort, Kootenay Boundary and Thompson Cariboo Shuswap were both significantly below the provincial average with 67.15% and 71.59% non-smokers, respectively. Among female respondents, Northeast (70.07%) was significantly below the provincial average for females, along with Central Vancouver Island and Northwest, where approximately 76% of females were non-smokers. In Richmond (90.56%) and Vancouver (89.04%), females were significantly more likely to be non-smokers than the provincial average for all females in BC.

Cohorts for both youth and older respondents had the highest rates for non-smoking in comparison to the mid-age cohort, with significantly high values of 89.83% for youth and 89.93% for older respondents. There were no

HSDAs that showed a significant difference to the provincial average in either the youth or older respondent cohorts. However, when compared to the mid-age cohort, there were notable differences: eight HSDAs had significantly more non-smoking youth and 12 HSDAs had significantly more non-smokers in the oldest cohort.

Geographically, there was a spread of more than 10 percentage points for each of the age cohorts, and the youth cohort showed the largest variation with a spread of 23 percentage points. A clear trend of consistently lower rates of non-smoking was apparent in the northern and interior HSDAs, with the exception of East Kootenay, for all respondents, and two of the northernmost HSDAs for the oldest cohort. The southwest lower mainland, with the exception of older respondents in Vancouver, tended towards higher rates of non-smoking.

There were no significant differences for BC respondents between 2005 and 2007/8. In comparison to the national rates for non-smoking in 2007/8, British Columbians were significantly more likely to be non-smokers. This significant difference was the case for males, females, and the mid-age cohorts. The youngest and oldest cohorts were also more likely to be non-smokers than their peers across Canada, but this difference was not significant.

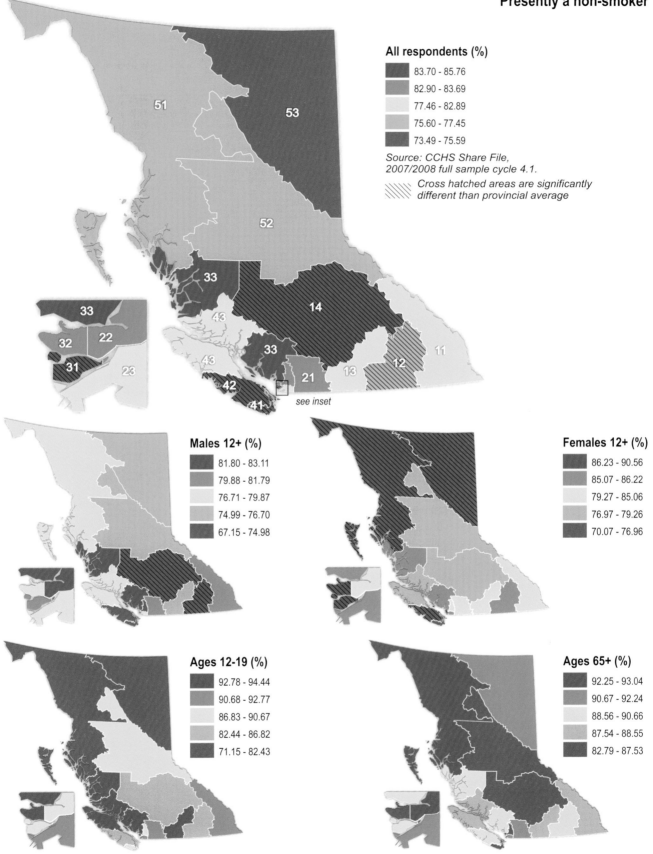

Presently a non-smoker

All respondents (%)

- 83.70 - 85.76
- 82.90 - 83.69
- 77.46 - 82.89
- 75.60 - 77.45
- 73.49 - 75.59

Source: CCHS Share File, 2007/2008 full sample cycle 4.1.

Cross hatched areas are significantly different than provincial average

Males 12+ (%)

- 81.80 - 83.11
- 79.88 - 81.79
- 76.71 - 79.87
- 74.99 - 76.70
- 67.15 - 74.98

Females 12+ (%)

- 86.23 - 90.56
- 85.07 - 86.22
- 79.27 - 85.06
- 76.97 - 79.26
- 70.07 - 76.96

Ages 12-19 (%)

- 92.78 - 94.44
- 90.68 - 92.77
- 86.83 - 90.67
- 82.44 - 86.82
- 71.15 - 82.43

Ages 65+ (%)

- 92.25 - 93.04
- 90.67 - 92.24
- 88.56 - 90.66
- 87.54 - 88.55
- 82.79 - 87.53

Student presently non-smoker

The Student Satisfaction Survey asked grade 7, 10, and 12 students whether they smoked cigarettes "every day," "occasionally," or "not a all." The results provide a more detailed look geographically at responses that were provided in the CCHS 4.1 analysis. This is a new indicator for this Atlas.

All students in grade 7

In 2008/9, 94.94% of student respondents in grade 7 indicated that they were presently non-smokers – one percentage point fewer than in 2007/8. Females (95.8%) were more likely than males (94.2%) to be non-smokers. All students in Central Coast responded that they were non-smokers, while only 88.81% in New Westminster indicated that they were non-smokers. The highest number of non-smoking responses were found in parts of the urban lower mainland, the central southeast, and parts of the northern interior of BC, with outliers in Haida Gwaii and Nisga'a in the northwest and Sooke on Vancouver Island. Relatively low numbers of non-smokers were evident in the central interior, the extreme northwest and southeast, and parts of the southern coastal areas.

All students in grade 10

In 2008/9, 83.87% of grade 10 students indicated they were non-smokers, a marginal increase over 2007/8. Females (84.3%) were again more likely to be non-smokers than males (83.4%). In the Gulf Islands, 91.67% of students responded they were non-smokers, compared with 59.09% in Vancouver Island West. Most of the north and interior had relatively low percentages for non-smokers, with the exception of Bulkley Valley, Okanagan Similkameen, and Okanagan Skaha. By contrast, school districts in the extreme southwest had relatively high percentages of students who did not smoke. On Vancouver Island, there was a wide range with a couple of school districts in the top quintile and one in the lowest quintile.

All students in grade 12

Students in the highest grade had the lowest average non-smoking responses (79.96%) of the three grades. Female students had substantially higher responses (82.1%) of non-smoking when compared to males (77.8%). The 2008/9 provincial average was lower (0.6 of a percentage point) than in 2007/8. Gulf Islands had the highest percentage of non-smokers (88.64%) compared with the lowest percentage (55.88%) for Vancouver Island West. While there were some similarities to the grade 10 pattern, particularly with higher percentages of students in the urban southwest who did not smoke, the rest of the province had a mixture of relatively high and low values, as did Vancouver Island.

School District	All students grade 7 (%)	All students grade 10 (%)	All students grade 12 (%)
49 Central Coast	100.00	71.43	80.00
50 Haida Gwaii/Queen Charlotte	98.21	77.50	63.64
38 Richmond	97.98	87.25	84.96
10 Arrow Lakes	97.67	81.97	84.78
60 Peace River North	97.07	74.42	77.00
19 Revelstoke	96.67	72.46	74.39
34 Abbotsford	96.60	85.29	81.54
62 Sooke	96.30	75.47	76.45
91 Nechako Lakes	96.21	72.77	66.67
36 Surrey	96.13	85.33	83.07
51 Boundary	96.08	71.43	61.90
84 Vancouver Island West	96.00	59.09	55.88
41 Burnaby	95.98	87.34	80.97
37 Delta	95.96	86.01	80.29
43 Coquitlam	95.95	88.14	85.68
42 Maple Ridge-Pitt Meadows	95.78	84.28	78.13
48 Howe Sound	95.64	77.51	80.34
83 North Okanagan-Shuswap	95.57	75.38	77.95
85 Vancouver Island North	95.54	78.26	74.07
67 Okanagan Skaha	95.48	84.88	75.67
71 Comox Valley	95.20	86.99	75.34
45 West Vancouver	95.16	88.41	84.01
72 Campbell River	95.06	85.63	74.57
75 Mission	95.02	78.71	74.12
47 Powell River	95.00	82.72	80.75
8 Kootenay Lake	94.95	78.31	78.48
74 Gold Trail	94.79	72.00	76.00
73 Kamloops/Thompson	94.78	77.54	72.14
59 Peace River South	94.74	77.60	77.33
58 Nicola-Similkameen	94.71	78.40	69.63
33 Chilliwack	94.68	86.77	78.25
79 Cowichan Valley	94.58	85.41	82.11
63 Saanich	94.57	84.73	76.65
6 Rocky Mountain	94.55	79.08	63.64
82 Coast Mountains	94.49	81.48	72.43
81 Fort Nelson	94.44	72.55	80.00
22 Vernon	94.44	78.00	78.21
39 Vancouver	94.34	89.27	85.28
68 Nanaimo-Ladysmith	94.27	78.09	74.30
61 Greater Victoria	94.19	83.43	79.38
35 Langley	94.13	85.87	79.21
52 Prince Rupert	93.98	74.74	74.39
54 Bulkley Valley	93.96	86.19	80.26
23 Central Okanagan	93.88	80.08	80.47
20 Kootenay-Columbia	93.49	80.41	72.64
44 North Vancouver	93.46	83.46	83.09
28 Quesnel	93.44	79.59	75.00
27 Cariboo-Chilcotin	93.26	81.48	78.54
46 Sunshine Coast	93.13	83.24	76.24
70 Alberni	92.41	80.56	77.88
5 Southeast Kootenay	92.35	79.25	74.61
53 Okanagan Similkameen	91.71	83.97	84.25
57 Prince George	91.64	82.81	74.09
69 Qualicum	91.13	84.59	82.86
78 Fraser-Cascade	90.37	86.84	79.59
64 Gulf Islands	90.32	91.67	88.64
40 New Westminster	88.81	80.05	79.26
87 Stikine	Msk	Msk	Msk
92 Nisga'a	Msk	Msk	Msk
British Columbia	**94.94**	**83.87**	**79.96**

Msk: Data masked for privacy

Student presently non-smoker

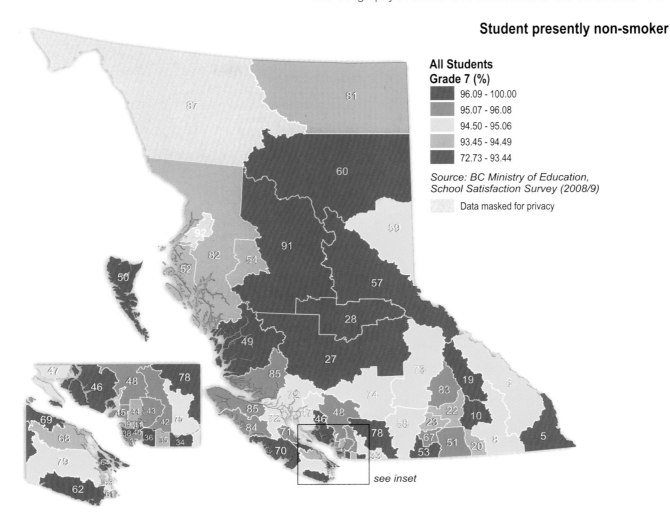

**All Students
Grade 7 (%)**

- 96.09 - 100.00
- 95.07 - 96.08
- 94.50 - 95.06
- 93.45 - 94.49
- 72.73 - 93.44

*Source: BC Ministry of Education,
School Satisfaction Survey (2008/9)*

Data masked for privacy

see inset

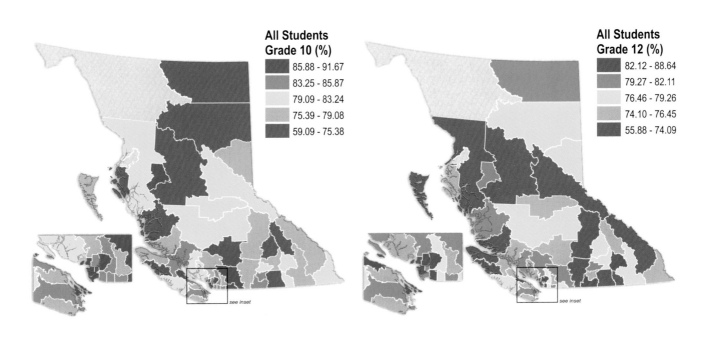

**All Students
Grade 10 (%)**

- 85.88 - 91.67
- 83.25 - 85.87
- 79.09 - 83.24
- 75.39 - 79.08
- 59.09 - 75.38

see inset

**All Students
Grade 12 (%)**

- 82.12 - 88.64
- 79.27 - 82.11
- 76.46 - 79.26
- 74.10 - 76.45
- 55.88 - 74.09

see inset

BC Healthy Living Alliance tobacco cessation initiatives

BCHLA produced the *Tobacco Reduction Strategy* (BCHLA, 2007d) in order to help guide tobacco reduction initiatives. This was funded as part of the $25.2 million grant provided by the Ministry of Health in 2005. It outlined a number of tobacco reduction initiatives based on best and emerging 'promising practices.' Research evidence indicated that the best group for the programs to target was young adults aged between 19 and 29 years. This would not only target the group with the highest rate of smoking in BC (those aged 20 to 24 years), but it would also help to address the significant gap in tobacco control in the province for that age group.

The objectives set out were to prevent youth and adults from starting to use tobacco, to encourage and assist tobacco users to quit their use of tobacco products, and to protect British Columbians from second-hand smoke.

These five tobacco reduction initiatives were chosen:

1. Tobacco-free Workplaces, led by the Canadian Cancer Society, BC and Yukon Division, which supported employees at 59 worksites to quit smoking.

2. Tobacco-free Post-secondary Institutions, led by the BC Lung Association, which established tobacco cessation programs in 10 post-secondary institutions and technical schools, and worked with these education establishments to develop and implement tobacco-free campus policies.

3. Smoke-free Housing, led by the Heart and Stroke Foundation, BC and Yukon, which produced a toolkit outlining how to implement smoke-free policies in multi-unit dwellings, and educating and engaging 8,200 housing providers to introduce smoke-free policies.

4. Community Detailing, led by the BC Lung Association, which partnered with over 1,000 businesses through the use of a marketing technique known as 'detailing' to promote smoking cessation information.

5. Targeted Education, led by the Heart and Stroke Foundation, BC and Yukon, which worked with professors on nine campuses to challenge students in senior level marketing classes to design a multi-media tobacco education campaign that was later developed and launched in 10 BC communities.

Community	Community
1 Abbotsford	19 Penticton
2 Aldergrove	20 Prince George
3 Burnaby	21 Quesnel
4 Campbell River	22 Radium
5 Castlegar	23 Richmond
6 Chilliwack	24 Salmon Arm
7 Cloverdale	25 Summerland
8 Courtenay	26 Surrey
9 Cranbrook	27 Terrace
10 Dawson Creek	28 Trail
11 Fort St. John	29 Tsawwassen
12 Kamloops	30 Vancouver
13 Kelowna	31 Vernon
14 Langley	32 Victoria
15 Nanaimo	33 West Vancouver
16 Nelson	34 Westbank
17 New Westminster	35 White Rock
18 North Vancouver	36 Williams Lake

The table and adjacent map show the reach throughout the province of the tobacco reduction initiatives, which took place from 2007 until 2010, when funding ran out. Programs were initiated in nearly 40 communities throughout the province.

BC Healthy Living Alliance tobacco cessation initiatives

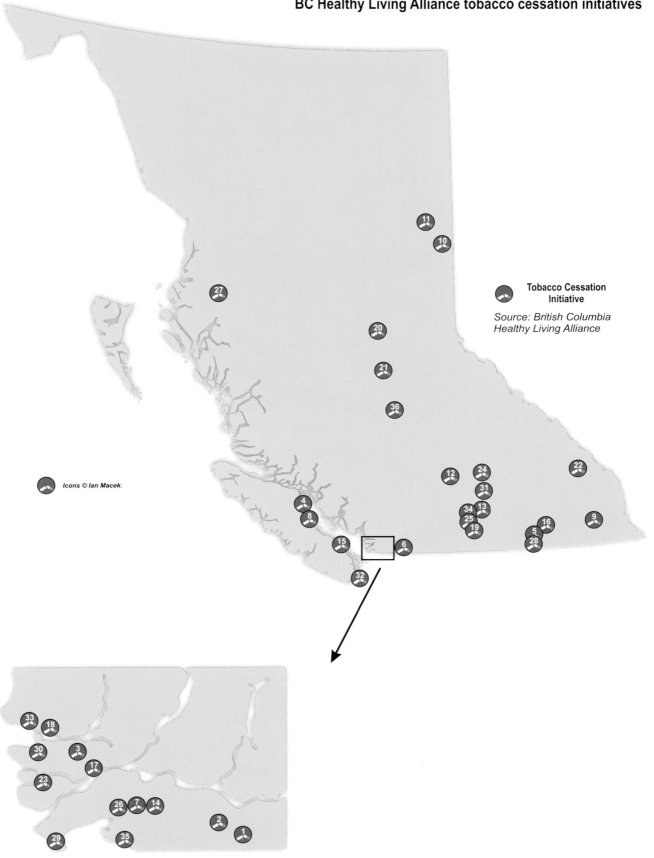

Tobacco Cessation
Initiative

*Source: British Columbia
Healthy Living Alliance*

Icons © Ian Macek.

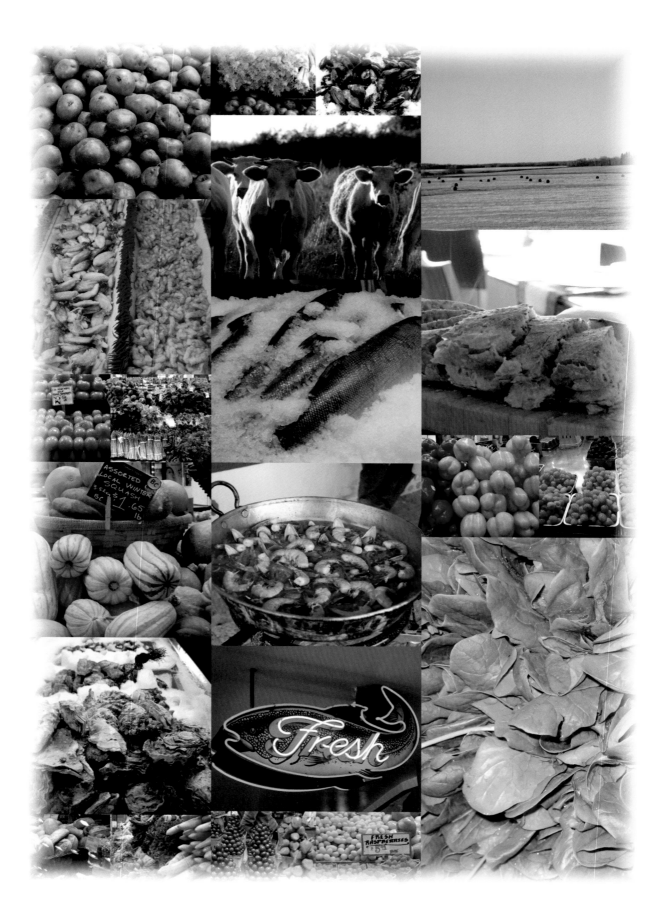

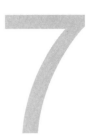

The Geography of Food Security and Nutrition

Introduction

Healthy, nutritious food is fundamental to wellness. The food we eat "defines, to a great extent, our health, growth, and development, and ability to function well in a complex world. Poor nutrition, especially low fruit and vegetable intake, is related to some of the leading risks of chronic diseases in developed nations: high blood pressure, cholesterol, overweight (obesity), and diabetes" (WHO, 2000; Sorhaindo & Feinstein, 2006).

"Eating a variety of nutrient-rich, high quality foods with the right proportions of fat, protein, carbohydrates, fibre, vitamins, minerals, and other dietary constituents provides our bodies with what they need for optimal growth and development" (Kendall, 2006, p. 1). A healthy diet promotes positive physical and psychological development and maintenance through every stage of the life course. It helps to build the body's resilience to illness and reduces the risk of developing chronic diseases.

Food security is viewed as a key determinant of health (Ostry, 2010a), and in BC is regarded as a core public health function (Pederson, 2006). According to Bellows and Hamm (2003): "Community food security exists when all citizens obtain a safe, personally acceptable, nutritional diet through a sustainable food system that maximizes healthy choices, community self-reliance, and equal access for everyone. This definition implies:

- The ability to acquire food is assured;

- Food is obtained in a manner that upholds human dignity;

- Food is safe, nutritionally adequate, and personally and culturally acceptable;

- Food is sufficient in quality and quantity to sustain healthy growth and development, and to prevent illness and disease; and

- Food is produced, processed, and distributed in a manner that does not compromise the land, air, or water for future generations" (Food Security Standing Committee, 2004).

The UN Food and Agriculture Organization (FAO) defines food security as existing "when all people, at all times, have physical and economic access to sufficient, safe, and nutritious food to meet their dietary needs and food preferences for an active and healthy life" (FAO, 1996). The BC Ministry of Health has adopted this broad approach to food security and encourages "local, provincial, and national policies to support local food systems" (Pederson, 2006). Nevertheless, food banks in BC served nearly 95,000 individuals in March 2010, an increase of 5% compared with the same month in the previous year (Kravitz, 2010). Relative to the US, Canada still does well when it comes to household food security (Nord & Hopwood, 2008).

Today, public interest in nutrition and food security (ranging from worries broadly about the sustainability and safety of systems of agricultural production to the desire for information on the links between vitamin intake and specific diseases) is very high (Ostry, 2006). With growing concerns about a host of food security issues that have emerged in the past decade (e.g., "mad cow" disease cases in Western Canada and bird flu, both with major potential for adverse health and economic impacts), and with increasing publicity and concern about an obesity epidemic, especially among children, government and regional health authorities have also begun to pay attention to food security (Rideout & Ostry, 2006). There is also increasing interest in food security issues in relation to climatic change (Ostry, 2010b) and, as we noted in the first Atlas, precipitation and temperature have shown important changes in the last decade or so that may impact food production in BC.

There is growing concern about increasing food prices, not only in BC but worldwide (Royal Bank of Canada, 2011). High food prices are becoming the most significant barrier to healthy eating and, because of fairly high levels of income inequality in BC (see Chapter 5), contribute to regional variation in food security across BC (Dieticians of Canada & Community Nutritionists Council of BC, 2009). Within BC, because there are many small and remote communities, access to inexpensive and fresh fruits and vegetables is a major problem. In 2009, the Produce Availability in Remote Communities Initiative was introduced to help deal with these issues. Initiatives included the development of community gardens in First Nations communities, and sustainable programs that addressed barriers to vegetable and fruit availability in other remote communities (Ministry of Agriculture and Lands & Ministry of Healthy Living and Sports, 2009).

Substantial modifications and expansions have been made to this section of the Atlas compared with the first edition. Based on the 2007 revised school guidelines, foods sold in the "Not Recommended" and "Choose Least" categories were eliminated from all elementary schools by January 2008, and from middle and secondary schools by September 2008 (Ministry of Education & Ministry of Healthy Living and Sport, 2010). This policy change obviated the need and utility of mapping variability in school nutrition policies in this current edition.

In this edition, we have added indicators related to the food production and food safety system as these are fundamental to food security. In addition, an indicator on alcohol consumption has been added, along with several indicators related to food content. The revised scope and expansion in the number of indicators and maps reflect recent policy changes in the province, as well as growing interest in issues of nutrition and food security as it affects health and wellness.

A suite of 85 maps for food security and nutrition has been selected, and these illustrate how nutrition and food security vary across the province. Many indicators provide patterns by gender and for different age cohorts. What follows is the presentation of maps that describe select indicators of nutrition and food security for much of BC's population. They have been divided into four major groups for description purposes, although there is overlap between the groups.

Food production, potential and safety

The first group of 18 maps provides a variety of indicators related to food production and safety and uses information from a variety of sources, particularly the 2006 Agricultural Census. Census-based maps follow the BC Regional

Districts administrative boundaries. The first three maps provide information on key climatic factors, such as growing degree days and key frost indicators. This is followed by information on the allocation of Agricultural Land Reserve (ALR), lands specifically set aside for farming, and the distribution and size of farms. The relationship between settlement patterns and the need for suitable land for growing food has resulted in major settlements being built on the best agricultural land in BC (Smith, 1998; Katz, 2009) and, as noted in Chapter 4, this settlement is highly concentrated. Only about 1% of soils in BC have the highest capability for growing crops, and most of that is in the lower mainland, southern part of Vancouver Island, and Okanagan Valley (SmartGrowth BC, nd). In total, BC has only about 1.4% of Canada's "dependable" agricultural land as defined by the Canada Land Inventory (Hofmann et al., 2005).

The next indicator considered in this group of maps provides information on the three major types of farming undertaken in each Regional District. These are followed by six maps that provide information on greenhouse and organic farming. The final map in this group illustrates the location of meat processing plants throughout BC. Overall, BC farmers produced just less than half (48%) of all foods consumed in the province in 2001, but only one-third of the recommended consumption by Canada's *Food Guide to Healthy Eating* (as referenced in Ministry of Agriculture and Lands, 2006). By 2008, the proportion of food imported was 45% (Ostry, 2010a).

Food security

The second group of maps is based on survey information, and describes several features of food security. In total, there are 18 maps in this section. The first three maps of this group are based on information from McCreary AHS IV, and provide information on students who were never hungry when going to bed. The next 15 maps are based on data from CCHS 4.1. These describe survey responses to questions on food access, preference, and affordability. A derived variable of overall food security is provided, developed by Statistics Canada from CCHS 4.1 responses to a large number of questions (Statistics Canada, nd). Age and gender differences are mapped at the HSDA level for all CCHS 4.1 responses.

The next five maps are focused on alcohol consumption, which has been shown to have certain benefits for cardiovascular health, and researchers have concluded that moderate alcohol intake is not only associated with a reduced risk of heart disease, but may actually improve heart health (Ronksley et al., 2011; Brien et al., 2011). Moderate intake of wine as part of the so-called

"Mediterranean diet" is an important dimension of the diet's healthy effects (Trichopoulou et al., 2009). However, while some research shows healthful effects of moderate alcohol consumption, there is still a debate about the impact of various kinds and amounts of alcohol on health. There are clearly many harmful effects (Kendall, 2008b), and daily drinkers may also become heavy drinkers. Alcohol consumption can be addictive, and there are many studies showing a link between heavy consumption and certain cancers. What most researchers agree on is that binge drinking, viewed as five alcoholic drinks or more at a session, is unhealthy. Our map on this topic focuses on those who do not binge drink, thus taking a wellness approach to this issue. Maps show variations at the HSDA level for gender and different age cohorts.

Food content and consumption

The next group of 46 maps provides data related to food content and consumption patterns. Most of the data are from CCHS 4.1, though several of the indicators are from McCreary AHS IV. All are at the HSDA level. Some of the maps provide information on the extent to which respondents choose or avoid certain food based on their knowledge of its salt, caloric, fat, or cholesterol content, while others focus on students' consumption of fruits and vegetables and their breakfast habits, on school days. The high levels of consumption of salt by Canadians has been recognized as a major health concern (Sodium Working Group, 2010). In addition, breakfast on school days is essential to health and a nutritious breakfast is important for learning (Murphy, 2007). Yet the most recent published survey of child nutrition habits across Canada, by Breakfast for Learning (2007), indicated that only about 50% of children had the minimum daily servings of fruits and vegetables, and many skip breakfast unless it is made for them.

Community food outlets and healthy eating programs

In keeping with our desire to move to a broader framing of nutrition and food security, we provide three maps of the location, size, and distribution of farmers markets, community gardens, and initiatives implemented by BCHLA to support ActNow BC.

Farmers markets are scattered throughout the province. These are outlets where local farmers sell their produce directly to consumers. The development of farmers markets may be important in establishing more direct contact between producers and consumers. Direct access to consumers for farmers may lower their costs and make their operations more viable, and increase opportunities

for basic public education about food production in BC.

Community gardens have been growing in importance, especially in urban areas. They provide an opportunity for individuals to grow their own food, socialize with others, trade produce, and learn more about growing food close to home. The establishment of these public gardens has grown over the past few years, as has urban farming, and using waste land, such as roof tops, to grow food for local consumption.

The final map shows where the BCHLA has focused its efforts to encourage healthy eating throughout BC (BCHLA, 2007b; 2010).

Growing season

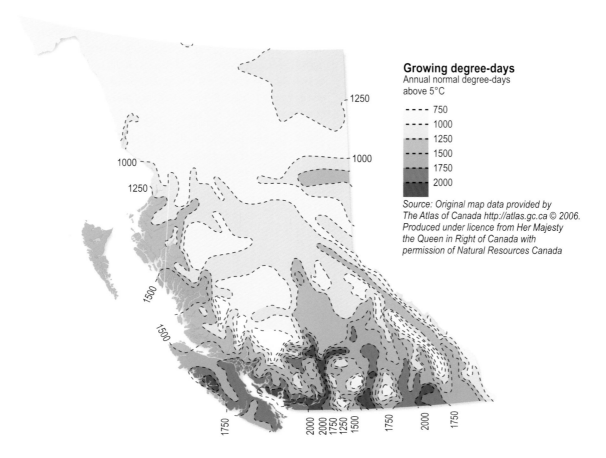

Growing degree-days
Annual normal degree-days
above 5°C

- - - - 750
- - - - 1000
- - - - 1250
- - - - 1500
- - - - 1750
- - - - 2000

*Source: Original map data provided by
The Atlas of Canada http://atlas.gc.ca © 2006.
Produced under licence from Her Majesty
the Queen in Right of Canada with
permission of Natural Resources Canada*

Crops need a certain amount of energy in order to thrive, otherwise growth and development will cease. Researchers have determined that air temperature is a dominant factor in determining crop development (Yang et al., 1995). Also, frosts can ruin crops that are in the ground. The three maps presented here are closely related, and important in determining crop planting, production, and harvesting. The first map shows growing degree-days, which is the annual sum of normal degree-days above 5°C in the growing season (Natural Resources Canada, 2006). The two maps opposite show the average date of the last frost in spring and the average date of the first frost in autumn. The data are based on averages for the 1941 to 1970 period, so they will have changed somewhat due to recently recorded climate changes. These indicators are new to the Atlas.

Not surprisingly, the three maps have very similar patterns. A higher number of growing degree-days is more common in the southwest of the province and the southern Fraser, central Okanagan, and eastern Columbia valleys, which have around 2,000 degree-days or more, while much of

the north has 1,000 or less growing degree-days. The last frost in spring occurs in April on the west coast and lower Fraser Valley, and as late as June in parts of the north and eastern sections of the province. The first frost in autumn occurs as late as November along the west coast and as early as September throughout the north, east, and higher elevation areas in central BC. Steep gradients or changes tend to run southwest to northeast, with earlier and later frosts occurring in the east and north.

Growing season

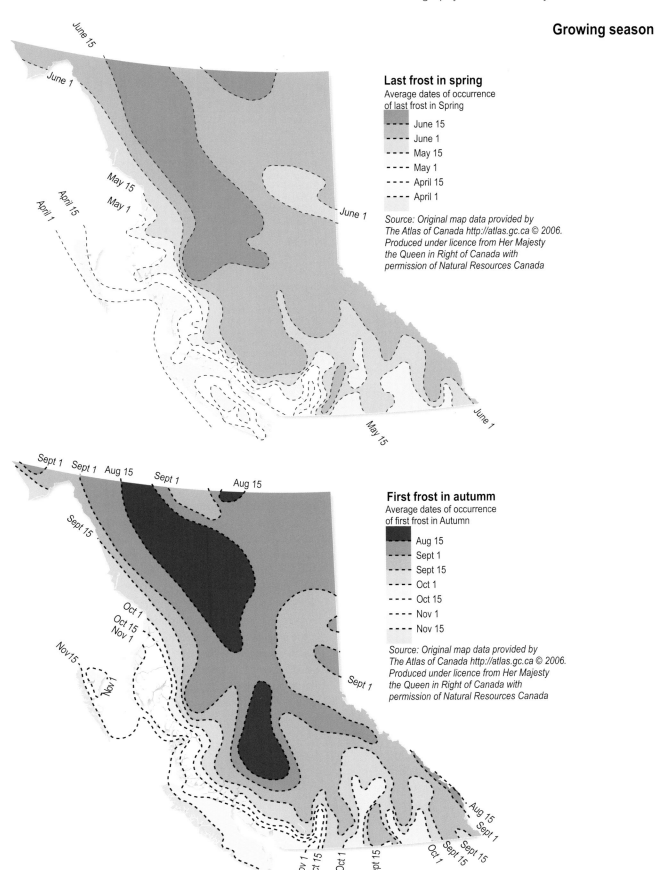

Last frost in spring
Average dates of occurrence
of last frost in Spring

- - - - June 15
- - - - June 1
- - - - May 15
- - - - May 1
- - - - April 15
- - - - April 1

*Source: Original map data provided by
The Atlas of Canada http://atlas.gc.ca © 2006.
Produced under licence from Her Majesty
the Queen in Right of Canada with
permission of Natural Resources Canada*

First frost in autumm
Average dates of occurrence
of first frost in Autumn

- - - - Aug 15
- - - - Sept 1
- - - - Sept 15
- - - - Oct 1
- - - - Oct 15
- - - - Nov 1
- - - - Nov 15

*Source: Original map data provided by
The Atlas of Canada http://atlas.gc.ca © 2006.
Produced under licence from Her Majesty
the Queen in Right of Canada with
permission of Natural Resources Canada*

Farming resources

Food security includes measures of farming resources and the assets that help to make up that security. Three measures are included in the table and maps opposite, which provide information at the regional district level. The first looks at the land put aside in the Agricultural Land Reserve (ALR), in which agriculture is recognized as the priority use and farming is encouraged, and non-agricultural uses are controlled (Agricultural Land Commission, 2009). These lands were established in 1974 with approximately 4,700,000 hectares. Over the years, nearly 140,000 hectares have been removed and just over 180,000 have been added. The ALR provides about half of BC's food production (Ostry, 2010a). The second measure shows where the province's farms are concentrated, while the third provides the average size of farms in each regional district.

ALR as percent of region's land

Just over 5% of the province was in the ALR in 2009 and protected primarily for farming. Greater Vancouver had the highest percentage (17.82%) of its land protected this way, followed by Comox Valley, Thompson-Nicola, Peace River, and Cariboo, all with more than 10% of the regional districts protected in the ALR. At the other extreme, Kitimat-Stikine, Northern Rockies, Central Coast, Mount Waddington, and Stikine had much less than 1% of their land so protected. Geographically, the north, northwestern, and north and central coastal parts of the province have relatively little land in the ALR, while much of the interior, including the Peace River, have above average allocations.

Percent of province's farms

Based on the 2006 Census of Agricultural Profiles, BC had a total of almost 20,000 farms (8.7% of all farms in Canada). The highest percentage of farms was found in the southwest of the province. Greater Vancouver and Fraser Valley each had approximately 13% of the province's farms, with the next in importance being Peace River (8.56%). Seven regional districts had well below 1% of BC's farms in their regions, while East Kootenay and Kootenay Boundary each had about 2% of the farms in BC. Overall geographical patterns were somewhat similar to those for the ALR.

Average size of farms

The average farm size in BC was 142.89 hectares, almost twice the average size of Canadian farms as a whole.

Regional District	Percent in ALR	Farms (% of total)	Average size (ha)
15 Greater Vancouver	17.82	13.19	15.67
25 Comox Valley	12.99	2.50	25.93
33 Thompson-Nicola	12.51	6.10	399.15
55 Peace River	12.38	8.56	521.18
41 Cariboo	11.13	5.85	419.03
1 East Kootenay	9.62	1.99	247.25
35 Central Okanagan	9.05	5.12	26.75
21 Nanaimo	8.87	2.32	17.97
37 North Okanagan	8.25	6.18	62.45
7 Okanagan-Similkameen	7.60	8.17	52.59
53 Fraser-Fort George	7.32	3.13	173.88
17 Capital	6.95	4.99	13.69
5 Kootenay Boundary	6.44	1.98	135.87
9 Fraser Valley	5.15	12.94	22.05
19 Cowichan Valley	5.05	3.53	16.51
51 Bulkley-Nechako	4.71	4.46	307.55
3 Central Kootenay	2.74	2.83	48.64
47 Skeena-Queen Charlotte	2.20	N/A	N/A
27 Powell River	1.81	0.43	19.08
39 Columbia-Shuswap	1.69	3.14	66.58
31 Squamish-Lillooet	1.51	0.65	151.82
23 Alberni-Clayoquot	1.12	0.45	35.63
29 Sunshine Coast	1.06	0.48	9.03
26 Strathcona	1.02	2.50	25.93
49 Kitimat-Stikine	0.62	0.68	88.86
59 Northern Rockies	0.52	0.15	247.27
45 Central Coast	0.18	0.16	83.72
43 Mount Waddington	0.08	N/A	N/A
57 Stikine	0.00	N/A	N/A
British Columbia	**5.05**	**100.00**	**142.89**

N/A: No data

Four regional districts in BC had an average farm size in excess of 300 hectares, based on the 2006 census. These were (units in hectares): Peace River (521.18); Cariboo (419.03); Thompson-Nicola (399.15); and Bulkley-Nechako (307.55). At the other extreme, the smallest average farm sizes were in Sunshine Coast (9.03), Capital (13.69), Greater Vancouver (15.67), Cowichan Valley (16.51), Nanaimo (17.97), and Powell River (19.08). Geographically, the smallest average farms were clustered in the southwest of the province, including Vancouver Island, while the largest ones were found in the northern two-thirds of BC. Some caution is required in interpreting the patterns based on the 2006 census because data were not available for three regional districts.

Farming resources

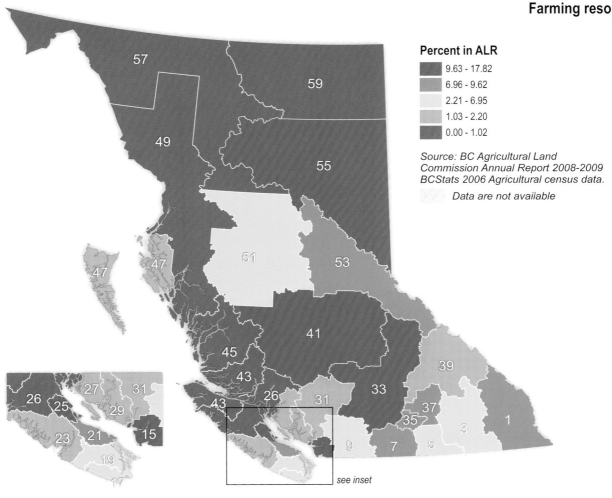

Percent in ALR

- 9.63 - 17.82
- 6.96 - 9.62
- 2.21 - 6.95
- 1.03 - 2.20
- 0.00 - 1.02

Source: BC Agricultural Land Commission Annual Report 2008-2009 BCStats 2006 Agricultural census data.

Data are not available

see inset

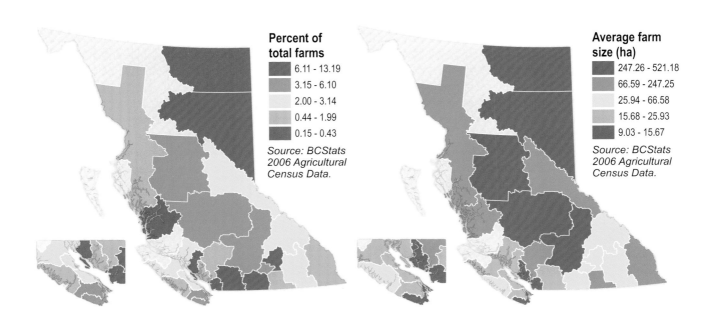

Percent of total farms

- 6.11 - 13.19
- 3.15 - 6.10
- 2.00 - 3.14
- 0.44 - 1.99
- 0.15 - 0.43

Source: BCStats 2006 Agricultural Census Data.

Average farm size (ha)

- 247.26 - 521.18
- 66.59 - 247.25
- 25.94 - 66.58
- 15.68 - 25.93
- 9.03 - 15.67

Source: BCStats 2006 Agricultural Census Data.

Distribution of farms by farm size

The province has a large variety of farm types and sizes. By way of background, according to the 2006 agriculture census, there were nearly 20,000 farms in the province with an average size of just over 350 acres. In total, the census indicated that more than 7,000,000 acres were in farming of one type or another. While the total gross annual revenue generated in 2005 was over $2.6 billion, just under half of all farms had total annual gross receipts of less than $10,000, while less than 6% generated gross annual revenue of over $500,000.

Percent of farms less than 10 acres

In total, more than 5,300 farms, or just over one quarter (26.88%) of all BC farms, had a size of less than 10 acres. Geographically, the regions with the highest percentage of smaller farms of this nature occurred in the southwest corner of the province, particularly in the lower mainland, southern and eastern parts of Vancouver Island, and parts of the Okanagan in the southern interior. These were all clustered in and around the major population sections of the province. Of particular note, Sunshine Coast had over two thirds (67.71%) of its farms in this size category, while more than half of the farms in Capital fell into this category. Greater Vancouver, Nanaimo, Cowichan Valley, Okanagan-Similkameen, Central Okanagan, and Fraser Valley all had more than one third of their farms in this size category. At the other extreme, Peace River, Bulkley-Nechako, Cariboo, and Fraser-Fort George had less than 10% of their farms in this smallest category.

Percent of farms 10 to 69 acres

This is the most common farm size category in BC, including just over 7,250 farms (36.54%). While there are some similarities in geographical patterns with those in the smallest farm category, more than half of the farms in Central Okanagan (53.98%) and Okanagan-Similkameen (51.39%), and more than 45% of farms in Central Kootenay, Cowichan Valley, Fraser Valley, Powell River, Comox Valley, Strathcona, and North Okanagan fell into this size category. Again, the more northern and central interior regions of the province had one quarter or less of their farms in this category.

Percent of farms 70 to 239 acres

Only about 3,600 farms (18.01%) in the province were in this size category. Geographically, as might be expected, patterns were reversed from those evident in the two smaller size categories. Those regions with the greatest

Regional District	< 10 acres (%)	10 - 69 acres (%)	70 - 239 acres (%)	240+ acres (%)
29 Sunshine Coast	67.71	23.96	6.25	2.08
17 Capital	51.56	38.95	6.96	2.52
15 Greater Vancouver	46.98	40.95	9.28	2.79
21 Nanaimo	39.70	42.30	13.88	4.12
19 Cowichan Valley	37.43	47.14	12.29	3.14
7 Okanagan-Similkameen	37.20	51.39	5.68	5.74
35 Central Okanagan	36.48	53.98	6.78	2.75
9 Fraser Valley	33.81	46.32	16.52	3.35
27 Powell River	32.94	47.06	16.47	3.53
25 Comox Valley	31.79	46.08	17.30	4.83
26 Strathcona	31.79	46.08	17.30	4.83
23 Alberni-Clayoquot	26.97	43.82	19.10	10.11
5 Kootenay Boundary	24.23	32.40	19.64	23.72
3 Central Kootenay	23.84	47.69	17.79	10.68
37 North Okanagan	23.06	46.13	19.23	11.57
45 Central Coast	18.75	31.25	31.25	18.75
49 Kitimat-Stikine	17.16	34.33	25.37	23.13
31 Squamish-Lillooet	15.50	40.31	24.03	20.16
39 Columbia-Shuswap	15.22	43.91	28.21	12.66
1 East Kootenay	13.92	25.06	24.56	36.46
59 Northern Rockies	13.33	16.67	20.00	50.00
33 Thompson-Nicola	12.30	32.29	25.76	29.64
53 Fraser-Fort George	7.25	20.13	33.17	39.45
41 Cariboo	4.83	18.88	31.38	44.91
51 Bulkley-Nechako	4.40	10.61	32.62	52.37
55 Peace River	1.65	5.30	27.43	65.63
43 Mount Waddington	N/A	N/A	N/A	N/A
47 Skeena-Queen Charlotte	N/A	N/A	N/A	N/A
57 Stikine	N/A	N/A	N/A	N/A
British Columbia	26.88	36.54	18.01	18.56

N/A: No data

percentage of their farms in this mid-size category were found away from the main population areas, and were mainly in the northern and central interior parts of the province. Four regional districts – Fraser Fort-George, Bulkley-Nechako, Cariboo, and Central Coast – had more than 30% of their farms in this size category.

Percent of farms 240 or more acres

Nearly 3,700 farms (18.56%) fell into this largest size category, and the geographical distribution was quite similar to that for the 70 to 239 acre group. The areas with the largest percentage of their farms in this category were distant from the higher population density parts of the southwest parts of the province. Peace River, Bulkley-Nechako, and Northern Rockies all had half or more of their farms in this highest acreage category. As might be expected, at the other extreme, Sunshine Coast, Capital, Central Okanagan, and Greater Vancouver had less than 3% of their farms in this size category.

Distribution of farms by farm size

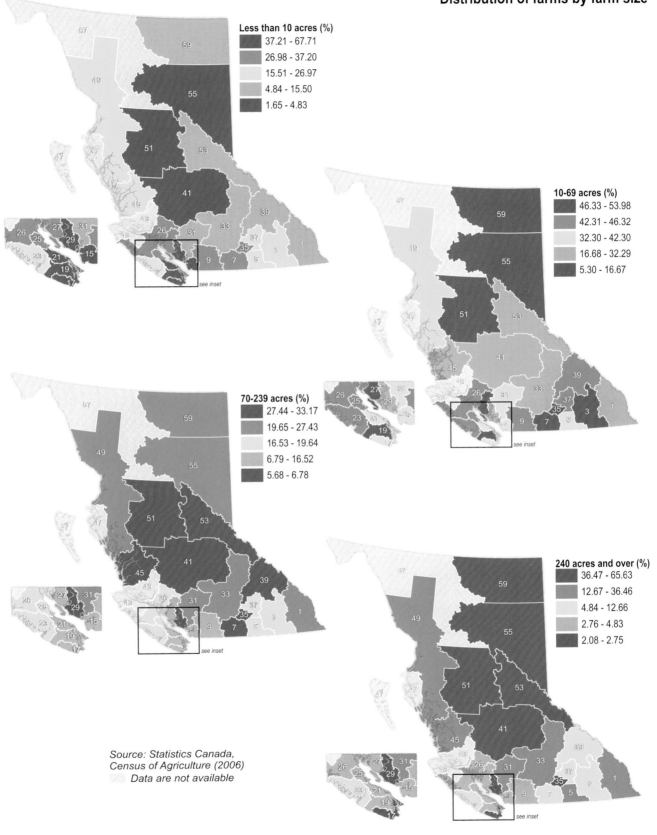

Less than 10 acres (%)
- 37.21 - 67.71
- 26.98 - 37.20
- 15.51 - 26.97
- 4.84 - 15.50
- 1.65 - 4.83

10-69 acres (%)
- 46.33 - 53.98
- 42.31 - 46.32
- 32.30 - 42.30
- 16.68 - 32.29
- 5.30 - 16.67

70-239 acres (%)
- 27.44 - 33.17
- 19.65 - 27.43
- 16.53 - 19.64
- 6.79 - 16.52
- 5.68 - 6.78

240 acres and over (%)
- 36.47 - 65.63
- 12.67 - 36.46
- 4.84 - 12.66
- 2.76 - 4.83
- 2.08 - 2.75

Source: Statistics Canada,
Census of Agriculture (2006)
Data are not available

Predominant farm types

Farm production in BC is an important indicator of food security, and local food production is a key component of food security (Ostry, 2010a). In 1946, BC imported only 3% of its food requirements, and this rose to 60% in the 1970s and is currently at about 45%. Ostry (2010a) has noted that "Dairy is the most 'local' food industry in the province. That is, most dairy products are produced in BC and import and export markets are small. A somewhat similar pattern exists for live animals and meats. In contrast, fishing has dynamic imports, exports and within BC production. Vegetables, fruits and nuts lie between these extremes" (p. 20).

The table and map opposite provide information on the top dominant farming types in each regional district, based on the 2006 agricultural census. The top three types of farming, based on the number of farms in each district, are included here. This is a new indicator for this Atlas.

More than one-fifth (21.05%) of all farms in BC were involved in beef cattle ranching and farming, including feedlots, while 16.11% of farms were involved in fruit and tree nut farming, 15.14% in horse and other equine production, and 10.22% in hay farming. Among the 26 regional districts for which data were available, all had at least two of these top four as their predominant farming types, while 17 had three of these as their predominant farming types.

Fraser Valley had dairy cattle and milk production as a dominant farming type, along with nursery and tree production, while Greater Vancouver, Capital, Nanaimo, and Sunshine Coast also had nursery and tree production as one of their top three farming types. Alberni-Clayquot, Powell River, and Northern Rockies had livestock combo farming as a dominant type, while Central Coast had fruit and vegetable farming as a dominant type.

For Canada as a whole, the key farming types in order of importance, based on the number of farms involved, are beef cattle ranching and farming, including feedlots, followed by grain farming, hay farming, oilseed farming, and horse and other equine production.

Predominant farm types

1	Beef cattle ranching and farming, including feedlots	5	Nursery and tree production
2	Fruit and tree nut farming	6	Livestock combo farming
3	Horse and other equine production	7	Dairy cattle and milk production
4	Hay farming	8	Fruit and vegetable combo farming

Regional District		Farm type
1	East Kootenay	134
3	Central Kootenay	124
5	Kootenay Boundary	134
7	Okanagan-Similkameen	231
9	Fraser Valley	275
15	Greater Vancouver	325
17	Capital	235
19	Cowichan Valley	312
21	Nanaimo	135
23	Alberni-Clayoquot	136
25	Comox Valley	132
26	Strathcona	132
27	Powell River	261
29	Sunshine Coast	523
31	Squamish-Lillooet	134
33	Thompson-Nicola	134
35	Central Okanagan	234
37	North Okanagan	134
39	Columbia-Shuswap	134
41	Cariboo	134
43	Mount Waddington	N/A: No Data
45	Central Coast	183
47	Skeena-Queen Charlotte	N/A: No Data
49	Kitimat-Stikine	134
51	Bulkley-Nechako	143
53	Fraser-Fort George	143
55	Peace River	143
57	Stikine	N/A: No Data
59	Northern Rockies	436
British Columbia		**123**

Predominant farm types

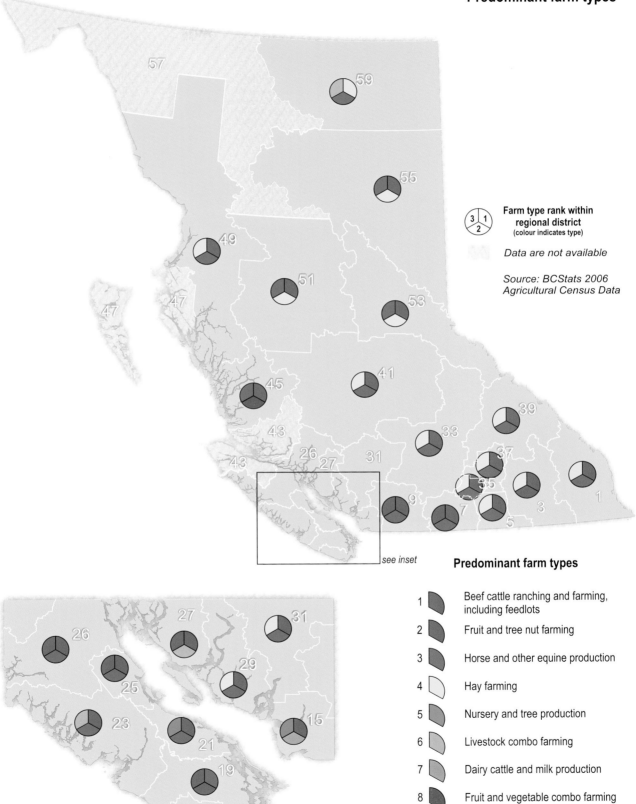

Farm type rank within
regional district
(colour indicates type)

Data are not available

*Source: BCStats 2006
Agricultural Census Data*

Predominant farm types

1   Beef cattle ranching and farming, including feedlots

2   Fruit and tree nut farming

3   Horse and other equine production

4   Hay farming

5   Nursery and tree production

6   Livestock combo farming

7   Dairy cattle and milk production

8   Fruit and vegetable combo farming

Greenhouse farming

It has been estimated that greenhouse farming produces over one-fifth of the total value of BC agriculture on less than 0.01% of BC's ALR (BC Agricultural Council, 2007). Greenhouses produce edible products (tomatoes, cucumbers, peppers, etc.) for 10 months of the year. Because of long living, healthy plants, and innovative crop management, greenhouses are able to produce up to 20 times the harvest as the same area of land producing field crops. No herbicides are used for growing vegetables because of biological pest control methods (BC Greenhouse Growers Association, 2007). Between 1993 and 2006, BC greenhouse production has grown from about 640,000 square metres (Ministry of Agriculture, Food and Fisheries, 2003) to nearly 5.3 million square metres in 2006.

According to the 2006 agricultural census, more than one-fifth (20.84%) of all farms reporting greenhouse production were from BC, and represented 24.10% of all the area in production in Canada. Three indicators are presented here to show the relative importance of greenhouse production, most of which is consumed locally. These are all new to this Atlas.

Percent of regional district farms with greenhouses

Nearly 6 in every 100 (5.90%) farms reported greenhouse production in 2006 in BC. The range throughout the province was quite considerable: Sunshine Coast had 20.83% of its farms with greenhouse production, compared with only 1.00% in Peace River. Greenhouse farming was most dominant as a type of farming in the coastal part of the province, including parts of Vancouver Island, and Greater Vancouver. Northern Rockies in the extreme northeast of the province was an outlier, with 16.67% of farms reporting greenhouse production. Much of the interior had less than the average percentage of farms reporting greenhouse production.

Percent of BC farms with greenhouses

While greenhouse farming occurs throughout the province, there is a heavy concentration of production in Greater Vancouver (23.68%) and Fraser Valley (13.76%) on the mainland, and in Capital (11.20%) on the southern tip of Vancouver Island. These regions all contain large urban populations. Geographically, the eastern, northern, and central and north coastal regions of the province have relatively low percentages of the BC farms with greenhouse production.

Regional District	% of RD farms	% of BC farms	Average size (sq. m.)
29 Sunshine Coast	20.83	1.71	336
59 Northern Rockies	16.67	0.43	162
27 Powell River	16.47	1.20	305
25 Comox Valley	13.88	5.90	632
26 Strathcona	13.88	5.90	632
17 Capital	13.22	11.20	1013
21 Nanaimo	11.71	4.62	N/A
15 Greater Vancouver	10.58	23.68	11,718
23 Alberni-Clayoquot	10.11	0.77	N/A
45 Central Coast	9.38	0.26	212
49 Kitimat-Stikine	8.96	1.03	440
19 Cowichan Valley	8.14	4.87	826
3 Central Kootenay	7.12	3.42	446
9 Fraser Valley	6.27	13.76	7,366
5 Kootenay Boundary	4.85	1.62	477
31 Squamish-Lillooet	4.65	0.51	775
39 Columbia-Shuswap	4.49	2.39	189
1 East Kootenay	3.80	1.28	930
41 Cariboo	3.79	3.76	1,615
53 Fraser-Fort George	3.54	1.88	8,978
51 Bulkley-Nechako	3.27	2.48	1,220
35 Central Okanagan	3.05	2.65	1,328
7 Okanagan-Similkameen	2.96	4.10	2,702
33 Thompson-Nicola	2.81	2.91	907
37 North Okanagan	2.04	2.14	764
55 Peace River	1.00	1.45	336
43 Mount Waddington	N/A	N/A	N/A
47 Skeena-Queen Charlotte	N/A	N/A	N/A
57 Stikine	N/A	N/A	N/A
British Columbia	**5.90**	**100.00**	**4,553**

N/A: No data

Average size (square metres) of farm greenhouse production

For those farms with greenhouses, the average size in greenhouse production varied greatly throughout the province. Greater Vancouver had the greatest average size in greenhouse production (11,717 square metres), followed by Fraser-Fort George (8,978 square metres) and Fraser Valley (7,366 square metres). At the other extreme, Northern Rockies had an average size of only 162 square metres in greenhouse production, followed by Columbia-Shuswap (189 square metres) and Central Coast (212 square metres).

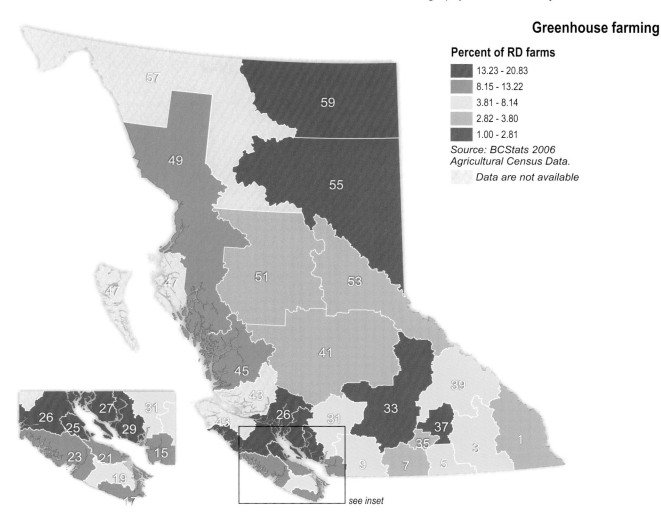

Greenhouse farming

Percent of RD farms

- 13.23 - 20.83
- 8.15 - 13.22
- 3.81 - 8.14
- 2.82 - 3.80
- 1.00 - 2.81

Source: BCStats 2006 Agricultural Census Data.

Data are not available

see inset

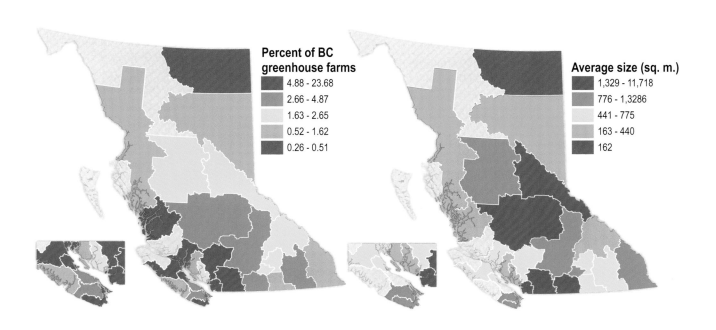

Percent of BC greenhouse farms

- 4.88 - 23.68
- 2.66 - 4.87
- 1.63 - 2.65
- 0.52 - 1.62
- 0.26 - 0.51

Average size (sq. m.)

- 1,329 - 11,718
- 776 - 1,3286
- 441 - 775
- 163 - 440
- 162

Organic farming

Organic farming is a type of food production that promotes the sustainable health and productivity of the ecosystem – soil, plants, animals, and people. Organic foods are farmed in an environmentally sustainable and socially responsible way, focusing on soil regeneration, water conservation, and animal welfare. Organic farmers use quality compost, cover crops (such as nitrogen-rich alfalfa), and crop rotation to nourish soil naturally, and to allow it to rest and regenerate. Produce is grown without synthetic pesticides, herbicides, fertilizers, or GMOs (genetically modified organisms). Animals are never fed the by-products of other animals, and are not kept constantly caged indoors, without access to fresh air.

With more than 20% of all Canadian farms that reported organic production in the 2006 Census of Agriculture, British Columbia has more organic farms than any other province in the country. More than 16% of all farms in the province reported that they were involved in organic production. Most organic farming, however, has not been certified by the Certified Organic Associations of BC. In 2006, 525 farms were producing certified or transitional organic products, and the most popular products were fruit, vegetables, or animals/animal products. The table and maps opposite use data from the 2006 census for all farms that reported organic production, regardless of certification status.

Farms reporting organic products

Organic farms were often involved in several types of products, although the main ones involved fruit, vegetable, and animal products. All areas in BC had organic production of one kind or another. Powell River had the highest percentage of farms in organic production, with nearly one half (48.24%) of its farms reporting such practices, while over a third (35.02%) of Capital farms also reported organic production. Those regions with more than one quarter of farms indicating organic production techniques all were clustered on Vancouver Island or neighbouring areas on the mainland in the southwest of BC, but not in the urban lower mainland part of the province. There were two outliers to this pattern: both Central Coast and Central Kootenay also had more than a quarter of their farms reporting organic production. At the other extreme, Fraser Valley and Peace River had less than 10% of their farms producing organically.

Regional District	All organic farms (%)	Organic fruit/vegetable farms (%)	Organic animal/animal products farms (%)
27 Powell River	48.24	70.73	60.98
17 Capital	35.02	66.57	53.31
25 Comox Valley	31.59	49.68	62.42
26 Strathcona	31.59	49.68	62.42
23 Alberni-Clayoquot	29.21	38.46	76.92
29 Sunshine Coast	29.17	75.00	39.29
45 Central Coast	28.13	66.67	44.44
19 Cowichan Valley	27.71	41.24	65.46
31 Squamish-Lillooet	26.36	44.12	41.18
21 Nanaimo	25.81	44.54	66.39
3 Central Kootenay	25.80	55.17	50.34
49 Kitimat-Stikine	24.63	48.48	51.52
59 Northern Rockies	23.33	14.29	57.14
5 Kootenay Boundary	20.41	35.00	57.50
39 Columbia-Shuswap	17.63	27.27	72.73
15 Greater Vancouver	15.74	44.66	54.85
53 Fraser-Fort George	15.46	25.00	67.71
33 Thompson-Nicola	14.78	25.14	69.83
7 Okanagan-Similkameen	14.56	78.81	20.76
41 Cariboo	13.28	14.94	77.27
37 North Okanagan	13.20	35.80	49.38
1 East Kootenay	13.16	17.31	59.62
35 Central Okanagan	12.29	52.80	43.20
51 Bulkley-Nechako	11.06	12.24	66.33
55 Peace River	9.30	5.70	57.59
9 Fraser Valley	8.96	38.26	56.09
43 Mount Waddington	N/A	N/A	N/A
47 Skeena-Queen Charlotte	N/A	N/A	N/A
57 Stikine	N/A	N/A	N/A
British Columbia	**16.29**	**42.76**	**56.22**

N/A: No data

Farms reporting organic fruit, vegetable, or greenhouse products

Of those farms reporting organic production, four of every ten (42.76%) indicated they had been involved in fruit, vegetable, or greenhouse produce. Powell River had the highest percentage, with 70.73% of its organic farms involved in fruit, vegetable, or greenhouse production, while two thirds of the organic farms in Central Coast and Capital were also involved in such production. The lowest percentages were found in the north and interior farms, particularly Peace River, Bulkley-Nechako, and Northern Rockies, which each had less than 15% of organic farms in this type of production.

Farms reporting organic animal or animal products

More than half (56.22%) of all farms reporting organic production indicated that they had been involved in organic animal or animal products. Cariboo, Alberni-Clayoquot, and Columbia-Shuswap (all more than 70%) had the highest percentage of organic farms involved in this type of production. Geographically, the highest percentage areas were in the central and northern interior parts of the province, as well as most of Vancouver Island.

Organic farming

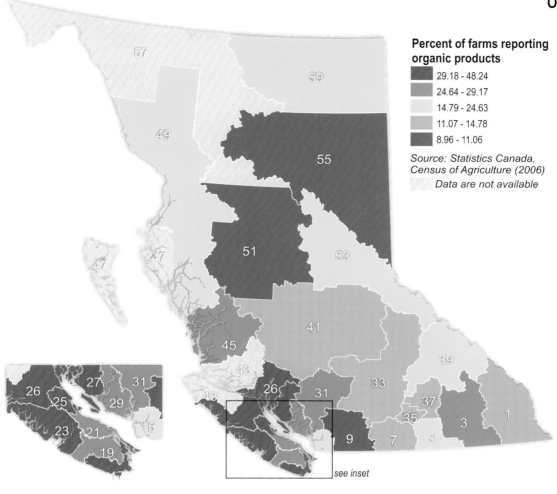

Percent of farms reporting
organic products

- 29.18 - 48.24
- 24.64 - 29.17
- 14.79 - 24.63
- 11.07 - 14.78
- 8.96 - 11.06

*Source: Statistics Canada,
Census of Agriculture (2006)*

Data are not available

see inset

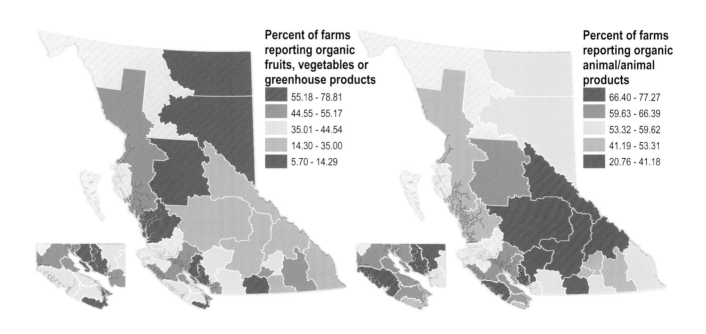

Percent of farms
reporting organic
fruits, vegetables or
greenhouse products

- 55.18 - 78.81
- 44.55 - 55.17
- 35.01 - 44.54
- 14.30 - 35.00
- 5.70 - 14.29

Percent of farms
reporting organic
animal/animal
products

- 66.40 - 77.27
- 59.63 - 66.39
- 53.32 - 59.62
- 41.19 - 53.31
- 20.76 - 41.18

Meat processing plants

Meat, including poultry, is high in protein and moisture, and is subject to micro-organisms or pathogens that can cause diseases in individuals (BC Centre for Disease Control (BCCDC), 2011). To ensure food safety, it has proven necessary to inspect animals prior to and during the slaughter process. It has been a requirement in BC that all meat sold in the province is inspected.

Food processing facilities have the responsibility to ensure that meat products are safe. Since September 2007, slaughter and processing of meats for sale in BC can only take place in provincially or federally licensed abattoirs. Within BC, there are different classes of licences available for meat slaughter and processing as follows: Class A is for the purposes of general slaughter and processing (cut and wrap services), and Class B is for slaughter only. In addition, there is a Class C license which enabled slaughter operators to become fully licensed. This is being phased out.

In April 2010, new classes of licences were introduced in response to concerns related to the ability to provide local food production in small, rural areas of BC. Class D allows on-farm slaughter of up to 25,000 pounds of produce annually for direct sale to consumers, or retail sales to secondary food establishments within the boundaries of the regional district where the meat was produced. Class D licences are only available in nine provincially designated regional districts.

Class E allows on-farm slaughter of up to10,000 pounds annually for direct sale to consumers in the regional district in which the meat is produced, and operators are only permitted to slaughter their own animals (Ministry of Healthy Living and Sport, 2010).

By early 2011, licences had been made available to producers along the BC coastal areas in the Bella Coola Valley (9), Haida Gwaii (9), and Powell River (12). More were expected in 2011, particularly in the Sechelt area and Kitimat Stikine.

The table and map opposite are based on data from the BCCDC (2011), and show only the larger licensed meat slaughter and processing plants in BC. While there is a total of 56 Class A, B, and C licensed facilities in the province, only 3 have the ability to slaughter and process both red meat and poultry. A further 24 are licensed to slaughter and process red meat, and 8 have transitional licences for these activities. There are 15 facilities with licences to slaughter and process poultry only, and a

Community		Community	
1	Darfield	29	70 Mile House
2	Redstone	30	Grassy Plains
3	Westholme	31	Kelowna
4	150 Mile House	32	Kelowna
5	Agassiz	33	Lower Nicola
6	Big Lake	34	Quesnel
7	Chilliwack	35	Terrace
8	Courtenay	36	Black Creek
9	Cranbrook	37	Black Creek
10	Creston	38	Chilliwack
11	Dawson Creek	39	Cowichan Bay
12	Duncan	40	Cranbrook
13	Duncan	41	Dawson Creek
14	Enderby	42	Farmington
15	Fort St. John	43	Keremeos
16	Gabriola	44	Pinantan Lake
17	Kamloops	45	Port Alberni
18	Nanaimo	46	Pritchard
19	Nanaimo	47	Qualicum
20	Pitt Meadows	48	Quesnel
21	Prince George	49	Richmond
22	Salmon Arm	50	Salmon Arm
23	Saturna Island	51	Burns Lake
24	Surrey	52	Kelowna
25	Telkwa	53	Quesnel
26	Vanderhoof	54	Terrace
27	Victoria	55	Terrace
28	100 Mile House	56	Vanderhoof

further 6 facilities with transitional licenses. Geographically, facilities are available on the southeastern part of Vancouver Island, parts of the Fraser Valley on the mainland, and throughout the interior, especially the Okanagan Valley, and in the Dawson Creek area in the northeast. Six mobile units are also available in Cranbrook, Fort St John, Quesnel, Burns Lake, Kamloops, and Kelowna.

Meat processing plants

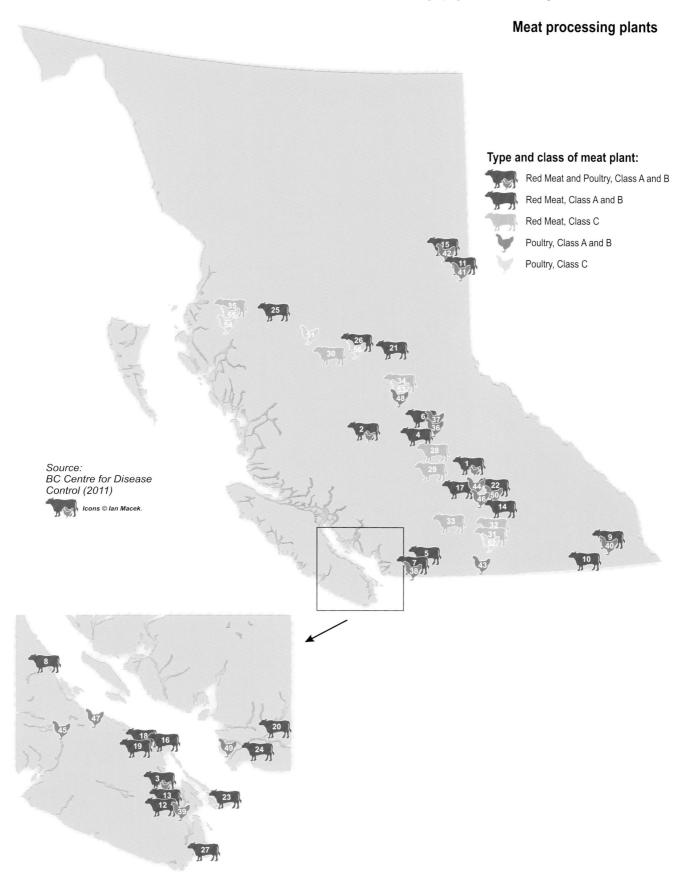

Type and class of meat plant:

Red Meat and Poultry, Class A and B

Red Meat, Class A and B

Red Meat, Class C

Poultry, Class A and B

Poultry, Class C

Source:
BC Centre for Disease
Control (2011)

Icons © Ian Macek.

Youth who never go to bed hungry because there is not enough food at home

While there are many dimensions to food security, as indicated earlier in the Atlas, being without hunger at the end of the day is an important component. The McCreary AHS IV asked student respondents: *"Some young people go to bed hungry because there is not enough food at home. How often does this happen to you. Always, often, sometimes, rarely, never?"*

Nearly nine out of every ten student respondents (89.11%) indicated that they had never gone to bed hungry because there was not enough food at home. Geographically, there was not a great deal of variation throughout the province, and less than five percentage points separated HSDAs. Kootenay Boundary (91.03%) had the highest percentage, and Richmond (86.56%) had the lowest percentage of students who indicated that they never went to bed hungry because of a lack of food at home. Richmond was significantly lower than the provincial average for this indicator. Geographically, higher values for student respondents who never went to bed hungry because of a lack of food in the house tended to occur in the urban lower mainland parts of the province (with the exception of Richmond), as well as Kootenay Boundary.

While the provincial difference between genders was very small, it was significant. Male students (88.30%) were significantly less likely to have never gone to bed hungry than female students (89.89%). Among male students, the highest percentage value of never having gone to bed hungry occurred in Kootenay Boundary (91.49%), and this HSDA was significantly higher than the provincial average for male students. Richmond, with a value of 84.93%, was significantly lower than average. Overall, the lowest values were evident in parts of the lower mainland (Richmond and Vancouver) and Central Vancouver Island.

Among female students, there was a six percentage point range between the highest and lowest value HSDAs. North Shore/Coast Garibaldi (92.11%) had the highest value for female students, and this was also significantly higher than the provincial average for females. East Kootenay, with the lowest value of 86.12%, and North Vancouver Island (86.33%) were both significantly lower than the provincial average for female students. Geographically, the pattern for female student respondents was quite similar to that for all students combined.

Health Service Delivery Area	All students (%)		Males (%)		Females (%)
12 Kootenay Boundary		91.03	▨	91.49	■ 90.61
33 North Shore/Coast Garibaldi		90.73	■	89.30	▨ 92.11
22 Fraser North		90.38	■	89.33	■ 91.41
21 Fraser South/Fraser East		89.89		89.19	90.51
32 Vancouver		88.87	■	87.06	90.41
41 South Vancouver Island		88.70		88.27	89.11
14 Thompson Cariboo Shuswap		88.65		88.33	89.18
51 Northwest		88.65	■	87.36	89.82
52 Northern Interior		88.54	■	88.86	88.43
13 Okanagan		88.28		87.96	88.59
42 Central Vancouver Island		87.37	■	85.79	88.97
43 North Vancouver Island	■	86.87		87.47	▨ 86.33
11 East Kootenay	■	86.65		87.24	▨ 86.12
31 Richmond	▨	86.56	▨	84.93	■ 88.28
53 Northeast		N/A		N/A	N/A
British Columbia		**89.11**		**88.30†**	**89.89**

† Male rate is significantly different than female rate.
Crosshatched HSDAs are significantly different than the provincial average.
N/A: No data

Youth who never go to bed hungry because there is not enough food at home

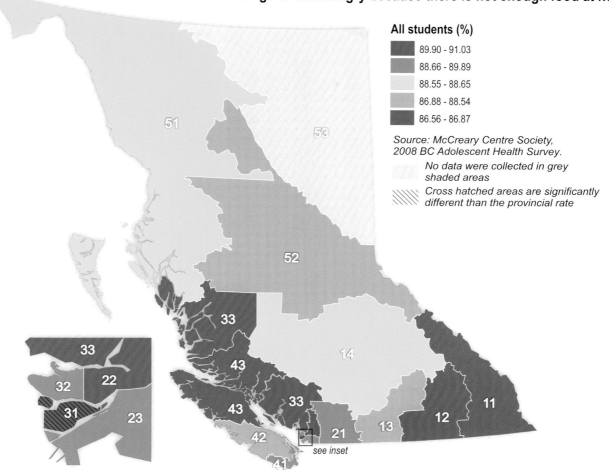

All students (%)

- 89.90 - 91.03
- 88.66 - 89.89
- 88.55 - 88.65
- 86.88 - 88.54
- 86.56 - 86.87

Source: McCreary Centre Society, 2008 BC Adolescent Health Survey.

No data were collected in grey shaded areas

Cross hatched areas are significantly different than the provincial rate

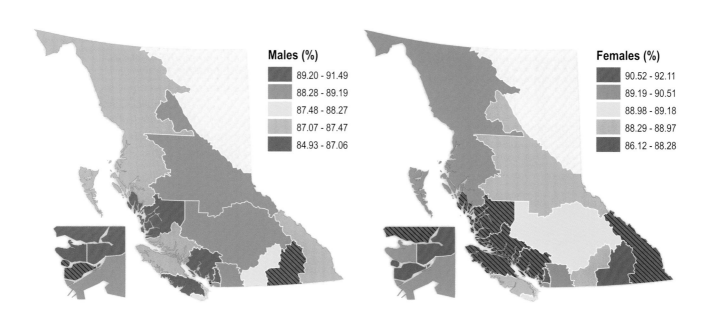

Males (%)

- 89.20 - 91.49
- 88.28 - 89.19
- 87.48 - 88.27
- 87.07 - 87.47
- 84.93 - 87.06

Females (%)

- 90.52 - 92.11
- 89.19 - 90.51
- 88.98 - 89.18
- 88.29 - 88.97
- 86.12 - 88.28

Always had enough of the kinds of food they wanted to eat in the past 12 months

Health Service Delivery Area	All respondents 12+ (%)	Males 12+ (%)	Females 12+ (%)	Ages 12-19 (%)	Ages 20-64 (%)	Ages 65+ (%)
31 Richmond	94.42	94.00	94.82	91.27	94.95	94.02
33 North Shore/Coast Garibaldi	93.81	94.23	93.41	93.13	92.85	98.40‡
43 North Vancouver Island	92.28	95.78	88.79	93.36	92.07	92.44
23 Fraser South	91.86	89.84	93.79	91.02	91.92	92.31
21 Fraser East	91.06	91.59	90.55	88.22	90.82	94.44
13 Okanagan	90.39	91.48	89.35	90.02	88.59	96.13‡
41 South Vancouver Island	89.81	89.82	89.79	84.16	89.32	94.57‡
14 Thompson Cariboo Shuswap	89.59	91.64	87.46	80.18	89.32	96.98‡
22 Fraser North	89.53	89.92	89.14	90.44	88.15	96.85‡
51 Northwest	89.44	88.72	90.22	85.86	89.20	95.34
12 Kootenay Boundary	89.17	91.04	87.33	84.85	87.52	97.70‡
53 Northeast	89.10	89.57	88.59	90.34	88.23	94.26
11 East Kootenay	88.84	91.57	86.11	94.02	87.02	93.35
42 Central Vancouver Island	88.64	89.16	88.12	81.16	87.51	96.79‡
32 Vancouver	86.54	85.83	87.23	81.99	86.24	90.66
52 Northern Interior	85.77	86.06	85.45	84.88	84.93	91.92
British Columbia (2007/8)	**89.98**	**90.05**	**89.90**	**87.86**	**89.29**	**94.64‡**
British Columbia (2005)	**89.65**	**90.79***	**88.56**	**84.33†**	**89.34**	**95.39‡**

Crosshatching beside the 2007/8 provincial rate indicates it is significantly different than the 2005 rate, while crosshatched HSDAs are significantly different than the 2007/8 provincial rate.
E interpret data with caution (16.67 ≤ coefficient of variation ≤ 33.3).

* Males differ significantly from females.
†12-19 age cohort differs significantly from the 20-64 age cohort.
‡ 65+ age cohort differs significantly from the 20-64 age cohort.
F data suppressed (n < 10, or coefficient of variation > 33.3).

British Columbia/Canada Cohort Comparison 2007/2008

Canada ■   British Columbia ▨
Ⱦ 95% confidence limits of estimate

The CCHS evaluated access to acceptable foods by asking respondents *"Which of the following statements best describes the food eaten in your household in the past 12 months? Would you say: you always had enough of the kinds of food they wanted to eat; you had enough food but not always the kind of food you desired; sometimes you did not have enough food; or, often you didn't have enough to eat."* The indicator used here reports the percentage of respondents who answered they always had enough of the kinds of food they wanted.

In BC, 89.98% reported always having had enough of the desired foods. Richmond and North Shore/Coast Garibaldi (both over 93%) were significantly higher, while Northern Interior (85.77%) was significantly lower than the provincial average.

For both males and females in BC, about nine out of every ten respondents reported always having had enough desired foods and there was no significant difference between genders, in contrast to 2005. For females, Fraser South and Richmond (both above 93%) were significantly higher than the provincial female average. For males, only North Vancouver Island (95.78%) was significantly higher than the provincial average for males.

For the youth cohort, 87.86% of respondents always had enough of the kinds of food they wanted to eat. There were no significant differences at the HSDA level, although East Kootenay (94.02%) had the highest value and Thompson Cariboo Shuswap (80.18%.) had the lowest. There were no significant differences between the youth cohort and the mid age cohort provincially or for any

HSDA. However, in 2005, youth were significantly lower than their mid-age counterparts.

Older respondents in BC (94.64%) were significantly more likely than the mid-age cohort to always have had access to desired foods. This was also the case for nearly half of all HSDAs. North Shore/Coast Garibaldi was the only HSDA that stood out for the older respondent group, with a significantly high value of 98.4%.

There was a modest spread of 10 percentage points or less for all cohorts. Higher values were generally evident along the south and central coastal HSDAs, except for older respondents, and lower values were seen predominantly in both the interior and Vancouver.

For the BC samples, there were no significant differences between 2005 and 2007/8, although the youth cohort had improved substantially between the two samples, and the significant difference apparent between genders in 2005 had disappeared in the 2007/8 sample. Comparing BC to the national averages for 2007/8, most cohorts were not significantly different; for the female cohorts, however, BC respondents had a significantly higher value than Canadian females as a whole.

Always had enough of the kinds of food they wanted to eat in the past 12 months

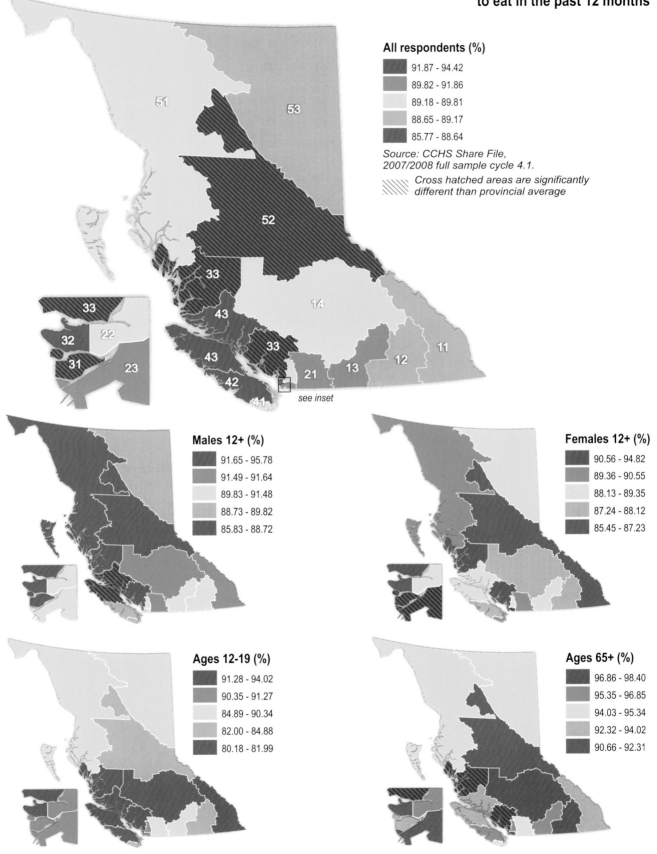

All respondents (%)

- 91.87 - 94.42
- 89.82 - 91.86
- 89.18 - 89.81
- 88.65 - 89.17
- 85.77 - 88.64

Source: CCHS Share File, 2007/2008 full sample cycle 4.1.

Cross hatched areas are significantly different than provincial average

Males 12+ (%)

- 91.65 - 95.78
- 91.49 - 91.64
- 89.83 - 91.48
- 88.73 - 89.82
- 85.83 - 88.72

Females 12+ (%)

- 90.56 - 94.82
- 89.36 - 90.55
- 88.13 - 89.35
- 87.24 - 88.12
- 85.45 - 87.23

Ages 12-19 (%)

- 91.28 - 94.02
- 90.35 - 91.27
- 84.89 - 90.34
- 82.00 - 84.88
- 80.18 - 81.99

Ages 65+ (%)

- 96.86 - 98.40
- 95.35 - 96.85
- 94.03 - 95.34
- 92.32 - 94.02
- 90.66 - 92.31

Household was always able to afford balanced meals in the past 12 months

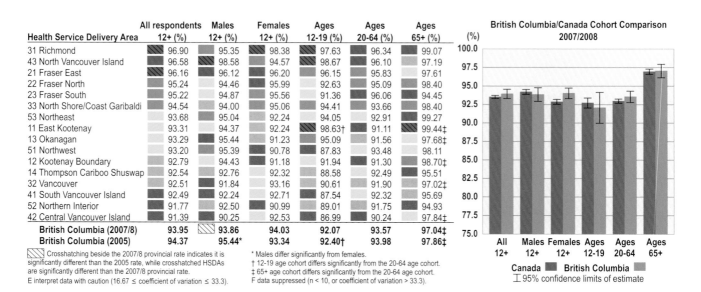

Health Service Delivery Area	All respondents 12+ (%)	Males 12+ (%)	Females 12+ (%)	Ages 12-19 (%)	Ages 20-64 (%)	Ages 65+ (%)
31 Richmond	96.90	95.35	98.38	97.63	96.34	99.07
43 North Vancouver Island	96.58	98.58	94.57	98.67	96.10	97.19
21 Fraser East	96.16	96.12	96.20	96.15	95.83	97.61
22 Fraser North	95.24	94.46	95.99	92.63	95.09	98.40
23 Fraser South	95.22	94.87	95.56	91.36	96.06	94.45
33 North Shore/Coast Garibaldi	94.54	94.00	95.06	94.41	93.66	98.40
53 Northeast	93.68	95.04	92.24	94.05	92.91	99.27
11 East Kootenay	93.31	94.37	92.24	98.63†	91.11	99.44‡
13 Okanagan	93.29	95.44	91.23	95.09	91.56	97.68‡
51 Northwest	93.20	95.39	90.78	87.83	93.48	98.11
12 Kootenay Boundary	92.79	94.43	91.18	91.94	91.30	98.70‡
14 Thompson Cariboo Shuswap	92.54	92.76	92.32	88.58	92.49	95.51
32 Vancouver	92.51	91.84	93.16	90.61	91.90	97.02‡
41 South Vancouver Island	92.49	92.24	92.71	87.54	92.32	95.69
52 Northern Interior	91.77	92.50	90.99	89.01	91.75	94.93
42 Central Vancouver Island	91.39	90.25	92.53	86.99	90.24	97.84‡
British Columbia (2007/8)	**93.95**	93.86	94.03	92.07	93.57	97.04‡
British Columbia (2005)	**94.37**	95.44*	93.34	92.40†	93.98	97.86‡

Crosshatching beside the 2007/8 provincial rate indicates it is significantly different than the 2005 rate, while crosshatched HSDAs are significantly different than the 2007/8 provincial rate.
E interpret data with caution (16.67 ≤ coefficient of variation ≤ 33.3).

* Males differ significantly from females.
† 12-19 age cohort differs significantly from the 20-64 age cohort.
‡ 65+ age cohort differs significantly from the 20-64 age cohort.
F data suppressed (n < 10, or coefficient of variation > 33.3).

British Columbia/Canada Cohort Comparison 2007/2008

Canada ■   British Columbia ▨
⊥ 95% confidence limits of estimate

Being able to afford a nutritionally balanced meal is important to ensuring individuals maintain a healthy body weight and receive the nutrients needed to lead a healthy life. The CCHS asked respondents: *"You and your household members couldn't afford to eat balanced meals. In the last 12 months was that often true, sometimes true, or never true?"* Within BC, 93.95% of respondents were always able to afford balanced meals, and respondents in Fraser East and Richmond (both over 96%), were significantly more likely to be able to afford balanced meals than the provincial average.

In contrast to 2005, males and females had very similar values for this variable (approximately 94%). For male respondents, North Vancouver Island (98.58%) was significantly higher than the provincial average, while for females Richmond (98.38%) had significantly more respondents who were always able to afford balanced meals than the average for females.

Provincially, the youth cohort had the lowest value for this variable, with only 92.07% reporting that their household was always able to afford balanced meals; however, in contrast to 2005, this was not significantly low when compared to the mid-age cohort. Only one HSDA (East Kootenay) had a significantly high value for youth in comparison to the mid-age group. When compared to the provincial average, youth in East Kootenay, Richmond, and North Vancouver Island (above 97%) all had significantly higher than average values.

Always being able to afford a balanced meal increased consistently with age, and the older respondents (97.04%)

in BC had significantly higher values than the mid-age cohort. This was also the case for older respondents in East Kootenay, Kootenay Boundary, Okanagan, Vancouver, and Central Vancouver Island. In comparison to the provincial average, older respondents in East Kootenay stood out with a significantly high value of 99.44%.

Geographically, there was a relatively small spread of 10 or less percentage points for each cohort. The spread was greatest for youth (10 percentage points). For all respondents, lower values were seen in the interior, while higher values were clustered along the south and central coastal areas, with the exception of Vancouver and South and Central Vancouver Island. A similar pattern appeared for female respondents, and to a large degree for youth respondents as well.

When compared to the 2005 CCHS results, British Columbians had lower values in all cohorts except females, and the 2007/8 male cohort was significantly lower than the 2005 sample. Comparing BC respondents to their Canadian peers, values were quite similar for 2007/8, although the BC female cohort was significantly higher than the Canadian sample.

Household was always able to afford balanced meals in the past 12 months

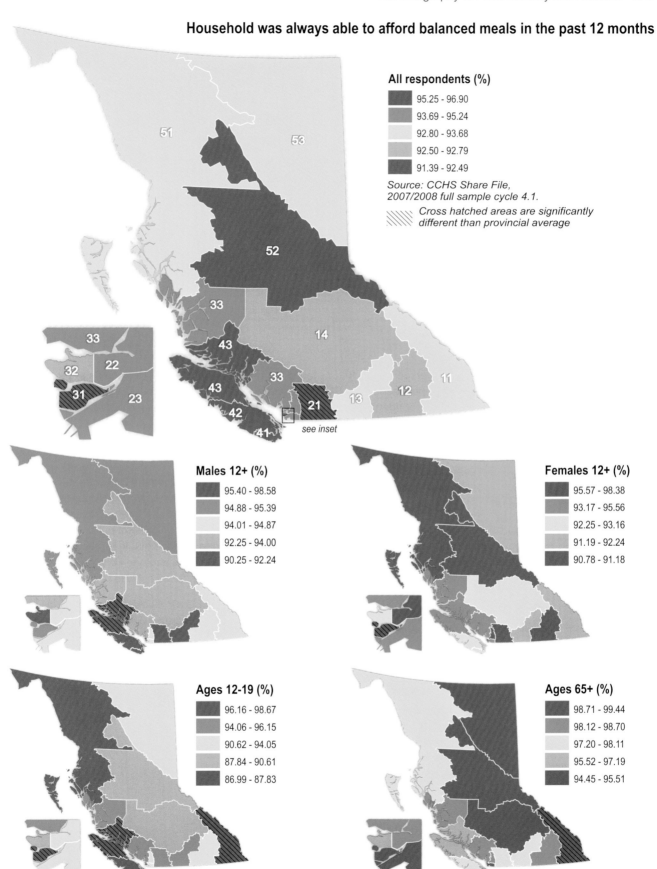

All respondents (%)

- 95.25 - 96.90
- 93.69 - 95.24
- 92.80 - 93.68
- 92.50 - 92.79
- 91.39 - 92.49

Source: CCHS Share File, 2007/2008 full sample cycle 4.1.

Cross hatched areas are significantly different than provincial average

Males 12+ (%)

- 95.40 - 98.58
- 94.88 - 95.39
- 94.01 - 94.87
- 92.25 - 94.00
- 90.25 - 92.24

Females 12+ (%)

- 95.57 - 98.38
- 93.17 - 95.56
- 92.25 - 93.16
- 91.19 - 92.24
- 90.78 - 91.18

Ages 12-19 (%)

- 96.16 - 98.67
- 94.06 - 96.15
- 90.62 - 94.05
- 87.84 - 90.61
- 86.99 - 87.83

Ages 65+ (%)

- 98.71 - 99.44
- 98.12 - 98.70
- 97.20 - 98.11
- 95.52 - 97.19
- 94.45 - 95.51

Food security

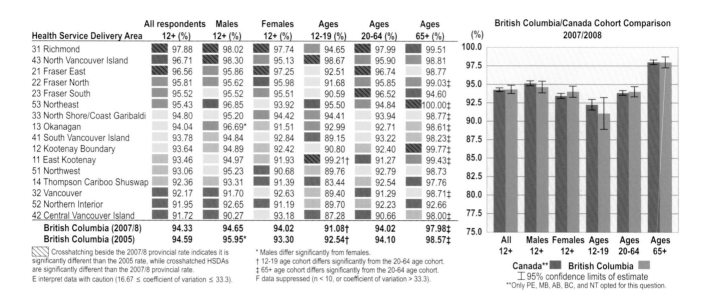

Health Service Delivery Area	All respondents 12+ (%)	Males 12+ (%)	Females 12+ (%)	Ages 12-19 (%)	Ages 20-64 (%)	Ages 65+ (%)
31 Richmond	97.88	98.02	97.74	94.65	97.99	99.51
43 North Vancouver Island	96.71	98.30	95.13	98.67	95.90	98.81
21 Fraser East	96.56	95.86	97.25	92.51	96.74	98.77
22 Fraser North	95.81	95.62	95.98	91.68	95.85	99.03‡
23 Fraser South	95.52	95.52	95.51	90.59	96.52	94.60
53 Northeast	95.43	96.85	93.92	95.50	94.84	100.00‡
33 North Shore/Coast Garibaldi	94.80	95.20	94.42	94.41	93.94	98.77‡
13 Okanagan	94.04	96.69*	91.51	92.99	92.71	98.61‡
41 South Vancouver Island	93.78	94.84	92.84	89.15	93.22	98.23‡
12 Kootenay Boundary	93.64	94.89	92.42	90.80	92.40	99.77‡
11 East Kootenay	93.46	94.97	91.93	99.21†	91.27	99.43‡
51 Northwest	93.06	95.23	90.68	89.76	92.79	98.73
14 Thompson Cariboo Shuswap	92.36	93.31	91.39	83.44	92.54	97.76
32 Vancouver	92.17	91.70	92.63	89.40	91.29	98.71‡
52 Northern Interior	91.95	92.65	91.19	89.70	92.23	92.66
42 Central Vancouver Island	91.72	90.27	93.18	87.28	90.66	98.00‡
British Columbia (2007/8)	**94.33**	**94.65**	**94.02**	**91.08†**	**94.02**	**97.98‡**
British Columbia (2005)	**94.59**	**95.95***	**93.30**	**92.54†**	**94.10**	**98.57‡**

Crosshatching beside the 2007/8 provincial rate indicates it is significantly different than the 2005 rate, while crosshatched HSDAs are significantly different than the 2007/8 provincial rate.
E interpret data with caution (16.67 ≤ coefficient of variation ≤ 33.3).

* Males differ significantly from females.
† 12-19 age cohort differs significantly from the 20-64 age cohort.
‡ 65+ age cohort differs significantly from the 20-64 age cohort.
F data suppressed (n < 10, or coefficient of variation > 33.3).

British Columbia/Canada Cohort Comparison 2007/2008

Canada** ■   British Columbia ▨
I 95% confidence limits of estimate
**Only PE, MB, AB, BC, and NT opted for this question.

Food security is a measure of how well a person is able to access safe, nutritional, and culturally acceptable foods. The following indicates the percentage of respondents who reported a good level of food security based on information derived from 18 separate CCHS questions (Statistics Canada, nd). In BC, 94.33% of all respondents were food secure. Richmond (97.88%) was significantly higher than the provincial average, as was Fraser East (96.56%).

While there was very little difference between genders, Okanagan males were significantly higher than their female counterparts. Compared to the provincial average for males, both Richmond and North Vancouver Island had significantly high values of over 98%. For females, Richmond and Fraser East (both over 97%) were significantly more likely to be food secure than the female provincial average.

Being food secure increased consistently with age in BC. Only 91.08% of youth respondents indicated they were food secure, which was significantly lower than those in the mid-age cohort. This significant difference was not reflected at the HSDA level, and in contrast, youth respondents in East Kootenay were significantly more likely to be food secure than their mid-age counterparts. Comparing HSDA values to the provincial average for youth, North Vancouver Island and East Kootenay stood out with significantly high values above 98%.

Of older respondents in BC, 97.98% indicated they were food secure. This was significantly higher than those in the mid-age cohort, and this significant trend was also

found in nine individual HSDAs. When compared to the provincial average, older respondents in Kootenay Boundary and Northeast both stood out with significantly high values above 99%.

Geographically, there was a modest spread of 11 percentage points or less for all cohorts. For all respondents, there was a cluster of high values in the southwest, with the exception of Vancouver, while a diagonal band of low scores was seen across the province from the northwest corner to the southeast. This grouping of low scores was particularly notable for the female cohort. North Vancouver Island and Richmond had consistently high scores for all cohorts.

When compared to the 2005 CCHS sample data, being food secure in BC had decreased in every cohort, except females; however, these differences were not significant. British Columbians had very similar values of food security for all cohorts when compared to Canada as a whole for 2007/8.

Food security

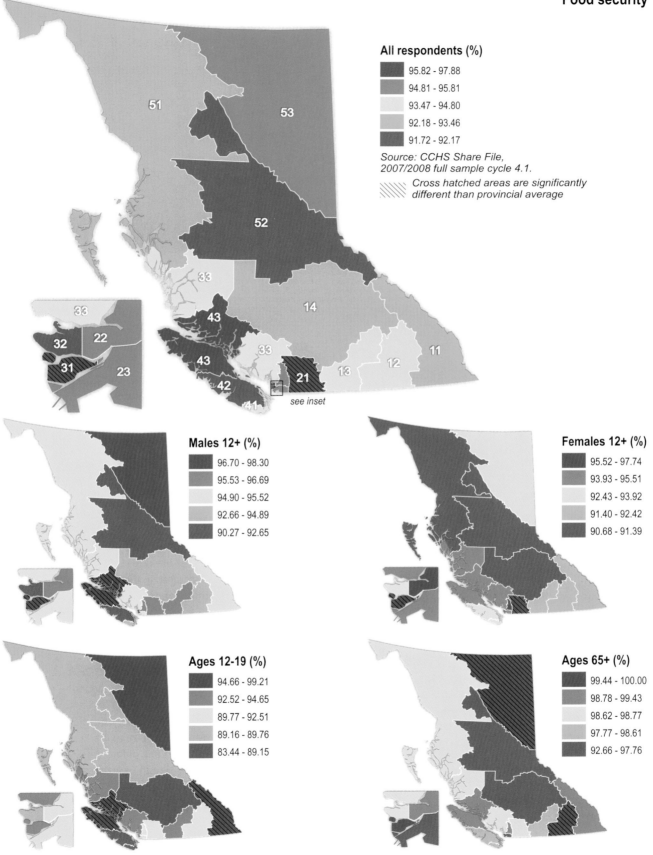

All respondents (%)
- 95.82 - 97.88
- 94.81 - 95.81
- 93.47 - 94.80
- 92.18 - 93.46
- 91.72 - 92.17

Source: CCHS Share File, 2007/2008 full sample cycle 4.1.

Cross hatched areas are significantly different than provincial average

Males 12+ (%)
- 96.70 - 98.30
- 95.53 - 96.69
- 94.90 - 95.52
- 92.66 - 94.89
- 90.27 - 92.65

Females 12+ (%)
- 95.52 - 97.74
- 93.93 - 95.51
- 92.43 - 93.92
- 91.40 - 92.42
- 90.68 - 91.39

Ages 12-19 (%)
- 94.66 - 99.21
- 92.52 - 94.65
- 89.77 - 92.51
- 89.16 - 89.76
- 83.44 - 89.15

Ages 65+ (%)
- 99.44 - 100.00
- 98.78 - 99.43
- 98.62 - 98.77
- 97.77 - 98.61
- 92.66 - 97.76

Did not binge drink in the past 12 months

Health Service Delivery Area	All respondents 12+ (%)	Males 12+ (%)	Females 12+ (%)	Ages 12-19 (%)	Ages 20-64 (%)	Ages 65+ (%)
31 Richmond	75.26	65.41*	84.79	77.87	71.46	91.68‡
22 Fraser North	71.12	64.33*	77.83	85.49†	65.03	93.47‡
32 Vancouver	69.48	61.33*	77.30	86.16†	63.96	91.30‡
23 Fraser South	68.99	58.59*	79.00	78.69†	63.91	87.38‡
21 Fraser East	68.77	59.57*	77.62	74.49	63.15	89.02‡
13 Okanagan	64.72	54.96*	73.97	74.82†	54.67	91.33‡
52 Northern Interior	61.64	51.48*	71.97	62.41	56.61	91.36‡
42 Central Vancouver Island	60.95	53.36*	68.36	61.79	53.35	85.41‡
41 South Vancouver Island	60.57	49.25*	70.55	72.56†	51.57	89.94‡
14 Thompson Cariboo Shuswap	60.48	53.40*	67.56	64.97	53.98	84.61‡
43 North Vancouver Island	59.84	50.84*	68.61	72.95	50.11	88.26‡
51 Northwest	59.51	53.29	66.27	76.46†	52.81	79.71‡
33 North Shore/Coast Garibaldi	59.29	51.66*	66.53	74.20†	51.48	82.17‡
53 Northeast	58.61	46.65*	71.11	57.15E	55.06	89.72‡
12 Kootenay Boundary	54.13	37.11*	71.63	59.54E	44.85	87.06‡
11 East Kootenay	52.07	43.58*	60.79	57.04	45.16	78.48‡
British Columbia (2007/8)	65.69	56.68*	74.41	75.31†	59.26	88.76‡
British Columbia (2005)	63.04	52.83*	72.91	70.51†	56.59	88.19‡

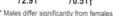 Crosshatching beside the 2007/8 provincial rate indicates it is significantly different than the 2005 rate, while crosshatched HSDAs are significantly different than the 2007/8 provincial rate.
E interpret data with caution (16.67 ≤ coefficient of variation ≤ 33.3).

* Males differ significantly from females.
†12-19 age cohort differs significantly from the 20-64 age cohort.
‡ 65+ age cohort differs significantly from the 20-64 age cohort.
F data suppressed (n < 10, or coefficient of variation > 33.3).

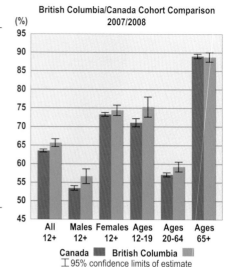

British Columbia/Canada Cohort Comparison 2007/2008

Canada ■ British Columbia ▨
⊥ 95% confidence limits of estimate

High risk drinking can contribute to an increased risk of injury or accident in the short-term, or cirrhosis of the liver, increased risk of some cancers, heart disease, or stroke in the long-term. The CCHS asked participants, *"How often in the past 12 months have you had 5 or more drinks on one occasion?"*. Such drinking behaviour is referred to as binge drinking. The following presents the percentage of respondents who answered that they did not binge drink.

Nearly two-thirds (65.69%) of BC respondents indicated they did not binge drink in the past 12 months. Respondents in Richmond and Fraser North (both above 71%) were significantly less likely to binge drink, while seven HSDAs were significantly more likely to binge drink.

There was a significant difference between genders for binge drinking behaviour. Among females, 74.41% were not binge drinkers, compared to only 56.68% of males. In all but one HSDA (Northwest), females were significantly more likely not to binge drink than their male counterparts.

Among male respondents, Fraser North and Richmond (both above 64%) were significantly less likely to be binge drinkers, while East Kootenay, Kootenay Boundary, and South Vancouver Island (all below 50%) were significantly more likely to binge drink. For females, Richmond (84.79%) had significantly more non-binge drinkers compared to females provincially, while East Kootenay, North Shore/Coast Garibaldi, and Northwest (all below 67%) had significantly fewer.

Within BC, youth (75.31%) were significantly more likely not to binge drink than the mid-age cohort. This significant

difference was also found in seven HSDAs. Compared to the youth provincial average, Fraser North and Vancouver (both over 85%) were significantly less likely to have participated in binge drinking in the past 12 months.

For the older cohort in BC, 88.76% of the respondents were non-binge drinkers, significantly more than the mid-age cohort. This significant difference was evident in every HSDA. Provincially, older respondents in Fraser North (93.47%) were significantly more likely to be non-binge drinkers, while those in East Kootenay (78.48%) were significantly less likely.

Geographically, there was a spread of 15 percentage points or more for each of the age cohorts. For all cohorts, high values occurred in the southwest mainland regions and eastward as far as Okanagan, while lower values were seen in East Kootenay and Kootenay Boundary.

Within BC, there was an increase in non-binge drinking for all cohorts when compared to the 2005 CCHS results, with a significant difference seen for all respondents, males, and the mid-age cohorts. For the 2007/8 sample, compared to Canadian respondents, British Columbians were more likely to be non binge-drinkers in all cohorts except the older cohort, and this difference was significant for all respondents, males, youth, and the mid-age cohorts.

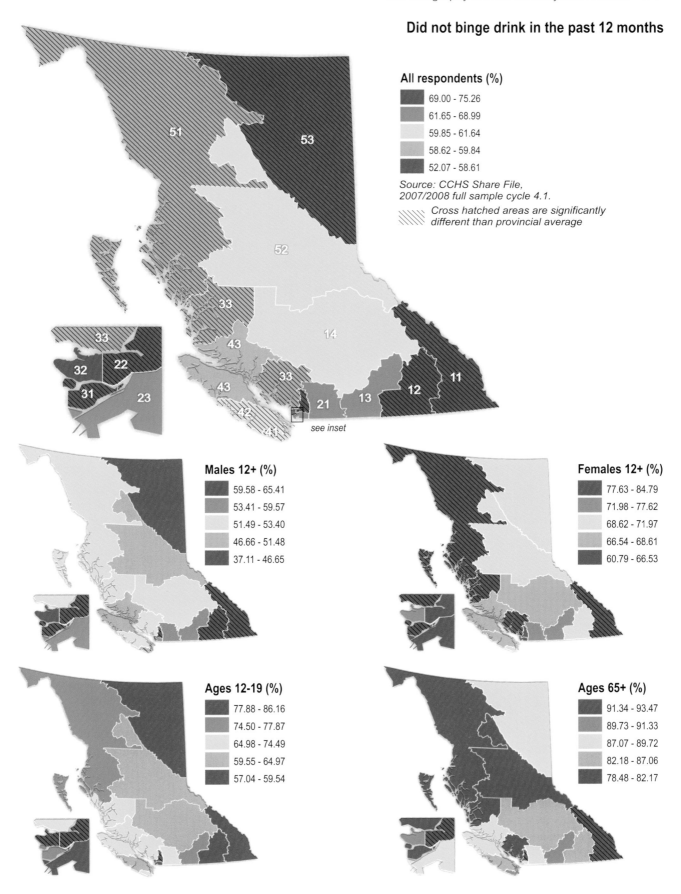

Did not binge drink in the past 12 months

All respondents (%)
- 69.00 - 75.26
- 61.65 - 68.99
- 59.85 - 61.64
- 58.62 - 59.84
- 52.07 - 58.61

Source: CCHS Share File, 2007/2008 full sample cycle 4.1.

Cross hatched areas are significantly different than provincial average

Males 12+ (%)
- 59.58 - 65.41
- 53.41 - 59.57
- 51.49 - 53.40
- 46.66 - 51.48
- 37.11 - 46.65

Females 12+ (%)
- 77.63 - 84.79
- 71.98 - 77.62
- 68.62 - 71.97
- 66.54 - 68.61
- 60.79 - 66.53

Ages 12-19 (%)
- 77.88 - 86.16
- 74.50 - 77.87
- 64.98 - 74.49
- 59.55 - 64.97
- 57.04 - 59.54

Ages 65+ (%)
- 91.34 - 93.47
- 89.73 - 91.33
- 87.07 - 89.72
- 82.18 - 87.06
- 78.48 - 82.17

Avoids certain foods because of the calorie content

Health Service Delivery Area	All respondents 12+ (%)	Males 12+ (%)	Females 12+ (%)	Ages 12-19 (%)	Ages 20-64 (%)	Ages 65+ (%)
33 North Shore/Coast Garibaldi	59.84	55.17	64.06	30.29E†	62.26	69.33
22 Fraser North	54.38	46.31*	62.17	42.41	56.46	52.34
31 Richmond	54.17	46.74	61.00	32.19E†	59.87	40.79‡
32 Vancouver	51.45	44.78*	57.94	39.04	53.20	48.19
13 Okanagan	51.22	39.98*	61.81	33.92†	53.41	53.24
23 Fraser South	50.96	42.25*	59.28	35.22†	54.04	47.85
41 South Vancouver Island	50.87	37.38*	63.00	32.52E†	54.30	46.19
53 Northeast	47.00	35.00*	59.41	30.64E	49.74	48.50E
52 Northern Interior	46.95	34.99*	59.06	34.69	48.46	51.24
42 Central Vancouver Island	46.45	37.38*	54.90	34.38	48.74	45.38
12 Kootenay Boundary	46.43	37.09*	55.93	35.61E	50.53	36.73
11 East Kootenay	46.18	34.56*	57.50	26.41E†	49.17	47.10
14 Thompson Cariboo Shuswap	45.87	30.46*	60.52	43.60	46.34	45.39
51 Northwest	45.00	37.35*	52.92	19.68E†	50.80	38.48E
21 Fraser East	44.67	32.54*	56.47	27.33†	48.35	41.69
43 North Vancouver Island	41.68	34.24	48.53	34.75E	43.74	37.80
British Columbia (2007/8)	**50.59**	**41.21***	**59.52**	**35.13†**	**53.25**	**48.67‡**

No comparable 2005 data available

Crosshatching beside the 2007/8 provincial rate indicates it is significantly different than the 2005 rate, while crosshatched HSDAs are significantly different than the 2007/8 provincial rate.
E interpret data with caution (16.67 ≤ coefficient of variation ≤ 33.3).

* Males differ significantly from females.
† 12-19 age cohort differs significantly from the 20-64 age cohort.
‡ 65+ age cohort differs significantly from the 20-64 age cohort.
F data suppressed (n < 10, or coefficient of variation > 33.3).

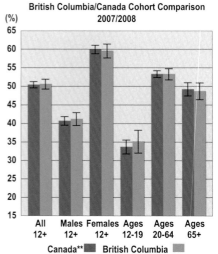

British Columbia/Canada Cohort Comparison 2007/2008

Canada** ■ British Columbia ■
⊥ 95% confidence limits of estimate
**Only PE, MB, AB, BC, and NT opted for this question

High calorie consumption is often related to unintended weight gain. Avoiding certain foods with high calorie content is an important wellness asset. The CCHS asked respondents *"Do you avoid certain foods because of the calorie content?"* About half (50.59%) of all BC participants responded in the affirmative. At the HSDA level, North Shore/Coast Garibaldi (59.84%) was significantly higher than the provincial average, while both Fraser East (44.67%) and North Vancouver Island (41.68%) were significantly lower.

With nearly a 20 percentage point difference between them, males (41.21%) were significantly less likely than females (59.52%) to avoid certain foods because of the calorie content. This significant difference between males and females was evident in all but three HSDAs. Female respondents in North Vancouver Island (48.53%) were significantly less likely than females provincially to avoid certain foods because of the calorie content. For male respondents, North Shore/Coast Garibaldi (55.17%) was significantly above, while Thompson Cariboo Shuswap and Fraser East (both below 33%) were significantly below the male provincial average.

In BC, 35.13% of youth avoided certain foods because of the calorie content – significantly lower than the mid-age cohort. This significant difference from the mid-age cohort was also found in eight of the 16 HSDAs. There were no HSDAs for the youth cohort with significantly higher or lower values than the provincial youth average. Results for the youth cohort should be interpreted with caution because eight of the 16 HSDAs had low sample sizes or

high coefficients of variation.

For older respondents, 48.67% of respondents avoided certain foods because of the calorie content. This was significantly lower than the mid-age cohort. At the HSDA level, only Richmond stood out, with a significantly lower value for older respondents than their mid-age counterparts. Comparing HSDAs to the provincial average for older respondents, North Shore/Coast Garibaldi was significantly higher at 69.33%, and no HSDA was significantly lower.

Geographically, there was a spread of more than 18 percentage points for each age cohort, with the largest variation occurring in the oldest cohort (over 32 percentage points). Clusters of high values were seen in the lower mainland HSDAs for all respondents as well as for males, and to a lesser degree for females and older respondents.

No comparable data from the 2005 CCHS survey were available. Values for the BC cohorts were very similar to those for their Canadian peers for the 2007/8 samples. Canadian values are based on a limited number of provinces/territories; therefore, caution in interpreting these comparisons is advised.

Avoids certain foods because of the calorie content

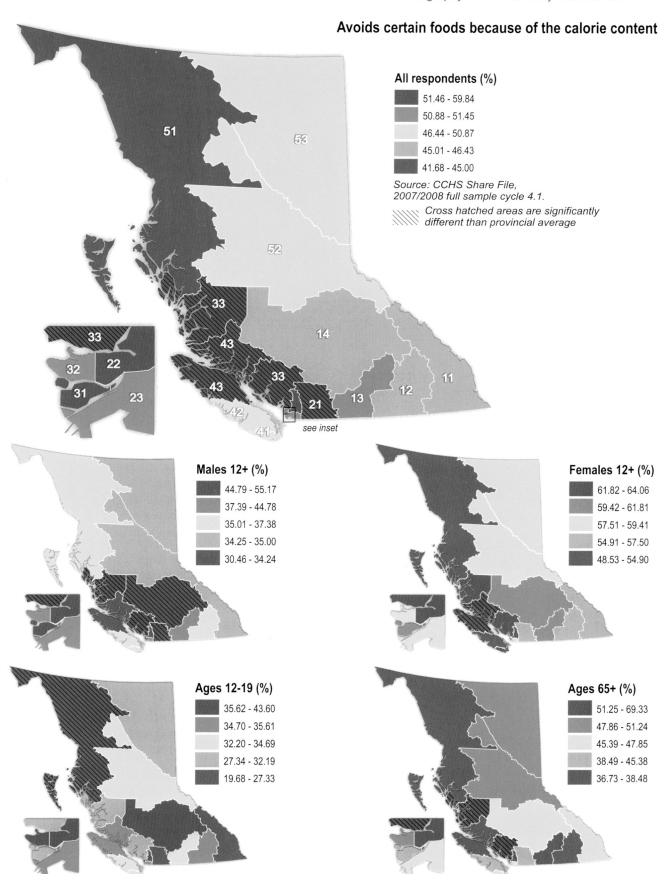

All respondents (%)

- 51.46 - 59.84
- 50.88 - 51.45
- 46.44 - 50.87
- 45.01 - 46.43
- 41.68 - 45.00

Source: CCHS Share File, 2007/2008 full sample cycle 4.1.

Cross hatched areas are significantly different than provincial average

Males 12+ (%)

- 44.79 - 55.17
- 37.39 - 44.78
- 35.01 - 37.38
- 34.25 - 35.00
- 30.46 - 34.24

Females 12+ (%)

- 61.82 - 64.06
- 59.42 - 61.81
- 57.51 - 59.41
- 54.91 - 57.50
- 48.53 - 54.90

Ages 12-19 (%)

- 35.62 - 43.60
- 34.70 - 35.61
- 32.20 - 34.69
- 27.34 - 32.19
- 19.68 - 27.33

Ages 65+ (%)

- 51.25 - 69.33
- 47.86 - 51.24
- 45.39 - 47.85
- 38.49 - 45.38
- 36.73 - 38.48

Avoids certain foods because of the cholesterol content

Health Service Delivery Area	All respondents 12+ (%)	Males 12+ (%)	Females 12+ (%)	Ages 12-19 (%)	Ages 20-64 (%)	Ages 65+ (%)
31 Richmond	58.89	53.81	63.59	26.70E†	63.21	61.15
33 North Shore/Coast Garibaldi	55.13	56.88	53.54	22.01E†	56.63	71.06‡
22 Fraser North	53.36	52.42	54.27	29.60E†	55.14	63.50
32 Vancouver	51.34	45.31*	57.22	30.75†	51.45	63.94‡
41 South Vancouver Island	49.81	45.95	53.27	29.26E†	50.99	55.75
13 Okanagan	48.35	47.45	49.19	14.42E†	48.50	65.68‡
12 Kootenay Boundary	48.19	45.58	50.85	25.15E†	50.45	53.29
51 Northwest	47.50	42.98	52.22	17.44E†	51.66	57.91
14 Thompson Cariboo Shuswap	47.01	41.63*	52.13	23.52E†	47.73	59.83‡
23 Fraser South	46.58	46.31	46.84	18.79E†	49.86	53.31
42 Central Vancouver Island	45.37	39.70	50.67	18.34E†	47.40	54.04
43 North Vancouver Island	45.12	46.29	44.05	33.21E	43.29	61.14
21 Fraser East	44.97	42.96	46.92	23.40E†	46.64	54.19
11 East Kootenay	44.37	37.99	50.59	F	46.51	51.78
52 Northern Interior	41.92	38.64	45.24	20.85E†	43.82	54.16
53 Northeast	41.64	36.90	46.54	F	46.17	39.65E
British Columbia (2007/8)	**49.26**	**46.54***	**51.85**	**23.63†**	**50.95**	**59.50‡**

No comparable 2005 data available

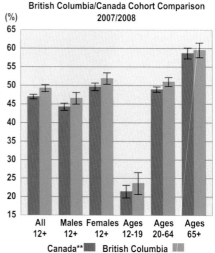

British Columbia/Canada Cohort Comparison 2007/2008

Canada** British Columbia
⊥ 95% confidence limits of estimate
**Only PE, MB, AB, BC, and NT opted for this question

Crosshatching beside the 2007/8 provincial rate indicates it is significantly different than the 2005 rate, while crosshatched HSDAs are significantly different than the 2007/8 provincial rate.
E interpret data with caution (16.67 ≤ coefficient of variation ≤ 33.3).

* Males differ significantly from females.
†12-19 age cohort differs significantly from the 20-64 age cohort.
‡ 65+ age cohort differs significantly from the 20-64 age cohort.
F data suppressed (n < 10, or coefficient of variation > 33.3).

Cholesterol is a type of fat and too much can increase the risk of heart disease and stroke. When the CCHS asked BC participants if they avoid certain foods because of cholesterol content, just under half (49.26%) responded in the affirmative. The highest percentage were in Richmond and North Shore/Coast Garibaldi (both over 55%), where respondents had significantly high values when compared to the provincial average, while Northern Interior and Northeast (both under 42%) were significantly lower.

In BC, female respondents (51.85%) were significantly more likely than males (46.54%) to avoid certain foods because of cholesterol content. Significantly fewer males than females also avoided cholesterol in Thompson Cariboo Shuswap and Vancouver. For females, Richmond (63.59%) was significantly higher while Northern Interior (45.24%) was significantly lower than the BC average for females. For males, North Shore/Coast Garibaldi (56.88%) had a significantly higher than average value, while East Kootenay, Northern Interior, and Northeast (all below 38%) were significantly lower than the provincial male average.

Avoiding foods because of the cholesterol content increased consistently with age in BC. Youth (23.63%) were significantly less likely to avoid cholesterol than the mid-age cohort. This significant difference was also apparent for all HSDAs, except North Vancouver Island. It should be noted that East Kootenay and Northeast did not have enough respondents to present data, and all other HSDAs, except Vancouver, had a small sample size, or high coefficient of variation in respondents, so results

should be interpreted with caution.

Nearly six out of every ten (59.5%) older respondents in BC indicated they avoided foods because of cholesterol – significantly more than in the mid-age cohort. Okanagan, Thompson Cariboo Shuswap, Vancouver, and North Shore/Coast Garibaldi were also significantly higher than their mid-age cohort counterparts. Comparing individual HSDAs to the provincial average for this older age cohort, only North Shore/Coast Garibaldi was significantly different, with a high value of 71.06%.

Geographically, there was a spread of more than 17 percentage points for each of the age cohorts, with the largest variation occurring in the oldest cohort. Consistently lower values were seen along the eastern border. Higher values were clustered in the lower mainland for all cohorts. Males and older respondents also had clusters of high values along the south and central coast, including the mainland regions, as well as North Vancouver Island.

No comparable data from the 2005 CCHS survey were available. For the 2007/8 sample, British Columbia respondents had consistently higher averages in every cohort than Canadian respondents, and these differences were significant for both the mid-age and all respondent cohorts. Canadian values are based on a limited number of provinces/territories; therefore, caution in interpreting these comparisons is advised.

Avoids certain foods because of the cholesterol content

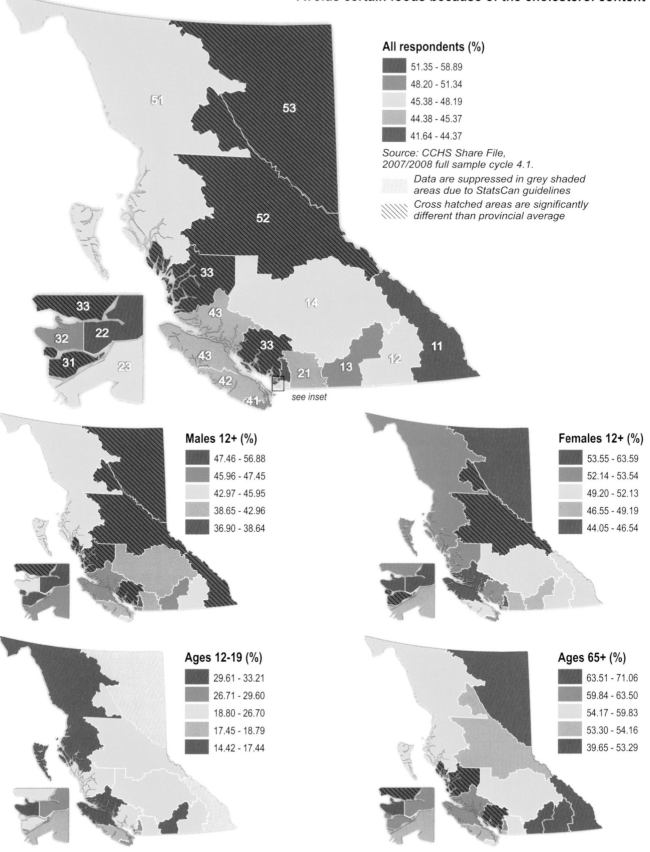

All respondents (%)

- 51.35 - 58.89
- 48.20 - 51.34
- 45.38 - 48.19
- 44.38 - 45.37
- 41.64 - 44.37

Source: CCHS Share File, 2007/2008 full sample cycle 4.1.

Data are suppressed in grey shaded areas due to StatsCan guidelines

Cross hatched areas are significantly different than provincial average

Males 12+ (%)

- 47.46 - 56.88
- 45.96 - 47.45
- 42.97 - 45.95
- 38.65 - 42.96
- 36.90 - 38.64

Females 12+ (%)

- 53.55 - 63.59
- 52.14 - 53.54
- 49.20 - 52.13
- 46.55 - 49.19
- 44.05 - 46.54

Ages 12-19 (%)

- 29.61 - 33.21
- 26.71 - 29.60
- 18.80 - 26.70
- 17.45 - 18.79
- 14.42 - 17.44

Ages 65+ (%)

- 63.51 - 71.06
- 59.84 - 63.50
- 54.17 - 59.83
- 53.30 - 54.16
- 39.65 - 53.29

Avoids certain foods because of the fat content

Health Service Delivery Area	All respondents 12+ (%)	Males 12+ (%)	Females 12+ (%)	Ages 12-19 (%)	Ages 20-64 (%)	Ages 65+ (%)
31 Richmond	74.85	65.03*	83.88	44.10†	79.32	75.04
32 Vancouver	73.92	67.04*	80.57	65.60	74.42	76.04
33 North Shore/Coast Garibaldi	73.35	70.71	75.73	41.88E†	76.88	79.21
41 South Vancouver Island	73.08	68.02*	77.64	52.94†	76.32	70.25
22 Fraser North	69.64	61.76*	77.24	51.70†	72.38	68.83
13 Okanagan	69.10	62.30*	75.52	41.00†	71.78	75.27
12 Kootenay Boundary	68.07	64.93	71.28	39.89E†	71.56	71.43
21 Fraser East	67.92	56.79*	78.72	44.68†	71.19	71.31
14 Thompson Cariboo Shuswap	67.26	56.79*	77.25	64.58	67.24	69.15
23 Fraser South	66.33	61.23*	71.21	43.62†	69.07	71.46
43 North Vancouver Island	65.98	56.87*	74.40	46.95E	68.75	67.44
52 Northern Interior	65.71	60.86	70.62	46.70†	67.65	75.20
51 Northwest	64.30	59.63	69.15	37.60E†	68.59	69.48
42 Central Vancouver Island	63.52	56.41*	70.16	49.96	65.00	66.24
11 East Kootenay	62.49	55.83	68.97	24.76E†	68.33	63.66
53 Northeast	59.16	51.64*	66.94	39.11E†	63.09	56.07
British Columbia (2007/8)	**69.25**	**62.43***	**75.75**	**48.59†**	**71.78**	**71.79**

No comparable 2005 data available

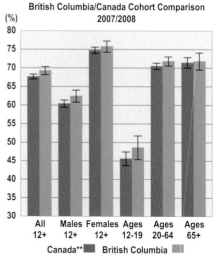

British Columbia/Canada Cohort Comparison 2007/2008

Canada** ■ British Columbia ▮
⊥ 95% confidence limits of estimate
**Only PE, MB, AB, BC, and NT opted for this question

▧ Crosshatching beside the 2007/8 provincial rate indicates it is significantly different than the 2005 rate, while crosshatched HSDAs are significantly different than the 2007/8 provincial rate.
E interpret data with caution (16.67 ≤ coefficient of variation ≤ 33.3).

* Males differ significantly from females.
†12-19 age cohort differs significantly from the 20-64 age cohort.
‡ 65+ age cohort differs significantly from the 20-64 age cohort.
F data suppressed (n < 10, or coefficient of variation > 33.3).

Consuming too much fat can make one more likely to put on weight, and a diet high in saturated fats can raise the level of cholesterol in the blood, increasing the risk of developing heart disease. Avoiding foods with a high fat content is an important wellness asset. Nearly seven out of every ten (69.25%) British Columbians responded in the affirmative when asked: *"Do you avoid certain foods because of the fat content?"* Respondents in Richmond and Vancouver (both above 73%) were significantly more likely than the provincial average to avoid certain foods based on fat content, while those in East Kootenay, Central Vancouver Island, and Northeast (all below 64%) were significantly less likely to do so.

Males (62.43%) in BC were significantly less likely than females (75.75%) to avoid food based on fat content. This significant difference between male and female respondents was evident in 11 of the 16 HSDAs. For females, compared to the provincial average, Richmond (83.88%) stood out as being significantly high, while Northeast (66.94%) was significantly low. For males, North Shore/Coast Garibaldi (70.71%) was significantly high, while Northeast (51.64%) was significantly lower than the provincial male average.

For youth in BC, 48.59% of respondents reported avoiding certain foods because of the fat content. This was significantly lower than the mid-age cohort. In fact, youth in 12 HSDAs were significantly lower than their mid-age counterparts. Compared to the provincial average for youth, respondents in Thompson Cariboo Shuswap and Vancouver were significantly higher than average, with

over 64% of respondents avoiding certain foods due to fat content, while East Kootenay (24.76%) was significantly lower. Some caution is required in interpreting the youth data because several HSDAs had small sample sizes or high coefficients of variation.

For older respondents, 71.79% indicated they avoided foods because of the fat content. This was nearly identical to the provincial average for the mid- age cohort (71.78%). No HSDA was significantly different from the provincial average for the older age cohort.

Geographically, there was a spread of more than 15 percentage points in all age cohorts, with the largest variation occurring in the youth cohort (over 40 percentage points). For the all respondents cohort, there was a cluster of lower values in the three northernmost HSDAs and a cluster of higher values in the southwest, including South Vancouver Island and most of the lower mainland. Similar patterns were evident with the female cohort, but other cohorts did not have any notable geographic patterns.

No comparable data were available from the 2005 CCHS survey. While British Columbian respondents had consistently higher values than their Canadian counterparts for all cohorts for the 2007/8 samples, none of these differences were significant. Canadian values are based on a limited number of provinces/territories; therefore, caution in interpreting these comparisons is advised.

Avoids certain foods because of the fat content

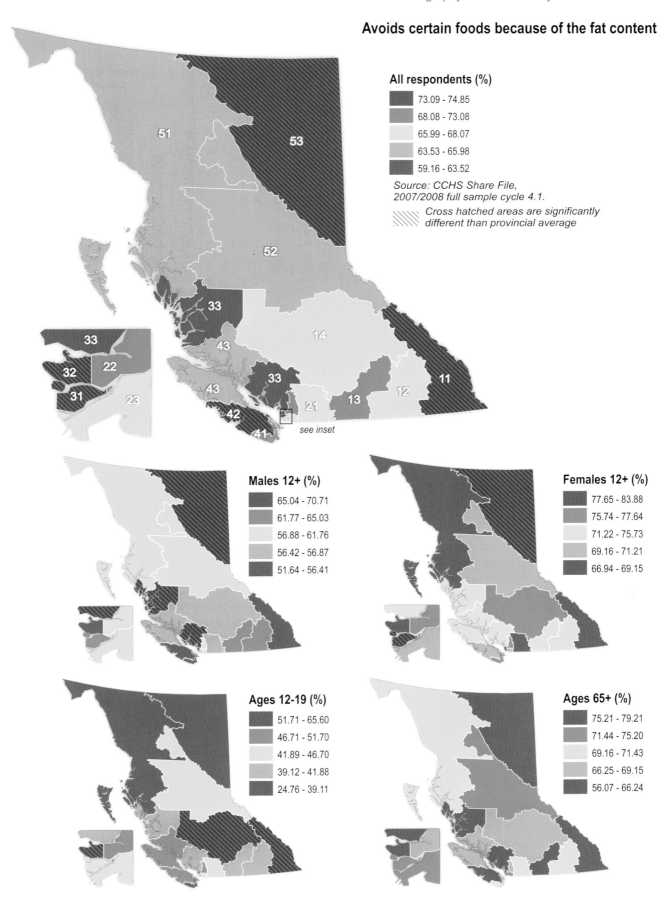

All respondents (%)

- 73.09 - 74.85
- 68.08 - 73.08
- 65.99 - 68.07
- 63.53 - 65.98
- 59.16 - 63.52

Source: CCHS Share File, 2007/2008 full sample cycle 4.1.

Cross hatched areas are significantly different than provincial average

Males 12+ (%)

- 65.04 - 70.71
- 61.77 - 65.03
- 56.88 - 61.76
- 56.42 - 56.87
- 51.64 - 56.41

Females 12+ (%)

- 77.65 - 83.88
- 75.74 - 77.64
- 71.22 - 75.73
- 69.16 - 71.21
- 66.94 - 69.15

Ages 12-19 (%)

- 51.71 - 65.60
- 46.71 - 51.70
- 41.89 - 46.70
- 39.12 - 41.88
- 24.76 - 39.11

Ages 65+ (%)

- 75.21 - 79.21
- 71.44 - 75.20
- 69.16 - 71.43
- 66.25 - 69.15
- 56.07 - 66.24

Chooses certain foods because of the low fat content

Health Service Delivery Area	All respondents 12+ (%)	Males 12+ (%)	Females 12+ (%)	Ages 12-19 (%)	Ages 20-64 (%)	Ages 65+ (%)
41 South Vancouver Island	71.39	65.90*	76.37	38.88†	75.66	70.92
33 North Shore/Coast Garibaldi	70.97	68.71	73.01	30.84E†	75.14	79.98
13 Okanagan	70.47	63.79*	76.75	39.34†	72.73	79.62
32 Vancouver	70.02	65.02*	74.85	51.49†	71.80	70.50
31 Richmond	68.63	63.43	73.45	35.64E†	72.90	71.74
12 Kootenay Boundary	67.40	61.14	73.80	39.76E†	72.19	65.21
42 Central Vancouver Island	67.10	61.43	72.37	51.06	69.61	67.69
22 Fraser North	66.44	59.96*	72.69	53.70	68.45	65.50
14 Thompson Cariboo Shuswap	65.63	56.78*	74.13	52.59	67.63	65.56
23 Fraser South	65.47	59.86*	70.86	31.76†	70.40	68.26
51 Northwest	64.54	58.12	71.22	36.75E†	69.15	69.02
21 Fraser East	64.27	53.06*	75.16	43.74†	66.44	70.47
11 East Kootenay	64.18	56.38*	71.77	39.53E†	67.49	67.10
43 North Vancouver Island	63.61	55.66	71.00	48.99E	64.38	70.50
52 Northern Interior	62.46	55.23*	69.81	42.50†	63.69	77.88‡
53 Northeast	60.63	53.04*	68.47	40.11E†	63.94	63.51
British Columbia (2007/8)	**67.46**	**61.22***	**73.41**	**42.71†**	**70.43**	**70.77**
No comparable 2005 data available						

Crosshatching beside the 2007/8 provincial rate indicates it is significantly different than the 2005 rate, while crosshatched HSDAs are significantly different than the 2007/8 provincial rate.
E interpret data with caution (16.67 ≤ coefficient of variation ≤ 33.3).

* Males differ significantly from females.
†12-19 age cohort differs significantly from the 20-64 age cohort.
‡ 65+ age cohort differs significantly from the 20-64 age cohort.
F data suppressed (n < 10, or coefficient of variation > 33.3).

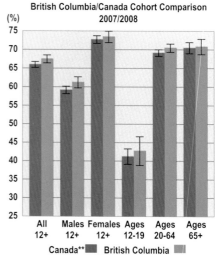

British Columbia/Canada Cohort Comparison 2007/2008

Canada** ■ British Columbia ■
⊥ 95% confidence limits of estimate
**Only PE, MB, AB, BC, and NT opted for this question

While the previous indicator looked at the avoidance of certain food because of fat content, another CCHS question asked participants if they consciously chose certain foods because of the low fat content. Choosing food with a low fat content can lead to a healthier diet and is an important wellness asset. In BC, 67.46% of respondents chose certain foods because of the low fat content. Northeast (60.63%) was the only HSDA with significantly fewer than average respondents who chose foods based on a low fat content.

Consistent with the previous indicator, males (61.22%) were significantly less likely than females (73.41%) to choose foods because of low fat content. This trend of significantly lower values for males was evident in 10 of 16 HSDAs. Compared to the provincial average, males in North Shore/Coast Garibaldi (68.71%) had a significantly high value, while those in Fraser East (53.06%) were significantly lower. For females, no HSDAs were significantly different from the provincial average.

For youth in BC, 42.71% of respondents chose foods because of the low fat content. This was significantly lower than the mid-age cohort. This significant difference was also evident in 12 HSDAs, but it should be noted that six HSDAs had small sample sizes or high coefficients of variation, and caution in interpretation is required.

Among older respondents, 70.77% reported choosing certain foods because of the low fat content. The Northern Interior was the only HSDA with a significantly higher value for older respondents compared to the mid-age cohort. Comparing HSDA rates to the provincial average

for older respondents, North Shore/Coast Garibaldi (79.98%) was significantly higher.

Geographically, there was a spread of more than 10 percentage points for each age cohort, with the largest variation seen in the youth cohort (more than 22 percentage points). The patterns for this indicator were very similar to those seen in the avoidance of fatty food indicator, with a notable grouping of lower values in the three northernmost regions for all respondents and females, and a wide range of spatial variability in high and low scores among the various cohorts.

No comparable data were available from the 2005 CCHS survey. There were no significant differences between the national and provincial values for this variable for the 2007/8 survey for any of the cohorts. Canadian values are based on a limited number of provinces/territories; therefore, caution in interpreting these comparisons is advised.

Chooses certain foods because of the low fat content

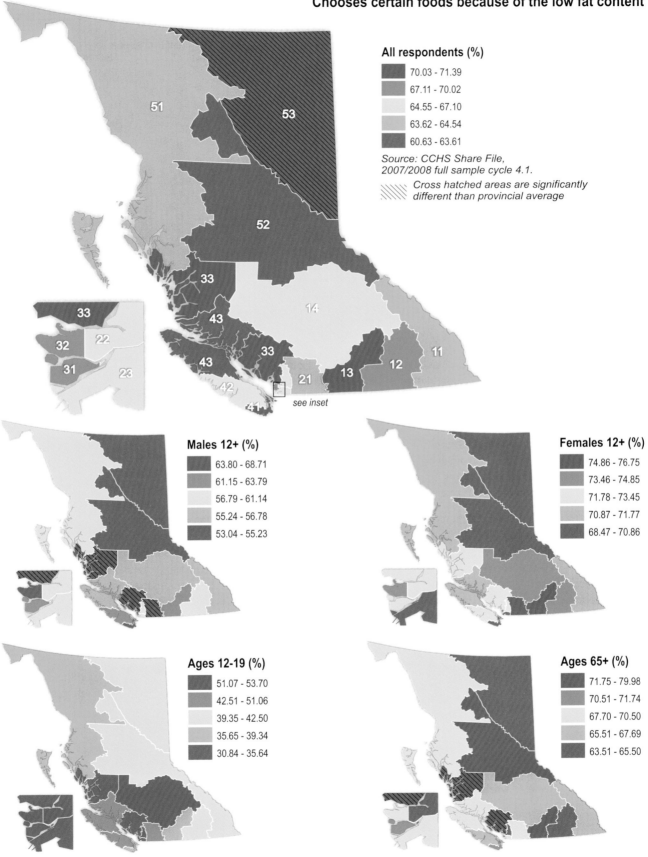

All respondents (%)

- 70.03 - 71.39
- 67.11 - 70.02
- 64.55 - 67.10
- 63.62 - 64.54
- 60.63 - 63.61

*Source: CCHS Share File,
2007/2008 full sample cycle 4.1.*

*Cross hatched areas are significantly
different than provincial average*

Males 12+ (%)

- 63.80 - 68.71
- 61.15 - 63.79
- 56.79 - 61.14
- 55.24 - 56.78
- 53.04 - 55.23

Females 12+ (%)

- 74.86 - 76.75
- 73.46 - 74.85
- 71.78 - 73.45
- 70.87 - 71.77
- 68.47 - 70.86

Ages 12-19 (%)

- 51.07 - 53.70
- 42.51 - 51.06
- 39.35 - 42.50
- 35.65 - 39.34
- 30.84 - 35.64

Ages 65+ (%)

- 71.75 - 79.98
- 70.51 - 71.74
- 67.70 - 70.50
- 65.51 - 67.69
- 63.51 - 65.50

Avoids certain foods because of the salt content

Health Service Delivery Area	All respondents 12+ (%)	Males 12+ (%)	Females 12+ (%)	Ages 12-19 (%)	Ages 20-64 (%)	Ages 65+ (%)
31 Richmond	59.44	52.24*	66.06	26.92E†	62.81	66.96
33 North Shore/Coast Garibaldi	58.02	53.84*	61.79	16.34E†	60.28	76.51‡
41 South Vancouver Island	52.87	44.45*	60.48	25.31E†	52.61	68.74‡
32 Vancouver	52.63	48.07*	57.06	34.95†	52.77	63.08
11 East Kootenay	52.06	40.22*	63.64	31.10E†	51.76	68.06‡
42 Central Vancouver Island	51.93	48.21	55.41	20.90E†	54.34	61.58
22 Fraser North	51.86	45.74*	57.78	26.82E†	53.60	63.44
14 Thompson Cariboo Shuswap	51.72	41.31*	61.59	27.28E†	53.72	59.61
13 Okanagan	51.59	47.64	55.31	20.37E†	50.24	72.50‡
12 Kootenay Boundary	51.56	43.94	59.33	24.39E†	52.93	62.73
43 North Vancouver Island	50.14	44.98	54.89	32.43E	50.21	62.05
23 Fraser South	49.87	45.32	54.23	24.29E†	50.72	68.29‡
21 Fraser East	49.39	43.37	55.24	25.92E†	50.22	63.91‡
52 Northern Interior	48.62	39.76*	57.58	26.71E†	49.85	66.58‡
51 Northwest	47.17	37.50*	57.24	13.59E†	51.59	60.17
53 Northeast	43.43	33.11*	54.03	F	46.51	51.36
British Columbia (2007/8)	**51.94**	**45.93***	**57.68**	**25.38†**	**52.96**	**66.23‡**
No comparable 2005 data available						

⬚ Crosshatching beside the 2007/8 provincial rate indicates it is significantly different than the 2005 rate, while crosshatched HSDAs are significantly different than the 2007/8 provincial rate.
E interpret data with caution (16.67 ≤ coefficient of variation ≤ 33.3).

* Males differ significantly from females.
† 12-19 age cohort differs significantly from the 20-64 age cohort.
‡ 65+ age cohort differs significantly from the 20-64 age cohort.
F data suppressed (n < 10, or coefficient of variation > 33.3).

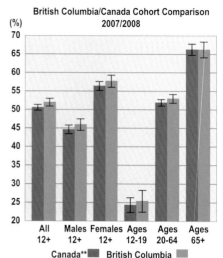

British Columbia/Canada Cohort Comparison 2007/2008

Canada**■   British Columbia ■
⊥ 95% confidence limits of estimate
**Only PE, MB, AB, BC, and NT opted for this question

Excessive salt intake can raise blood pressure increasing the risk of heart disease and stroke. Avoiding foods with a high salt content can lead to a healthier diet and is an important wellness asset. The CCHS asked: *"Do you avoid certain foods because of the salt content?"* Over half (51.94%) of those questioned in BC responded in the affirmative. Richmond and North Shore/Coast Garibaldi, both with values above 58%, had significantly more respondents who avoided foods because of the salt content, while Northeast (43.43%) had significantly fewer.

Males (45.93%) in BC were significantly less likely than their female counterparts (57.68%) to avoid salty foods. This significant difference was also seen in nine individual HSDAs. Males in North Shore/Coast Garibaldi (53.84%) were significantly more likely than the provincial male average to avoid foods because of the salt content, while those in Northeast (33.11%) were significantly less likely.

Avoiding food because of the salt content increased consistently with age. Youth (25.38%) in BC were significantly less likely than the mid-age cohort to avoid salty foods. This significant difference was reflected in all HSDAs where appropriate data were available, except North Vancouver Island; however, caution in interpreting these results is required as the sample sizes for nearly all HSDAs in the youth cohort were small. Northwest (13.59%) was the only HSDA that was significantly lower than the youth provincial average.

Among older respondents, 66.23% avoided salty foods, which was significantly more than the mid-age cohort. There were seven HSDAs in which older respondents

were significantly more likely than their mid-age counterparts to avoid foods because of the salt content. Compared to the provincial average for this cohort, respondents in North Shore/Coast Garibaldi (76.51%) were significantly more likely to avoid salty foods, while those in Northeast (51.36%) were significantly less likely to do so.

Geographically, there was a spread of over 16 percentage points for all age cohorts, with both the youth and older cohorts having spreads of over 21 percentage points. Excluding the youth cohort, Northeast had a low value of salt avoidance among all cohorts, while North Shore/Coast Garibaldi had consistently higher values for all cohorts. Generally, lower values of salt avoidance were seen in the northern regions, while higher values were seen in the south and central coastal and lower mainland HSDAs and in various HSDAs in the southern interior.

There were no comparable data available from the 2005 CCHS survey. For the 2007/8 samples, BC respondents and their Canadian peers had similar values for all cohorts. Canadian values are based on a limited number of provinces/territories; therefore, caution in interpreting these comparisons is advised.

Avoids certain foods because of the salt content

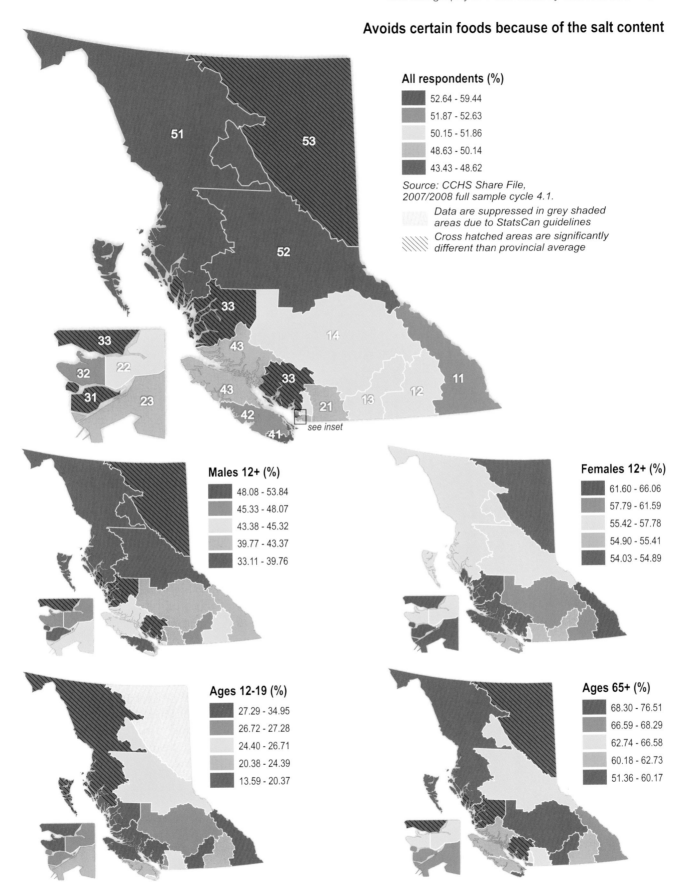

All respondents (%)

- 52.64 - 59.44
- 51.87 - 52.63
- 50.15 - 51.86
- 48.63 - 50.14
- 43.43 - 48.62

Source: CCHS Share File, 2007/2008 full sample cycle 4.1.

Data are suppressed in grey shaded areas due to StatsCan guidelines

Cross hatched areas are significantly different than provincial average

Males 12+ (%)

- 48.08 - 53.84
- 45.33 - 48.07
- 43.38 - 45.32
- 39.77 - 43.37
- 33.11 - 39.76

Females 12+ (%)

- 61.60 - 66.06
- 57.79 - 61.59
- 55.42 - 57.78
- 54.90 - 55.41
- 54.03 - 54.89

Ages 12-19 (%)

- 27.29 - 34.95
- 26.72 - 27.28
- 24.40 - 26.71
- 20.38 - 24.39
- 13.59 - 20.37

Ages 65+ (%)

- 68.30 - 76.51
- 66.59 - 68.29
- 62.74 - 66.58
- 60.18 - 62.73
- 51.36 - 60.17

Avoids foods for content reasons

Health Service Delivery Area	All respondents 12+ (%)	Males 12+ (%)	Females 12+ (%)	Ages 12-19 (%)	Ages 20-64 (%)	Ages 65+ (%)
32 Vancouver	84.74	80.05*	89.30	75.68	85.74	84.07
41 South Vancouver Island	83.80	76.85*	90.06	62.99†	86.23	84.74
31 Richmond	83.75	76.80*	90.13	58.73†	87.58	82.62
12 Kootenay Boundary	82.80	75.93*	89.81	57.55E†	86.07	85.23
43 North Vancouver Island	82.79	73.12*	91.73	68.36	84.25	86.61
33 North Shore/Coast Garibaldi	82.64	79.53	85.46	53.46†	86.03	87.60
42 Central Vancouver Island	79.34	74.40	83.96	60.10†	82.59	79.07
13 Okanagan	78.84	74.00*	83.41	54.30†	79.81	88.66‡
22 Fraser North	78.56	72.72*	84.22	63.17†	80.07	83.03
21 Fraser East	78.53	69.69*	87.14	51.80†	81.44	86.22
14 Thompson Cariboo Shuswap	78.46	68.79*	87.64	69.63	79.33	80.67
23 Fraser South	78.00	71.79*	83.95	54.81†	80.73	83.62
52 Northern Interior	76.40	71.59	81.26	57.66†	77.88	88.72‡
51 Northwest	75.38	68.04*	83.03	44.89†	80.41	80.53
11 East Kootenay	74.43	64.87*	83.74	42.94E†	77.97	81.11
53 Northeast	68.13	58.60*	77.92	48.45E	71.12	72.62
British Columbia (2007/8)	**80.21**	**74.02***	**86.12**	**59.74†**	**82.42**	**84.21**

No comparable 2005 data available

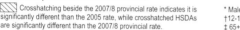 Crosshatching beside the 2007/8 provincial rate indicates it is significantly different than the 2005 rate, while crosshatched HSDAs are significantly different than the 2007/8 provincial rate.
E interpret data with caution (16.67 ≤ coefficient of variation ≤ 33.3)

* Males differ significantly from females.
† 12-19 age cohort differs significantly from the 20-64 age cohort.
‡ 65+ age cohort differs significantly from the 20-64 age cohort.
F data suppressed (n < 10, or coefficient of variation > 33.3).

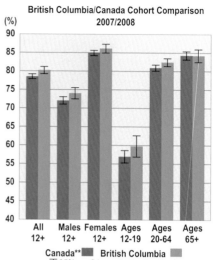

British Columbia/Canada Cohort Comparison 2007/2008

Canada** ■   British Columbia ▨
⊥ 95% confidence limits of estimate
**Only PE, MB, AB, BC, and NT opted for this question

A healthy diet is integral to the achievement of overall good health and well-being. This indicator is based on the preceding questions related to food content. The following represents the percentage of respondents who avoided foods for one or more content reasons.

More than eight out of every ten (80.21%) British Columbians indicated they avoided certain food for one or more content reasons. Respondents in Vancouver and South Vancouver Island (both above 83%) were significantly more likely than the provincial average to avoid foods for content reasons. Meanwhile, East Kootenay and Northeast (both less than 75%) were significantly less likely to do so.

Females (86.12%) were significantly more likely than males (74.02%) to avoid foods for content reasons. This significant difference was also seen in 13 of the 16 HSDAs. For males, Vancouver (80.05%) was significantly higher than the provincial male average, while East Kootenay (64.87%) and Northeast (58.6%) were significantly lower. For females, respondents in North and South Vancouver Island (both above 90%) were significantly more likely than their female peers provincially to avoid certain foods for content reasons, while those in Northeast (77.92%) were significantly less likely.

Youth were by far the least likely group in the province to avoid foods for content reasons, with only 59.74% indicating they avoided certain foods. This was significantly lower than the mid-age group. This significant difference from the mid-age cohort was seen in all but four HSDAs. Provincially, Vancouver (75.68%) was the only

HSDA with a significantly higher value than the youth provincial average.

For older respondents, 84.21% avoided certain foods for content reasons. At the provincial level, there was no significant difference from the mid-age group; however at the HSDA level, both Okanagan and Northern Interior were significantly more likely than their mid-age counterparts to avoid certain foods.

Geographically, there was a spread of 16 or more percentage points in each age cohort, with the largest variation occurring in the youth cohort (32 percentage points). For all cohorts, lower values of food avoidance were seen in the northern and interior areas of the province, with a few exceptions. Higher values tended to be concentrated in the south and particularly in the southwest regions of the province.

No comparable data from the 2005 CCHS survey were available. Compared to the national average for this variable, British Columbians in all cohorts were more likely to avoid foods for content reasons; however, the only significant difference was seen in the all respondents cohort. Canadian values are based on a limited number of provinces/territories; therefore, caution in interpreting these comparisons is advised.

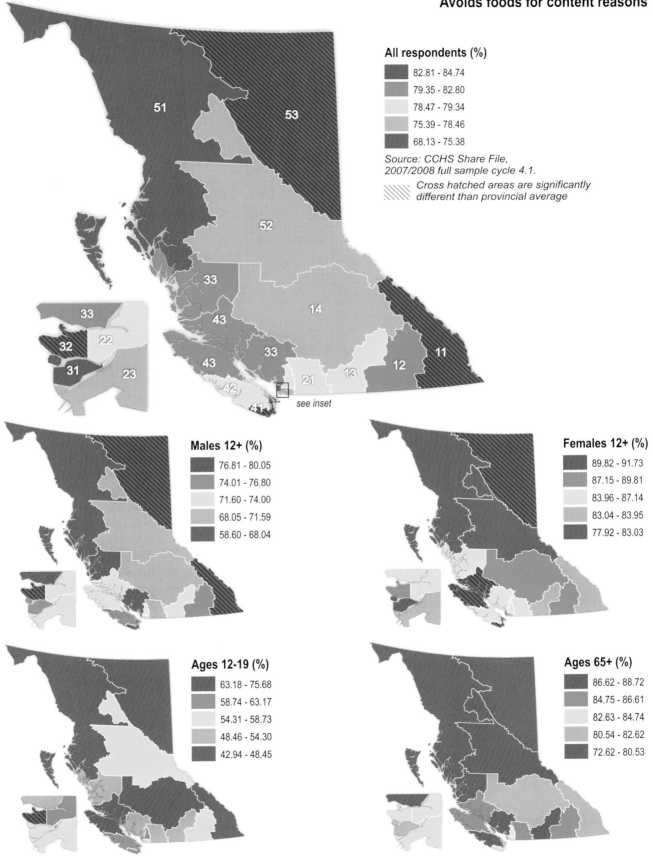

Avoids foods for content reasons

All respondents (%)

- 82.81 - 84.74
- 79.35 - 82.80
- 78.47 - 79.34
- 75.39 - 78.46
- 68.13 - 75.38

*Source: CCHS Share File,
2007/2008 full sample cycle 4.1.*

*Cross hatched areas are significantly
different than provincial average*

Males 12+ (%)

- 76.81 - 80.05
- 74.01 - 76.80
- 71.60 - 74.00
- 68.05 - 71.59
- 58.60 - 68.04

Females 12+ (%)

- 89.82 - 91.73
- 87.15 - 89.81
- 83.96 - 87.14
- 83.04 - 83.95
- 77.92 - 83.03

Ages 12-19 (%)

- 63.18 - 75.68
- 58.74 - 63.17
- 54.31 - 58.73
- 48.46 - 54.30
- 42.94 - 48.45

Ages 65+ (%)

- 86.62 - 88.72
- 84.75 - 86.61
- 82.63 - 84.74
- 80.54 - 82.62
- 72.62 - 80.53

Eats fruits and vegetables five or more times or servings a day

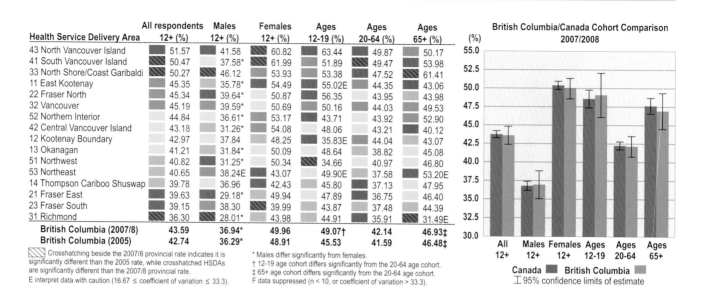

Health Service Delivery Area	All respondents 12+ (%)	Males 12+ (%)	Females 12+ (%)	Ages 12-19 (%)	Ages 20-64 (%)	Ages 65+ (%)
43 North Vancouver Island	51.57	41.58	60.82	63.44	49.87	50.17
41 South Vancouver Island	50.47	37.58*	61.99	51.89	49.47	53.98
33 North Shore/Coast Garibaldi	50.27	46.12	53.93	53.38	47.52	61.41
11 East Kootenay	45.35	35.78*	54.49	55.02E	44.35	43.06
22 Fraser North	45.34	39.64*	50.87	56.35	43.95	43.98
32 Vancouver	45.19	39.59*	50.69	50.16	44.03	49.53
52 Northern Interior	44.84	36.61*	53.17	43.71	43.92	52.90
42 Central Vancouver Island	43.18	31.26*	54.08	48.06	43.21	40.12
12 Kootenay Boundary	42.97	37.84	48.25	35.83E	44.04	43.07
13 Okanagan	41.21	31.84*	50.09	48.64	38.82	45.08
51 Northwest	40.82	31.25*	50.34	34.66	40.97	46.80
53 Northeast	40.65	38.24E	43.07	49.90E	37.58	53.20E
14 Thompson Cariboo Shuswap	39.78	36.96	42.43	45.80	37.13	47.95
21 Fraser East	39.63	29.18*	49.94	47.89	36.75	46.40
23 Fraser South	39.15	38.30	39.99	43.87	37.48	44.39
31 Richmond	36.30	28.01*	43.98	44.91	35.91	31.49E
British Columbia (2007/8)	**43.59**	**36.94***	**49.96**	**49.07†**	**42.14**	**46.93‡**
British Columbia (2005)	**42.74**	**36.29***	**48.91**	**45.53**	**41.59**	**46.48‡**

▨ Crosshatching beside the 2007/8 provincial rate indicates it is significantly different than the 2005 rate, while crosshatched HSDAs are significantly different than the 2007/8 provincial rate.
E interpret data with caution (16.67 ≤ coefficient of variation ≤ 33.3).

* Males differ significantly from females.
† 12-19 age cohort differs significantly from the 20-64 age cohort.
‡ 65+ age cohort differs significantly from the 20-64 age cohort.
F data suppressed (n < 10, or coefficient of variation > 33.3).

British Columbia/Canada Cohort Comparison 2007/2008

Canada ■ British Columbia ▦
⊥ 95% confidence limits of estimate

Canadian nutrition guidelines recommend a high intake of fruits and vegetables to maintain a healthy diet. The CCHS asked participants to indicate the number of times per day they consumed fruits and vegetables. The following presents respondents who ate fruits and vegetables five or more times or servings daily – indicating a healthy intake of fruits and vegetables.

More than four in every ten (43.59%) British Columbians reported they ate fruits and vegetables five or more times daily. Respondents in South Vancouver Island and North Shore/Coast Garibaldi (both over 50%) were significantly more likely to consume a healthy amount of fruits and vegetables, while Richmond (36.30%) consumed significantly lower than the provincial average.

Healthy fruit and vegetable consumption for males and females showed a clear difference between the genders. At the provincial level, 49.96% of females had a healthy fruit and vegetable intake, significantly higher than their male counterparts (36.94%). This significant difference was also found in 10 HSDAs.

For males, healthy fruit and vegetable consumption ranged from a significant high of 46.12% for North Shore/Coast Garibaldi to a significant low of 28.01% in Richmond. For females, North and South Vancouver Island had significantly high values (both over 60%) of healthy fruit and vegetable consumption, while Fraser South (39.99%) was significantly lower than the provincial average for female respondents.

Within BC, 49.07% of youth respondents reported a

healthy consumption of fruits and vegetables, significantly higher than the provincial average for the mid-age cohort, but there were no significant differences between youth and the mid-age cohort for any individual HSDA. Northwest (34.66%) was significantly lower than the provincial average for the youth cohort.

For older respondents, 46.93% reported a healthy intake of fruits and vegetables. This was significantly higher than the provincial average for the mid-age cohort, but there were no significant differences between older respondents and the mid-age cohort for any individual HSDA. Healthy fruit and vegetable consumption for North Shore/Coast Garibaldi (61.41%) was significantly higher, while Richmond (31.49%) was significantly lower than the provincial average for older respondents.

There was a 15 to 20 percentage point spread among HSDAs. Geographically, parts of the southern lower mainland had low levels, while parts of Vancouver Island and North Shore/Coast Garibaldi had higher than average levels of healthy fruit and vegetable consumption.

There were no significant differences for BC respondents between 2005 and 2007/8. In comparison to the national average, British Columbians had very similar levels of fruit and vegetable consumption for all cohorts in 2007/8.

Eats fruits and vegetables five or more times or servings a day

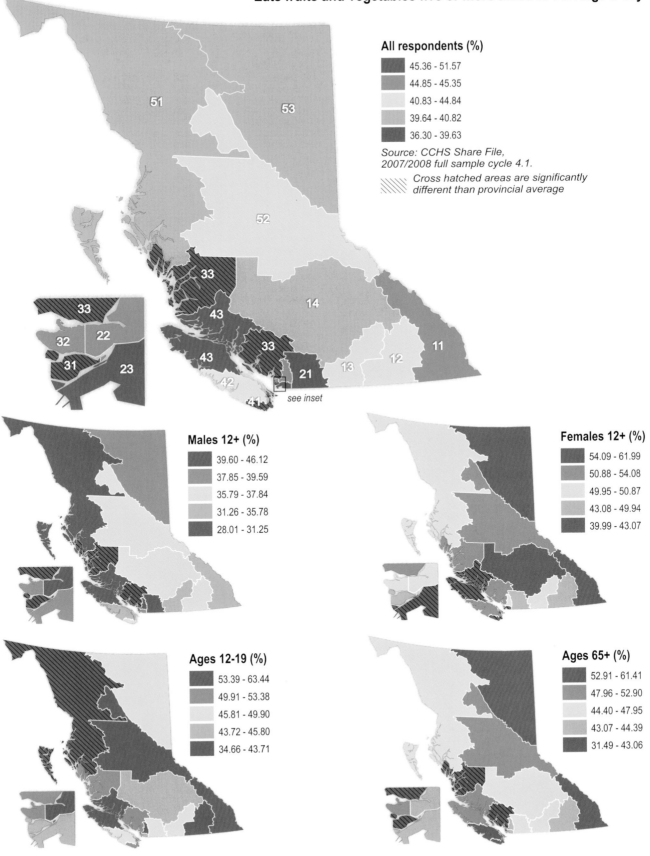

All respondents (%)

- 45.36 - 51.57
- 44.85 - 45.35
- 40.83 - 44.84
- 39.64 - 40.82
- 36.30 - 39.63

Source: CCHS Share File, 2007/2008 full sample cycle 4.1.

Cross hatched areas are significantly different than provincial average

Males 12+ (%)

- 39.60 - 46.12
- 37.85 - 39.59
- 35.79 - 37.84
- 31.26 - 35.78
- 28.01 - 31.25

Females 12+ (%)

- 54.09 - 61.99
- 50.88 - 54.08
- 49.95 - 50.87
- 43.08 - 49.94
- 39.99 - 43.07

Ages 12-19 (%)

- 53.39 - 63.44
- 49.91 - 53.38
- 45.81 - 49.90
- 43.72 - 45.80
- 34.66 - 43.71

Ages 65+ (%)

- 52.91 - 61.41
- 47.96 - 52.90
- 44.40 - 47.95
- 43.07 - 44.39
- 31.49 - 43.06

Students eating five or more servings of fruits and vegetables in the past 24 hours

The Student Satisfaction Survey asked students about their nutritious eating patterns, and provides some more detail than the CCHS question on the previous page. The table and maps provide results from the 2008/9 survey for those who indicated they had five or more servings of fruits and vegetables in the previous 24 hours.

All students grade 7

Overall, 47.38% of grade 7 students in 2008/9 responded that they had five or more servings of fruits and vegetables in the previous 24 hours. Results among school districts varied substantially: less than 30% of students in Central Coast and Fort Nelson compared with more than 60% of students in Stikine and Revelstoke responded that they had five or more servings in the previous 24 hours. Much of the central interior, north, and coastal parts of BC had below average values, while there was a dominant cluster of well above average values in the southeast.

All students grade 10

Four in every ten students (40.72%) had five or more servings of fruits and vegetables in the previous 24 hours. Less than three in every ten student respondents in Stikine, Nicola-Similkameen, Nisga'a, and Peace River South compared with five in every ten students in Central Coast, West Vancouver, Sunshine Coast, and Revelstoke reported five or more servings. Most of the north, with the exception of Fort Nelson, and interior, as well as some school districts in the lower mainland had below average values, while higher values were clustered in the southwest of the province, north of the Fraser River, and southern part of Vancouver Island.

All students grade 12

While the average for this grade was 38.93%, half or more of the students in Arrow Lakes, North Okanagan-Shuswap, and Gulf Islands responded that they had five or more servings of fruits and vegetables in the past 24 hours. At the other extreme, one-third or less of students in Central Coast, Vancouver Island West, Peace River North, Nechako Lakes, Cariboo-Chilcotin, and Mission did so. Much of the north and interior of BC had lower than average values, while above average values were clustered in the southeast, south coast, and south Vancouver Island regions of the province.

School District	All students grade 7 (%)	All students grade 10 (%)	All students grade 12 (%)
87 Stikine	63.64	26.67	Msk
19 Revelstoke	61.96	50.75	39.02
63 Saanich	54.23	49.78	45.33
10 Arrow Lakes	53.49	40.98	52.17
6 Rocky Mountain	53.33	40.82	35.06
28 Quesnel	52.65	37.41	37.50
69 Qualicum	52.38	45.54	46.12
23 Central Okanagan	52.06	43.76	43.34
46 Sunshine Coast	51.70	50.55	42.31
35 Langley	51.44	37.94	37.70
8 Kootenay Lake	50.79	41.55	45.74
68 Nanaimo-Ladysmith	50.78	40.63	39.25
38 Richmond	50.72	39.22	34.95
45 West Vancouver	50.55	50.00	46.19
62 Sooke	50.44	43.66	40.65
5 Southeast Kootenay	50.00	43.20	36.08
75 Mission	49.66	41.94	33.33
54 Bulkley Valley	49.18	39.23	37.50
67 Okanagan Skaha	49.07	41.75	40.74
41 Burnaby	48.95	39.68	36.49
42 Maple Ridge-Pitt Meadows	48.63	41.66	37.85
37 Delta	48.47	41.45	42.59
40 New Westminster	48.40	45.72	40.96
58 Nicola-Similkameen	48.40	27.16	37.50
44 North Vancouver	48.07	46.27	44.33
39 Vancouver	48.00	38.96	35.05
61 Greater Victoria	47.97	46.97	45.66
43 Coquitlam	47.61	45.16	41.68
73 Kamloops/Thompson	47.23	44.23	38.80
48 Howe Sound	47.16	42.74	44.94
71 Comox Valley	46.95	44.63	44.44
22 Vernon	46.79	40.10	36.55
34 Abbotsford	46.66	36.18	36.63
50 Haida Gwaii/Queen Charlotte	46.43	32.50	45.45
36 Surrey	46.18	36.46	34.73
92 Nisga'a	46.15	23.08	Msk
27 Cariboo-Chilcotin	45.82	35.76	33.17
70 Alberni	45.21	33.33	35.48
59 Peace River South	44.74	29.60	37.16
20 Kootenay-Columbia	43.56	40.07	42.26
91 Nechako Lakes	43.30	37.97	32.59
33 Chilliwack	43.12	42.45	39.58
74 Gold Trail	42.71	41.58	41.33
83 North Okanagan-Shuswap	42.62	42.93	50.00
82 Coast Mountains	42.49	37.32	38.52
52 Prince Rupert	41.35	40.31	33.94
51 Boundary	41.18	33.78	32.14
79 Cowichan Valley	41.17	38.86	42.29
47 Powell River	40.14	42.59	41.12
72 Campbell River	39.55	41.09	38.46
57 Prince George	38.76	38.70	35.56
78 Fraser-Cascade	38.06	40.00	38.38
60 Peace River North	38.03	36.79	30.05
85 Vancouver Island North	37.17	40.00	41.98
53 Okanagan Similkameen	36.07	30.57	42.52
64 Gulf Islands	35.11	44.83	51.14
84 Vancouver Island West	32.00	31.82	32.35
81 Fort Nelson	29.17	45.10	36.67
49 Central Coast	23.08	53.33	30.00
British Columbia	**47.38**	**40.72**	**38.93**

Msk: Data masked for privacy

Students eating five or more servings of fruits and vegetables in the past 24 hours

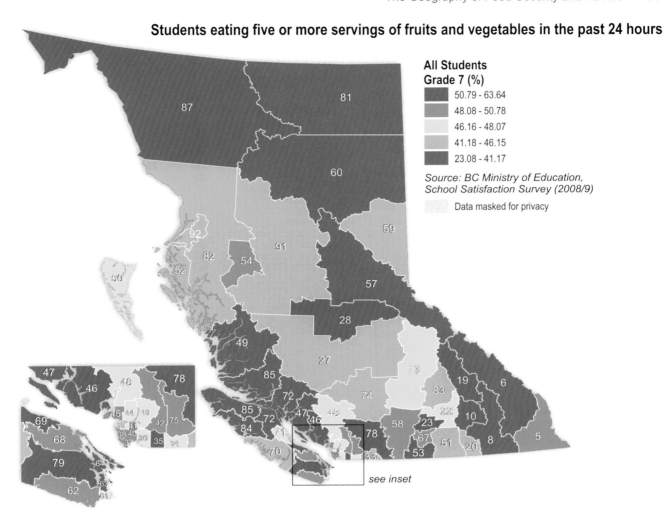

**All Students
Grade 7 (%)**
- 50.79 - 63.64
- 48.08 - 50.78
- 46.16 - 48.07
- 41.18 - 46.15
- 23.08 - 41.17

*Source: BC Ministry of Education,
School Satisfaction Survey (2008/9)*

Data masked for privacy

see inset

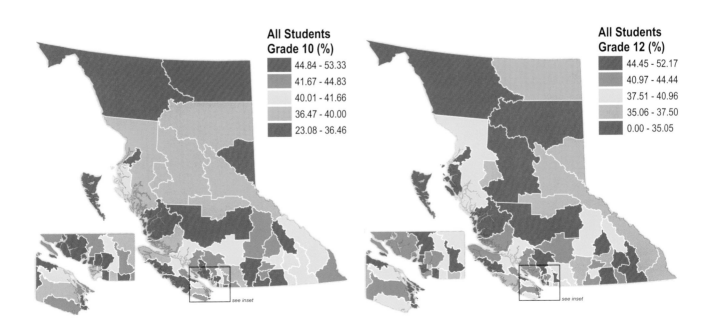

**All Students
Grade 10 (%)**
- 44.84 - 53.33
- 41.67 - 44.83
- 40.01 - 41.66
- 36.47 - 40.00
- 23.08 - 36.46

**All Students
Grade 12 (%)**
- 44.45 - 52.17
- 40.97 - 44.44
- 37.51 - 40.96
- 35.06 - 37.50
- 0.00 - 35.05

Youth who always eat breakfast on school days

Breakfast is viewed as the most important meal of the day, and is particularly so for young people. It prepares them to be able to concentrate and focus in the school setting, thus improving their ability to learn and comprehend.

The McCreary AHS IV asked the question *"How often do you eat breakfast on school days? Never, sometimes, always."* On average, 52.66% of BC student respondents indicated that they always ate breakfast on school days. This percentage was significantly higher than in 2003, when less than half the students (49.56%) indicated they always had breakfast on school days. There was a range of over 10 percentage points between the highest and lowest HSDAs, much bigger than the 6 percentage range evident in 2003. Student respondents in North Shore/Coast Garibaldi (58.03%) were significantly more likely, while those in Northern Interior (46.80%) were significantly less likely than the provincial average to always have breakfast on school days.

There were significant differences between genders. The provincial average for male student respondents was 57.13%, compared to only 48.58% for female respondents. This gender difference was consistent for every HSDA, and the difference was significant for eight of the individual HSDAs. The biggest difference, which was also significant, was in Okanagan, where there was a 15 percentage point spread between male and female students.

Among male students, the range in responses went from a high of 62.48% in Okanagan to a low of 52.40% in Northern Interior. Two HSDAs, Okanagan and South Vancouver Island (61.65%), were significantly higher than the provincial average for male students. At nearly 15 percentage points, the range in responses among HSDAs for female students was much higher than that for male students. North Shore/Coast Garibaldi (55.53%) was significantly higher than the provincial average for female students, while Northern Interior (41.03%) was significantly lower.

Throughout the province, students in South Vancouver Island and the urban lower mainland HSDAs, with the exception of Fraser South/Fraser East, were more likely to always eat breakfast on school days, while those in the northern part of the province, parts of the interior, and Vancouver Island tended to have lower percentages of students always eating breakfast.

Health Service Delivery Area	All students (%)	Males (%)	Females (%)
33 North Shore/Coast Garibaldi	58.03	60.69	55.53
41 South Vancouver Island	55.45	61.65†	49.31
22 Fraser North	55.05	58.79†	51.46
32 Vancouver	54.52	58.63	51.48
13 Okanagan	54.28	62.48†	47.10
31 Richmond	53.39	55.33	51.48
12 Kootenay Boundary	52.81	57.07	48.97
21 Fraser South/Fraser East	50.76	54.58†	47.42
43 North Vancouver Island	50.69	54.81	47.40
51 Northwest	50.52	54.34	46.85
14 Thompson Cariboo Shuswap	50.42	56.43†	44.69
11 East Kootenay	50.21	57.17†	44.09
42 Central Vancouver Island	49.98	53.91†	45.97
52 Northern Interior	46.80	52.40†	41.03
53 Northeast	N/A	N/A	N/A
British Columbia	**52.66**	**57.13†**	**48.58**

† Male rate is significantly different than female rate.
Crosshatched HSDAs are significantly different than the provincial average.
N/A: No data

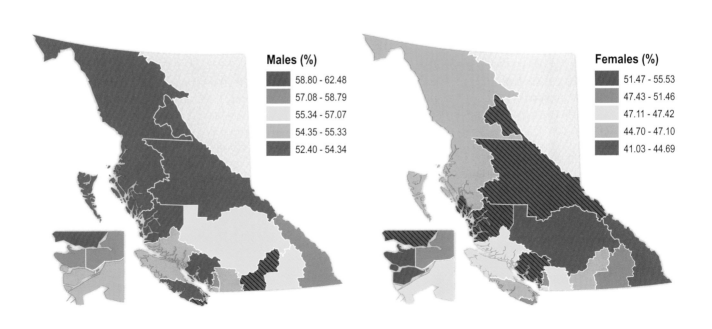

Youth who always eat breakfast on school days

All students (%)

▓	54.53 - 58.03
▓	52.82 - 54.52
▓	50.70 - 52.81
▓	50.22 - 50.69
▓	46.80 - 50.21

Source: McCreary Centre Society,
2008 BC Adolescent Health Survey.

No data were collected in grey
shaded areas

Cross hatched areas are significantly
different than the provincial rate

Males (%)

▓	58.80 - 62.48
▓	57.08 - 58.79
▓	55.34 - 57.07
▓	54.35 - 55.33
▓	52.40 - 54.34

Females (%)

▓	51.47 - 55.53
▓	47.43 - 51.46
▓	47.11 - 47.42
▓	44.70 - 47.10
▓	41.03 - 44.69

Farmers' markets

Farmers' markets in British Columbia have been growing steadily over the years, from 60 known markets in 2000 to 100 in 2006 and approximately 130 in operation throughout the province by 2009 (Connell et al., 2006; BC Association of Farmers' Markets (BCAFM), 2010). Prior to 2000, farmers' markets in BC operated independently, but since then they have been represented as part of the BC Association of Farmers' Markets.

From a wellness perspective, farmers' markets can benefit both food producers and consumers alike. From the producer perspective, farmers' markets contribute to the economic well-being of local agricultural communities, providing a viable, local source of income. A study in 2006 found that farmers' markets in BC contributed as much as $65.3 million to local economies each year through direct profits of market vendors, as well as from profits of the local businesses that supply those vendors (Connell et al., 2006).

From the consumer perspective, farmers' markets "can play an integral role in providing nutrition education and access to healthy foods" (Fisher, 1999, p. 12) at a reasonable price, create a good social atmosphere where consumers can connect with producers, and can help to promote a strong sense of community

Community	Community	Community
1 100 Mile House	44 Kamloops	87 Salmon Arm
2 Abbotsford	45 Kamloops	88 Salmon Arm
3 Abbotsford	46 Kelowna	89 Saltspring Island
4 Aldergrove	47 Ladner	90 Sechelt
5 Armstrong	48 Lake Country	91 Sidney
6 Ashcroft	49 Langford	92 Silverton
7 Barriere	50 Langley	93 Smithers
8 Bella Coola	51 Lytton	94 Sooke
9 Blind Bay	52 Maple Ridge	95 Sorrento
10 Burnaby	53 Mayne island	96 Squamish
11 Campbell River	54 McBride	97 Stevenston
12 Central Saanich	55 Merrit	98 Summerland
13 Chase	56 Metchosin	99 Sun Peaks
14 Cherryville	57 Mission	100 Surrey
15 Chilliwack	58 Nanaimo	101 Surrey
16 Clearwater	59 Nanaimo	102 Terrace
17 Colwood	60 Nanaimo	103 Terrace
18 Comox	61 Nanaimo	104 Texada Island
19 Coquitlam	62 Naramata	105 Tlell
20 Cranbrook	63 Nelson	106 Vancouver
21 Creston	64 New Denver	107 Vancouver
22 Crofton	65 New Westminster	108 Vancouver
23 Dawson Creek	66 North Saanich	109 Vancouver
24 Duncan	67 North Vancouver	110 Vancouver
25 Dunster	68 Oliver	111 Vancouver
26 Enderby	69 Osoyoos	112 Vancouver
27 Errington	70 Parksvile	113 Vancouver
28 Esquimalt	71 Peachland	114 Vanderhoof
29 Falkland	72 Pemberton	115 Vanderhoof
30 Fernie	73 Pender Island	116 Vernon
31 Fort St. James	74 Penticton	117 Vernon
32 Fort St. John	75 Port Alberni	118 Victoria
33 Fort Steele	76 Port Moody	119 Victoria
34 Gabriola Island	77 Powell River	120 Victoria
35 Gibsons	78 Prince Rupert	121 Victoria
36 Golden	79 Quadra Island	122 Wasa
37 Grand Forks	80 Quadra Island	123 West Vancouver
38 Hazelton	81 Qualicum Beach	124 Whistler
39 Hope	82 Queen Charlotte City	125 Whistler
40 Hornby Island	83 Quesnel	126 Whistler
41 Invermere	84 Quesnel	127 White Rock
42 Jaffray	85 Revelstoke	128 Williams Lake
43 Kamloops	86 Rossland	129 Winlaw

(Feagan et al., 2004; Oberholtzer & Grow, 2003; Brown & Miller, 2008). Many farmers' products at these markets are pesticide free, and have been organically produced (BCAFM, 2010).

Improving consumer access to fresh fruits and vegetables is particularly important where affordable healthy food is absent. Farmers' markets improve food access and variety for residents and reduce the cost of living, either by providing lower cost foods or by reducing the need for transportation to access food (Larsen & Gilliland, 2009; Tarasuk, 2005). Farmers' markets can be important wellness assets as they help to increase food security in communities, which in turn enables individuals to meet their dietary needs to lead healthy lives.

Based on 2009 data, the table and map opposite indicates farmers' markets may have up to 180 individual vendors, or as few as six. The largest ones were found in the Okanagan valley, southern part of Vancouver Island, and the southern part of the lower mainland of the province. Vancouver, with a total of eight farmers' markets, had the most, while Victoria and Nanaimo, on Vancouver Island both had four farmers' markets.

Farmers' markets

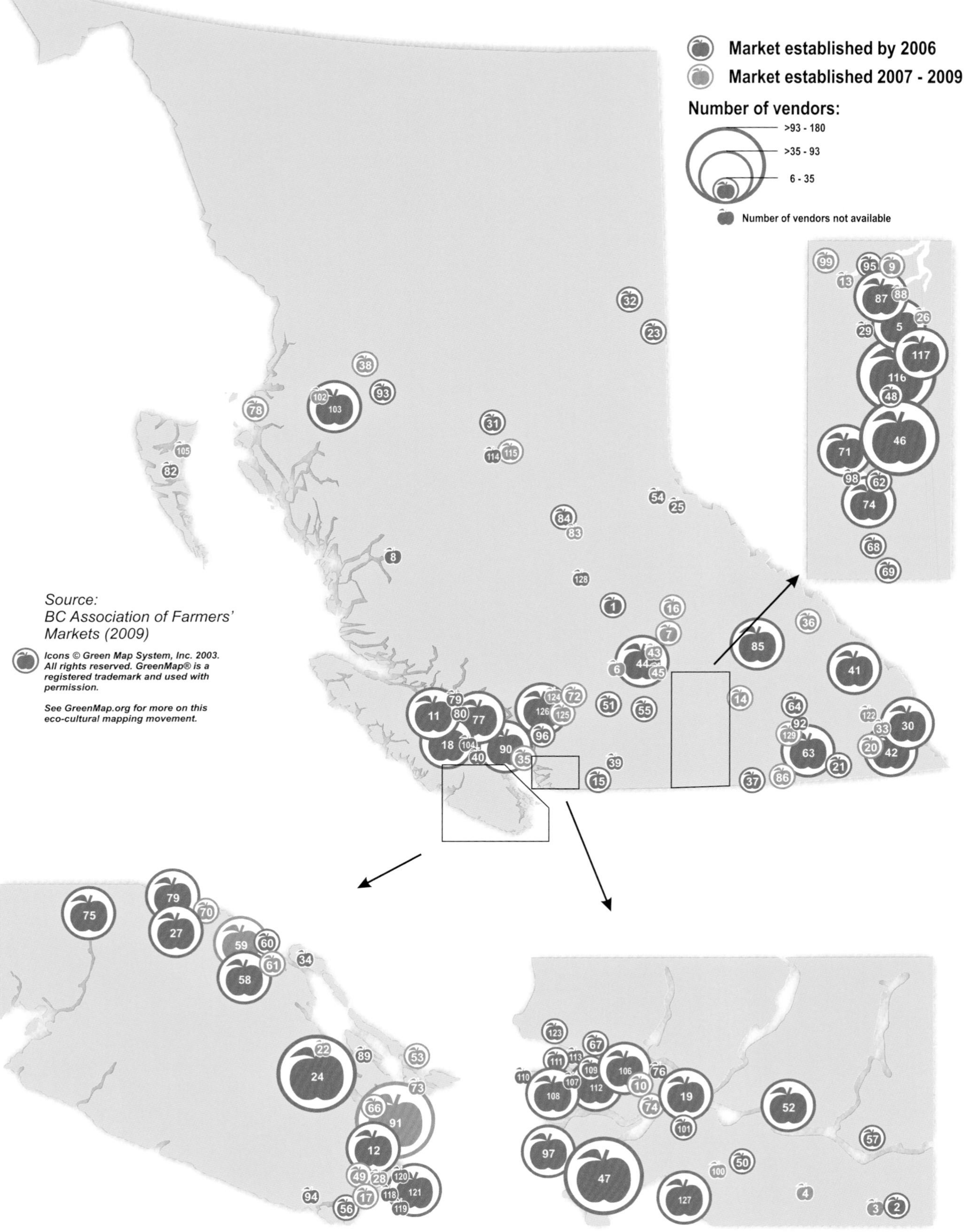

Market established by 2006
Market established 2007 - 2009

Number of vendors:
>93 - 180
>35 - 93
6 - 35

Number of vendors not available

Source:
BC Association of Farmers'
Markets (2009)

Icons © Green Map System, Inc. 2003.
All rights reserved. GreenMap® is a
registered trademark and used with
permission.

See GreenMap.org for more on this
eco-cultural mapping movement.

Community gardens

Community gardens are shared spaces that provide residents an opportunity to grow their own nutritious food, usually in small plots known as allotments within community gardens. These spaces are an important resource in both urban areas where people live in high density housing with little or no adequate gardening space, and remote areas where individuals lack access to healthy fresh food. They provide a means to access culturally acceptable foods (Wakefield, 2007), and serve as gathering places for members of the community to connect and to share food knowledge, and perhaps produce. Community gardens have also been used for low-income groups to obtain fresh fruits and vegetables at low cost, and in some cases have been a means of social enterprise by selling excess food to others.

In addition to direct benefits like food security and access, there are many health benefits from community gardening, including improved nutrition, physical activity, and social and psychological well-being (Blair et al., 1991; Myers, 1998; Nutbeam, 1998; Armstrong, 2000; Brown & Jameton, 2000; Hanna & Oh, 2000; Milligan et al., 2004; Wakefield, 2007; Blake & Cloutier-Fisher, 2009). Community gardens have also improved community capital, contributed to development of social networks, beautified communities, and reduced crime (Armstrong, 2000; Hancock, 2001), as well as promoted intergenerational interaction. They can also promote participants to become more active in other community activities or issues (Kurtz, 2001; Twiss et al., 2003; Milligan et al., 2004; Wakefield et al., 2007).

Based on information from the Ministry of Agriculture and Lands (2008), more than 70 communities in BC in 2008 had at least one community garden, with the largest numbers in Vancouver and Victoria (see table and map opposite). Numbers are expected to grow; as food prices rise, community gardens in urban, rural, and remote areas will become increasingly important to ensuring food security in BC.

The benefits of community gardens have been widely acknowledged in BC (Ostry, 2010a), from the City of Vancouver's *2010 Challenge* which called for 2,010 new community gardening plots to be created as an Olympic legacy in the city (City of Vancouver, 2010), to the provincial government's 2009/10 Produce Availability Initiative, which included grants for community gardens in remote First Nations communities to increase access to healthy foods in those areas. Grants were also offered to

Community	Community
1 100 Mile House	37 Matsqui
2 Abbotsford	38 Merritt
3 Agassiz	39 Mission
4 Alkali Lake	40 Moberly Lake
5 Anahim Lake	41 Nakusp
6 Avola	42 Nanaimo
7 Barriere	43 New Westminster
8 Bella Coola	44 North Saanich
9 Burnaby	45 North Vancouver
10 Burns Lake	46 Parksville
11 Canim Lake	47 Peachland
12 Canoe Creek	48 Pemberton
13 Castlegar	49 Penticton Indian Band
14 Chase	50 Pitt Meadows
15 Chemainus	51 Port Coquitlam
16 Clearwater	52 Port Edward
17 Colwood	53 Port Moody
18 Coquitlam	54 Prince George
19 Courtenay	55 Quesnel
20 Cranbrook	56 Revelstoke
21 Creston	57 Richmond
22 Dawson Creek	58 Sechelt
23 Duncan	59 Smithers
24 Grasmere	60 Soda Creek
25 Hazelton	61 Squamish
26 Houston	62 Surrey
27 Invermere	63 Vancouver
28 Kamloops	64 Vanderhoof
29 Kaslo	65 Victoria
30 Kelowna	66 Wells
31 Kimberley	67 West Vancouver
32 Ladysmith	68 Westbank
33 Langley	69 Whistler
34 Lone Butte	70 Williams Lake
35 Mackenzie	71 Winfield
36 Maple Ridge	72 Xeni Gwet'in

communities to build gardens as part of the BC Healthy Living Alliance Community Capacity Building Strategy to promote healthy living. Community gardens have also expanded into schools to educate students about the importance of healthy eating, and will be an area of development during the new *Think & Eat Green @ School Project*, run by the University of BC and the Vancouver School Board, aiming to connect Vancouver K–12 students to food and sustainability issues while helping schools lighten their ecological footprint and reduce greenhouse gas emissions.

Community gardens

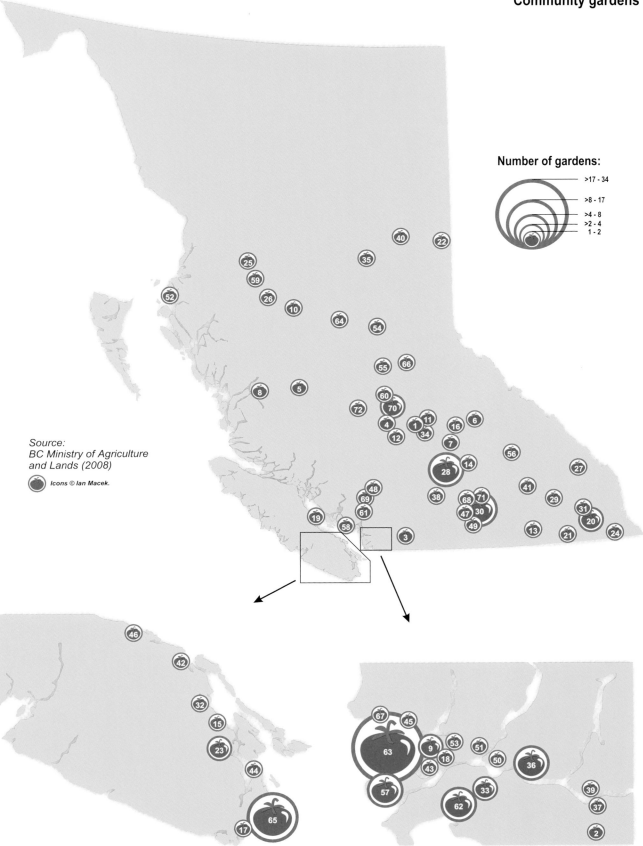

Number of gardens:

>17 - 34
>8 - 17
>4 - 8
>2 - 4
1 - 2

Source:
BC Ministry of Agriculture
and Lands (2008)

Icons © Ian Macek.

BC Healthy Living Alliance healthy eating initiatives

In order to help guide a series of healthy eating initiatives, BCHLA developed and produced the *Healthy Eating Strategy* (BCHLA, 2007b). It outlined a number of initiatives based on best and emerging 'promising practices,' and looked at existing evidence to choose where programs should be targeted. It was determined that targeting those BC families with parents between the ages of 35 and 54 years with young children would have the greatest impact on healthy eating. The focus was specifically on vegetable and fruit consumption and a reduction in unhealthy food choices. Targeting these families was also seen to have the maximum potential to reach vulnerable families, including those that were low income, food insecure, Aboriginal, and/or new immigrants.

The objectives set out by the BCHLA were: to build skills and knowledge that would lead to greater consumption of vegetables and fruit for individuals in BC; to improve access to vegetables and fruit for all British Columbians; and to decrease British Columbians' access to, and consumption of unhealthy food and beverage choices.

	Community		Community		Community
1	Abbotsford	36	Heiltsuk Nation	70	Prince Rupert
2	Agassiz	37	Hope	71	Qualicum
3	Alert Bay	38	Houston	72	Quesnel
4	Babine	39	Ittatsoo	73	Revelstoke
5	Barriere	40	Kamloops	74	Richmond
6	Bella Bella	41	Kelowna	75	Saanich
7	Burnaby	42	Kent	76	Seabird Island
8	Burns Lake	43	Kimberley		Band
9	Canoe Creek	44	Kitimat	77	Simpcw First Nation
10	Cawston	45	Kuper Island	78	Skidegate
11	Chehailis Indian	46	Ladysmith	79	Smithers
	Band	47	Lake Babine	80	Sooke
12	Chemainus	48	Lantzville	81	Squamish
13	Cherryville	49	Lillooet	82	Stellat'en First
14	Chetwynd	50	Malahat		Nation
15	Colwood	51	Maple Ridge	83	Stewart
16	Coquitlam	52	Masset	84	Summerland
17	Courtenay	53	Mission	85	Surrey
18	Cranbrook	54	Nanaimo	86	Takla Lake
19	Crawford Bay	55	Nanoose	87	Taylor
20	Creston	56	Nazko First Nation	88	Terrace
21	Dawson Creek	57	New Aiyansh Village	89	Tofino
22	Daylu Dena Council		Government	90	Trail
23	Delta	58	New Westminster	91	Tsawout First Nation
24	Esquimalt	59	North Cowichan		Band
25	Fernie	60	North Vancouver	92	Ucluelet
26	Fort Fraser	61	Oliver	93	Vancouver
27	Fort St. James	62	Parksville	94	Vernon
28	Fort St. John	63	Pauquachin First	95	Vernon
29	Fraser Lake		Nation	96	Victoria
30	Gibsons	64	Penticton	97	West Moberly First
31	Gitanmaax	65	Pitt Meadows		Nation
32	Gitwangak	66	Port Alberni	98	West Vancouver
33	Granisle	67	Port Coquitlam	99	White Rock
34	Haida Gwaii	68	Powell River	100	Wickaninnish
35	Hazelton	69	Prince George	101	Williams Lake

Five healthy eating initiatives were introduced:

1. Farm to School Salad Bar, led by the Public Health Association of BC, which provided fresh, locally grown produce delivered directly to schools and BC children at least twice a week.

2. Food Skills for Families, led by the Canadian Diabetes Association, which developed four targeted food skills curricula aimed at Aboriginal, South Asian, newcomer, and low income families.

3. School Guidelines Support, led by Dietitians of Canada, which supported faster and easier implementation of the *Guidelines for Food and Beverage Sales in BC Schools* (Ministry of Education, 2010b) by helping schools identify and serve healthier choices.

4. Sip Smart! BC, led by the BC Pediatric Society and the Heart and Stroke Foundation, BC & Yukon, which created an education module for long-term use by BC teachers aimed at reducing the consumption of sugar sweetened beverages by children in grades 4 to 6.

5. Stay Active Eat Healthy – Healthy Food and Beverage Sales in Local Recreation Facilities and Local Government Buildings, led by the BC Recreation and Parks Association and the Union of BC Municipalities. Supports for local government buildings and recreation facilities to voluntarily adopt the sale of healthy food and beverages, and provided grants to support implementation in local governments and Aboriginal communities (BCHLA, 2010).

The table and adjacent map, which are new to this Atlas, represent the reach throughout the province of the healthy eating initiatives, which took place from 2007 to 2010, when funding ran out. More than 100 communities were involved in the various initiatives, including 6 regional districts, and 15 First Nations local governments.

BC Healthy Living Alliance healthy eating initiatives

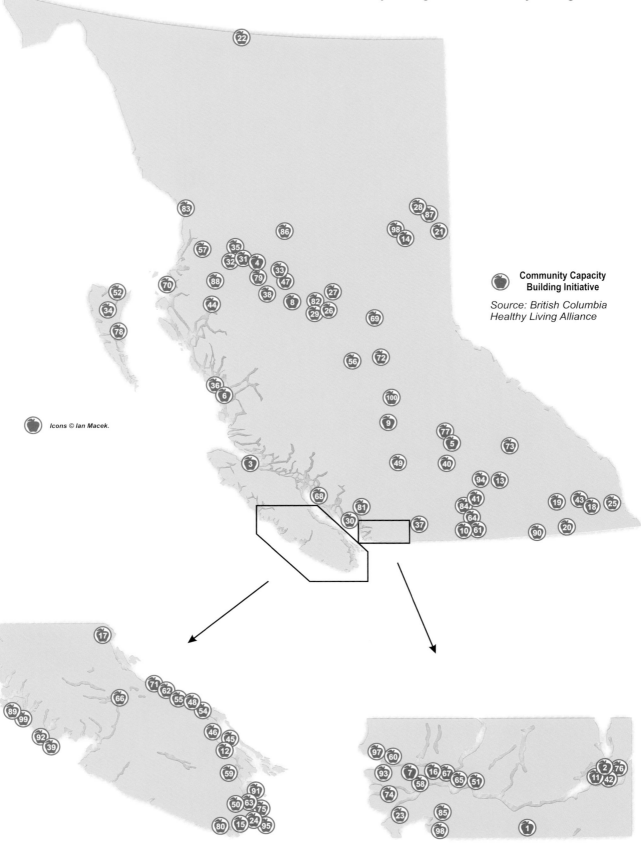

Community Capacity
Building Initiative

*Source: British Columbia
Healthy Living Alliance*

Icons © Ian Macek.

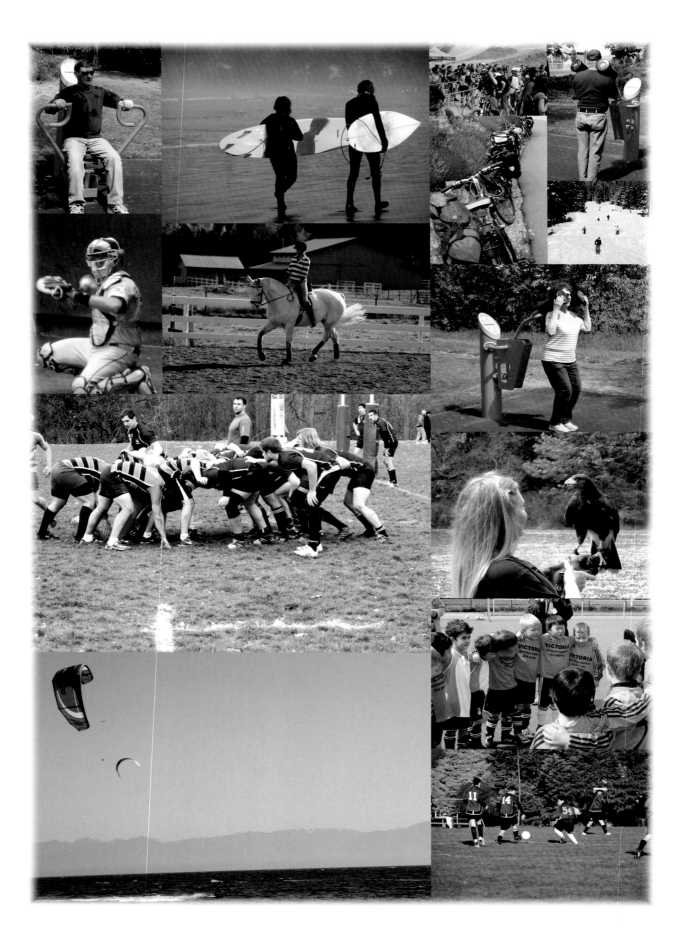

The Geography of Physical Activity

Participation in fitness activities and sports play an important role in increasing health status and reducing illness and health care costs, and increasing physical activity was one of the key pillars of ActNow BC. A lack of physical exercise is related to many disease risk factors (BC Select Standing Committee on Health, 2004). Although the process is not well understood, regular physical activity appears to be a protective factor (or wellness asset) for several chronic conditions, including heart disease, obesity, high blood pressure, diabetes, osteoporosis, stroke, depression, and some types of cancer (Kendall, 2006; Gilmour, 2007; Bryan & Katzmarzyk, 2011). Physical activity also maintains physical strength and flexibility, and there is evidence that higher levels of physical activity have health benefits and "the more activity, the greater the health benefit" (Colley et al., 2011b).

The economic impact of physical inactivity was estimated at $5.3 billion, or 2.6% of total health care costs in Canada in 2001 (Katzmarzyk & Janssen, 2004). Thanks in part to the province's temperate climate and abundant recreational opportunities, adult British Columbians are one the most active populations in all of Canada during their leisure time (Gilmour, 2007; McKee et al., 2009a).

The World Health Organisation (2010) recommends that adults should engage in at least 150 minutes per week of moderate-to-vigorous physical activity, through sessions lasting at least 10 minutes (Colley et al., 2011a). Physical activity is not limited to traditional forms of exercise such as running, walking, swimming, or sport, but can include daily activities such as gardening, or housecleaning (Sharrat & Hearst, 2007). Some Canadians also incorporate activity into their daily commutes with active transportation in the form of walking or cycling, although these latter activities tend to be undertaken by younger

members of the population (Cragg et al., 2006; Gilmour, 2007; Butler et al., 2007).

Recent results from the Canadian Health Measures Survey (CHMS), based on actual physical activity measurements rather than just questionnaire surveys, indicated that only 15% of Canadian adults engaged in at least 150 minutes of moderate-to-vigorous physical activity per week (Colley et al., 2011a), and this sedentary behaviour and physical inactivity has resulted in increasing levels of adult overweight and obesity (Shields & Tremblay, 2008). For adults as a whole, it has been estimated that 25% of those over the age of 18 years in Canada are obese, and the rates as a whole have been increasing (Public Health Agency of Canada (PHAC), 2009b). Analysis suggests that the total cost of obesity was estimated to be $4.3 billion in 2001 (Katzmarzyk & Janssen, 2004), and this amount was likely an underestimate of the overall economic cost of excess weight in Canada as it did not include the costs for those who were overweight but not obese (PHAC, 2009b).

In a recent Canadian study, physical inactivity was the most strongly associated factor with obesity at the population level (Public Health Agency of Canada & Canadian Institute for Health Information, 2011).

The benefits of physical activity are multifold in the early years of life. For young children, physical activity has been found to have an important impact on growth and maturation. Further, recreation and play are key elements for healthy childhood development, promoting the acquisition of key motor skills, social skills, and creativity (Active Healthy Kids Canada (AHKC), 2010). In addition, physically activity for young children is important to avoid issues of overweight and obesity. For youth, research has shown that recreation activities reduce boredom and associated risky behaviour (Torjman, 2004; AHKC, 2011).

Despite these benefits, concern has been expressed about the increasing levels of inactivity among children and youth in Canada, and in BC in particular (BC Select Standing Committee on Health, 2006). Indeed, in Canada overall, sports participation of children aged 5 to 14 was lowest in BC and Quebec in 2005 (Clark, 2008). For children and adolescents aged 5 to 17 years, health benefits accrue with moderate-to-vigorous physical activity of 1 hour each day, and they should engage in vigorous physical activity at least 3 days a week. Based on results from the CHMS, only 9% of boys and 4% of girls engaged in at least 1 hour of moderate-to-vigorous physical activity on at least 6 days a week (Colley et al., 2011b). This has raised increasing concerns about early problems of overweight and obesity (BC Select Standing Committee on Health, 2006; Ostry, 2010b; Ministry of Health Services, 2010). As AHKC (2010, p. 2) noted:

- Obesity in infancy persists through the preschool years.

- Children who become obese before the age of 6 years are likely to be obese later in childhood.

- Obese children have a 25-50% increased risk of being obese as adults. It is estimated that overweight 2 to 5 year-olds are four times as likely to be overweight as adults.

Further, "National data show that 15.2% of 2-5-year-olds are overweight and 6.3% are obese." There has also been a disturbing trend of rising obesity in Canadian youth, due in part to a lack of physical activity and increasing levels of sedentary behaviour (Shields, 2006). The results from the CHMS confirm the continuing trend of declining physical activity, especially as children move into their adolescent and teen years (Tremblay et al., 2007; 2011). Overall, there is growing evidence that "the health of Canadian children has deteriorated in the past few decades" related in part to increased sedentary behaviours of children (6 out of 10 waking hours are devoted to sedentary activities) and increasing levels of obesity (Colley et al., 2011b, p. 1).

For seniors, recreation and active living prolong independent functioning by compressing the impairment and disease period typically associated with aging. The strengthening of muscles and enhancement of bone density reduces osteoporosis and improves balance, thus reducing the potential for falls. However, despite the clear benefits of physical activity in the senior years, older adults are the most inactive demographic group in Canada (Torjman, 2004; Public Health Agency of Canada, 2006). In BC, nearly half of the senior population is inactive. Common barriers to physical activity for seniors include

long term illness or disability, lack of interest or motivation, fear of injury, lack of energy, time, and physical skills, with the first two being most common (Canadian Fitness and Lifestyle Research Institute (CFLRI), 2007a).

Leisure time activities alone may not be adequate for individuals to meet health-promoting levels of physical activity, although most prevention and research efforts are directed at this area. Those who are physically active at work are at lower risk of chronic disease. Additionally, those with active occupations tend to be physically active in their leisure time, while those who are sedentary at work are more likely to be sedentary during leisure time, demonstrating an interdependent relationship between these two realms of physical activity (Probart et al., 2008).

Approximately two-thirds of Canadians spend about half of their waking hours at work, and so the workplace becomes an important venue for promoting health and wellness (ActNow BC, 2009). The Public Health Agency of Canada encourages businesses to promote physical activity in the workplace (PHAC, 2007). Further, over 80% of Canadian workplaces recognize some degree of employer responsibility for employee physical activity, but there has been little improvement in workplace support for employee physical activity over time (CFLRI, 2007b). What we can say is that in Canada, women workers generally have better access to programs and facilities at or close to work than male workers (Virtue et al., 2010), and this may be one of the reasons that obesity among male workers in Canada has increased at a faster rate than for female workers (Park, 2009). It is also worth noting that BC women workers have better access to programs and facilities at or close to work than Canadian women workers as a whole (Virtue et al., 2010).

The 65 maps provided in this chapter are based on a diversity of data sources, and several of the indicators are new to this edition of the Atlas, while others from the first edition have not been repeated. Action Schools! BC and Active Communities maps have been excluded, as over 90% of the eligible schools (91%) and all school districts now have these programs, and most of the province's population resided in the 226 communities that were covered by the Active Communities program before funding was discontinued. Community recreation facilities, centres, and playing fields have also been dropped as there have been no updates to these surveys since the first edition, and the parks map has not been repeated because there has been little change to the system. Others excluded are transit because of little change, and Hearts in Motion walking clubs, which have actually been reduced in number, although walking trails available have been mapped elsewhere (http://www.walkbc.ca/map).

The first 25 maps provide information at the HSDA level on the key leisure time physical activities—walking, gardening and yard work, swimming, home exercise, bicycling—as recorded through CCHS 4.1. These are all important behaviours that maintain or improve health and wellness. Next are three maps from the Student Satisfaction Survey at the school district level that look at participation in physical exercise. It is worth noting that BC introduced physical activity requirements for school children starting in September 2008. Kindergarten to grade 9 students were required to do 30 minutes of daily physical activity as part of their educational program, and grade 10 to 12 students were required to document and report a minimum of 150 minutes per week of physical activity at a moderate to vigorous intensity at school, home, and/or in the community (Ministry of Education & ActNow BC, 2008). The next three maps, also based on the Student Satisfaction Survey, provide information on where students usually do physical activity, either within school or outside of the school setting. Research suggests that physical activity outside of the school environment may be more successful in reducing obesity levels of school children (Harris et al., 2009). This is followed by five maps based on responses to CCHS 4.1 related to accessibility to a gym or physical fitness facilities at or near to work, an important asset for wellness.

The next group of 22 maps provides a picture of sport club membership in BC, based on data provided to us at the HSDA level by 2010 Legacies Now. Sport club membership is an important wellness asset as clubs provide an opportunity for physical activity, as well as the opportunity for socializing. The first three maps in this group provide patterns for all sports club memberships for the BC population as a whole (age 4 to 80 years), and for males and females separately, and are mapped as rates per 1,000 population. Caution is required as some individuals will be members of more than one sports club and so rates are likely overstated to some extent. These maps are followed by maps of the most popular sports—soccer, athletics, golf, artistic gymnastics, hockey, baseball, curling, tennis, equestrian, softball, figure skating, lacrosse, and cross-country skiing.

The next five maps are based on a derived variable developed from the CCHS 4.1 that provides a physical activity index score. The index is based on respondents' answers to several questions related to the frequency, duration, and intensity of their participation in certain activities. For each leisure time activity, an average daily energy expenditure was calculated. Respondents were then classified as Active if their average daily energy expenditure was 3 kcal/kg/day (e.g., walking an hour a day or jogging 20 minutes a day), Moderately Active with an

energy expenditure between 2.9 and 1.5 kcal/kg/day (e.g., walking 30 to 60 minutes a day, or taking an hour-long exercise class three times a week), and Inactive below 1.5 kcal/day (e.g., walking less than half an hour each day) (Gilmour, 2007).

The final two maps provide information about programs developed specifically to support the original physical activity goal of ActNow BC. These include seniors parks and LocalMotion projects.

Walked for exercise in the past three months

Health Service Delivery Area	All respondents 12+ (%)	Males 12+ (%)	Females 12+ (%)	Ages 12-19 (%)	Ages 20-64 (%)	Ages 65+ (%)
11 East Kootenay	83.76	80.71	86.74	74.34	86.89	76.94
41 South Vancouver Island	82.63	75.13*	89.38	74.47	84.42	79.73
12 Kootenay Boundary	80.88	72.16*	89.78	72.54	82.86	78.20
51 Northwest	80.50	77.99	83.09	79.65	83.25	63.49‡
42 Central Vancouver Island	78.55	74.30	82.48	65.01†	82.03	74.22
43 North Vancouver Island	77.36	69.91	84.27	73.79	79.42	71.12
52 Northern Interior	76.44	71.57*	81.36	76.90	77.65	67.21
13 Okanagan	74.77	71.83	77.55	59.63	75.90	79.10
14 Thompson Cariboo Shuswap	73.69	65.63*	81.34	83.53	73.70	66.96
21 Fraser East	73.69	65.78*	81.45	67.21	76.25	67.36
32 Vancouver	72.35	67.67*	76.91	51.30†	72.98	81.77
53 Northeast	72.01	67.23	77.02	63.50	73.49	72.37
33 North Shore/Coast Garibaldi	71.98	69.66	74.11	56.34	72.73	79.35
23 Fraser South	70.34	66.21	74.32	58.20†	72.00	71.95
22 Fraser North	67.81	62.50*	72.82	45.38†	70.76	69.87
31 Richmond	67.22	61.34	72.62	59.99	67.17	73.12
British Columbia (2007/8)	**73.53**	**68.40***	**78.42**	**61.63†**	**75.07**	**74.65**
British Columbia (2005)	**72.82**	**65.68***	**79.69**	**63.96†**	**74.14**	**73.36**

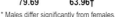

Crosshatching beside the 2007/8 provincial rate indicates it is significantly different than the 2005 rate, while crosshatched HSDAs are significantly different than the 2007/8 provincial rate.
E interpret data with caution (16.67 ≤ coefficient of variation ≤ 33.3).

* Males differ significantly from females.
† 12-19 age cohort differs significantly from the 20-64 age cohort.
‡ 65+ age cohort differs significantly from the 20-64 age cohort.
F data suppressed (n < 10, or coefficient of variation > 33.3).

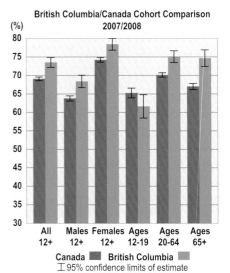

British Columbia/Canada Cohort Comparison 2007/2008

Canada ■   British Columbia ▨
⊥ 95% confidence limits of estimate

Walking is one of the simplest ways to meet Health Canada's recommended guidelines for physical activity. It requires no special equipment or gym memberships, and a person can integrate physical activity into a daily commute simply by opting to walk rather than use inactive forms of transportation. The CCHS asked participants if they had walked for exercise in the past three months. In BC, 73.53% responded in the affirmative. Respondents in East Kootenay, Kootenay Boundary, South Vancouver Island, Central Vancouver Island, and Northwest (all above 78%) were significantly more likely than the provincial average to walk for exercise. Fraser North and Richmond were significantly lower than the provincial average (both below 68%).

Within BC, females (78.42%) were significantly more likely than males (68.40%) to walk for exercise. This was also the case for seven individual HSDAs. For females at the HSDA level, respondents in East Kootenay, Kootenay Boundary, and South Vancouver Island (all above 86%) were significantly more likely to walk for exercise than the provincial average. For males, East Kootenay and the Northwest (both above 77%) also had significantly more walkers than the provincial average.

Provincially, 61.63% of youth respondents reported walking for exercise in the past 3 months. This was significantly lower than the mid-age cohort. At the HSDA level, youth in Fraser North, Fraser South, Vancouver, and Central Vancouver Island were significantly less likely than their mid-age counterparts to report walking for exercise. Thompson Cariboo Shuswap, South Vancouver Island,

and Northwest (all above 74%) all had significantly higher walking participation, while Fraser North (45.38%) was significantly lower than the provincial average for youth.

Older respondents in BC (74.65%) reported high rates of walking. Northwest was the only HSDA where seniors had a significantly lower level of walking than the mid-age cohort. There were no HSDAs that had a significantly different rate than the provincial average for the older respondent cohort.

Geographically, there were major differences throughout the province, with a spread of 15 to 30 percentage points. Consistently lower levels of walking for exercise occurred in the urban lower mainland, except for older respondents in Vancouver and North Shore/Coast Garibaldi. While the northern and central regions of the province had relatively low rates for most cohorts, there was a cluster of high values for youth in those areas. The southern interior of the province had a cluster of HSDAs with higher participation for all but the youth cohort.

There were no significant differences for any of the BC cohorts between 2005 and 2007/8. When compared to Canadian respondents, British Columbians in all cohorts, except for youth, were significantly more likely than their Canadian counterparts to walk for exercise.

Walked for exercise in the past three months

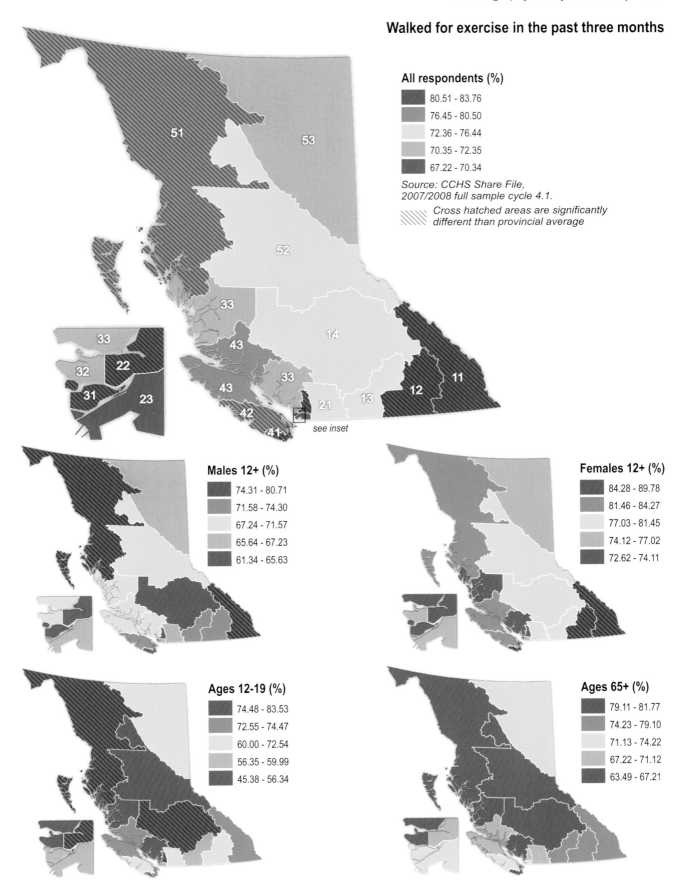

All respondents (%)

- 80.51 - 83.76
- 76.45 - 80.50
- 72.36 - 76.44
- 70.35 - 72.35
- 67.22 - 70.34

Source: CCHS Share File, 2007/2008 full sample cycle 4.1.

Cross hatched areas are significantly different than provincial average

Males 12+ (%)

- 74.31 - 80.71
- 71.58 - 74.30
- 67.24 - 71.57
- 65.64 - 67.23
- 61.34 - 65.63

Females 12+ (%)

- 84.28 - 89.78
- 81.46 - 84.27
- 77.03 - 81.45
- 74.12 - 77.02
- 72.62 - 74.11

Ages 12-19 (%)

- 74.48 - 83.53
- 72.55 - 74.47
- 60.00 - 72.54
- 56.35 - 59.99
- 45.38 - 56.34

Ages 65+ (%)

- 79.11 - 81.77
- 74.23 - 79.10
- 71.13 - 74.22
- 67.22 - 71.12
- 63.49 - 67.21

Did gardening or yard work in the past three months

Health Service Delivery Area	All respondents 12+ (%)	Males 12+ (%)	Females 12+ (%)	Ages 12-19 (%)	Ages 20-64 (%)	Ages 65+ (%)
12 Kootenay Boundary	71.67	79.42*	63.74	53.90	74.63	70.93
52 Northern Interior	64.74	67.12	62.34	42.34†	69.43	58.77
11 East Kootenay	63.23	67.06	59.50	39.84E†	68.11	58.60
14 Thompson Cariboo Shuswap	60.06	62.39	57.85	41.18E	63.39	58.61
43 North Vancouver Island	58.85	57.32	60.28	F	64.92	57.24
42 Central Vancouver Island	56.54	60.33	53.04	39.08E†	60.90	51.42
41 South Vancouver Island	55.20	57.13	53.47	37.38†	58.68	50.65
53 Northeast	53.10	52.01	54.24	45.72E	56.24	37.74‡
51 Northwest	52.60	52.10	53.11	32.33E†	56.62	51.44
21 Fraser East	52.42	51.34	53.47	35.08E†	57.76	42.19‡
13 Okanagan	49.80	57.19*	42.84	27.90E†	54.06	47.55
33 North Shore/Coast Garibaldi	41.81	45.32	38.60	20.33E†	44.87	42.79
23 Fraser South	39.13	46.57*	31.96	19.49†	42.22	39.47
22 Fraser North	32.43	32.43	32.43	8.65E†	36.37	29.74
31 Richmond	29.46	32.52	26.66	15.36E†	31.72	28.44E
32 Vancouver	17.82	18.57	17.09	5.22E†	18.03	24.48
British Columbia (2007/8)	42.76	45.61*	40.05	24.62†	45.46	42.69
British Columbia (2005)	47.18	49.94*	44.51	30.89†	49.85	46.93

Crosshatching beside the 2007/8 provincial rate indicates it is significantly different than the 2005 rate, while crosshatched HSDAs are significantly different than the 2007/8 provincial rate.
E interpret data with caution (16.67 ≤ coefficient of variation ≤ 33.3).

* Males differ significantly from females.
† 12-19 age cohort differs significantly from the 20-64 age cohort.
‡ 65+ age cohort differs significantly from the 20-64 age cohort.
F data suppressed (n < 10, or coefficient of variation > 33.3).

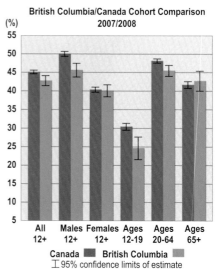

British Columbia/Canada Cohort Comparison 2007/2008

Canada ■   British Columbia ■
⊥ 95% confidence limits of estimate

Gardening and yard work are great forms of functional exercise. When the CCHS asked if respondents had done gardening or yard work in the past 3 months, less than half of all respondents (42.76%) in BC responded in the affirmative. While most HSDAs were significantly higher, Fraser North, Richmond, and Vancouver were significantly lower than the provincial average.

For BC as a whole, males (45.61%) were significantly more likely than females (40.05%) to have done gardening or yard work in the past 3 months. This pattern of significantly higher values for males was also seen at the individual HSDA level in Kootenay Boundary, Okanagan, and Fraser South.

In comparison to the provincial average for females, Fraser North, Fraser South, Richmond, and Vancouver (all below 33%) were significantly less likely to have done gardening or yard work in the past 3 months. Aside from these significantly low areas, only two HSDAs, Okanagan and North Shore/Coast Garibaldi, were not significantly higher than the provincial average for females. For male respondents, half of the HSDAs were significantly higher, while Fraser North, Richmond, and Vancouver were significantly lower than the provincial average for males.

Youth responses require cautious interpretation because of small sample sizes. Provincially, only 24.62% of youth respondents reported doing gardening or yard work in the past 3 months, significantly lower than the provincial average for the mid-age cohort, and this difference was significant for nine of the individual HSDAs. At the HSDA level, Kootenay Boundary, South Vancouver Island, and

Northern Interior (all above 37%) were significantly higher, while Fraser North and Vancouver (both below 9%) were significantly lower than the provincial average for youth.

For older respondents, 42.69% had done gardening and yard work in the past 3 months. While this was not significantly different than the mid-age cohort, Fraser East and Northeast older respondents were significantly less likely than their mid-age peers to have participated in gardening or yard work. East Kootenay, Kootenay Boundary, Thompson Cariboo Shuswap, and Northern Interior (all above 58%) were significantly higher, while Fraser North, Richmond, and Vancouver (all below 30%) were significantly lower than the provincial average for older respondents.

Throughout the province there were major geographical variations, with a spread of approximately 50 percentage points for all cohorts. The interior parts of BC and, to a lesser extent, Vancouver Island, had higher values, while the urban southwest mainland had much lower values.

All BC cohorts showed a significant decline between 2005 and 2007/8, except for the older age cohort. Compared to Canadian peers, British Columbians were significantly less likely to participate in gardening or yard work, and the male, youth, and mid-age cohorts in particular were significantly lower than their peers nationally.

Did gardening or yard work in the past three months

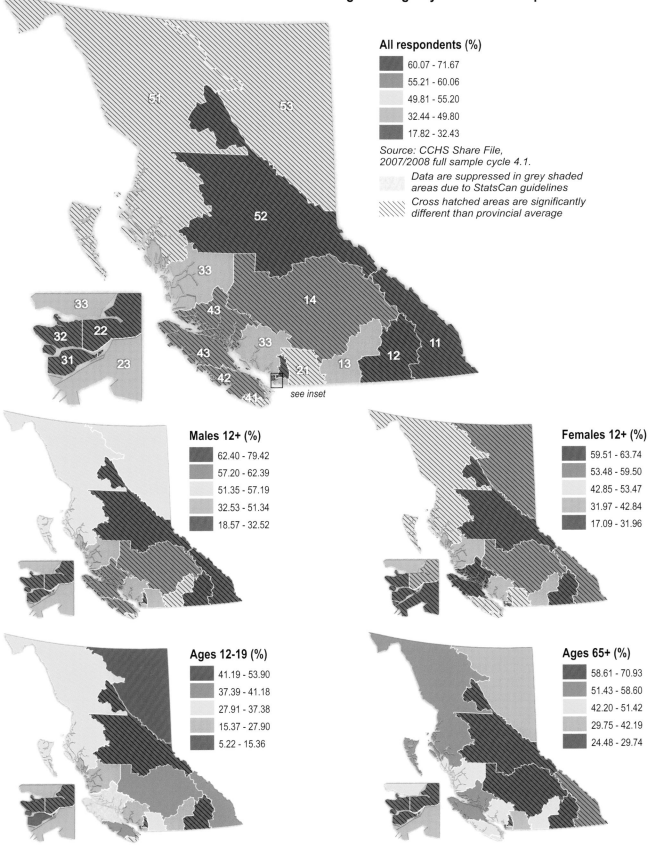

All respondents (%)

- 60.07 - 71.67
- 55.21 - 60.06
- 49.81 - 55.20
- 32.44 - 49.80
- 17.82 - 32.43

Source: CCHS Share File, 2007/2008 full sample cycle 4.1.

Data are suppressed in grey shaded areas due to StatsCan guidelines

Cross hatched areas are significantly different than provincial average

Males 12+ (%)

- 62.40 - 79.42
- 57.20 - 62.39
- 51.35 - 57.19
- 32.53 - 51.34
- 18.57 - 32.52

Females 12+ (%)

- 59.51 - 63.74
- 53.48 - 59.50
- 42.85 - 53.47
- 31.97 - 42.84
- 17.09 - 31.96

Ages 12-19 (%)

- 41.19 - 53.90
- 37.39 - 41.18
- 27.91 - 37.38
- 15.37 - 27.90
- 5.22 - 15.36

Ages 65+ (%)

- 58.61 - 70.93
- 51.43 - 58.60
- 42.20 - 51.42
- 29.75 - 42.19
- 24.48 - 29.74

Went swimming in the past three months

Health Service Delivery Area	All respondents 12+ (%)	Males 12+ (%)	Females 12+ (%)	Ages 12-19 (%)	Ages 20-64 (%)	Ages 65+ (%)
12 Kootenay Boundary	36.56	35.61	37.54	61.82†	37.63	16.68E‡
53 Northeast	32.50	27.70	37.53	49.98	32.28	F
41 South Vancouver Island	31.46	30.05	32.73	52.75†	33.13	12.69E‡
13 Okanagan	30.10	33.49	26.90	66.37†	29.82	11.92E‡
11 East Kootenay	29.08	26.41	31.68	63.56†	28.47	F
42 Central Vancouver Island	29.06	29.79	28.38	63.70†	28.77	9.80E‡
33 North Shore/Coast Garibaldi	28.09	31.90	24.61	54.84†	25.29	22.34
14 Thompson Cariboo Shuswap	27.98	27.15	28.76	55.83†	27.44	11.43E‡
52 Northern Interior	27.72	30.18	25.23	44.82†	27.72	F
21 Fraser East	26.37	26.87	25.89	56.80†	25.04	8.29E‡
43 North Vancouver Island	24.73	22.01E	27.25	55.04E	22.75	12.35E
51 Northwest	23.76	26.01	21.43	44.48†	22.54	F
23 Fraser South	23.00	24.75	21.30	37.43†	23.63	6.46E‡
32 Vancouver	22.12	20.60	23.60	36.42E	22.31	11.77E‡
22 Fraser North	21.76	18.90	24.46	33.90E	22.50	6.58E‡
31 Richmond	18.38	15.98	20.59	45.93†	15.03	14.78E
British Columbia (2007/8)	**25.64**	**25.51**	**25.77**	**47.88†**	**25.37**	**10.85‡**
British Columbia (2005)	**25.49**	**26.29**	**24.72**	**47.43†**	**24.98**	**10.23‡**

Crosshatching beside the 2007/8 provincial rate indicates it is significantly different than the 2005 rate, while crosshatched HSDAs are significantly different than the 2007/8 provincial rate.
E interpret data with caution (16.67 ≤ coefficient of variation ≤ 33.3).

* Males differ significantly from females.
† 12-19 age cohort differs significantly from the 20-64 age cohort.
‡ 65+ age cohort differs significantly from the 20-64 age cohort.
F data suppressed (n < 10, or coefficient of variation > 33.3).

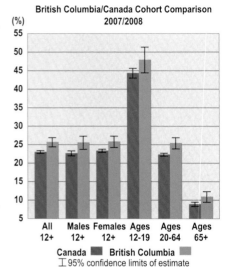

British Columbia/Canada Cohort Comparison 2007/2008

Canada ■   British Columbia ▨
⊥ 95% confidence limits of estimate

The likelihood of an individual to take up swimming for exercise depends not only on the ability to swim, but also on the availability and accessibility of suitable swimming facilities. Furthermore, there are usually user fees associated with this form of recreation which may restrict the participation of people with limited incomes. These factors may help explain why only a quarter (25.64%) of all respondents in BC reported having gone swimming in the past 3 months when the question was posed by the CCHS. Kootenay Boundary, South Vancouver Island, and Northeast were significantly higher (all over 31%) than the provincial average (25.64%), while Richmond (18.38%) was significantly lower than average.

Swimming participation for males and females province-wide was fairly similar, with about 25% of both genders reporting having gone swimming in the past 3 months. There was no significant difference between male and female swimming participation for any individual HSDA.

At the HSDA level, female respondents in Kootenay Boundary, South Vancouver Island, and Northeast (all above 32%) were significantly more likely to swim in comparison to females provincially. For males, no HSDA was significantly higher, but Fraser North and Richmond (both below 19%) were significantly below the provincial male average for swimming.

The youth cohort in BC was by far the most likely to participate in swimming, with an average value of 47.88% provincially. Overall, youth were significantly more likely to swim than the mid-age cohort, and within almost every HSDA for which adequate data were available. At the

HSDA level, youth in the Okanagan (66.37%) were significantly more likely to swim than youth provincially.

Data for older respondents were not very reliable because of high coefficients of variations or small sample sizes. Only about 1 in 10 older respondents reported swimming in the past 3 months, significantly lower than that of the mid-age cohort, a trend repeated for nearly every HSDA. Only North Shore/Coast Garibaldi had a rate significantly higher than the provincial average for older respondents.

Geographically, high and low rates for all cohorts were scattered and varied throughout the province for the different cohorts. However, there was a consistent cluster of lower participation in the urban southwest mainland of the province, while greater swimming values were found in parts of the interior and Vancouver Island.

There were no significant differences between the 2005 and 2007/8 sample cohorts in BC. In comparison to the Canadian averages, British Columbians on the whole were significantly more likely to take part in swimming activities, and this significant difference was also evident for the male, female, and mid-age cohorts. The youth and older respondent cohorts, however, were not significantly different from the national cohorts.

Went swimming in the past three months

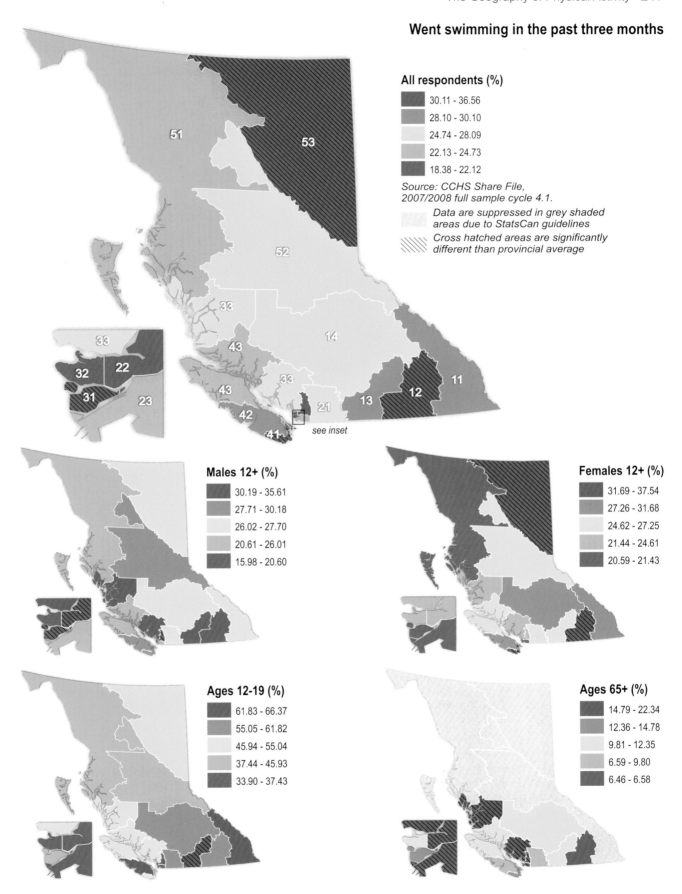

All respondents (%)

- 30.11 - 36.56
- 28.10 - 30.10
- 24.74 - 28.09
- 22.13 - 24.73
- 18.38 - 22.12

*Source: CCHS Share File,
2007/2008 full sample cycle 4.1.*

Data are suppressed in grey shaded
areas due to StatsCan guidelines

Cross hatched areas are significantly
different than provincial average

Males 12+ (%)

- 30.19 - 35.61
- 27.71 - 30.18
- 26.02 - 27.70
- 20.61 - 26.01
- 15.98 - 20.60

Females 12+ (%)

- 31.69 - 37.54
- 27.26 - 31.68
- 24.62 - 27.25
- 21.44 - 24.61
- 20.59 - 21.43

Ages 12-19 (%)

- 61.83 - 66.37
- 55.05 - 61.82
- 45.94 - 55.04
- 37.44 - 45.93
- 33.90 - 37.43

Ages 65+ (%)

- 14.79 - 22.34
- 12.36 - 14.78
- 9.81 - 12.35
- 6.59 - 9.80
- 6.46 - 6.58

Exercised at home in the past three months

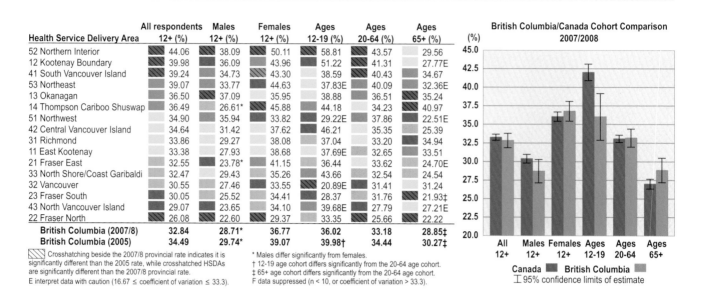

Health Service Delivery Area	All respondents 12+ (%)	Males 12+ (%)	Females 12+ (%)	Ages 12-19 (%)	Ages 20-64 (%)	Ages 65+ (%)
52 Northern Interior	44.06	38.09	50.11	58.81	43.57	29.56
12 Kootenay Boundary	39.98	36.09	43.96	51.22	41.31	27.77E
41 South Vancouver Island	39.24	34.73	43.30	38.59	40.43	34.67
53 Northeast	39.07	33.77	44.63	37.83E	40.09	32.36E
13 Okanagan	36.50	37.09	35.95	38.88	36.51	35.24
14 Thompson Cariboo Shuswap	36.49	26.61*	45.88	44.18	34.23	40.97
51 Northwest	34.90	35.94	33.82	29.22E	37.86	22.51E
42 Central Vancouver Island	34.64	31.42	37.62	46.21	35.35	25.39
31 Richmond	33.86	29.27	38.08	37.04	33.20	34.94
11 East Kootenay	33.38	27.93	38.68	37.69E	32.65	33.51
21 Fraser East	32.55	23.78*	41.15	36.44	33.62	24.70E
33 North Shore/Coast Garibaldi	32.47	29.43	35.26	43.66	32.54	24.54
32 Vancouver	30.55	27.46	33.55	20.89E	31.41	31.24
23 Fraser South	30.05	25.52	34.41	28.37	32.37	21.93‡
43 North Vancouver Island	29.07	23.65	34.10	39.68E	27.79	27.21E
22 Fraser North	26.08	22.60	29.37	33.35	25.66	22.22
British Columbia (2007/8)	**32.84**	**28.71***	**36.77**	**36.02**	**33.18**	**28.85‡**
British Columbia (2005)	**34.49**	**29.74***	**39.07**	**39.98†**	**34.44**	**30.27‡**

⬚ Crosshatching beside the 2007/8 provincial rate indicates it is significantly different than the 2005 rate, while crosshatched HSDAs are significantly different than the 2007/8 provincial rate.
E interpret data with caution (16.67 ≤ coefficient of variation ≤ 33.3).

* Males differ significantly from females.
† 12-19 age cohort differs significantly from the 20-64 age cohort.
‡ 65+ age cohort differs significantly from the 20-64 age cohort.
F data suppressed (n < 10, or coefficient of variation > 33.3).

Regular physical activity plays an important role in maintaining a healthy body and increasing health and wellness. Exercising at home is a relatively easy way to achieve physical exercise outcomes. When asked whether they had exercised at home in the past 3 months, 32.84% of respondents in BC answered positively. Northern Interior, Kootenay Boundary, and South Vancouver Island (all above 39%) were significantly higher than the provincial average, while Fraser North (26.08%) was significantly lower.

In BC, males (28.71%) were significantly less likely than females (36.77%) to have exercised at home. This significant gender difference was also evident in Thompson Cariboo Shuswap and Fraser East. For males, Northern Interior and Okanagan (both above 37%) were significantly higher than the provincial male average, while Fraser North (22.60%) was significantly lower. For females, Fraser North (29.37%) was also significantly lower than the provincial female average, while female respondents in Northern Interior, Thompson Cariboo Shuswap, and South Vancouver Island (all above 43%) were significantly higher.

Exercising at home decreased consistently with age in BC. For youth, 36.02% of respondents indicated they had exercised at home in the past 3 months. Again, Northern Interior (58.81%) was significantly higher than the provincial average for this cohort, and Vancouver (20.89%) was significantly lower. Among youth respondents, some caution in interpretation is required because of small sample sizes for some HSDAs.

For older respondents, 28.85% indicated they exercised at home. This was significantly lower than the mid-age cohort. This significant difference was also evident in Fraser South. Comparing HSDAs to the provincial average for this cohort, older respondents in Thompson Cariboo Shuswap and Okanagan (both above 35%) were significantly high, while Fraser North and Fraser South (both below 23%) were significantly low. Among older respondents, some caution in interpretation is required because of small sample sizes for some HSDAs.

Geographically, there was a spread of approximately 18 percentage points for each of the age cohorts, except the youth cohort, with a spread of 37 percentage points, showing a large geographic variation across the province. Again, caution in interpretation is recommended due to small sample sizes or large coefficients of variation. Generally, lower levels of home exercising occurred in urban areas of the lower mainland in the southwest of the province, while higher levels occurred in the north and interior of the province, as well as South Vancouver Island.

When compared to the 2005 CCHS data, exercising at home in BC had decreased in all cohorts; however, this difference was not significant. For the 2007/8 sample, Canadian values were quite similar to those for BC, except for the youth cohort: BC youth were significantly less likely to have exercised at home compared to their Canadian peers.

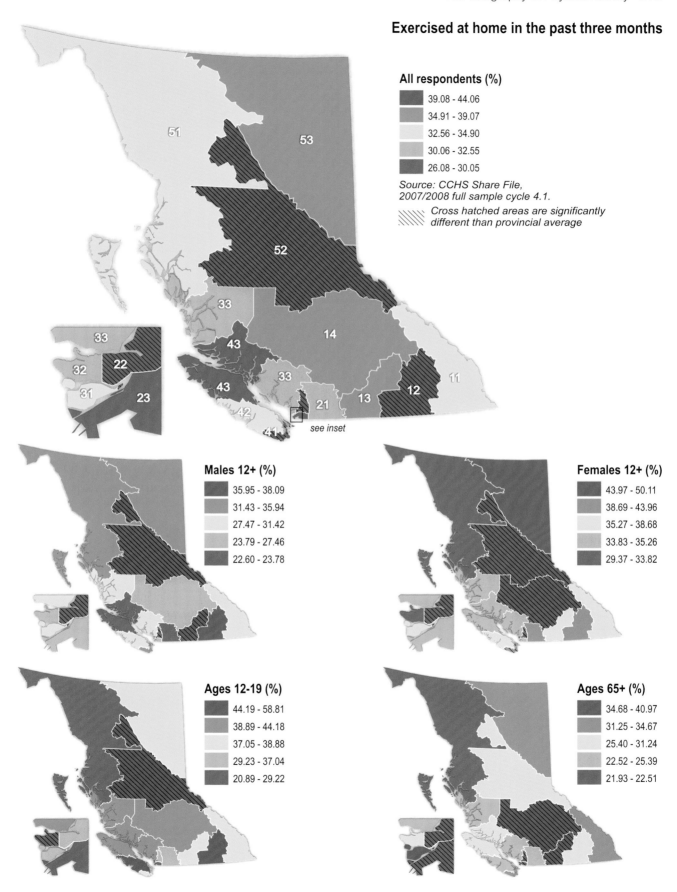

Exercised at home in the past three months

All respondents (%)

- 39.08 - 44.06
- 34.91 - 39.07
- 32.56 - 34.90
- 30.06 - 32.55
- 26.08 - 30.05

*Source: CCHS Share File,
2007/2008 full sample cycle 4.1.*

*Cross hatched areas are significantly
different than provincial average*

Males 12+ (%)

- 35.95 - 38.09
- 31.43 - 35.94
- 27.47 - 31.42
- 23.79 - 27.46
- 22.60 - 23.78

Females 12+ (%)

- 43.97 - 50.11
- 38.69 - 43.96
- 35.27 - 38.68
- 33.83 - 35.26
- 29.37 - 33.82

Ages 12-19 (%)

- 44.19 - 58.81
- 38.89 - 44.18
- 37.05 - 38.88
- 29.23 - 37.04
- 20.89 - 29.22

Ages 65+ (%)

- 34.68 - 40.97
- 31.25 - 34.67
- 25.40 - 31.24
- 22.52 - 25.39
- 21.93 - 22.51

Bicycled in the past three months

Health Service Delivery Area	All respondents 12+ (%)	Males 12+ (%)	Females 12+ (%)	Ages 12-19 (%)	Ages 20-64 (%)	Ages 65+ (%)
33 North Shore/Coast Garibaldi	28.19	32.60	24.17	46.33	29.66	9.23E‡
11 East Kootenay	26.87	31.05	22.80	48.86†	27.73	8.10E‡
43 North Vancouver Island	26.42	31.47	21.74	49.98E	27.58	F
41 South Vancouver Island	26.37	31.66	21.61	47.44†	27.42	10.27E‡
52 Northern Interior	26.02	31.18	20.80	44.24†	25.71	F
51 Northwest	24.75	30.13	19.20	58.48†	21.33	F
13 Okanagan	23.72	27.07	20.56	45.09†	25.09	8.08E‡
42 Central Vancouver Island	23.72	27.00	20.68	63.19†	22.22	5.92E‡
12 Kootenay Boundary	23.34	28.34	18.24	43.46E	23.90	F
14 Thompson Cariboo Shuswap	22.63	24.19	21.15	35.17	24.70	F
32 Vancouver	21.49	27.26*	15.87	31.15	23.03	5.52E‡
53 Northeast	21.42	20.81	22.06E	49.70E†	17.69	F
23 Fraser South	18.97	23.75*	14.37	34.45†	18.80	5.99E‡
21 Fraser East	18.57	22.53	14.68	43.65†	17.09	F
22 Fraser North	18.50	20.13	16.97	31.62†	19.02	F
31 Richmond	18.15	21.12	15.41	39.83E†	17.45	F
British Columbia (2007/8)	**22.04**	**26.00***	**18.27**	**41.03†**	**22.39**	**6.55‡**
British Columbia (2005)	**22.94**	**27.85***	**18.20**	**46.27†**	**22.35**	**6.94‡**

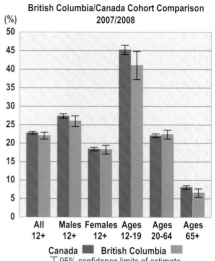

British Columbia/Canada Cohort Comparison 2007/2008

Canada ■   British Columbia ▨
⊥ 95% confidence limits of estimate

▨ Crosshatching beside the 2007/8 provincial rate indicates it is significantly different than the 2005 rate, while crosshatched HSDAs are significantly different than the 2007/8 provincial rate.
E interpret data with caution (16.67 ≤ coefficient of variation ≤ 33.3).

* Males differ significantly from females.
†12-19 age cohort differs significantly from the 20-64 age cohort.
‡ 65+ age cohort differs significantly from the 20-64 age cohort.
F data suppressed (n < 10, or coefficient of variation > 33.3).

Bicycling is an enjoyable recreational activity and an efficient form of active transportation. Cycling commuters are able to effectively integrate physical activity into a portion of their day that may otherwise have been spent sitting in a car. Of all British Columbian respondents to the CCHS, 22.04% had bicycled in the past 3 months. Respondents in North Shore/Coast Garibaldi and South Vancouver Island (both with cycling rates over 26%) reported significantly high levels of bicycling in comparison to the provincial average, while Richmond (only 18.15%) was significantly below average.

Bicycling was significantly more common among the male cohort than it was in the female cohort provincially, with 26% of males compared to 18.27% of females reporting having bicycled in the past 3 months. Male respondents in Fraser South and Vancouver were significantly more likely to cycle than their female counterparts within those HSDAs. There were no HSDAs in which females were significantly more likely than males to cycle, and there were no significant differences when comparing individual HSDAs to the provincial averages for either males or females.

The youth cohort in BC had the highest rates of cycling compared to any other cohort, and at 41.03% had almost double the bicycling rate of the mid-age cohort, a significant difference. Youth in 11 HSDAs had significantly higher rates of bicycling than the mid-age cohorts within those areas. Comparing the HSDA youth rates to the provincial youth average, both Central Vancouver Island and Northwest (both above 58%) had significantly higher

values of bicycling, and no HSDA was significantly below the provincial average for youth.

Older respondents provincially had by far the lowest bicycling rate at only 6.55%, significantly below that of the mid-age cohort. However, data were only available for seven HSDAs for this cohort, and all had relatively high coefficients of variation. Comparisons are therefore not possible.

Generally, there was a modest 10 to 15 percentage spread in values among cohorts. In examining the maps for this indicator, with the exception of North Shore/Coast Garibaldi there were consistently lower values for bicycling in the south western urban mainland areas, as well as Fraser East. Higher values were more likely in East Kootenay and parts of Vancouver Island.

There were no significant differences for any of the BC cohorts between the 2005 and 2007/8 samples, and British Columbians did not show any significant differences when compared to Canadian cohorts for bicycling in 2007/8.

Bicycled in the past three months

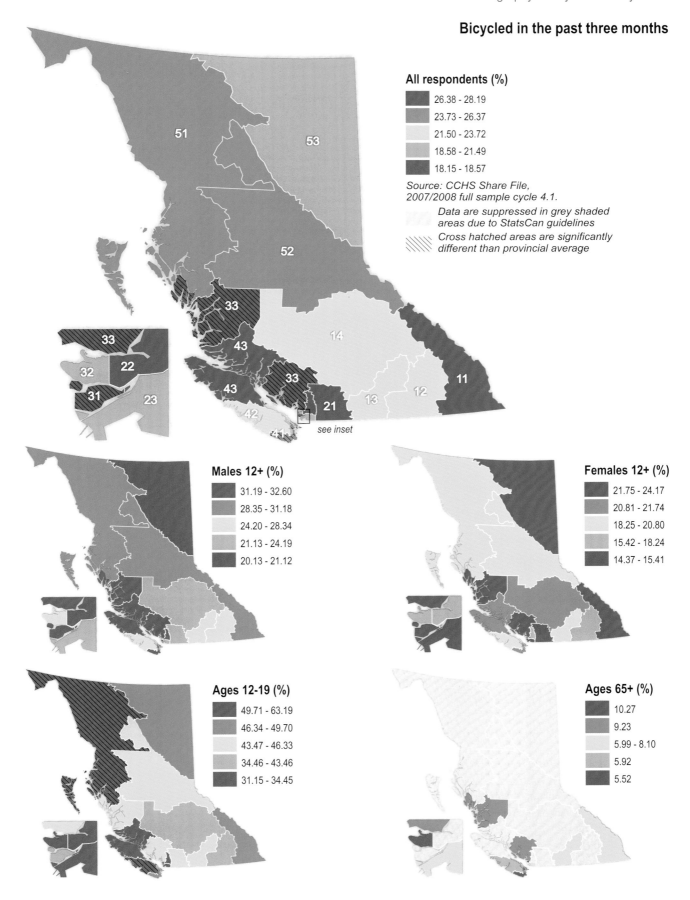

All respondents (%)

- 26.38 - 28.19
- 23.73 - 26.37
- 21.50 - 23.72
- 18.58 - 21.49
- 18.15 - 18.57

*Source: CCHS Share File,
2007/2008 full sample cycle 4.1.*

Data are suppressed in grey shaded
areas due to StatsCan guidelines

Cross hatched areas are significantly
different than provincial average

see inset

Males 12+ (%)

- 31.19 - 32.60
- 28.35 - 31.18
- 24.20 - 28.34
- 21.13 - 24.19
- 20.13 - 21.12

Females 12+ (%)

- 21.75 - 24.17
- 20.81 - 21.74
- 18.25 - 20.80
- 15.42 - 18.24
- 14.37 - 15.41

Ages 12-19 (%)

- 49.71 - 63.19
- 46.34 - 49.70
- 43.47 - 46.33
- 34.46 - 43.46
- 31.15 - 34.45

Ages 65+ (%)

- 10.27
- 9.23
- 5.99 - 8.10
- 5.92
- 5.52

Students that exercised or participated in physical activities for at least 30 minutes on 5 or more of the past 7 days

The Student Satisfaction Survey asked how many days in the past week (7 days) they had participated for at least 30 minutes in activities that made them sweat and breathe hard (e.g., soccer, running, dancing, bicycling, or similar aerobic activity). This new indicator for the Atlas provides analysis of those students who said they participated in physical activities on 5 or more days in the past week. It should be noted that self-reported physical activity is often over-reported by children and youth (Colley, et al., 2011b).

Grades 3/4

Provincially, close to seven in every ten (68.79%) grades 3/4 respondents in 2008/9 indicated that they exercised quite vigorously on at least 5 of the past 7 days. However, there was a 30 percentage point difference among school districts. Revelstoke had 88.71% of students that indicated they had exercised 5 or more days, compared to only 58.57% in Peace River North, and Vancouver and Kootenay-Columbia (both below 61%). Geographically, there were clusters of school districts in the southern interior, parts of the south coast, and western central parts of the province with relatively high values, and outliers in the extreme northeast and southeast of the province and on western Vancouver Island. In contrast, much of the northern and central interior had below average values.

Grade 7

Students in this grade had a marginally lower participation value (67.58%) than those in grades 3/4. The range among school districts went from a high of 92.22% in Revelstoke, to a low of 30.77% in Central Coast and 38.46% in Nisga'a. While there are some similarities in geographical patterns with the grades 3/4 students, the differences are perhaps more striking. Most of the northern half of the province had below average values, with the exception of Nechako Lakes (77.67%) and Peace River South (74.87%), while many school districts in the southeastern part of the province were above average, but again there were major exceptions, particularly North Okanagan-Shuswap (61.47%) and Vernon (62.99%).

Grade 10

The provincial average for grade 10 students (53.29%) was 14 percentage points lower than the grade 7 average. North Okanagan-Shuswap (78.28%) had the highest average among school districts for grade 10 students, while Vancouver Island West (27.27%) had the lowest average value, followed by Nisga'a (30.77%). Geographical patterns were very different from both grade 3/4 and grade 7 students. And there were no clear regional clusters of school districts with similar values, except for the majority of the Vancouver Island school districts, which were above average; however, Cowichan Valley and Vancouver Island West were both lower than average.

School District	All students grades 3/4 (%)	All students grade 7 (%)	All students grade 10 (%)
19 Revelstoke	88.71	92.22	50.72
81 Fort Nelson	81.97	61.11	48.15
49 Central Coast	81.25	30.77	53.33
78 Fraser-Cascade	78.10	67.41	61.40
58 Nicola-Similkameen	76.67	60.43	43.21
67 Okanagan Skaha	75.52	64.34	49.03
91 Nechako Lakes	74.75	77.66	63.14
47 Powell River	74.11	75.69	52.17
84 Vancouver Island West	74.07	64.00	27.27
54 Bulkley Valley	74.00	66.48	54.10
74 Gold Trail	73.91	68.75	54.90
37 Delta	73.90	73.51	52.66
46 Sunshine Coast	73.79	72.83	47.85
51 Boundary	73.39	84.31	45.27
34 Abbotsford	73.07	74.47	58.56
50 Haida Gwaii/Queen Charlotte	72.97	71.43	47.50
48 Howe Sound	72.96	73.00	53.01
44 North Vancouver	72.73	68.14	51.64
69 Qualicum	72.70	72.64	68.20
82 Coast Mountains	72.52	66.30	53.82
5 Southeast Kootenay	72.46	65.89	59.32
22 Vernon	72.31	62.99	55.91
53 Okanagan Similkameen	72.02	62.09	57.32
42 Maple Ridge-Pitt Meadows	71.61	69.22	53.45
61 Greater Victoria	71.43	71.25	62.35
8 Kootenay Lake	71.43	72.87	52.19
62 Sooke	71.20	67.43	59.16
28 Quesnel	71.01	68.01	52.74
72 Campbell River	70.88	52.72	63.51
87 Stikine	70.59	54.55	46.67
38 Richmond	70.55	68.13	49.67
70 Alberni	70.50	77.47	58.99
23 Central Okanagan	70.50	71.06	43.77
36 Surrey	70.45	66.33	55.13
64 Gulf Islands	70.13	63.83	61.90
75 Mission	69.87	64.48	54.30
63 Saanich	69.81	77.97	63.24
40 New Westminster	69.38	65.83	56.84
41 Burnaby	68.71	65.92	49.34
35 Langley	68.61	68.59	50.98
71 Comox Valley	67.92	70.71	62.89
43 Coquitlam	67.35	66.60	54.70
6 Rocky Mountain	66.96	81.33	59.69
68 Nanaimo-Ladysmith	66.89	68.70	56.98
10 Arrow Lakes	66.67	72.09	58.33
59 Peace River South	66.67	74.87	49.80
52 Prince Rupert	66.67	65.67	54.97
73 Kamloops/Thompson	66.43	74.97	61.45
83 North Okanagan-Shuswap	66.34	61.47	78.28
27 Cariboo-Chilcotin	65.77	72.04	65.56
45 West Vancouver	65.69	71.27	47.94
57 Prince George	65.03	63.78	55.51
85 Vancouver Island North	64.89	64.04	66.09
33 Chilliwack	64.68	65.32	52.08
79 Cowichan Valley	64.15	64.50	50.73
20 Kootenay-Columbia	60.53	69.61	62.75
39 Vancouver	60.48	59.04	35.58
60 Peace River North	58.57	62.33	56.48
92 Nisga'a	Msk	38.46	30.77
British Columbia	**68.79**	**67.58**	**53.29**

Msk: Data masked for privacy

Students that exercised or participated in physical activities for at least 30 minutes on 5 or more of the past 7 days

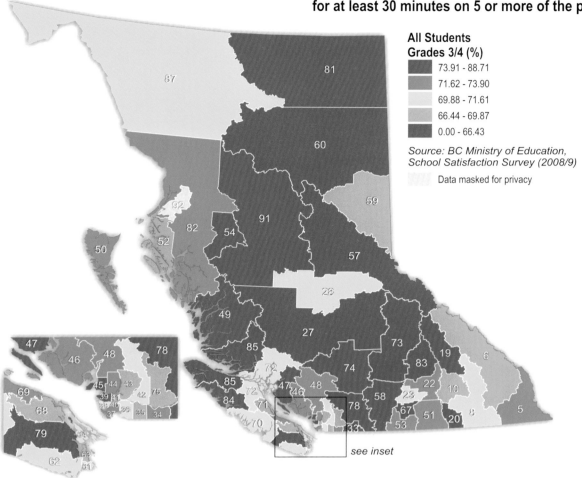

**All Students
Grades 3/4 (%)**

- 73.91 - 88.71
- 71.62 - 73.90
- 69.88 - 71.61
- 66.44 - 69.87
- 0.00 - 66.43

*Source: BC Ministry of Education,
School Satisfaction Survey (2008/9)*

Data masked for privacy

see inset

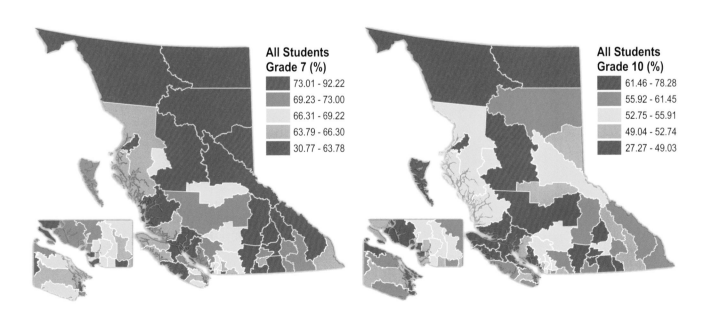

**All Students
Grade 7 (%)**

- 73.01 - 92.22
- 69.23 - 73.00
- 66.31 - 69.22
- 63.79 - 66.30
- 30.77 - 63.78

**All Students
Grade 10 (%)**

- 61.46 - 78.28
- 55.92 - 61.45
- 52.75 - 55.91
- 49.04 - 52.74
- 27.27 - 49.03

Students that usually do physical activity within school

Opportunities to undertake physical activity represent an important wellness asset. For some children, the school may be the only or key resource available to them for participating in physical exercise and activities. The Student Satisfaction Survey asked students where they usually did physical activity. *"Within school"* responses included: in my regular classroom, in my PE classes, in school teams or clubs, at class trips to recreation centres, and in other activities at school. *"Outside of school"* responses included: with clubs or sports teams in the community, at recreation centres, with other groups or organizations, and on my own. This is a new indicator for the Atlas, and those who indicated that they usually did their physical activity within schools in 2008/9 are analysed in the table and maps opposite.

Grades 3/4

More than half (53.22%) of all respondents in these grades indicated that they usually did physical activity within the school setting in 2008/9, leaving 46.78% of students who usually did physical activity outside the school setting. Within school values ranged from a high of 75.00% in Stikine to 47.30% in Powell River and 47.32% in West Vancouver. Higher values were found primarily outside the lower mainland and southern coastal region, with negative outliers in Revelstoke (48.10%) and Central Okanagan (50.79%), and positive outliers in Mission (58.31%), and Burnaby, Richmond, and Surrey (all about 55%).

Grade 7

Just half (50.13%) of the grade 7 respondents indicated that they did physical activity within school, indicating that 49.87% usually did physical activity outside of school. Values ranged from a high of 69.57% in Central Coast to a low of 39.39% in Nisga'a. While the geographical patterns were somewhat similar to those for grades 3/4 respondents, the difference between the southwestern part of the province and the rest of the province was not as prominent. For example, Fort Nelson (44.03%) in the north had a low value, as did several school districts in the southeastern quadrant of the province. In contrast, New Westminster (53.98%) in the lower mainland was in the highest value quintile.

Grade 10

Just over four in every ten (43.26%) respondents in grade 10 indicated that the usual place for their physical activity was within school, with the remainder (56.74%) usually doing physical activity outside of school. Within school values varied from 55.56% in Vancouver Island West to

School District	All students grades 3/4 (%)	All students grade 7 (%)	All students grade 10 (%)
87 Stikine	75.00	53.33	47.06
49 Central Coast	70.37	69.57	45.45
74 Gold Trail	63.90	53.79	48.82
10 Arrow Lakes	60.80	49.15	48.02
82 Coast Mountains	58.76	52.47	37.58
53 Okanagan Similkameen	58.73	54.00	44.21
75 Mission	58.31	49.19	41.20
27 Cariboo-Chilcotin	58.02	54.04	41.62
51 Boundary	57.51	48.26	40.59
67 Okanagan Skaha	57.22	47.33	41.34
6 Rocky Mountain	56.94	48.93	42.06
91 Nechako Lakes	56.73	53.20	45.01
50 Haida Gwaii/Queen Charlotte	56.38	51.90	53.78
58 Nicola-Similkameen	55.92	45.61	45.09
22 Vernon	55.57	52.67	40.55
52 Prince Rupert	55.52	54.43	40.90
85 Vancouver Island North	55.51	51.84	44.03
41 Burnaby	55.47	55.34	45.58
73 Kamloops/Thompson	55.23	51.18	42.94
81 Fort Nelson	55.06	44.03	48.59
8 Kootenay Lake	55.04	46.06	46.78
38 Richmond	54.93	55.15	46.74
36 Surrey	54.81	53.24	44.39
79 Cowichan Valley	54.72	48.43	40.58
33 Chilliwack	54.70	50.37	37.77
72 Campbell River	54.41	44.11	37.09
57 Prince George	54.38	49.77	37.64
78 Fraser-Cascade	54.12	51.14	40.67
83 North Okanagan-Shuswap	53.95	46.77	47.71
60 Peace River North	53.90	53.62	40.60
70 Alberni	53.81	46.64	43.85
54 Bulkley Valley	53.15	49.01	50.29
59 Peace River South	53.09	51.16	33.00
62 Sooke	53.03	44.94	37.67
39 Vancouver	52.85	52.90	50.68
34 Abbotsford	52.44	47.64	45.01
63 Saanich	52.35	42.09	38.23
35 Langley	52.21	48.74	40.64
28 Quesnel	52.21	48.91	38.77
5 Southeast Kootenay	52.21	47.11	40.59
43 Coquitlam	51.98	48.85	44.44
46 Sunshine Coast	51.97	45.13	39.11
61 Greater Victoria	51.60	47.07	41.26
42 Maple Ridge-Pitt Meadows	51.59	48.08	42.99
37 Delta	51.58	49.87	42.53
68 Nanaimo-Ladysmith	51.40	51.60	41.56
20 Kootenay-Columbia	51.07	49.77	36.18
69 Qualicum	50.81	47.58	39.18
23 Central Okanagan	50.79	45.53	41.41
64 Gulf Islands	50.00	49.59	43.10
84 Vancouver Island West	50.00	52.24	55.56
71 Comox Valley	49.50	44.65	43.58
44 North Vancouver	49.11	45.89	41.51
40 New Westminster	48.98	53.98	43.51
19 Revelstoke	48.10	44.95	42.25
48 Howe Sound	47.86	45.10	40.96
45 West Vancouver	47.32	47.14	41.73
47 Powell River	47.30	48.72	40.00
92 Nisga'a	Msk	39.39	32.79
British Columbia	**53.22**	**50.13**	**43.26**

Msk Data masked for privacy

lows of 32.79% in Nisga'a and 33.00% in Peace River South. Geographical patterns were quite different from those of the other grades. A cluster of low values was found in the eastern north central part of BC, as well as the north coastal region, although Haida Gwaii (53.78%) was an outlier in the top quintile.

Students that usually do physical activity within school

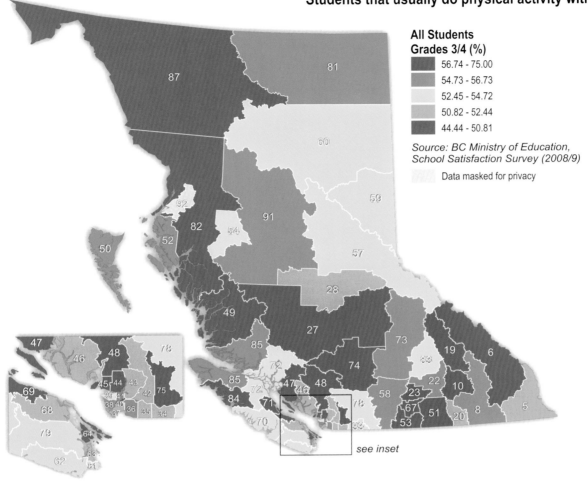

**All Students
Grades 3/4 (%)**

- 56.74 - 75.00
- 54.73 - 56.73
- 52.45 - 54.72
- 50.82 - 52.44
- 44.44 - 50.81

*Source: BC Ministry of Education,
School Satisfaction Survey (2008/9)*

Data masked for privacy

see inset

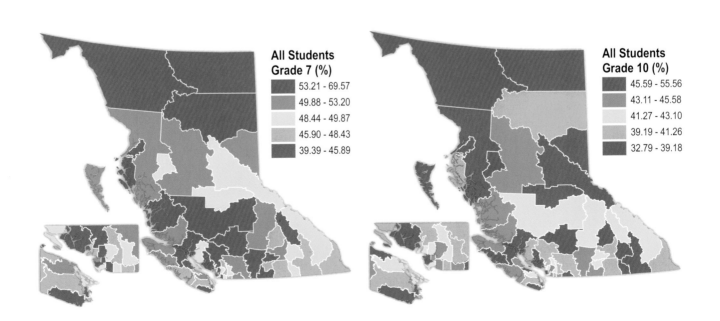

**All Students
Grade 7 (%)**

- 53.21 - 69.57
- 49.88 - 53.20
- 48.44 - 49.87
- 45.90 - 48.43
- 39.39 - 45.89

**All Students
Grade 10 (%)**

- 45.59 - 55.56
- 43.11 - 45.58
- 41.27 - 43.10
- 39.19 - 41.26
- 32.79 - 39.18

Has access to a gym or physical fitness facilities at or near work

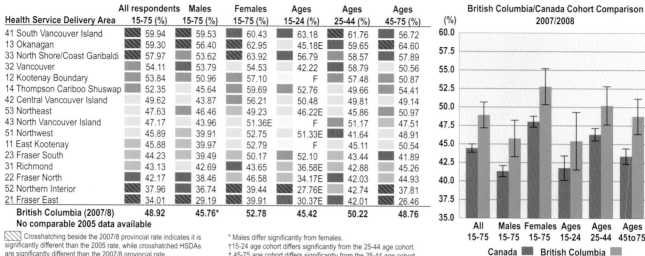

Health Service Delivery Area	All respondents 15-75 (%)	Males 15-75 (%)	Females 15-75 (%)	Ages 15-24 (%)	Ages 25-44 (%)	Ages 45-75 (%)
41 South Vancouver Island	59.94	59.53	60.43	63.18	61.76	56.72
13 Okanagan	59.30	56.40	62.95	45.18E	59.65	64.60
33 North Shore/Coast Garibaldi	57.97	53.62	63.92	56.79	58.57	57.89
32 Vancouver	54.11	53.79	54.53	42.22	58.79	50.56
12 Kootenay Boundary	53.84	50.96	57.10	F	57.48	50.87
14 Thompson Cariboo Shuswap	52.35	45.64	59.69	52.76	49.66	54.41
42 Central Vancouver Island	49.62	43.87	56.21	50.48	49.81	49.14
53 Northeast	47.63	46.46	49.23	46.22E	45.86	50.97
43 North Vancouver Island	47.17	43.96	51.36E	F	51.17	47.51
51 Northwest	45.89	39.91	52.75	51.33E	41.64	48.91
11 East Kootenay	45.88	39.97	52.79	F	45.11	50.54
23 Fraser South	44.23	39.49	50.17	52.10	43.44	41.89
31 Richmond	43.13	42.69	43.65	36.58E	42.88	45.26
22 Fraser North	42.17	38.46	46.58	34.17E	42.03	44.93
52 Northern Interior	37.96	36.74	39.44	27.76E	42.74	37.81
21 Fraser East	34.01	29.19	39.91	30.37E	42.01	26.46
British Columbia (2007/8)	**48.92**	**45.76***	**52.78**	**45.42**	**50.22**	**48.76**
No comparable 2005 data available						

Crosshatching beside the 2007/8 provincial rate indicates it is significantly different than the 2005 rate, while crosshatched HSDAs are significantly different than the 2007/8 provincial rate.
E interpret data with caution (16.67 ≤ coefficient of variation ≤ 33.3).

* Males differ significantly from females.
†15-24 age cohort differs significantly from the 25-44 age cohort.
‡ 45-75 age cohort differs significantly from the 25-44 age cohort.
F data suppressed (n < 10, or coefficient of variation > 33.3).

In response to the CCHS question *"At or near your place of work, do you have access to a gym or physical fitness facility?"* nearly half (48.92%) of respondents in BC aged 15-75 years who worked outside the home answered positively. Respondents in South Vancouver Island, Okanagan, and North Shore/Coast Garibaldi (all at, or above, 60%) were significantly more likely, while Northern Interior and Fraser East were significantly less likely than the provincial average to have access to such facilities.

Female respondents (52.78%) provincially were significantly more likely than male respondents (45.76%) to have proximate access to facilities, and while not significant, females in each HSDA had greater access than their male counterparts. For males, South Vancouver Island (59.53%) and Okanagan (56.40%) were significantly higher, while Fraser East (29.19%) was significantly lower than the provincial male average. For females, North Shore/Coast Garibaldi (63.92%) and Okanagan (62.95%) were significantly higher, while Fraser East and Northern Interior (both below 40%) were significantly lower than the BC average for females.

There were no significant differences between any of the age cohorts, either at the provincial level or for any individual HSDA. For the younger cohort (15-24 years), Northern Interior (27.76%) was significantly lower than the provincial average (45.42%) for this cohort, although caution is required in interpretation because of relatively high coefficients of variation for many of the youth values, while values for still other HSDAs were not reportable because of small sample sizes. For the older age (45-75 years) cohort, Okanagan (64.60%) was significantly higher, while Northern Interior (37.81%) and Fraser East (26.46%) were significantly lower than the provincial average (48.76%) for this age cohort.

Generally, there was a 20 to 30 percentage point range in values for all cohorts, indicating major geographic differences throughout the province. South Vancouver Island and North Shore Coast/Garibaldi were consistently above provincial averages for all cohorts, while Richmond, Fraser North, Northern Interior, and Fraser East were consistently below provincial averages for all cohorts.

There were no comparative CCHS data for 2005. For the 2007/8 CCHS samples, BC respondents had greater access to gyms or physical fitness facilities at or near work than their Canadian counterparts, and the difference was significant for all cohorts except for the youngest age (15-24 years) cohort.

Has access to a gym or physical fitness facilities at or near work

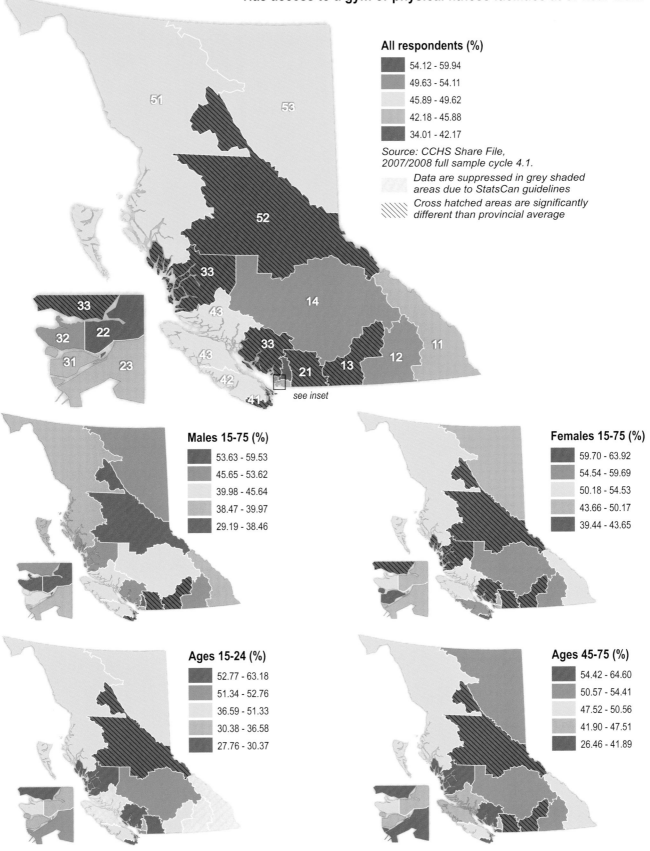

All respondents (%)

- 54.12 - 59.94
- 49.63 - 54.11
- 45.89 - 49.62
- 42.18 - 45.88
- 34.01 - 42.17

Source: CCHS Share File, 2007/2008 full sample cycle 4.1.

Data are suppressed in grey shaded areas due to StatsCan guidelines

Cross hatched areas are significantly different than provincial average

see inset

Males 15-75 (%)

- 53.63 - 59.53
- 45.65 - 53.62
- 39.98 - 45.64
- 38.47 - 39.97
- 29.19 - 38.46

Females 15-75 (%)

- 59.70 - 63.92
- 54.54 - 59.69
- 50.18 - 54.53
- 43.66 - 50.17
- 39.44 - 43.65

Ages 15-24 (%)

- 52.77 - 63.18
- 51.34 - 52.76
- 36.59 - 51.33
- 30.38 - 36.58
- 27.76 - 30.37

Ages 45-75 (%)

- 54.42 - 64.60
- 50.57 - 54.41
- 47.52 - 50.56
- 41.90 - 47.51
- 26.46 - 41.89

Sports club membership

2010 LegaciesNow provides data on membership in sports clubs funded by Sports BC. The data used in the following pages are based on sports club membership rates by HSDA. It is important to note that individuals could be members of more than one sports organization, so for the total club membership data shown in the table and maps opposite, there was likely some double counting. Nevertheless, the patterns that emerge are representative of sports club membership throughout the province.

Sports club membership rates are provided per 1,000 population between the ages of 4 and 80 years. Four years old is an estimate of the lower age limit for participation in organized sports. While 80 years of age may appear to be high for participation in many competitive sports, increasingly more seniors are participating in sports (Turcotte & Schellenberg, 2007). Membership in a sports club provides opportunities for participation in activities, as well as opportunities for attending social events and being connected with others, all important wellness assets.

Total sports club membership

Based on approximately 60 different sports activities, ranging from archery to wrestling, there were more than 600,000 members of sports clubs in BC in 2008/9. This represented a provincial membership rate of 140.10 per 1,000 population between the ages of 4 and 80 years. Geographically, Northern Interior had the highest overall rate in the province of 281.45 per 1,000 population, a figure that was twice the provincial rate. Northeast, Thompson Cariboo Shuswap, and North Shore/Coast Garibaldi all had rates greater than 200 per 1,000 population. At the other extreme, Fraser East had the lowest membership rate at 91.28 per 1,000 population, less than one-third of the rate of the highest HSDA.

Geographically, higher membership rates were generally found in the north (with the exception of Northwest), central interior, and in the southeast of the province, while the lower mainland area of the province (with the exception of North Shore/Coast Garibaldi) and parts of Vancouver Island had lower rates than the provincial average.

Total sports club membership for males

There were approximately 350,000 males in the province who were members of sports clubs in 2008/9. This represented an overall rate of 162.55 per 1,000 male population between the ages of 4 and 80 years. The

Health Service Delivery Area	Total membership rate	Male membership rate	Female membership rate
52 Northern Interior	281.45	286.59	276.05
53 Northeast	237.92	257.46	216.65
14 Thompson Cariboo Shuswap	237.63	262.00	212.95
33 North Shore/Coast Garibaldi	200.99	237.47	165.11
12 Kootenay Boundary	196.07	226.00	165.59
11 East Kootenay	179.73	204.48	154.53
51 Northwest	169.82	189.81	148.57
13 Okanagan	154.54	177.28	132.30
42 Central Vancouver Island	150.06	174.85	125.51
41 South Vancouver Island	137.71	173.82	102.93
43 North Vancouver Island	133.84	156.60	110.83
22 Fraser North	112.17	133.53	90.72
23 Fraser South	111.47	129.75	93.02
31 Richmond	105.30	137.38	74.22
32 Vancouver	102.07	117.69	86.39
21 Fraser East	91.28	106.32	75.87
British Columbia	**140.10**	**162.55**	**117.60**

Rate is per 1,000 population aged 4 to 80

highest rate was found in Northern Interior (286.59 per 1,000 population), while Thompson Cariboo Shuswap, Northeast, North Shore/Coast Garibaldi, Kootenay Boundary, and East Kootenay all had rates in excess of 200 per 1,000 population. Fraser East, with a rate of 106.32 per 1,000 population, had the lowest male membership rate. Geographical patterns were almost identical to those for the population as a whole.

Total sports membership for females

Approximately 250,000 females in the province were members of sports clubs in 2008/9, a rate of 117.60 per 1,000 female population between the ages of 4 and 80 years. Northern Interior again had the highest sports club membership rate, with 276.05 members per 1,000 female population. Two other HSDAs, Northeast and Thompson Cariboo Shuswap, had rates in excess of 200 per 1,000 population. Fraser East, with a rate of 75.87 per 1,000 population, had the lowest rate, and was approximately 25% of the rate recorded for Northern Interior. Overall geographical patterns were similar to those for the population as a whole, and to those for the male club membership population.

Sports club membership

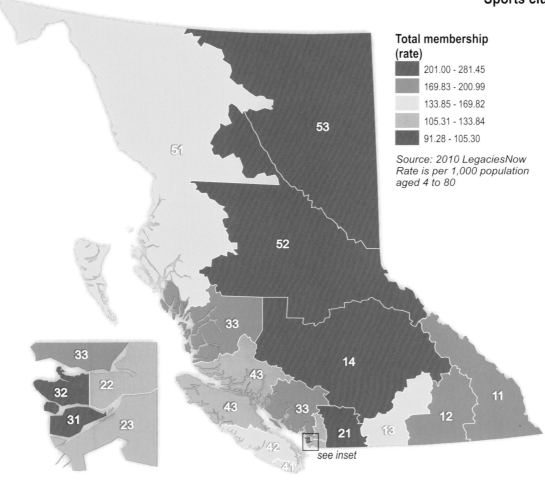

Total membership (rate)

- 201.00 - 281.45
- 169.83 - 200.99
- 133.85 - 169.82
- 105.31 - 133.84
- 91.28 - 105.30

*Source: 2010 LegaciesNow
Rate is per 1,000 population aged 4 to 80*

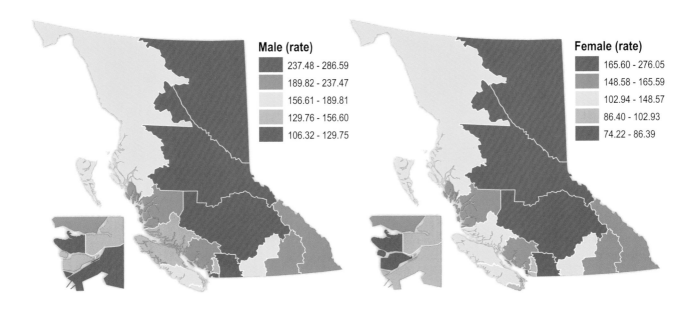

Male (rate)

- 237.48 - 286.59
- 189.82 - 237.47
- 156.61 - 189.81
- 129.76 - 156.60
- 106.32 - 129.75

Female (rate)

- 165.60 - 276.05
- 148.58 - 165.59
- 102.94 - 148.57
- 86.40 - 102.93
- 74.22 - 86.39

Soccer and athletics membership

Soccer club membership

Soccer is by far the most popular sports club membership in BC, with more than 113,000 registered club members in 2008/9. Nearly 4% of registered club members were 5 years old or younger, while nearly 70% were between the ages of 6 to 17 years. There were nearly twice as many members as the next most popular club membership (athletics).

Provincially, membership was higher for males at 31.41 per 1,000 male population between the ages of 4 and 80 years old, compared with 21.46 per 1,000 female population. Northern Interior was the only HSDA where female soccer club membership was higher than that for males.

For males, membership rates were highest in North Shore/Coast Garibaldi at 56.13 per 1,000 male population, followed by Northwest at 44.09 per 1,000 male population. This compared with only 19.46 per 1,000 male population for Northeast and 19.78 per 1,000 male population for Central Vancouver Island. Geographically, there were no clear patterns, with high and low values in the northern part of the province and also in the urban lower mainland

southwestern part of the province and on Vancouver Island.

For females, soccer club membership was again highest in North Shore/Coast Garibaldi at

Health Service Delivery Area	Soccer male (rate)	Soccer female (rate)
33 North Shore/Coast Garibaldi	56.13	44.69
51 Northwest	44.09	34.19
41 South Vancouver Island	38.91	16.50
22 Fraser North	38.16	24.57
13 Okanagan	35.46	28.10
23 Fraser South	32.60	22.26
12 Kootenay Boundary	32.07	22.28
14 Thompson Cariboo Shuswap	31.59	29.16
52 Northern Interior	30.19	33.90
11 East Kootenay	27.01	17.09
31 Richmond	23.95	12.55
43 North Vancouver Island	22.99	18.64
21 Fraser East	20.75	14.89
32 Vancouver	20.67	11.73
42 Central Vancouver Island	19.78	9.92
53 Northeast	19.46	15.75
British Columbia	**31.41**	**21.46**

44.69 per 1,000 female population between the ages of 4 and 80 years old, more than four times the club membership rate for Central Vancouver Island (9.92 per 1,000 female population). Overall, membership rates for females were higher in the northern part of the province with the exception of Northeast, while rates in the urban southwest were mixed with high rates already noted for North Shore/Coast Garibaldi and low rates for Vancouver and Richmond.

Athletics club membership

After soccer, athletics had the next most popular club membership in BC with more than 59,000 members. Rates for males, at 14.42 per 1,000 male population between the ages of 4 and 80 years old, were marginally higher than the rate for females (13.29 per 1,000 female population).

For males, Northern Interior, with a membership rate of 110.43 per 1,000 male population, had by far the highest athletics club membership rate, followed by Northeast and Thompson Cariboo Shuswap (both approximately 80 per 1,000 population). At the other extreme, East Kootenay, Kootenay Boundary, Northwest, and Fraser East all had rates of less than 1 per 1,000 male population. Geographically, membership rates were dominated by the north (excluding Northwest) and central interior HSDAs, while the lowest rates occurred in the extreme northwest and southeast of the province.

Overall, rates and geographical patterns were remarkably similar for females. Again, Northern Interior was dominant with a rate of 114.31 per 1,000 female population, followed by Northeast (82.02 per 1,000 population) and Thompson

Cariboo Shuswap (76.34 per 1,000 population), while the lowest membership HSDAs were the same as for males.

Health Service Delivery Area	Athletics male (rate)	Athletics female (rate)
52 Northern Interior	110.43	114.31
53 Northeast	80.73	82.02
14 Thompson Cariboo Shuswap	79.83	76.34
42 Central Vancouver Island	20.52	19.19
32 Vancouver	14.32	11.27
33 North Shore/Coast Garibaldi	7.34	6.63
23 Fraser South	5.90	5.27
31 Richmond	4.40	1.73
43 North Vancouver Island	3.00	3.65
41 South Vancouver Island	1.54	1.29
22 Fraser North	1.44	1.11
13 Okanagan	1.39	1.43
21 Fraser East	0.81	0.73
51 Northwest	0.48	0.79
12 Kootenay Boundary	0.42	1.28
11 East Kootenay	0.05	0.08
British Columbia	**14.42**	**13.29**

Soccer and athletics membership

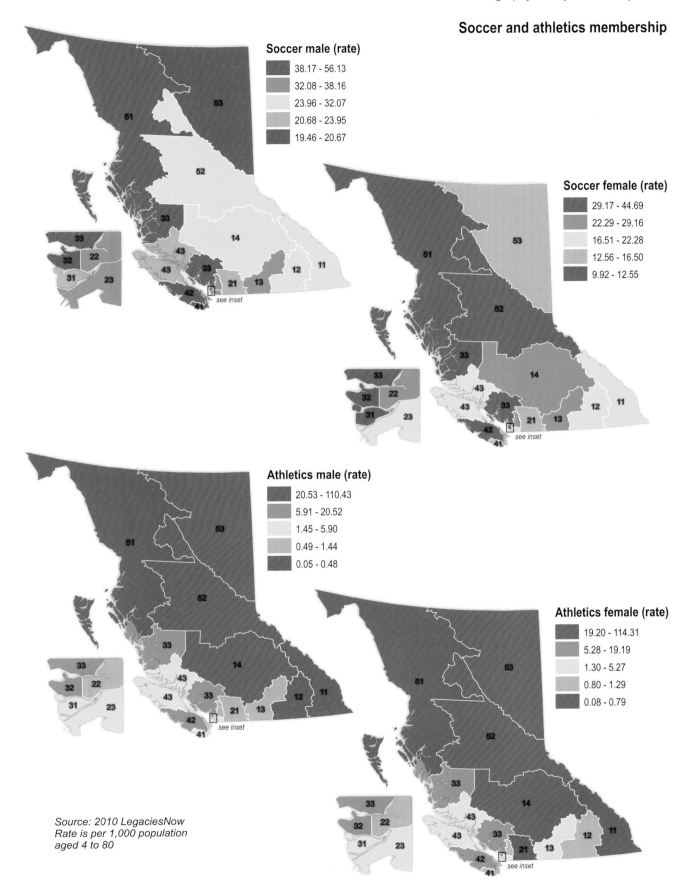

Soccer male (rate)
- 38.17 - 56.13
- 32.08 - 38.16
- 23.96 - 32.07
- 20.68 - 23.95
- 19.46 - 20.67

Soccer female (rate)
- 29.17 - 44.69
- 22.29 - 29.16
- 16.51 - 22.28
- 12.56 - 16.50
- 9.92 - 12.55

Athletics male (rate)
- 20.53 - 110.43
- 5.91 - 20.52
- 1.45 - 5.90
- 0.49 - 1.44
- 0.05 - 0.48

Athletics female (rate)
- 19.20 - 114.31
- 5.28 - 19.19
- 1.30 - 5.27
- 0.80 - 1.29
- 0.08 - 0.79

Source: 2010 LegaciesNow
Rate is per 1,000 population
aged 4 to 80

Golf and artistic gymnastics

Golf club membership

Golf had the third highest club membership in the province with more than 55,000 members in 2008/9. The membership rates were quite different between genders. The male membership rate of 18.68 per 1,000 male population between the ages of 4 to 80 years was more than twice the female membership rate of 7.03 per 1,000 female population. Male rates were consistently higher than those for females for every HSDA.

For males, the highest rates were found in East Kootenay (53.64 per 1,000 male population), and Kootenay Boundary and Richmond (both greater than 40 per 1,000 male population). The lowest membership rates (all less than 10 per 1,000 population) occurred in Fraser South, Fraser North, and Fraser East. East Kootenay had a membership rate more than seven times the rate for Fraser South, indicating a major geographical variation across the province. The lowest rates were clustered in the Fraser Valley in the southwest of the province, while the highest rates were in the Kootenay region in the southeast, along with Richmond in the urban southwest, which was an outlier in that region.

East Kootenay had the highest female membership rate at 24.21 per 1,000 female population, which was nearly twice that of the next highest HSDAs, Kootenay Boundary (13.91 per 1,000 population) and Richmond (13.05 per 1,000 population), and eight times the rates of the lowest HSDAs in the Fraser Valley region (all around 3 per 1,000 population). Overall, the geographical patterns were almost identical to the male patterns.

Health Service Delivery Area	Golf male (rate)	Golf female (rate)
11 East Kootenay	53.64	24.21
12 Kootenay Boundary	43.09	13.91
31 Richmond	41.17	13.05
53 Northeast	32.57	11.15
14 Thompson Cariboo Shuswap	29.71	11.81
41 South Vancouver Island	28.87	8.71
13 Okanagan	26.10	10.74
33 North Shore/Coast Garibaldi	24.53	9.22
51 Northwest	23.07	9.14
42 Central Vancouver Island	21.94	9.07
43 North Vancouver Island	18.95	8.12
52 Northern Interior	16.15	5.97
32 Vancouver	12.22	5.06
21 Fraser East	9.29	3.05
22 Fraser North	8.00	2.88
23 Fraser South	7.47	3.09
British Columbia	**18.68**	**7.03**

Artistic gymnastics club membership

Artistic gymnastics clubs ranked fifth in popularity in the province in 2008/9, with a membership of approximately 37,000. The provincial female rate of 11.56 per 1,000 female population between the ages of 4 and 80 years old was twice the rate for males (5.65 per 1,000 male population). Rates were consistently higher for females for every HSDA. Club membership was dominated by young members: more than 40% were below the age of 6 years and more than 43% were between the ages of 6 and 12 years.

For males, East Kootenay was dominant with a club membership rate of 12.52 per 1,000 male population between the ages of 4 and 80 years, twice the provincial rate and three times the rate of the lowest membership HSDAs (Richmond and North Shore/Coast Garibaldi, both 4 per 1,000 population or less). Geographically, the highest membership rates were found in the southeast and central interior of the province, with the lower rates in parts of the lower mainland and parts of Vancouver Island.

For females, the dominant membership rate was also found in East Kootenay. The rate of 31.10 per 1,000 female population was nearly three times the provincial rate, and nearly four times the rate of Fraser East (8.25 per 1,000 population). Geographically, the overall patterns were quite similar to those for males, although the northern HSDAs were relatively higher than for males.

Health Service Delivery Area	Artistic gymnastics male (rate)	Artistic gymnastics female (rate)
11 East Kootenay	12.52	31.10
14 Thompson Cariboo Shuswap	8.72	13.44
12 Kootenay Boundary	8.62	19.55
52 Northern Interior	6.79	18.64
41 South Vancouver Island	6.63	12.63
13 Okanagan	6.53	11.85
51 Northwest	6.12	15.15
53 Northeast	5.48	15.37
23 Fraser South	5.34	12.55
32 Vancouver	5.16	9.94
22 Fraser North	5.06	9.61
42 Central Vancouver Island	4.92	9.89
21 Fraser East	4.81	8.25
43 North Vancouver Island	4.47	9.69
31 Richmond	4.08	8.31
33 North Shore/Coast Garibaldi	3.64	8.45
British Columbia	**5.65**	**11.56**

Golf and artistic gymnastics

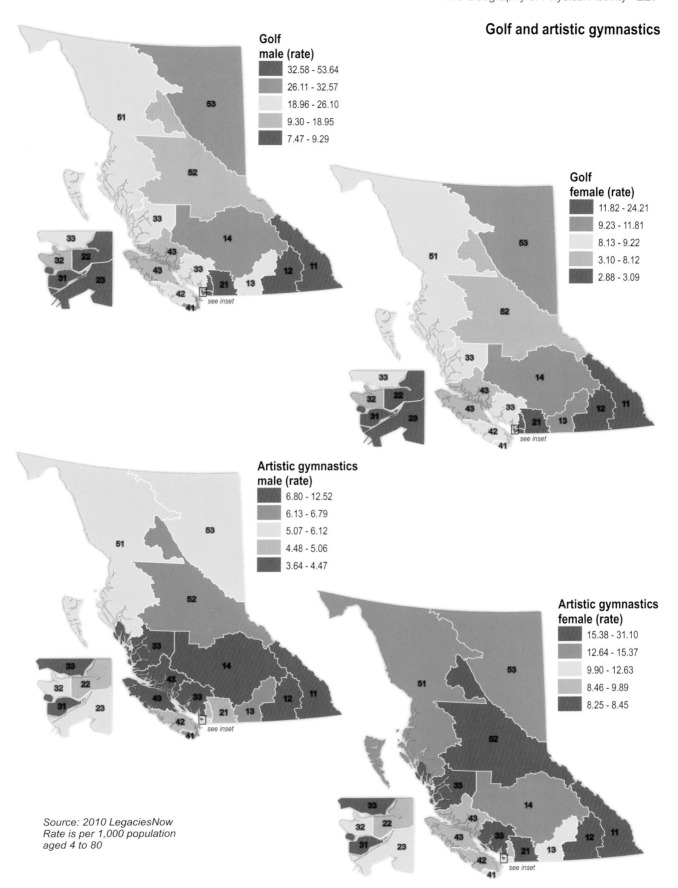

Golf male (rate)
- 32.58 - 53.64
- 26.11 - 32.57
- 18.96 - 26.10
- 9.30 - 18.95
- 7.47 - 9.29

Golf female (rate)
- 11.82 - 24.21
- 9.23 - 11.81
- 8.13 - 9.22
- 3.10 - 8.12
- 2.88 - 3.09

Artistic gymnastics male (rate)
- 6.80 - 12.52
- 6.13 - 6.79
- 5.07 - 6.12
- 4.48 - 5.06
- 3.64 - 4.47

Artistic gymnastics female (rate)
- 15.38 - 31.10
- 12.64 - 15.37
- 9.90 - 12.63
- 8.46 - 9.89
- 8.25 - 8.45

Source: 2010 LegaciesNow
Rate is per 1,000 population aged 4 to 80

Hockey team membership

Hockey, while not the most popular participation sport, is certainly the sport that is viewed is the key national sport in Canada. With respect to hockey club membership in BC, hockey ranks fourth after soccer, athletics, and golf.

In 2008/9, nearly 53,000 individuals in the province were members of a hockey club. Overall, this represented a rate of 12.34 per 1,000 population between the ages of 4 and 80 years old. Residents in Northeast had the highest membership rate with 27.94 per 1,000 population, while at the other extreme, Vancouver had a rate of only 3.72 per 1,000 population, a mere 13% of the rate in Northeast. Northwest, Kootenay Boundary, East Kootenay, North Vancouver Island, Thompson Cariboo Shuswap, and Northern Interior all had rates in excess of 20 per 1,000 population, while Fraser North and Richmond both had rates below 10 per 1,000 population.

Geographically, the northern and central interior, along with the southeastern parts of the province had the highest membership rates, while the lowest rates were clustered in the urban lower mainland part of BC.

Male hockey club membership

In 2008/9, nearly over 46,000 males were hockey club members. Club membership in the province was 21.57 per 1,000 male population ages 4 to 80 years old. Most members (74.4%) were between the ages of 6 to 17 years old. Again the Northeast had the highest membership rate with 45.03 per 1,000 population, a rate nearly seven times that of Vancouver (6.61 per 1,000 population). Northwest also had a high rate of over 40 per 1,000 population, while Richmond had a rate of less than 15 per 1,000 population. Geographically the pattern of membership were very similar to that of the total population.

Female hockey club membership

Approximately 6,600 females were members of hockey clubs in the province in 2008/9. This represented a rate of 3.09 per 1,000 female population between the ages of 4 to 80 years. As with the male membership, the majority (58.2%) were between the ages of 6 and 17 years. Northeast, with a rate of 9.34 per 1,000 female population, had the highest membership rate among HSDAs, followed by Northwest (8.89 per 1,000 population) and North Vancouver Island (7.03 per 1,000 population). With a rate of less than 1 per 1,000 female population, Vancouver had the lowest membership rate in the province. Low rates below 2 per 1,000 population were also recorded for Fraser North, Fraser South, and Fraser East.

Health Service Delivery Area	Total (rate)	Male (rate)	Female (rate)
53 Northeast	27.94	45.03	9.34
51 Northwest	25.51	41.16	8.89
12 Kootenay Boundary	21.60	36.67	6.25
11 East Kootenay	20.80	34.85	6.49
43 North Vancouver Island	20.65	34.13	7.03
14 Thompson Cariboo Shuswap	20.37	34.35	6.21
52 Northern Interior	20.19	33.89	5.84
33 North Shore/Coast Garibaldi	15.72	28.68	2.97
13 Okanagan	15.20	27.70	2.98
42 Central Vancouver Island	15.07	24.14	6.08
21 Fraser East	11.04	20.13	1.73
23 Fraser South	10.81	19.84	1.70
41 South Vancouver Island	10.01	16.74	3.52
22 Fraser North	9.87	18.03	1.68
31 Richmond	8.52	14.79	2.44
32 Vancouver	3.72	6.61	0.81
British Columbia	**12.34**	**21.57**	**3.09**

Geographical patterns for female membership rates were similar to those for males and for the population as a whole.

Hockey team membership

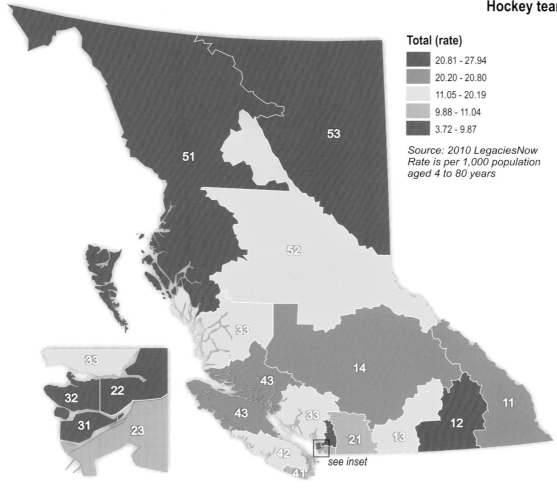

Total (rate)

- 20.81 - 27.94
- 20.20 - 20.80
- 11.05 - 20.19
- 9.88 - 11.04
- 3.72 - 9.87

Source: 2010 LegaciesNow
Rate is per 1,000 population
aged 4 to 80 years

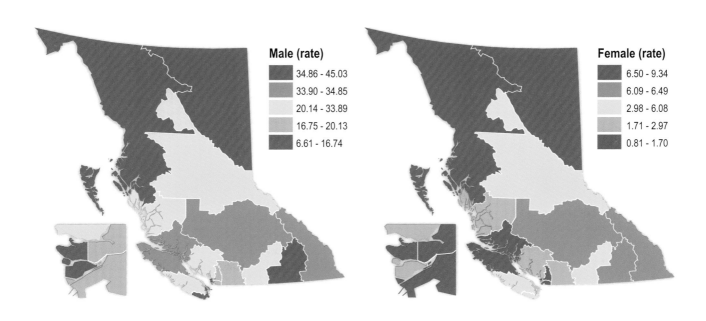

Male (rate)

- 34.86 - 45.03
- 33.90 - 34.85
- 20.14 - 33.89
- 16.75 - 20.13
- 6.61 - 16.74

Female (rate)

- 6.50 - 9.34
- 6.09 - 6.49
- 2.98 - 6.08
- 1.71 - 2.97
- 0.81 - 1.70

Other leading sports membership

Baseball club membership

Baseball is an outdoor sport and more than 29,000 individuals in BC were members of baseball clubs in 2008/9, a rate of 6.79 per 1,000 population between the ages of 4 and 80 years. Club membership was dominated by males, with over 90% of the total membership. Membership rates varied from a high of 14.11 per

Health Service Delivery Area	Baseball (rate)
33 North Shore/Coast Garibaldi	14.11
12 Kootenay Boundary	9.99
41 South Vancouver Island	9.76
42 Central Vancouver Island	8.48
43 North Vancouver Island	8.48
23 Fraser South	7.93
32 Vancouver	6.11
22 Fraser North	6.09
52 Northern Interior	5.67
13 Okanagan	5.63
21 Fraser East	4.03
31 Richmond	3.88
14 Thompson Cariboo Shuswap	3.83
11 East Kootenay	2.04
51 Northwest	0.01
53 Northeast	0.00
British Columbia	**6.79**

1,000 population in North Shore/Coast Garibaldi, to practically zero for Northwest and Northeast. Overall, rates were low over much of the north and in the extreme southeast of the province, while higher rates were found along much of the south and central coastal area of the province, including Vancouver Island, and also in Kootenay Boundary.

Tennis club membership

Tennis is both an outdoor and indoor game, and club membership in BC totalled more than 22,000 in 2008/9, for a rate of 5.17 per 1,000 population between the ages of 4 and 80 years. Membership was fairly evenly split between males (54%) and females (46%). Both Vancouver and North Shore/Coast Garibaldi

Health Service Delivery Area	Tennis (rate)
32 Vancouver	14.60
33 North Shore/Coast Garibaldi	14.08
41 South Vancouver Island	5.59
31 Richmond	5.40
22 Fraser North	3.62
43 North Vancouver Island	3.38
23 Fraser South	2.98
21 Fraser East	2.38
14 Thompson Cariboo Shuswap	1.88
42 Central Vancouver Island	1.46
13 Okanagan	1.26
12 Kootenay Boundary	0.62
11 East Kootenay	0.25
52 Northern Interior	0.12
51 Northwest	0.03
53 Northeast	0.00
British Columbia	**5.17**

had rates in excess of 14 per 1,000, while Kootenay Boundary, East Kootenay, and the three northern HSDAs all had rates below 1 per 1,000 population. Geographically, the north had the lowest rates, followed by the Kootenay and Okanagan regions, while parts of the urban lower mainland and South Vancouver Island had the higher club membership rates.

Curling club membership

Curling takes place indoors and approximately 26,000 individuals were club members in BC in 2008/9, a rate of 6.01 per 1,000 population between the ages of 4 and 80 years. Just over 60% of the membership was male. Kootenay Boundary led the province, with a rate of 19.29 per 1,000

Health Service Delivery Area	Curling (rate)
12 Kootenay Boundary	19.29
14 Thompson Cariboo Shuswap	15.53
11 East Kootenay	11.70
51 Northwest	10.06
13 Okanagan	9.92
42 Central Vancouver Island	9.49
43 North Vancouver Island	9.03
52 Northern Interior	7.02
41 South Vancouver Island	6.48
33 North Shore/Coast Garibaldi	6.27
21 Fraser East	4.88
23 Fraser South	4.22
31 Richmond	3.20
22 Fraser North	2.82
32 Vancouver	2.11
53 Northeast	0.72
British Columbia	**6.01**

population, while Northeast had a rate of only 0.72 per 1,000 population. There were some very distinctive overall regional trends in club membership. The urban lower mainland region had the lowest rates, along with Northeast, which was an outlier, while much of the southeast and south central interior parts of the province had the highest membership rates.

Equestrian club membership

Equestrian activities are primarily outdoor in nature, although grooming and care activities can also take place indoors. Of the approximate 21,000 members of equestrian clubs in BC in 2008/9, a rate of 4.95 per 1,000 population between the ages of 4 and 80 years, more than 75% were

Health Service Delivery Area	Equestrian (rate)
53 Northeast	12.75
52 Northern Interior	11.71
12 Kootenay Boundary	9.03
14 Thompson Cariboo Shuswap	8.46
51 Northwest	7.91
42 Central Vancouver Island	7.83
43 North Vancouver Island	7.69
13 Okanagan	7.08
21 Fraser East	6.50
41 South Vancouver Island	6.00
11 East Kootenay	5.91
23 Fraser South	4.40
33 North Shore/Coast Garibaldi	4.29
22 Fraser North	2.05
32 Vancouver	1.10
31 Richmond	0.98
British Columbia	**4.95**

females. The Northeast and Northern Interior both had rates of around 12 per 1,000 population, while Richmond, Vancouver, and Fraser North had rates of 2 or less per 1,000 population. Rates were higher in the north, central interior and Kootenay Boundary, while the lowest rates occurred in the urban lower mainland.

Other leading sports membership

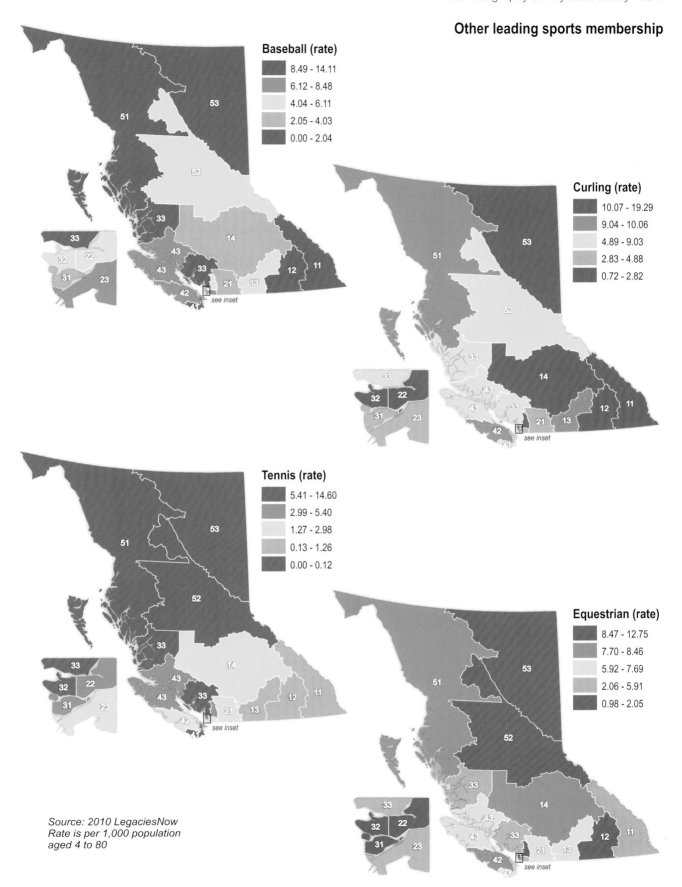

Baseball (rate)
- 8.49 - 14.11
- 6.12 - 8.48
- 4.04 - 6.11
- 2.05 - 4.03
- 0.00 - 2.04

Curling (rate)
- 10.07 - 19.29
- 9.04 - 10.06
- 4.89 - 9.03
- 2.83 - 4.88
- 0.72 - 2.82

Tennis (rate)
- 5.41 - 14.60
- 2.99 - 5.40
- 1.27 - 2.98
- 0.13 - 1.26
- 0.00 - 0.12

Equestrian (rate)
- 8.47 - 12.75
- 7.70 - 8.46
- 5.92 - 7.69
- 2.06 - 5.91
- 0.98 - 2.05

Source: 2010 LegaciesNow
Rate is per 1,000 population
aged 4 to 80

Other leading sports membership

Softball club membership

Softball, like baseball, is played outdoors, and in 2008/9, there were nearly 21,000 club members in BC and approximately 70% were females. The membership rate for the province as a whole was 4.83 per 1,000 population between the ages of 4 and 80 years. Northeast dominated the sport in terms of club

Health Service Delivery Area	Softball (rate)
53 Northeast	23.41
42 Central Vancouver Island	8.04
23 Fraser South	6.60
21 Fraser East	5.39
41 South Vancouver Island	5.31
51 Northwest	4.99
22 Fraser North	4.93
11 East Kootenay	4.79
12 Kootenay Boundary	4.65
33 North Shore/Coast Garibaldi	4.65
52 Northern Interior	4.63
14 Thompson Cariboo Shuswap	3.84
31 Richmond	3.75
43 North Vancouver Island	2.62
13 Okanagan	2.22
32 Vancouver	1.59
British Columbia	**4.83**

membership with a rate of 23.41 per 1,000 population, nearly five times the provincial rate, while at the other extreme, Vancouver had a rate of just 1.59 per 1,000 population. Geographically, there were no clear patterns, with higher rates in Northeast and parts of the Fraser Valley, as well as Central Vancouver Island and Northwest, while the lowest rates were found in Vancouver, Okanagan, and North Vancouver Island.

Lacrosse club membership

Lacrosse can be played both indoors and outdoors, and in 2008/9, BC had 16,000 club members, of which almost 90% were males. The provincial rate for club membership was 3.73 per 1,000 population between the ages of 4 and 80 years. Fraser North, with a rate of 8.17 per 1,000 population, or more than

Health Service Delivery Area	Lacrosse (rate)
22 Fraser North	8.17
42 Central Vancouver Island	5.89
41 South Vancouver Island	5.85
43 North Vancouver Island	3.55
21 Fraser East	3.52
23 Fraser South	3.42
52 Northern Interior	3.21
14 Thompson Cariboo Shuswap	3.20
53 Northeast	2.98
13 Okanagan	2.77
33 North Shore/Coast Garibaldi	2.60
51 Northwest	2.15
31 Richmond	1.89
11 East Kootenay	1.69
12 Kootenay Boundary	1.50
32 Vancouver	0.63
British Columbia	**3.73**

twice the provincial average, had the highest membership rate, while its neighbour, Vancouver, had a rate of less than 1 per 1,000 population. There were distinct regional trends, with the southeastern part of BC joining Vancouver with the lowest rates, while higher rates were found on Vancouver Island and Fraser North.

Figure skating club membership

Skating is primarily an indoor sport, although it can be outdoors during the winter season. Of nearly 18,000 members in BC in 2008/9, 76.4% were females. Provincially, the rate was 4.16 per 1,000 population between the ages of 4 and 80 years. Northeast had the highest membership rate, with 10.11 per 1,000 population, four

Health Service Delivery Area	Figure skating (rate)
53 Northeast	10.11
11 East Kootenay	8.61
12 Kootenay Boundary	8.43
51 Northwest	7.79
52 Northern Interior	7.71
13 Okanagan	7.29
33 North Shore/Coast Garibaldi	6.24
14 Thompson Cariboo Shuswap	4.15
43 North Vancouver Island	4.09
42 Central Vancouver Island	3.36
22 Fraser North	3.29
21 Fraser East	3.09
32 Vancouver	3.09
31 Richmond	2.90
23 Fraser South	2.66
41 South Vancouver Island	2.65
British Columbia	**4.16**

times the rate for South Vancouver Island (2.65 per 1,000 population). The north, south eastern and south central parts of the province all had rates above average, while the urban lower mainland (with the exception of North Shore/Coast Garibaldi) and South Vancouver Island had rates below the provincial average.

Cross-country skiing club membership

This winter outdoor sport had nearly 14,000 members in BC in 2008/9, for a provincial rate of 3.20 per 1,000 population between the ages of 4 and 80 years, with females (54%) slightly outnumbering males. Kootenay Boundary had the highest membership rate with 23.12 per 1,000 population, followed by Northern Interior, Northwest, and East

Health Service Delivery Area	Cross-country skiing (rate)
12 Kootenay Boundary	23.12
52 Northern Interior	15.64
51 Northwest	14.40
11 East Kootenay	13.41
14 Thompson Cariboo Shuswap	9.51
13 Okanagan	9.33
53 Northeast	6.16
43 North Vancouver Island	3.36
33 North Shore/Coast Garibaldi	3.15
32 Vancouver	0.81
22 Fraser North	0.35
42 Central Vancouver Island	0.19
23 Fraser South	0.14
41 South Vancouver Island	0.11
31 Richmond	0.09
21 Fraser East	0.05
British Columbia	**3.20**

Kootenay (all between 16 and 13 per 1,000 population). Seven HSDAs had rates of less than 1 per 1,000 population. The north and interior parts of BC all had above average rates, while the lower mainland and most of Vancouver Island had rates below average.

Other leading sports membership

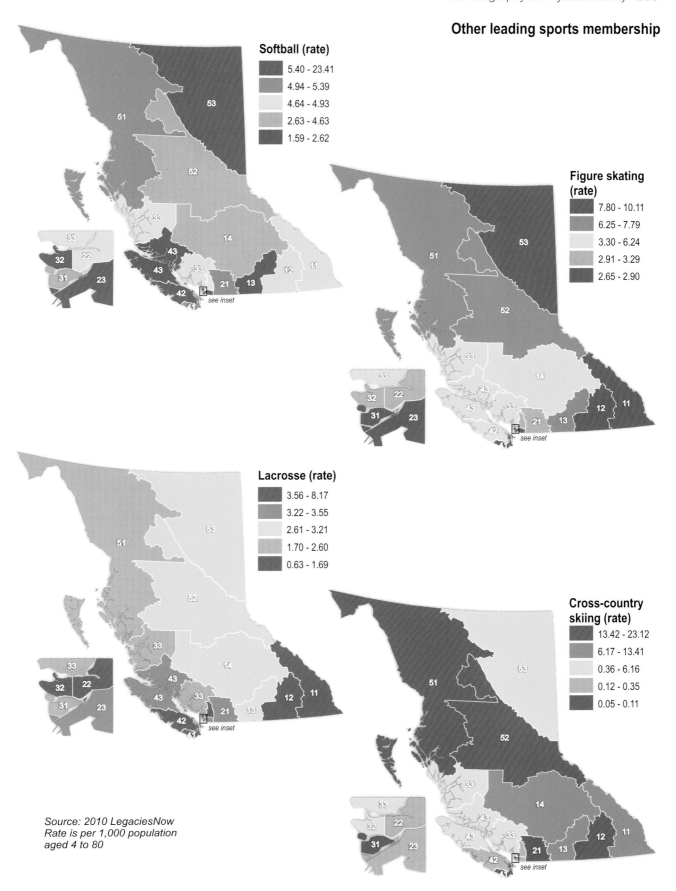

Softball (rate)
- 5.40 - 23.41
- 4.94 - 5.39
- 4.64 - 4.93
- 2.63 - 4.63
- 1.59 - 2.62

Figure skating (rate)
- 7.80 - 10.11
- 6.25 - 7.79
- 3.30 - 6.24
- 2.91 - 3.29
- 2.65 - 2.90

Lacrosse (rate)
- 3.56 - 8.17
- 3.22 - 3.55
- 2.61 - 3.21
- 1.70 - 2.60
- 0.63 - 1.69

Cross-country skiing (rate)
- 13.42 - 23.12
- 6.17 - 13.41
- 0.36 - 6.16
- 0.12 - 0.35
- 0.05 - 0.11

Source: 2010 LegaciesNow
Rate is per 1,000 population
aged 4 to 80

Active or moderately active leisure time physical activity index score

Health Service Delivery Area	All respondents 12+ (%)	Males 12+ (%)	Females 12+ (%)	Ages 12-19 (%)	Ages 20-64 (%)	Ages 65+ (%)
12 Kootenay Boundary	71.28	76.52	65.92	82.19	70.99	65.65
33 North Shore/Coast Garibaldi	65.34	66.04	64.69	77.00	64.56	60.84
41 South Vancouver Island	64.86	63.52	66.07	68.51	65.25	61.22
43 North Vancouver Island	62.20	59.28	64.91	78.49	62.26	50.86
52 Northern Interior	61.42	60.25	62.60	67.39	62.24	48.25
13 Okanagan	61.39	64.13	58.80	79.94†	59.18	58.77
11 East Kootenay	60.64	65.93	55.49	79.69†	59.87	50.86
42 Central Vancouver Island	59.09	59.41	58.79	73.88	58.64	52.02
14 Thompson Cariboo Shuswap	58.53	57.25	59.74	78.15†	57.89	48.01
51 Northwest	57.27	60.31	54.13	63.15	59.22	37.13‡
21 Fraser East	56.46	56.08	56.84	79.60†	54.80	45.65
32 Vancouver	55.66	56.62	54.72	74.06†	54.39	51.96
23 Fraser South	55.01	58.12	52.01	77.83†	53.79	41.31‡
53 Northeast	54.55	56.89	52.08	79.01†	51.92	39.72E
22 Fraser North	53.10	58.81*	47.71	64.49	53.53	40.48‡
31 Richmond	50.27	54.01	46.84	64.12†	47.47	54.41
British Columbia (2007/8)	**57.98**	**59.75***	**56.29**	**73.79†**	**57.08**	**50.88‡**
British Columbia (2005)	**59.14**	**60.32**	**58.00**	**73.81†**	**57.81**	**53.93‡**

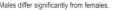

Crosshatching beside the 2007/8 provincial rate indicates it is significantly different than the 2005 rate, while crosshatched HSDAs are significantly different than the 2007/8 provincial rate.
E interpret data with caution (16.67 ≤ coefficient of variation ≤ 33.3).

* Males differ significantly from females.
† 12-19 age cohort differs significantly from the 20-64 age cohort.
‡ 65+ age cohort differs significantly from the 20-64 age cohort.
F data suppressed (n < 10, or coefficient of variation > 33.3).

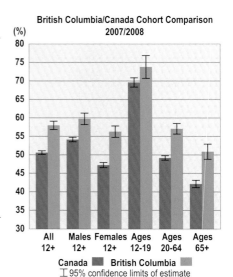

Physical activity is an important wellness asset that helps keep the body in shape and provides protection against numerous chronic conditions. The CCHS physical activity index is based on the frequency, duration, and intensity of participation in certain leisure time activities (Statistics Canada, nd). The information presented here is based on respondents in the Active and Moderately Active categories combined.

Nearly six out of every ten BC respondents (57.98%) were considered active or moderately active in their leisure time. Kootenay Boundary, North Shore/Coast Garibaldi, and South Vancouver Island respondents (all above 64%) were significantly more active, while those in Fraser North and Richmond (both below 54%) were significantly less active than the provincial average.

Males (59.75%) were significantly more likely than females (56.29%) to be physically active in their leisure time, although Fraser North was the only individual HSDA where males (58.81%) had a significantly higher average than females (47.41%).

Females in Kootenay Boundary, North Shore/Coast Garibaldi, South Vancouver Island, and North Vancouver Island (all above 64%) were significantly more likely than the female average to have a high level of physical activity, while those in Fraser North and Richmond were significantly less likely (both below 48%). For males, respondents in Kootenay Boundary and North Shore/Coast Garibaldi had significantly higher values than the BC male average (both above 66%).

BC youth respondents (73.79%) had a significantly higher average than their mid-age counterparts for high levels of physical activity in their leisure time. Youth in East Kootenay, Okanagan, Thompson Cariboo Shuswap, Fraser East, Fraser South, Richmond, Vancouver, and Northeast were all significantly more likely than their mid-age counterparts to report high levels of physical activity. There was no individual HSDA where youth values were significantly different from the provincial average.

Older respondents (50.88%) had a significantly lower average than their mid-age counterparts, as did three HSDAs: Fraser North, Fraser South, and Northwest. In Kootenay Boundary and South Vancouver Island (both above 61%), seniors were significantly higher than the provincial average, while Fraser North, Fraser South, and Northwest (all below 41%) were significantly lower.

Provincially, there was a 20 to 25 percentage point spread among HSDAs. Overall, Kootenay Boundary had a consistently high value. Lower averages were found in the southwest mainland of the province. For youth, a cluster of high physical activity was seen in the south east and south interior of the province.

There were no significant differences for any BC cohorts between 2005 and 2007/8. When compared to Canadian respondents, British Columbians were significantly more likely to engage in leisure time physical activity for all cohorts, except youth.

Active or moderately active leisure time physical activity index score

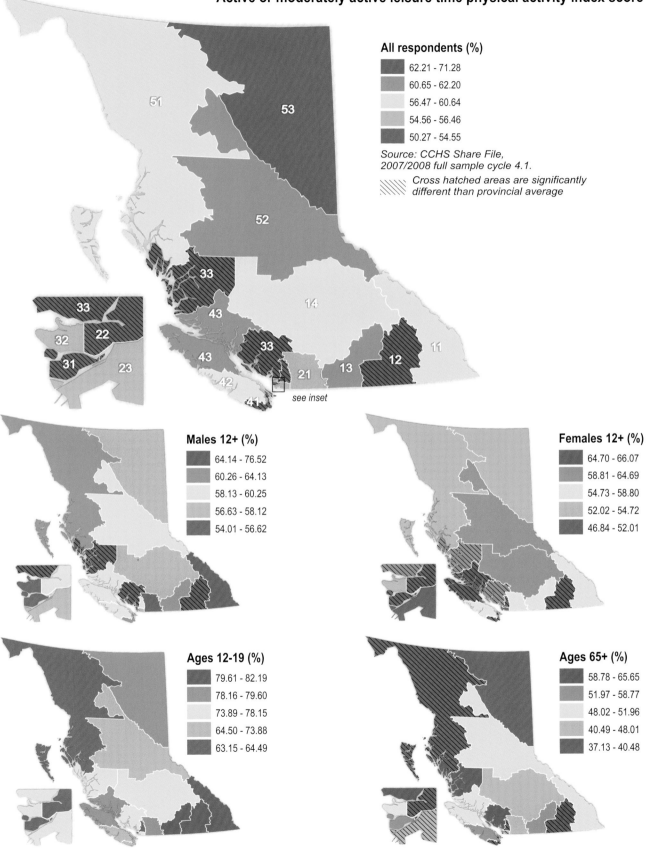

All respondents (%)

- 62.21 - 71.28
- 60.65 - 62.20
- 56.47 - 60.64
- 54.56 - 56.46
- 50.27 - 54.55

Source: CCHS Share File, 2007/2008 full sample cycle 4.1.

Cross hatched areas are significantly different than provincial average

Males 12+ (%)

- 64.14 - 76.52
- 60.26 - 64.13
- 58.13 - 60.25
- 56.63 - 58.12
- 54.01 - 56.62

Females 12+ (%)

- 64.70 - 66.07
- 58.81 - 64.69
- 54.73 - 58.80
- 52.02 - 54.72
- 46.84 - 52.01

Ages 12-19 (%)

- 79.61 - 82.19
- 78.16 - 79.60
- 73.89 - 78.15
- 64.50 - 73.88
- 63.15 - 64.49

Ages 65+ (%)

- 58.78 - 65.65
- 51.97 - 58.77
- 48.02 - 51.96
- 40.49 - 48.01
- 37.13 - 40.48

LocalMotion

The built environment can have a significant impact on population health and well-being (PHSA, 2008). Environments that have mixed land use and promote walking, cycling, and exercise are important in helping to encourage physical activity and thus reduce levels of overweight and obesity in the population. Increased physical activity, age- and ability-friendly infrastructure, and environmental factors such as pollution can have a considerable impact on population wellness.

The LocalMotion Program was a $40 million fund administered by the Ministry of Community and Rural Development and the Ministry of Transportation and Infrastructure to support the ActNow BC initiative, particularly related to improving community assets to increase levels of physical activity. The program helped local governments develop capital projects aimed at building bike paths, walkways, and greenways and building senior-friendly and disability-friendly communities by improving access to public amenities. Funds were also available for community playgrounds and activities in children's parks. All projects promoted physical activity, a reduction in car dependency, and in associated greenhouse gas emissions (Ministry of Community and Rural Development, 2010d).

Each grant covered 50 percent of the eligible project costs, with the other 50 percent coming from local governments. Grants were made available to local governments between 2007 and 2009, up to a maximum of $1 million per year, although several projects received funding over more than a year. In all, 34 projects were funded in 2007, 37 projects in 2008, and 51 projects in 2009, for a total of 122 projects in 86 communities throughout BC. The table and map opposite show the locations of the projects. This is a new indicator for the Atlas. While the majority of projects were relatively small in nature, approximately 10 percent received $1 million or more in government grants. Projects must be completed by March 31, 2012 (Ministry of Community and Rural Development, 2010d).

Community		Community	
1	Abbotsford	45	North Okanagan RD
2	Barriere	46	North Saanich
3	Burnaby	47	North Vancouver (City)
4	Campbell River	48	North Vancouver (District)
5	Capital RD	49	Northern Rockies RM
6	Castlegar	50	Oak Bay
7	Central Kootenay RD	51	Okanagan Similkameen RD
8	Central Saanich	52	Oliver
9	Chetwynd	53	Parksville
10	Chilliwack	54	Peachland
11	Columbia Shuswap RD	55	Pemberton
12	Colwood	56	Penticton
13	Comox	57	Pitt Meadows
14	Coquitlam	58	Port Alice
15	Cowichan Valley RD	59	Port Moody
16	Creston	60	Prince George
17	Dawson Creek	61	Prince Rupert
18	Delta	62	Princeton
19	Duncan	63	Qualicum Beach
20	Esquimalt	64	Quesnel
21	Fort St. John	65	Radium Hot Springs
22	Golden	66	Revelstoke
23	Grand Forks	67	Richmond
24	Harrison Hot Springs	68	Rossland
25	Hazelton	69	Saanich
26	Houston	70	Salmon Arm
27	Hudson's Hope	71	Sicamous
28	Invermere	72	Smithers
29	Kamloops	73	Sparwood
30	Kaslo	74	Squamish Lillooet RD
31	Kelowna	75	Surrey
32	Kimberley	76	Terrace
33	Kootenay Boundary RD	77	Vancouver
34	Langford (City)	78	Vanderhoof
35	Langley (District)	79	Vernon
36	Lillooet	80	Victoria
37	Lumby	81	View Royal
38	Maple Ridge	82	Warfield
39	Merritt	83	West Kelowna
40	Mission	84	West Vancouver
41	Nanaimo	85	White Rock
42	Nanaimo RD	86	Williams Lake
43	Nelson		
44	New Westminster		

LocalMotion

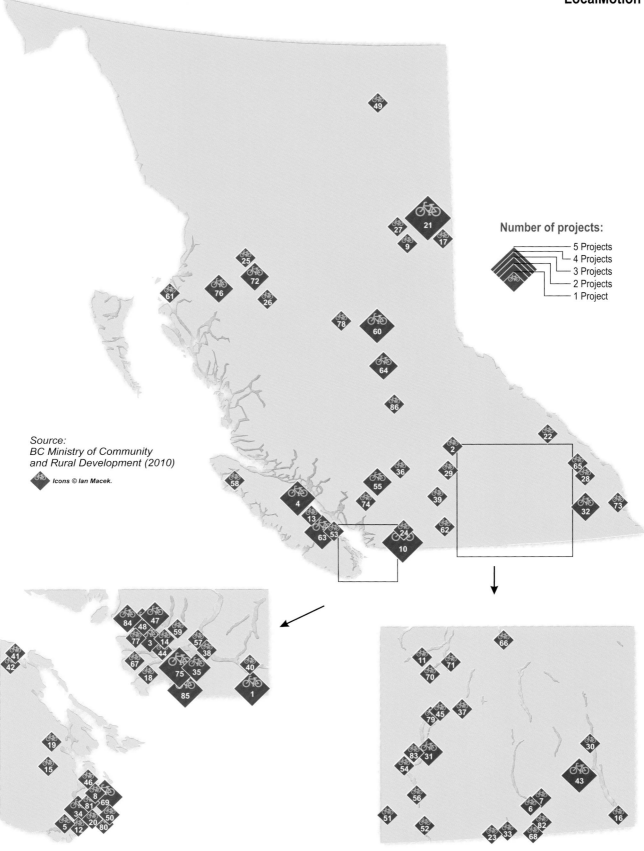

Number of projects:
5 Projects
4 Projects
3 Projects
2 Projects
1 Project

Source:
BC Ministry of Community
and Rural Development (2010)

Icons © Ian Macek.

Seniors community parks

	Community	Location
1	Abbotsford	Mill Lake Park
2	Burnaby	9523 Cameron Street (Cameron Recreation Complex)
3	Courtenay	358 Anderton Avenue (across from the Florence Filberg Centre)
4	Cranbrook	17 Avenue and Baker Street (next to the Cranbrook RecPlex)
5	Dawson Creek	Corner of 13th Street and 110 Avenue
6	Kamloops	Located along McArthur Island Parkway adjacent to Norbrock Stadium
7	Kelowna	1800 Parkinson Way (Parkinson Recreation Centre)
8	Nanaimo	6000 Oliver Road (adjacent to the new Oliver Woods Recreation Centre)
9	Nelson	2001 Lakeside Drive
10	North Cowichan	5847 Chesterfield Avenue (Cowichan Sportsplex)
11	North Vancouver	Located at the northern end of Parkgate Avenue just west of Mt. Seymour Road
12	Oak Bay	2291 Cedar Hill X Road (Henderson Recreation Centre)
13	Prince George	2121 Massey Place (Masich Place Stadium)
14	Richmond	Hugh Boyd Park
15	Sidney	10091 Resthaven Drive (Located on the grounds of the Sidney/North Saanich library)
16	Surrey	Located north of 83rd Avenue and west of 160th Street (adjacent to the Fleetwood Community Centre)
17	Terrace	4620 Park Avenue
18	Tsawwassen	5027 11A Avenue (Lions Wellness Park)
19	Vancouver	6210 Tisdall Street (Tisdall at 49th - Tisdall Park)

Announced in the 2008 throne speech, seniors community parks were designed as an ActNow BC initiative to help older adults stay and/or become more mobile, physically active, and remain healthy in their communities. The concept was inspired by the Lions Wellness Park, which became Canada's first seniors park when it opened in Tsawwassen.

The seniors parks provide specialized outdoor recreational equipment and activities designed to improve mobility, coordination, and balance specifically for seniors. In short, they provide an outdoor asset where seniors can do exercises like stretching, helping maintain strength and flexibility, which becomes increasingly important for seniors as they age. This is an important strategy to help to reduce injuries from falls. In addition, they provide a community resource for social interaction, not only with other seniors but with younger families, thus promoting intergenerational contacts and helping to keep seniors active in their communities. When individuals see assets provided by these parks they provide an opportunity to get moving and a challenge to increase fitness. These factors are all important for individual wellness and healthy living (http://www.actnowbc.ca/actnow_bc__seniors_community _parks).

A total of 19 seniors community parks have been developed in the first round throughout the province to support the wellness of seniors. This is a new indicator for the Atlas.

Funds for the purchase and installation of the equipment were provided by the province, while local governments provided land, site preparation, ongoing maintenance, and program delivery. Communities receiving provincial funding were selected based on regional representation and seniors population. As can be seen from the map opposite, most regions have a least one site, with concentrations in the lower mainland and southern part of Vancouver Island.

Seniors community parks

Location of seniors community parks
Source:
ActNow BC (2010)
Icons © Ian Macek.
1
2
3
4
5
6
7
8
9
10
11
12
13
14
15
16
17
18
19

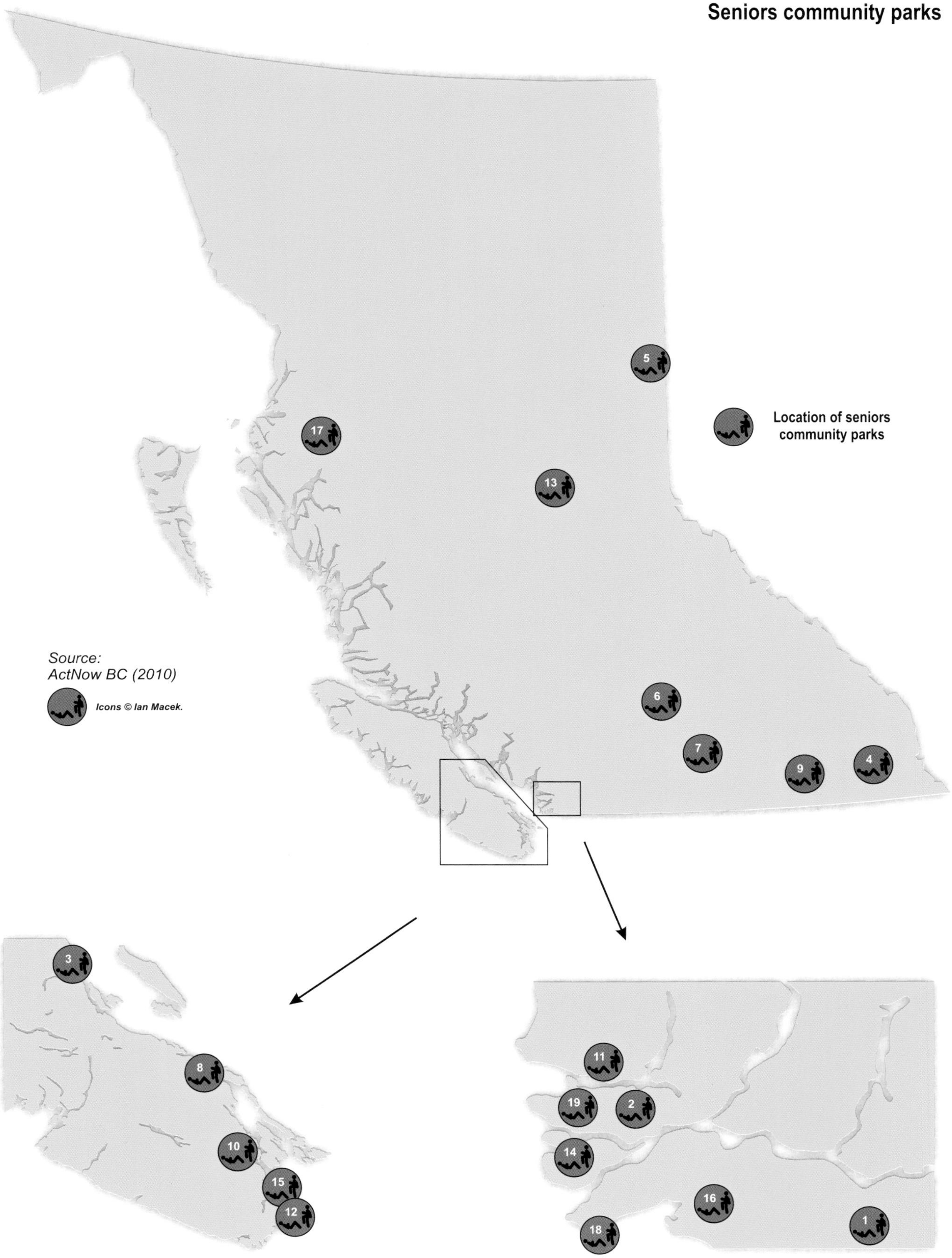

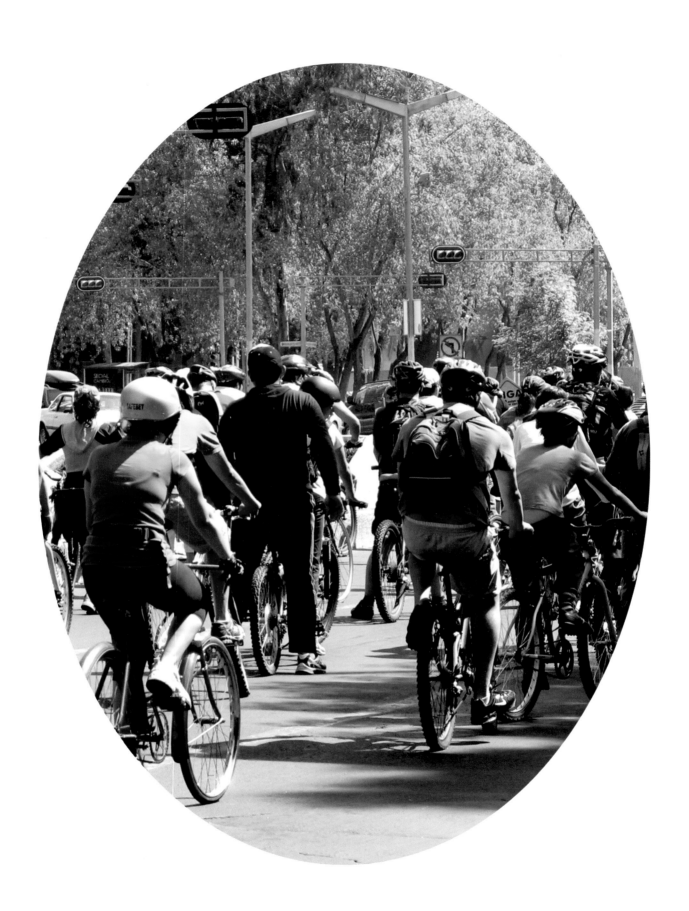

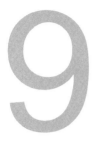

The Geography of Healthy Weight

One of the key pillars of ActNow BC involved reduction in the percentage of the population who were overweight. Our wellness approach is to look at those individuals who rate their weight as healthy. Healthy weight is related to a variety of factors, including individual factors such as healthy nutrition, avoiding unnecessarily high calorific foods and drinks (see Chapter 7), genetic and metabolic factors, and undertaking a healthy physical exercise regime and healthy leisure time activities (see Chapter 8), as well as environmental factors such as building and community design, and media advertising, especially for children (Vanasse et al., 2006; Wardle et al., 2008; Chronic Disease Prevention Alliance of Canada, 2009; Shields et al., 2008; Shields & Tremblay, 2008; Langlois et al., 2009; Ostry, 2010b; Ministry of Health Services, 2011; Public Health Agency of Canada & Canadian Institute for Health Information, 2011).

Healthy weight is a very important wellness asset for a variety of reasons. Research has shown that there are a variety of health and wellness factors related to being either underweight or overweight. For example, being overweight or obese has several key health risks, such as type 2 diabetes, hypertension cardiovascular disease, some types of cancer, osteoarthritis, gallbladder disease, functional limitations, and impaired fertility, among others (Kendall, 2006). Further, recent survey work has indicated that there has been a substantial increase in stigma related to being obese worldwide (Brewis et al., 2011), and self-esteem is lower among obese children in Canada (Wang et al., 2009).

There are several indicators available to measure healthy weight, and the measure that is most in use internationally is the Body Mass Index (BMI) although there are shortcomings in the measure. In self-reporting, height is often overestimated and weight is often underestimated. The measure also does not account for muscular or lean individuals (Elgar & Stewart, 2008; Shields et al., 2008; Kendall, 2006). BMI uses both weight and height measurements to compute a healthy body weight. The measure is based on kilograms per metre squared (weight and height, respectively). Any person aged 18 or over with a BMI lower than 25 but higher than 18.5 is considered to have a healthy body mass index (Kendall, 2006). Values below 18.5 are considered underweight, while those between 25 and 29.9 are considered overweight. Individuals with a BMI of 30 or more are considered obese. For those aged 17 or younger, a different measure is used (Cole et al., 2000) because of rapid changes in adolescence.

Healthy BMI has been shown to vary by province/territory, and BC had the highest proportion of its population with a healthy BMI for those aged 18 years and over (McKee et al., 2009). Pouliou and Elliott (2009) also found regional variations throughout Canada, with higher values of being overweight and obese found in the northern and Atlantic regions, and lower levels in southern and western regions of the country, while Lebel et al., (2009) have documented geographical variations in Quebec. Further, for both BC residents and Canada as a whole, the proportion with a healthy BMI was reduced with age until age 64, and then increased thereafter (Virtue et al., 2010).

A total of 16 maps are presented in this chapter. Two basic measures were used to consider healthy weight. BMI measures were based on self-identified height and weight from CCHS 4.1 for those aged 18 years and older, and from McCreary AHS IV for younger respondents. A second question, again from both data sets, related to whether or not respondents felt their weight was about right. Feeling that one's weight is about right is a useful measure to assess satisfaction with weight. Some caution in interpreting results is required as no data were available for McCreary AHS IV for Northeast.

Healthy body mass index based on self-reported height and weight

Health Service Delivery Area	All respondents 18+ (%)	Males 18+ (%)	Females 18+ (%)	Ages 20-34 (%)	Ages 35-64 (%)	Ages 65+ (%)
32 Vancouver	63.02	55.43*	70.46	66.36	61.18	56.86
31 Richmond	61.40	54.31	68.13	62.33	61.75	61.25
23 Fraser South	55.26	48.83*	61.61	66.47†	51.25	46.93
33 North Shore/Coast Garibaldi	54.57	46.47*	62.36	64.33	53.97	48.04
41 South Vancouver Island	51.90	44.06*	58.99	58.90†	44.99	54.87
22 Fraser North	51.66	44.59*	58.63	55.25	48.10	51.83
13 Okanagan	51.63	47.07	56.14	61.51	49.90	44.99
12 Kootenay Boundary	47.71	43.24	52.51	69.57†	40.82	42.85
21 Fraser East	46.69	40.52	52.84	50.63	44.69	41.97
43 North Vancouver Island	46.66	40.19	53.01	44.68E	44.18	46.30
14 Thompson Cariboo Shuswap	44.71	42.11	47.42	50.61	40.71	46.21
11 East Kootenay	44.55	30.39*	58.78	47.88	42.15	43.42
42 Central Vancouver Island	44.19	38.46	49.46	51.77	39.50	45.91
53 Northeast	39.44	33.98	45.65	49.75	34.32	25.43E
52 Northern Interior	38.01	32.24	44.03	40.19	35.44	31.10
51 Northwest	35.70	26.76*	45.77	39.23	33.92	35.79
British Columbia (2007/8)	**52.29**	**45.60***	**58.85**	**58.95†**	**49.07**	**48.57**
British Columbia (2005)	**50.82**	**44.66***	**57.03**	**59.21†**	**47.15**	**47.36**

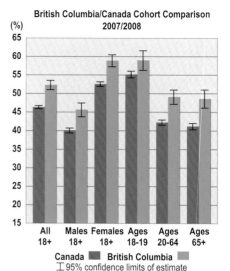

British Columbia/Canada Cohort Comparison 2007/2008

Canada ■   British Columbia ▨
⊥ 95% confidence limits of estimate

▨ Crosshatching beside the 2007/8 provincial rate indicates it is significantly different than the 2005 rate, while crosshatched HSDAs are significantly different than the 2007/8 provincial rate.
E interpret data with caution (16.67 ≤ coefficient of variation ≤ 33.3).

* Males differ significantly from females.
† 12-19 age cohort differs significantly from the 20-64 age cohort.
‡ 65+ age cohort differs significantly from the 20-64 age cohort.
F data suppressed (n < 10, or coefficient of variation > 33.3).

BMI calculations are complex for children and teens, and so BMI for younger respondents are included in the following pages.

Based on self-reported weight and height, over half (52,29%) of all respondents (aged 18 years and over) in British Columbia had a healthy body-mass index. Respondents in Richmond and Vancouver were significantly more likely than all respondents provincially to have a healthy BMI, whereas those in East Kootenay, Thompson Cariboo Shuswap, Central Vancouver Island, Northwest, Northern Interior, and Northeast (all below 45%) were significantly less likely.

There was a significant difference between males (45.6%) and females (58.85%) reporting a healthy BMI. Males in East Kootenay, Fraser North, Fraser South, Vancouver, North Shore/Coast Garibaldi, South Vancouver Island, and Northwest all had significantly lower rates of healthy BMI than their female counterparts in those HSDAs.

At the HSDA level, female respondents in Vancouver (70.46%) were significantly more likely than females provincially to have a healthy BMI, while females in Thompson Cariboo Shuswap, Central Vancouver Island, Northwest, Northern Interior, and Northeast (all below 50%) were significantly less likely. For males, Richmond and Vancouver (above 54%) had a significantly higher value of healthy BMI, while those in East Kootenay, Northwest, Northern Interior, and Northeast (below 33%) had a significantly lower value than the provincial average.

Provincially, younger respondents (age 20-34 years) were significantly more likely than the mid-age cohort (age 35-

64 years) to have reported a healthy BMI, and also at the HSDA level in Kootenay Boundary, Fraser South, and South Vancouver Island. Comparing younger respondents provincially to their peers within the individual HSDAs, no HSDA was significantly above average, but Northwest and Northern Interior (both below 41%) were significantly below average.

Older respondents (48.57%), both at the provincial level and for individual HSDAs, were not significantly different from the mid-age cohort with respect to a healthy BMI. There were no HSDAs in which the value for older respondents was significantly higher than the provincial average; however, older respondents in the three northern HSDAs (all below 36%) had significantly lower rates of healthy BMI than the provincial average for older respondents.

Geographically, the spread among HSDAs for most cohorts was close to 30 percentage points. Northern and some interior HSDAs had lower levels, while the lower mainland HSDAs reported higher levels of a healthy BMI.

There were no significant differences for any of the BC cohorts between the 2005 and 2007/8 samples. When compared to the respondents across the country, all age and gender cohorts in British Columbians were significantly more likely to report a healthy BMI.

Healthy body mass index based on self-reported height and weight

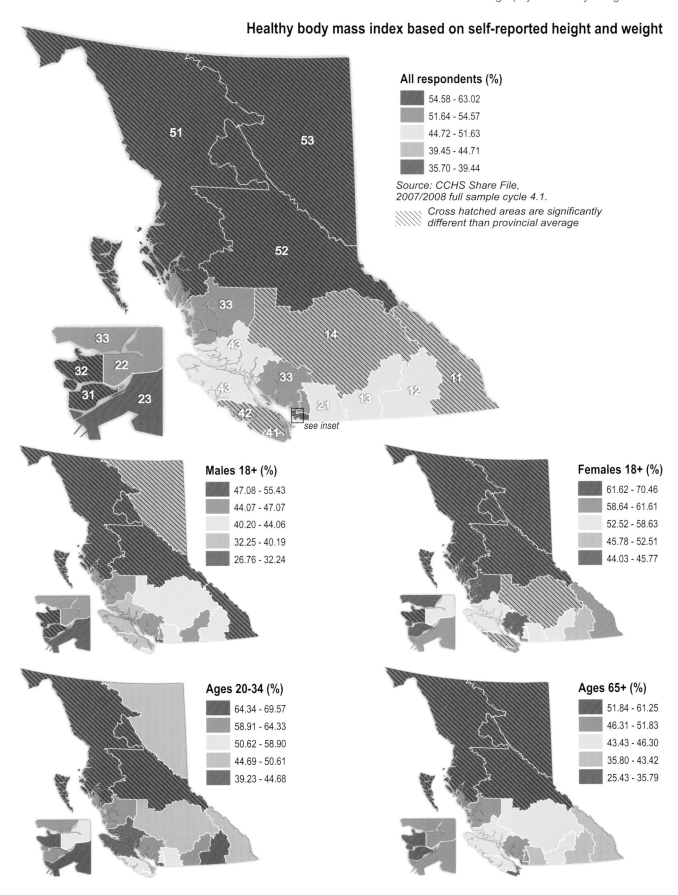

All respondents (%)

- 54.58 - 63.02
- 51.64 - 54.57
- 44.72 - 51.63
- 39.45 - 44.71
- 35.70 - 39.44

*Source: CCHS Share File,
2007/2008 full sample cycle 4.1.*

*Cross hatched areas are significantly
different than provincial average*

Males 18+ (%)

- 47.08 - 55.43
- 44.07 - 47.07
- 40.20 - 44.06
- 32.25 - 40.19
- 26.76 - 32.24

Females 18+ (%)

- 61.62 - 70.46
- 58.64 - 61.61
- 52.52 - 58.63
- 45.78 - 52.51
- 44.03 - 45.77

Ages 20-34 (%)

- 64.34 - 69.57
- 58.91 - 64.33
- 50.62 - 58.90
- 44.69 - 50.61
- 39.23 - 44.68

Ages 65+ (%)

- 51.84 - 61.25
- 46.31 - 51.83
- 43.43 - 46.30
- 35.80 - 43.42
- 25.43 - 35.79

Youth with healthy body mass index

As noted earlier, healthy weight is an important wellness indicator. This is particularly true for young people. Rising concern has been expressed about the increase in unhealthy weights among young people, particularly with respect to being overweight or obese. Young people with unhealthy weights also are likely to have unhealthy weights, and all the risk factors that accompany this condition, in adulthood.

The McCreary AHS IV asked students about their height and weight, from which the Body Mass Index (BMI) was calculated. It should be noted that the BMI calculation for young people is different from that for adults and a lot more complex (Cole et al., 2000).

Based on student self reports of their weight and height, nearly eight out of every ten respondents (78.42%) had a healthy BMI, a percentage almost identical to that reported for 2003. The difference among HSDAs ranged from 82.11% to 72.24%. Vancouver (82.11%) and North Shore/Coast Garibaldi (81.74%) were both significantly higher than the average for all students, while Northwest students (72.24%) were significantly lower than the provincial student average.

There were significant differences between genders. Provincially, female students (83.01%) had a significantly higher average percentage with healthy BMIs when compared to male students, provincially (73.57%). This difference between genders was consistent for all HSDAs, and for all but one HSDA (East Kootenay), the difference was significant.

Among the HSDAs for male students, the range in healthy weights varied from a high of 77.04% for South Vancouver Island (not significant) to a significant low of 66.26% for Northwest. The range for female student respondents among HSDAs varied from a significant high of 87.17% for Vancouver to a significant low of 78.40% for Northwest. North Shore/Coast Garibaldi (86.76%) was also significantly higher than the provincial average for female students.

It is worth noting that the lowest value HSDA for female students is higher than the highest value HSDA for males.

Geographically, the lower mainland urban HSDAs had higher percentages of students with healthy weights than the provincial average for all students and for male and female students (with the exception of Fraser South/Fraser East, which was lower than average), along

Health Service Delivery Area	All students (%)	Males (%)	Females (%)
32 Vancouver	82.11	75.58†	87.17
33 North Shore/Coast Garibaldi	81.74	76.72†	86.76
41 South Vancouver Island	79.81	77.04†	82.49
13 Okanagan	79.18	74.37†	83.53
31 Richmond	79.17	72.87†	85.62
22 Fraser North	78.59	74.46†	82.68
11 East Kootenay	78.37	76.76	79.87
21 Fraser South/Fraser East	77.83	72.99†	82.29
43 North Vancouver Island	77.04	70.31†	82.63
42 Central Vancouver Island	76.85	72.32†	81.53
12 Kootenay Boundary	76.47	71.25†	81.29
52 Northern Interior	76.26	71.85†	80.88
14 Thompson Cariboo Shuswap	75.94	70.89†	81.07
51 Northwest	72.24	66.26†	78.40
53 Northeast	N/A	N/A	N/A
British Columbia	**78.42**	**73.57†**	**83.01**

† Male rate is significantly different than female rate.
Crosshatched HSDAs are significantly different than the provincial average.
N/A: No data

with Okanagan in the interior of the province. By contrast, the northern HSDAs, Central and North Vancouver Island, and Kootenay Boundary and Thompson Cariboo Shuswap in the interior of the province had lower than average values.

Youth with healthy body mass index

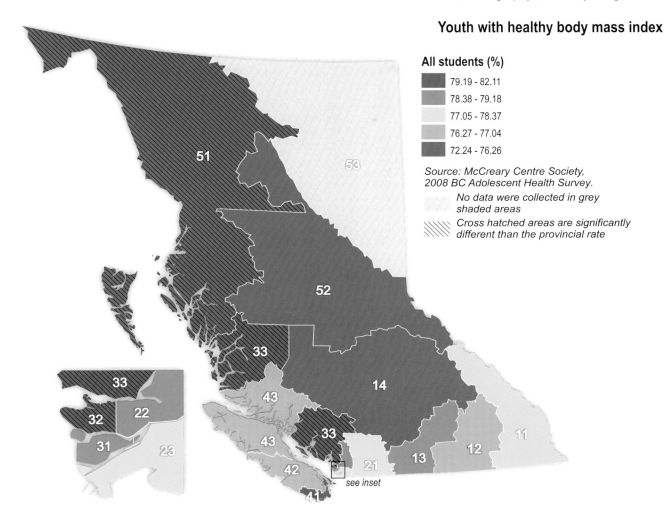

All students (%)

- 79.19 - 82.11
- 78.38 - 79.18
- 77.05 - 78.37
- 76.27 - 77.04
- 72.24 - 76.26

Source: McCreary Centre Society, 2008 BC Adolescent Health Survey.

No data were collected in grey shaded areas

Cross hatched areas are significantly different than the provincial rate

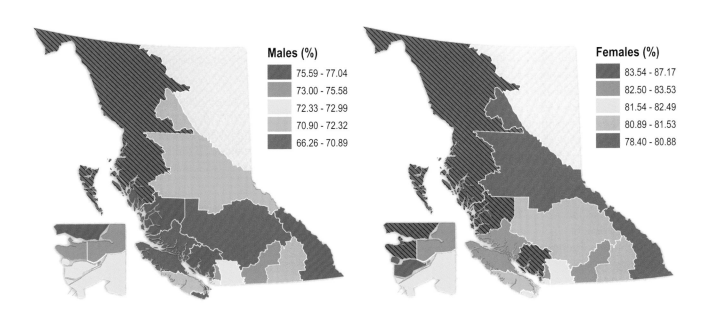

Males (%)

- 75.59 - 77.04
- 73.00 - 75.58
- 72.33 - 72.99
- 70.90 - 72.32
- 66.26 - 70.89

Females (%)

- 83.54 - 87.17
- 82.50 - 83.53
- 81.54 - 82.49
- 80.89 - 81.53
- 78.40 - 80.88

Weight is perceived to be just about right

Health Service Delivery Area	All respondents 12+ (%)	Males 12+ (%)	Females 12+ (%)	Ages 12-19 (%)	Ages 20-64 (%)	Ages 65+ (%)
32 Vancouver	62.17	61.64	62.69	72.48	61.09	62.58
23 Fraser South	60.75	67.59*	53.77	81.27†	59.62	48.72‡
33 North Shore/Coast Garibaldi	60.61	60.58	60.64	78.37	60.04	51.92
22 Fraser North	59.04	62.00	56.08	76.95†	56.95	56.67
21 Fraser East	57.28	64.51	50.01	79.51†	52.98	58.60
31 Richmond	55.80	58.73	52.95	62.51	53.57	62.40
12 Kootenay Boundary	55.53	60.13	50.60	81.69†	53.33	47.70
13 Okanagan	55.46	63.24*	47.91	83.22†	51.57	53.07
11 East Kootenay	54.46	53.72	55.23	91.47†	50.82	43.83
43 North Vancouver Island	54.43	61.34	47.58	74.03	52.98	47.59
14 Thompson Cariboo Shuswap	54.21	62.89*	45.31	79.24†	52.62	45.11
41 South Vancouver Island	54.14	55.83	52.59	77.37†	51.77	51.63
42 Central Vancouver Island	53.02	56.34	49.87	74.45†	49.43	52.88
51 Northwest	51.58	54.42	48.43	82.41†	45.71	53.80
52 Northern Interior	51.08	55.47	46.37	77.32†	47.80	44.55
53 Northeast	47.63	53.90	40.62	63.21	44.84	47.56
British Columbia (2007/8)	**57.49**	**61.36***	**53.66**	**77.51†**	**55.43**	**53.36**
British Columbia (2005)	**56.05**	**59.59***	**52.55**	**76.03†**	**53.23**	**54.31**

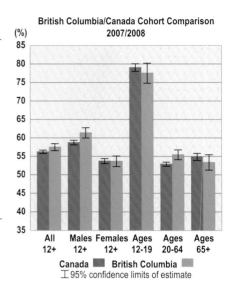

British Columbia/Canada Cohort Comparison 2007/2008

Canada ■ British Columbia ▨
⊥ 95% confidence limits of estimate

▧ Crosshatching beside the 2007/8 provincial rate indicates it is significantly different than the 2005 rate, while crosshatched HSDAs are significantly different than the 2007/8 provincial rate.
E interpret data with caution (16.67 ≤ coefficient of variation ≤ 33.3).

* Males differ significantly from females.
† 12-19 age cohort differs significantly from the 20-64 age cohort.
‡ 65+ age cohort differs significantly from the 20-64 age cohort.
F data suppressed (n < 10, or coefficient of variation > 33.3).

Identifying one's weight to be just about right is a useful measure of perceived wellness. The CCHS asked, *"Do you consider yourself: overweight, underweight or just about right?"* In BC, 57.49% of respondents identified with the "just about right" classification, indicating that over half of British Columbians feel they have a healthy weight. Values in most HSDAs were statistically similar to the provincial average, however Northwest, Northern Interior, and Northeast (all less than 52%) had values that were significantly below average.

At the provincial level, significantly more male respondents (61.36%) than female respondents (53.66%) identified as having a healthy weight. There were three HSDAs displaying this same trend: Okanagan, Thompson Cariboo Shuswap, and Fraser South.

Male respondents in Fraser South (67.59%) were significantly more likely than males provincially to report a healthy weight, while males in East Kootenay and Northwest (both below 55%) were significantly less likely to do so. Females in Vancouver (62.69%) were significantly more likely, and females in Northeast (40.62%) were significantly less likely, to report a healthy weight when compared to the average for female respondents in BC.

Among youth respondents, 77.51% reported having a healthy body weight – a significantly higher value than the mid-age cohort. Further, youth in 11 HSDAs were significantly more likely than the mid-age cohort to describe their body weight as being "just about right." In East Kootenay (91.47%), youth were significantly more

likely to report a healthy body weight than the youth provincial average.

For older respondents in BC, 53.36% identified their body weight as "just about right," statistically the same as the mid-age cohort. However, there was one HSDA, Fraser South, in which older respondents were significantly less likely to identify as having a healthy body weight than the mid-age cohort.

Geographically, there was a spread of over 14 percentage points for each of the cohorts, with the greatest variation occurring in the youth cohort (nearly 30 percentage points). The HSDAs with significantly low percentages of respondents reporting healthy weights were clustered in the north of the province. HSDAs with lower values for both males and females were located in the northern and central regions of the province, in a pattern similar to that of all respondents.

There were no significant differences for BC respondents between 2005 and 2007/8. When British Columbians' 2007/8 body weight perceptions were compared to their Canadian peers, males and the mid-age cohorts were significantly more likely to report weight as being "just about right."

Weight is perceived to be just about right

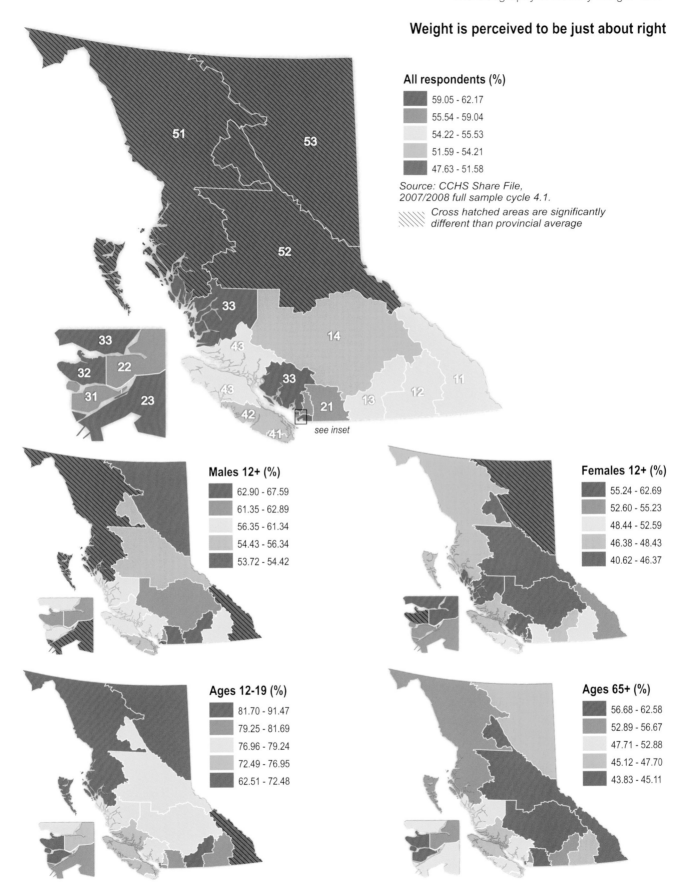

All respondents (%)

- 59.05 - 62.17
- 55.54 - 59.04
- 54.22 - 55.53
- 51.59 - 54.21
- 47.63 - 51.58

*Source: CCHS Share File,
2007/2008 full sample cycle 4.1.*

*Cross hatched areas are significantly
different than provincial average*

Males 12+ (%)

- 62.90 - 67.59
- 61.35 - 62.89
- 56.35 - 61.34
- 54.43 - 56.34
- 53.72 - 54.42

Females 12+ (%)

- 55.24 - 62.69
- 52.60 - 55.23
- 48.44 - 52.59
- 46.38 - 48.43
- 40.62 - 46.37

Ages 12-19 (%)

- 81.70 - 91.47
- 79.25 - 81.69
- 76.96 - 79.24
- 72.49 - 76.95
- 62.51 - 72.48

Ages 65+ (%)

- 56.68 - 62.58
- 52.89 - 56.67
- 47.71 - 52.88
- 45.12 - 47.70
- 43.83 - 45.11

Youth who think their weight is about right

For adolescents and others, perception of what they think about their own body can be an important emotional wellness asset and important from the perspective of self esteem. The McCreary AHS IV asked students *"How do you think of your body? Underweight, about the right weight, or overweight."*

Approximately two-thirds of all student respondents (66.90%) in BC indicated that they felt their body was about the right weight. This was significantly lower than the response to the measurement of a healthy Body Mass Index (78.42%). There were some differences among HSDAs in the province, with 69.81% of Kootenay Boundary student respondents feeling their body weight was about right, compared with only 63.09% of students in Richmond. Okanagan (69.66%) was the only HSDA where students were significantly higher, while both Richmond and Vancouver (63.28%) students were significantly lower than the provincial average. The results for Vancouver are in stark contrast to the BMI results reported earlier: Vancouver had the highest percentage of students with a healthy BMI.

There were significant differences for this indicator between genders. At the provincial level, male students (70.85%) were significantly more likely to think their body weight was about right, compared to only 63.24% of female student respondents. This gender differential was consistent in all regions of the province, and the difference was significant for nine of the HSDAs.

For male students, those who thought their body weight was about right ranged from a high of 75.10% in Okanagan to a low of 64.62% in Richmond. Both these HSDA results were significantly different from the provincial average for male student respondents.

The range in values for female student respondents went from a high of 67.31% in Kootenay Boundary to a low of only 58.34% in Vancouver. Vancouver female students were significantly lower than the provincial female student average. Again, this result is in stark contrast to the result which indicated that Vancouver had the highest percentage of female students with a healthy BMI, based on self assessment of weight and height.

Geographically, there was a tendency to find lower than average values of students who felt their body weight was about right in the urban lower mainland of the province, with the exception of North Shore/Coast Garibaldi, which was consistently above average. Other areas that were

Health Service Delivery Area	All students (%)	Males (%)	Females (%)
12 Kootenay Boundary	69.81	72.54	67.31
13 Okanagan	69.66	75.10†	64.85
41 South Vancouver Island	69.23	72.39†	66.17
33 North Shore/Coast Garibaldi	68.35	71.55†	65.25
14 Thompson Cariboo Shuswap	68.14	71.74†	64.82
42 Central Vancouver Island	67.92	72.57†	63.14
51 Northwest	67.92	69.54	66.20
52 Northern Interior	67.65	73.90†	61.21
11 East Kootenay	67.44	74.56†	61.14
22 Fraser North	66.67	69.22	64.18
43 North Vancouver Island	66.44	69.35	63.88
21 Fraser South/Fraser East	66.18	69.94†	62.80
32 Vancouver	63.28	69.68†	58.34
31 Richmond	63.09	64.62	61.55
53 Northeast	N/A	N/A	N/A
British Columbia	**66.90**	**70.85†**	**63.24**

† Male rate is significantly different than female rate.
Crosshatched HSDAs are significantly different than the provincial average.
N/A: No data

above average were found in the interior, especially Kootenay Boundary and Okanagan, and South Vancouver Island.

Again, it should be noted that data were not collected in the schools in Northeast, and the data for Fraser South and Fraser East have been combined because several school districts did not participate in the survey. Therefore some caution in the interpretation may be required.

Youth who think their weight is about right

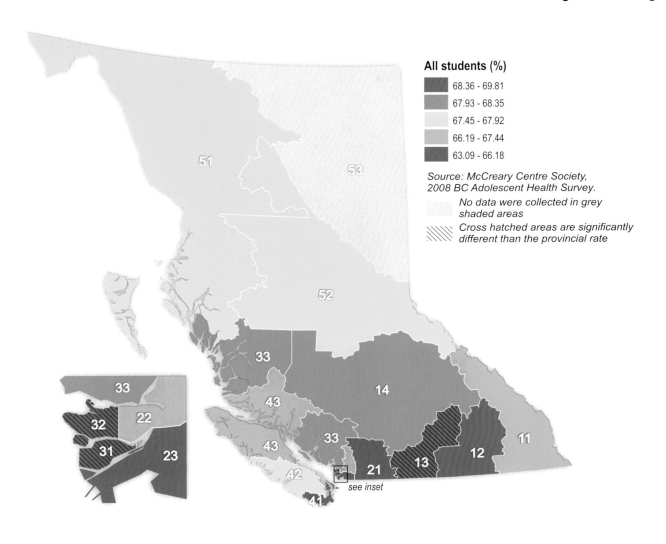

All students (%)

- 68.36 - 69.81
- 67.93 - 68.35
- 67.45 - 67.92
- 66.19 - 67.44
- 63.09 - 66.18

Source: McCreary Centre Society,
2008 BC Adolescent Health Survey.

No data were collected in grey
shaded areas

Cross hatched areas are significantly
different than the provincial rate

see inset

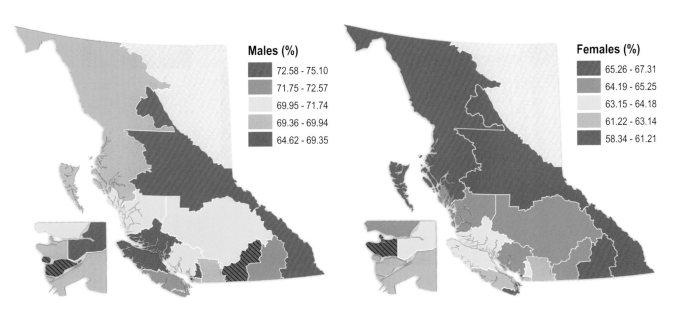

Males (%)

- 72.58 - 75.10
- 71.75 - 72.57
- 69.95 - 71.74
- 69.36 - 69.94
- 64.62 - 69.35

Females (%)

- 65.26 - 67.31
- 64.19 - 65.25
- 63.15 - 64.18
- 61.22 - 63.14
- 58.34 - 61.21

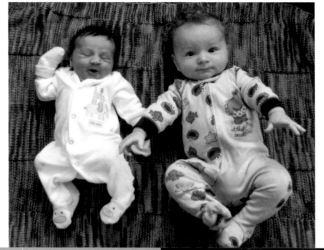

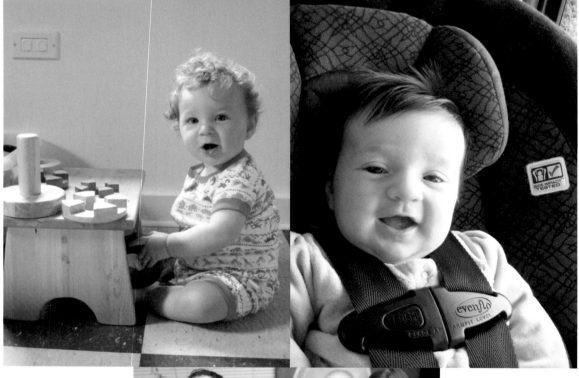

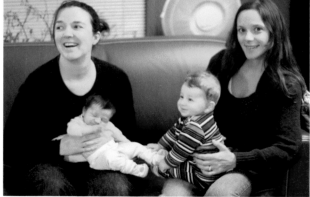

10

The Geography of Healthy Pregnancy and Birth

An important component of the ActNow BC initiative concerned healthy pregnancy and birth, and focused on discouraging the use of alcohol during pregnancy. We have taken a much broader perspective related to wellness indicators on healthy pregnancy and birth, and include a series of indicators that can result in improved health and wellness outcomes. There is substantial research that shows the importance of healthy beginnings for healthy child development and its impact on healthy adulthood. Having a good start in life is an important wellness asset.

Alcohol consumed in pregnancy can interfere with the ability of the fetus to get sufficient oxygen and nutrition to generate normal cell growth. Because fetal brain development occurs throughout pregnancy, alcohol consumption during pregnancy, as well as affecting learning skills and intelligence, can result in hyperactivity, attention and/or memory deficits, an inability to manage anger, speech and hearing difficulties, challenges with problem solving, and fully recognizing the consequences of actions (VON, Canada, 2011). Some effects are obvious, such as shortened eye slits, flattened midline ridge between nose and lip, flattened mid face, as well as a thin upper lip, but many are "invisible," at least initially.

Breastfed full-term infants have reduced risks for a variety of health problems, including lower respiratory tract diseases in the first year requiring hospitalization, gastrointestinal infections resulting in diarrhea and/or vomiting, acute ear infection, type 2 diabetes, Sudden Infant Death Syndrome, asthma, eczema, and childhood obesity, among others. Exclusive breastfeeding for long durations (at least the recommended 6 months) is also associated with better maternal health outcomes, and there is clear evidence that cervical and breast cancer is higher among those who have never breastfed (US Department of Health and Human Services, 2011). For

many mothers, breastfeeding gives a sense of bonding with newborns and reduces the risk of postpartum depression.

Not only does smoking by the mother affect the fetus, but concerns have been expressed about the damage second-hand smoke can cause. The BC Perinatal Registry Program Annual Report for 2007 noted that, based on the Maternity Experiences Survey report for 2006/7, nearly one-fifth of women respondents in BC reported living with a smoker during pregnancy (BC Reproductive Care Program, 2008).

This chapter contains a total of 12 maps. The first three maps focus on breastfeeding behaviour. Some of the data used here are different from those used in the first Atlas. We have used data from CCHS 4.1 rather than the BC Perinatal Registry (BCPR), as data are now only partly reported on a geographical basis in the BCPR annual reports, and only by place of birth delivery rather than place of residence of the mother. Breastfeeding behaviours are provided based on the last birth of the mother, and come from the 2007/8 CCHS 4.1. The next two maps look at non-smoking (BCPR) and alcohol-free behaviours (CCHS 4.1) during pregnancy, and these are followed by five maps related to pregnancies and births that were free of maternal and perinatal complications, healthy birth weight, full-term births, and healthiest age for pregnancy. These five indicators are then combined to provide a single indicator that shows babies born with the healthiest conditions, and a final map looks at infant mortality. These maps are based on data provided by the BC Vital Statistics Agency.

A few words are necessary with respect to the alcohol-free and breastfeeding indicators. Sample sizes for these two maps were small, so interpretation of results should be undertaken with caution.

Breastfed or tried to breastfeed baby

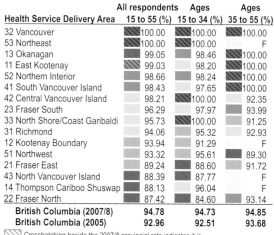

Health Service Delivery Area	All respondents 15 to 55 (%)	Ages 15 to 34 (%)	Ages 35 to 55 (%)
32 Vancouver	100.00	100.00	100.00
53 Northeast	100.00	100.00	F
13 Okanagan	99.05	98.46	100.00
11 East Kootenay	99.03	98.20	100.00
52 Northern Interior	98.66	98.24	100.00
41 South Vancouver Island	98.43	97.65	100.00
42 Central Vancouver Island	98.21	100.00	92.35
23 Fraser South	96.29	97.97	93.99
33 North Shore/Coast Garibaldi	95.73	100.00	91.25
31 Richmond	94.06	95.32	92.93
12 Kootenay Boundary	93.94	91.29	F
51 Northwest	93.32	95.61	89.30
21 Fraser East	89.24	88.60	91.72
43 North Vancouver Island	88.39	87.77	F
14 Thompson Cariboo Shuswap	88.13	96.04	F
22 Fraser North	87.42	84.60	93.14
British Columbia (2007/8)	**94.78**	**94.73**	**94.85**
British Columbia (2005)	**92.96**	**92.51**	**93.68**

Crosshatching beside the 2007/8 provincial rate indicates it is significantly different than the 2005 rate, while crosshatched HSDAs are significantly different than the 2007/8 provincial rate.
F data suppressed (n < 10, or coefficient of variation > 33.3).

British Columbia/Canada Cohort Comparison (%) 2007/2008

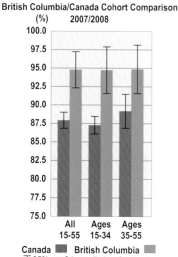

Canada ■   British Columbia ▤
⊥ 95% confidence limits of estimate

The advantages of breastfeeding have been long recognized in Canada (Ostry, 2005; 2006). A recent summary of the importance of breastfeeding statesl "Breast milk is uniquely suited to the human infant's nutritional needs and is a live substance with unparalleled immunological and anti-inflammatory properties that protect against a host of illnesses and diseases for both mothers and children" (US Department of Health and Human Services, 2011, p.1).

The CCHS asked females if they had breastfed or tried to breastfeed their last baby, even if only for a short time, and those between the ages of 15 and 55 years who responded positively are used in the table and maps opposite. For BC mothers as a whole, 94.78% responded positively to the question. This compared to only 87.90% for Canada as a whole, and this difference was significant. It should be noted that the latest published data from the BCPR, which is for 2006/7, reported that 69.2% used exclusively breast milk on leaving the hospital after birth, and a further 25.3% used a combination of breast milk and formula (BC Reproductive Care Program, 2008).

Among HSDAs, Vancouver and Northeast had 100% of respondents answer positively, as did over 99% of those in Okanagan and East Kootenay. All of these HSDAs, except Okanagan, were significantly higher than the provincial average. At the other extreme, Fraser East, North Vancouver Island, Thompson Cariboo Shuswap, and Fraser North were all below 90%. Among those in the 15 to 34 age cohort, 94.73% responded positively, significantly higher than the 87.27% for Canada as a

whole. Vancouver, Northeast, Central Vancouver Island, and North Shore/Coast Garibaldi (all 100%) were significantly higher than the provincial average for this age cohort. Fraser East, North Vancouver Island, and Fraser North were all below 90%. For the 35 to 55 age cohort, 100% positive responses occurred in Vancouver, Okanagan, East Kootenay, Northern Interior, and South Vancouver Island, while the remainder of the HSDAs were lower than the provincial average of 94.85% for this cohort. The provincial average was again significantly higher than the Canadian average (89.19%).

Geographically, there were no clear regional patterns.

It is interesting to note that the BC average was higher than every other province in Canada, and the difference was significant, except for Alberta. Further, every individual HSDA was higher in value than the Canadian average, except for Fraser North for the 15 to 55 and 15 to 34 age cohorts. Also, based on the Canadian Maternal Experience Survey for 2006/7, 97.0% of BC women respondents reported breastfeeding initiation, the highest of any province in Canada, and significantly higher than the Canadian average (90.3%). By 3 months, the rate of positive responses had fallen to 61.4% for exclusive breastfeeding, and to 19.2% by 6 months. Both values were the highest among provinces, and significantly higher than the Canadian averages (Public Health Agency of Canada, 2009c).

Breastfed or tried to breastfeed baby

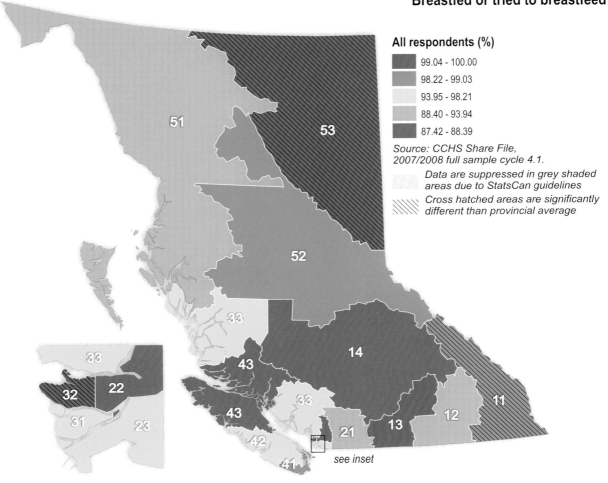

All respondents (%)

- 99.04 - 100.00
- 98.22 - 99.03
- 93.95 - 98.21
- 88.40 - 93.94
- 87.42 - 88.39

*Source: CCHS Share File,
2007/2008 full sample cycle 4.1.*

*Data are suppressed in grey shaded
areas due to StatsCan guidelines*

*Cross hatched areas are significantly
different than provincial average*

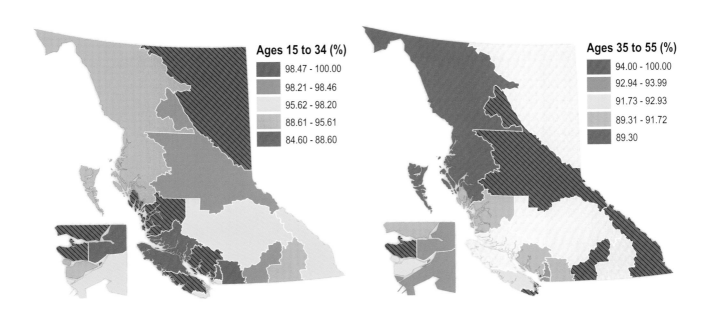

Ages 15 to 34 (%)

- 98.47 - 100.00
- 98.21 - 98.46
- 95.62 - 98.20
- 88.61 - 95.61
- 84.60 - 88.60

Ages 35 to 55 (%)

- 94.00 - 100.00
- 92.94 - 93.99
- 91.73 - 92.93
- 89.31 - 91.72
- 89.30

Healthiest mothers

Mother did not smoke during pregnancy

Smoking tobacco during pregnancy can affect the mother and the fetus. Tobacco smoke has many teratogens that can cause birth defects, and approximately 50 of the chemicals found in tobacco smoke are associated with cancer (Public Health Agency of Canada, 2011b). Also, intrauterine growth can be restricted resulting in lower birth weights, and there is an increase in the risk of prematurity, placental complications, stillbirths, miscarriage, and SIDS (Jensen, 2007).

Using data from the BCPR averaged for the 4 year period 2003/4 to 2006/7, 89.26% of all births were to mothers who had not smoked during pregnancy. This was an improvement from 88.01% for the 2000/1 to 2003/4 period. Among HSDAs, there was a 17 percentage point difference. The highest non-smoking values occurred in Richmond and Vancouver (both greater than 96%), while Northern Interior was less than 80%. Geographically, there were quite distinct patterns. The highest non-smoking values occurred in the lower mainland, while the

Health Service Delivery Area		Non smoker (%)
31 Richmond		96.91
32 Vancouver		96.25
33 North Shore/Coast Garibaldi		93.47
22 Fraser North		93.17
23 Fraser South		91.38
21 Fraser East		86.00
12 Kootenay Boundary		85.35
41 South Vancouver Island		85.28
13 Okanagan		85.19
51 Northwest		84.71
42 Central Vancouver Island		83.17
43 North Vancouver Island		82.93
11 East Kootenay		82.16
14 Thompson Cariboo Shuswap		81.96
53 Northeast		80.15
52 Northern Interior		79.95
British Columbia		**89.26**

lowest occurred in the central and northern interior and northeast of the province.

For comparative purposes, results from the CCHS for 2007/8 indicated that 83.74% of female respondents had not smoked during their last pregnancy, compared with 79.41% for their Canadian counterparts. Values improved generally with age.

Did not drink any alcohol during last pregnancy

It is known that consuming alcohol during pregnancy can impede the development of the fetus, especially brain development, which can affect learning skills and intelligence, among other things. It can result in what is known as Fetal Alcohol Spectrum Disorder (FASD).

As many as 9 in every 1,000 infants are born with FASD (Ministry of Children and Family Development, 2011) and there is "no known safe amount or safe time to drink alcohol during pregnancy" (Public Health Agency of Canada, 2011a).

Based on the 2007/8 CCHS, 93.36% of women between the ages of 15 and 55 gave a negative response to the question about consuming alcohol during their last pregnancy. This was marginally lower than the Canadian average (94.30%). Within BC, Richmond and Northern Interior (both above 98%) were significantly higher than average. At the other extreme, Okanagan, Thompson Cariboo Shuswap, and Northeast were all less than 89%. Younger female respondents (between the ages of 15 and 34) were more likely to be alcohol free in pregnancy (94.95%) than mothers between the ages of 35 and 55 (90.45%). This difference also occurred in the Canadian sample.

Health Service Delivery Area		All respondents aged 15 to 55 (%)
31 Richmond		100.00
52 Northern Interior		98.89
12 Kootenay Boundary		98.55
33 North Shore/Coast Garibaldi		96.60
43 North Vancouver Island		96.36
51 Northwest		95.56
42 Central Vancouver Island		94.77
32 Vancouver		94.53
41 South Vancouver Island		94.12
21 Fraser East		93.59
22 Fraser North		91.97
11 East Kootenay		91.42
23 Fraser South		90.00
13 Okanagan		88.77
14 Thompson Cariboo Shuswap		88.51
53 Northeast		88.26
British Columbia (2007/8)		**93.36**
No comparable 2005 data available		

Crosshatching beside the 2007/8 provincial rate indicates it is significantly different than the 2005 rate, while crosshatched HSDAs are significantly different than the 2007/8 provincial rate.

By comparison, based on the Canadian Maternal Experience Survey for 2006/7, slightly less than 8% of BC women respondents had reported consuming alcohol during the course of their pregnancy (Public Health Agency of Canada, 2009c).

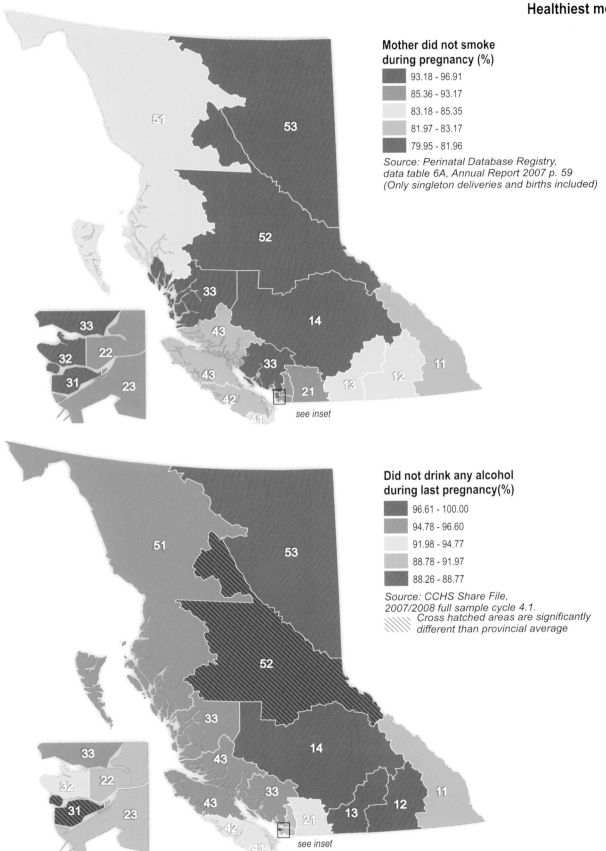

Healthiest mothers

Mother did not smoke
during pregnancy (%)

- 93.18 - 96.91
- 85.36 - 93.17
- 83.18 - 85.35
- 81.97 - 83.17
- 79.95 - 81.96

*Source: Perinatal Database Registry,
data table 6A, Annual Report 2007 p. 59
(Only singleton deliveries and births included)*

Did not drink any alcohol
during last pregnancy(%)

- 96.61 - 100.00
- 94.78 - 96.60
- 91.98 - 94.77
- 88.78 - 91.97
- 88.26 - 88.77

*Source: CCHS Share File,
2007/2008 full sample cycle 4.1.
Cross hatched areas are significantly
different than provincial average*

Births free of complications

Being free of maternal and perinatal complications are important wellness assets for both mother and child. They also reflect, in part, the lifestyle lived by the mother both pre- and post-conception. The information presented in the table and maps opposite has been provided by the BC Vital Statistics Agency and covers the five calendar years 2005 to 2009, in which 214,744 live births occurred. These data include only live births to BC women that occurred in the province, and location is based on the residence of the mother. Caution is required in interpreting the patterns because some births to BC mothers, especially those with complications, may have occured in neighbouring Alberta hospitals. This may affect the southeast and to a lesser extent the northeast of the province.

No maternal complications of pregnancy and delivery

There is a large variety of maternal complications that can occur in pregnancy and delivery. Nearly one-fifth of all complications are related to the need for assisted or surgical delivery, while another major complication involves maternal abnormality of pelvic organs (Vital Statistics Agency, 2010). Less than half (47.66%) of the 214,744 live births for the 2005 to 2009 period were free of maternal complications related to pregnancy and delivery, slightly lower than the 48.38% recorded for the 2001 to 2005 period. There was a range of almost 14 percentage points between the highest and lowest value HSDAs. Northeast and Kootenay Boundary (both above 57%) had the highest values, followed by East Kootenay, Fraser East, Northern Interior, and Northwest (all above 50%). The lowest value HSDAs were Central Vancouver Island and Fraser North (both below 45%). Geographically, new mothers in the northern half and southeastern part of the province were less likely to have complications, while mothers in parts of Vancouver Island and the lower mainland were more likely to have complications. Generally, the pattern was quite similar to that for the 2001 to 2005 period.

No perinatal complications affecting pregnancy and delivery

Approximately 80% of all perinatal complications include intrauterine hypoxia and birth asphyxia, disorders related to long gestation or high birth weight, and disorders related to short gestation (Vital Statistics Agency, 2010). Close to two-thirds (66.2%) of all live births in BC between 2005 and 2009 were free of any perinatal complications, and the range in values was over 14 percentage points. The HSDAs with the highest complication-free values

Health Service Delivery Area	Maternal (%)	Perinatal (%)
53 Northeast	57.87	66.38
12 Kootenay Boundary	56.98	65.66
11 East Kootenay	52.58	63.75
21 Fraser East	52.42	63.15
52 Northern Interior	52.08	58.97
51 Northwest	50.39	59.96
31 Richmond	48.79	73.20
14 Thompson Cariboo Shuswap	48.41	61.67
41 South Vancouver Island	47.17	64.22
23 Fraser South	47.00	68.59
13 Okanagan	46.93	65.15
43 North Vancouver Island	46.51	61.37
33 North Shore/Coast Garibaldi	46.18	68.29
32 Vancouver	45.92	70.87
22 Fraser North	44.77	66.84
42 Central Vancouver Island	44.16	59.78
British Columbia	**47.66**	**66.20**

were Richmond and Vancouver (both over 70.9%), while at the other extreme, Northwest, Central Vancouver Island, and Northern Interior all had values of 60% or less. Geographically, there were distinct regional patterns. The lower mainland urban HSDAs had above average values for being free of perinatal complications, while the north, with the exception of Northeast (66.4%) and North and Central Vancouver Island, had well below average values, along with Thompson Cariboo Shuswap in the central interior. Overall, values were very similar to the values provided in the original Atlas.

Births free of complications

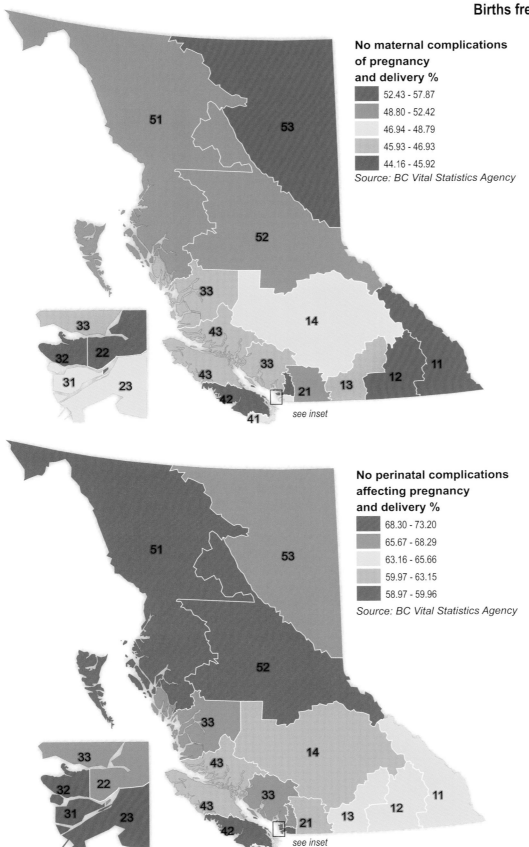

No maternal complications of pregnancy and delivery %

- 52.43 - 57.87
- 48.80 - 52.42
- 46.94 - 48.79
- 45.93 - 46.93
- 44.16 - 45.92

Source: BC Vital Statistics Agency

see inset

No perinatal complications affecting pregnancy and delivery %

- 68.30 - 73.20
- 65.67 - 68.29
- 63.16 - 65.66
- 59.97 - 63.15
- 58.97 - 59.96

Source: BC Vital Statistics Agency

see inset

Healthiest pregnancies

Having a healthy pregnancy and healthy birth outcome are important wellness indicators for both mother and child. A healthy start for a child is important in terms of future development. The table and maps opposite provide data related to three important indicators that increase the chances for the healthiest pregnancies and births. These include the best age range to conceive and give birth, the best range of birth weight for babies, and the full gestational development of the baby.

Full-term live births

Of the births in BC between 2005 and 2009, 91.7% were full-term babies (37 to 41 weeks of gestation). Full-term babies have fewer risk factors than premature babies or those who go well beyond normal term. There was a small range in values among HSDAs of only 3 percentage points. The highest value occurred in Northeast (93.56%), and Richmond (92.69%), while the lowest values occurred in Central Vancouver Island (90.50%) and Kootenay Boundary (91.01%). Values and patterns were very similar to those found in the 2001 to 2005 period.

Healthy birth weight

Babies born below a weight of 2,500 grams are viewed as low birth weight, and that condition increases the risks of relatively poor development and is responsible for about three quarters of all perinatal mortality and morbidity. Large babies, 4,500 grams or more, are referred to as macrosomic babies. Macrosomic deliveries have higher rates of complications due to diabetes, disproportion, shoulder dystocia, facial palsy, and infant asphyxia, as well as obstructed labour (Kierans et al., 2007). The healthiest birth weights therefore occur in the range of 2,500 to 4,499 grams. For the period 2005 to 2009, 92.33% of births fell within this range, a similar percentage to that noted for the 2001 to 2005 period. There was a very small variation among HSDAs of less than 2 percentage points. The highest values were found in Okanagan (93.05%), Northeast (93.04%), and Richmond (92.97%), while the lowest value was found in Northwest (91.35%).

Healthiest mother's age

The healthiest age to conceive and have a baby is between age 20 and 34 years. Teen pregnancies are associated with relatively high infant mortality rates, as are pregnancies for those over the age of 40 years (Vital Statistics Agency, 2010). Complications of pregnancy, including prematurity and restriction in intrauterine growth,

Health Service Delivery Area	Full-term live births (%)	Healthy birth weight (%)	Healthiest mother's age (%)
53 Northeast	93.56	93.04	82.55
31 Richmond	92.69	92.97	68.06
43 North Vancouver Island	92.27	91.99	77.60
13 Okanagan	92.23	93.05	79.21
21 Fraser East	92.02	92.44	82.45
23 Fraser South	91.95	91.95	78.41
11 East Kootenay	91.94	92.59	79.76
22 Fraser North	91.94	92.49	70.56
52 Northern Interior	91.75	91.87	81.04
33 North Shore/Coast Garibaldi	91.74	92.60	64.33
51 Northwest	91.48	91.35	76.89
41 South Vancouver Island	91.18	92.28	73.41
14 Thompson Cariboo Shuswap	91.17	92.30	80.35
32 Vancouver	91.12	92.37	63.79
12 Kootenay Boundary	91.01	91.80	78.99
42 Central Vancouver Island	90.50	91.94	77.80
British Columbia	**91.72**	**92.33**	**74.35**

are more common among teens and those 35 years or older. In addition, older pregnancies are more likely to result in maternal diabetes, hypertension, and/or hemorrhaging (Jensen, 2007).

For the period 2005 to 2009, 74.35% of all live births were to women in the healthiest age group of 20 to 34 years. This is a reduction of 1.5 percentage points when compared with 2001 to 2005 (75.94%). This change was due to the tendency for women to delay having children, rather than an increase in teen mothers (Vital Statistics Agency, 2010). Throughout the province, there is close to a 20 percentage point range between the highest value HSDA and the lowest: Northeast and Fraser East both have more than 82% of all births to mothers in the healthiest age group, while Vancouver and North Shore/Coast Garibaldi both have less than 65% of births to women in the 20 to 34 age group. Geographically, with the exception of Fraser South (78.41%), the lowest values were clustered in the extreme southwestern part of the province, including South Vancouver Island, while the higher values were found in the north (with the exception of Northwest) and interior of BC.

Healthiest pregnancies

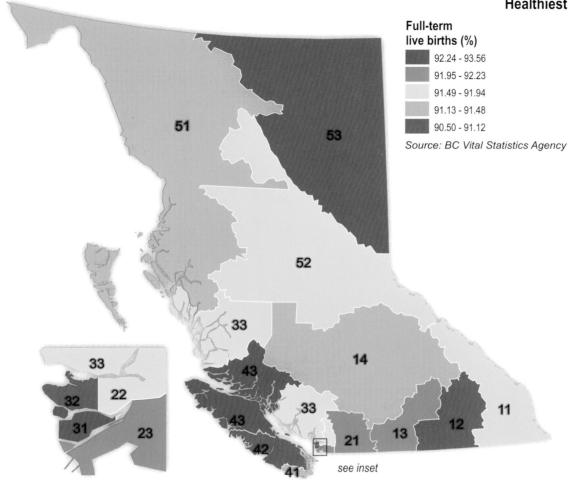

Full-term
live births (%)

- 92.24 - 93.56
- 91.95 - 92.23
- 91.49 - 91.94
- 91.13 - 91.48
- 90.50 - 91.12

Source: BC Vital Statistics Agency

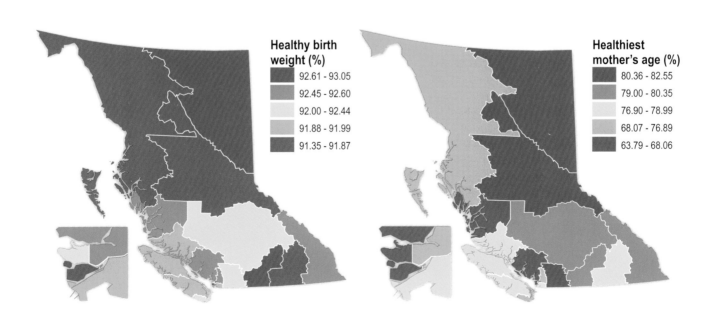

Healthy birth
weight (%)

- 92.61 - 93.05
- 92.45 - 92.60
- 92.00 - 92.44
- 91.88 - 91.99
- 91.35 - 91.87

Healthiest
mother's age (%)

- 80.36 - 82.55
- 79.00 - 80.35
- 76.90 - 78.99
- 68.07 - 76.89
- 63.79 - 68.06

Healthiest babies

Two key indicators are presented here. The first indicator, "babies with healthiest potential," combines several indicators already used. The second provides data on infant mortality rates throughout the province. All of the data were provided by the Vital Statistics Agency.

Babies with healthiest potential

The Vital Statistics Agency was able to combine information from several indicators for the period 2005 to 2009 to enable us to define a single indicator. The indicator combines the following characteristics: no maternal or perinatal complications; mother's age between 20 and 34 years; healthy birth weight between 2,500 and 4,499 grams; and full-term live births between 39 and 41 weeks gestation. These characteristics describe the potential for the healthiest babies, and therefore those with the best, immediate early development opportunities.

Between 2005 and 2009, less than three in every ten (28.4%) of live births in the province had all of the five characteristics noted above. There was a 10 percentage point range among HSDAs. Northeast had the highest value at 35.2%, while North Shore/Coast Garibaldi had the lowest, with only 25.3% of all live births.

Geographically, the northeast and southeast had above average values, all of Vancouver Island had below average values, and the remainder of the province was mixed. For example, while several lower mainland HSDAs (Fraser North, Vancouver, and North Shore/Coast Garibaldi) had relatively low values, others (Richmond, Fraser South) had above average values, and the north and interior were also mixed.

Infant mortality rate

One of the most recognized health and wellness indicators internationally is the infant mortality rate. This indicator gives the number of deaths in the first year of life as a rate per 1,000 live births. In the first edition of the Atlas, we calculated the percentage of newborns who survived the first year of life, which is the opposite of the infant mortality rate. However, the large majority of infants do survive, so using the survival rate did not provide a useful indicator, which is why we have used the more traditional infant mortality rate.

The infant mortality rate in BC for the period 2005 to 2009 was 3.87 per 1,000 live births. This is an improvement over the 4.24 per 1,000 live births for the period 2001 to 2005. Indeed, the infant mortality rate has been generally

Health Service Delivery Area	Healthiest % of live births	Mortality rate per 1,000 live births
53 Northeast	35.24	4.20
12 Kootenay Boundary	32.17	2.55
21 Fraser East	31.97	3.44
11 East Kootenay	31.58	4.07
31 Richmond	30.20	2.98
23 Fraser South	29.73	3.79
52 Northern Interior	29.41	4.09
13 Okanagan	28.66	3.36
51 Northwest	27.99	4.00
14 Thompson Cariboo Shuswap	27.84	4.59
41 South Vancouver Island	27.67	3.85
32 Vancouver	26.91	4.62
22 Fraser North	26.37	2.86
43 North Vancouver Island	26.34	4.77
42 Central Vancouver Island	25.70	5.74
33 North Shore/Coast Garibaldi	25.30	3.75
British Columbia	**28.37**	**3.87**

decreasing for decades in BC, and has been lower than the Canadian rate for at least the past 20 years. Although the overall infant mortality rate is low, there were major differences among HSDAs. The lowest infant mortality rate (highest survival rate) occurred in Kootenay Boundary (2.55 deaths per 1,000 live births), which was less than half the rate for Central Vancouver Island at 5.74 per 1,000 live births. Fraser North and Richmond also had relatively low infant mortality rates (both below 3 per 1,000 live births), while Thompson Cariboo Shuswap, Vancouver, and North Vancouver Island all had rates above 4.5 per 1,000 live births.

Geographically, rates were higher than average in the north and much of Vancouver Island. The lower mainland HSDAs had below average infant mortality rates, with the exception of Vancouver.

Healthiest babies

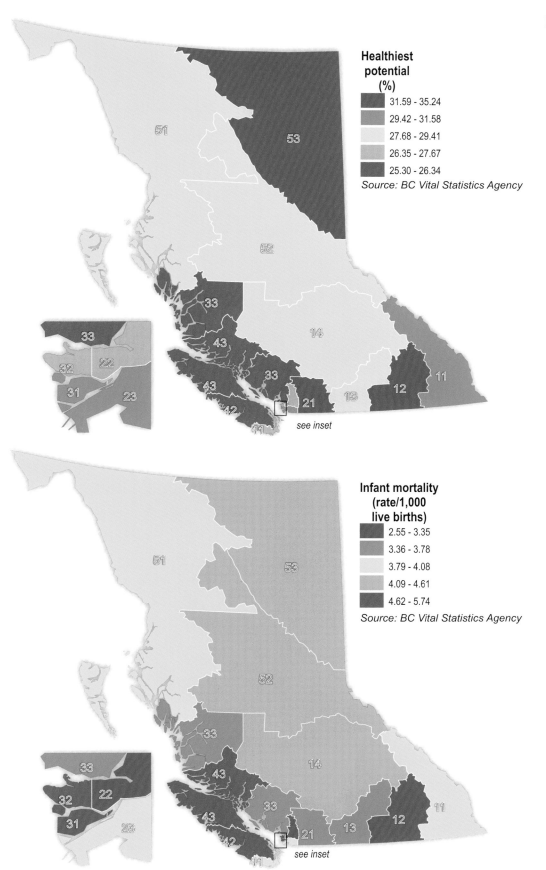

Source: BC Vital Statistics Agency

**Healthiest
potential
(%)**

31.59 - 35.24
29.42 - 31.58
27.68 - 29.41
26.35 - 27.67
25.30 - 26.34

**Infant mortality
(rate/1,000
live births)**

2.55 - 3.35
3.36 - 3.78
3.79 - 4.08
4.09 - 4.61
4.62 - 5.74

see inset

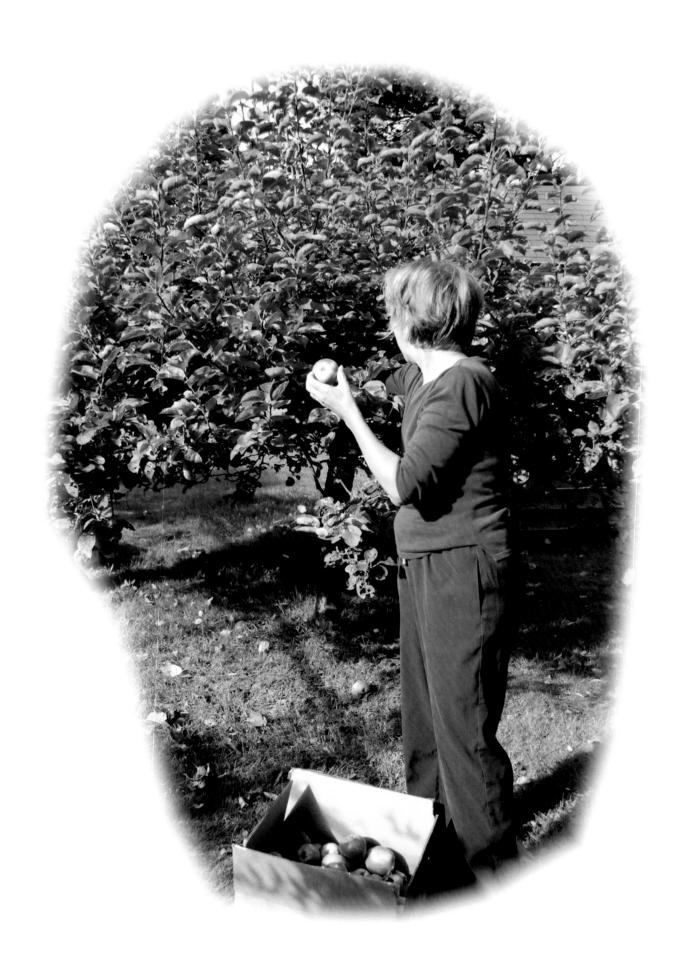

11

The Geography of Chronic-free Conditions

The ActNow BC program initiatives had, as a major focus, the reduction of chronic conditions and their impacts on individuals, the economy, and health care costs (ActNow BC, 2006; 2008). The second ActNow progress report noted "ActNow BC's approach is to focus on key risk factors for chronic disease and to lead and take integrated action to reduce these risk factors" (ActNow BC, 2010, p. iii).

This is a new section for the Atlas so that geographical variations in chronic-free conditions can be examined. While the previous Atlas reported on several of the indicators used in this chapter, we have expanded the number of indicators to give a more complete picture of the province in terms of being free of chronic conditions.

Many chronic conditions result in a reduction in life quality, whether the condition is a disease, a precursor for a disease, or a physical, mental, or other condition that interferes with the life. This is not to say that those with a chronic condition are necessarily unwell. Indeed, many with a chronic condition report a positive state of mind and well-being, and some without a chronic condition can experience a poor sense of well-being (Ryan & Deci, 2001). Many chronic conditions are related to smoking, poor nutrition, physical inactivity, and risky alcohol consumption.

This chapter contains a 50 maps based on CCHS 4.1. Ten indicators have maps for the total respondents, males and females separately, and younger and older populations. Because many chronic conditions are more common in older age groups, and might be entirely absent in the youngest age group for many HSDAs (McKee et al., 2010), the age cohorts in many of the indicators are different from those used elsewhere. The age cohorts used for cancer, diabetes, high blood pressure, heart disease, and arthritis or rheumatism were as follows: age

12 years and over; age 35-49 years (youngest); age 50-64 years (mid-age); 65 years and over (seniors). It is also important to note that seniors are significantly more likely to have two or more chronic conditions than younger age cohorts (Ramage-Morin et al., 2010).

The first 15 maps provide patterns related to being free of difficulties with regular, in-home, or outside activities.

The final 35 maps provide patterns related to being free of a variety of chronic diseases or their precursors as diagnosed by health professionals. Respondents were asked if they had ever been diagnosed with high blood pressure (hypertension) or cancer, or if they had arthritis or rheumatism, asthma, diabetes, or heart disease. Many of these are related to smoking (Patra et al., 2007), high salt ingestion (Sodium Working Group, 2010), and/or obesity conditions (Kendall, 2006). As we have noted earlier, obesity is often the outcome of physical inactivity and poor nutrition, among other factors. Deaths from cancer, cardiovascular, and cerebrovascular diseases were responsible for 17,800 deaths in BC in 2009, or 57% of all deaths in the province.

This group also includes information on being free of back problems. Back problems are common for a variety of reasons, and are often associated with a reduction in physical activity.

While diagnosis by a health professional is important, some conditions may not have been diagnosed. Therefore, it is highly likely that responses to these CCHS questions are actually underestimations of the conditions. For example, based on the Canadian Health Measures Survey, only 83.4% of those with high blood pressure were actually aware they had the condition, and this awareness increased with age (Wilkins et al., 2010). Consistent with our wellness perspective, we map the percentage of respondents that have never had any of these diagnoses.

Does not have difficulty with regular activities

Health Service Delivery Area	All respondents 12+ (%)	Males 12+ (%)	Females 12+ (%)	Ages 12-19 (%)	Ages 20-64 (%)	Ages 65+ (%)
31 Richmond	80.70	79.61	81.72	88.23	85.49	51.79‡
32 Vancouver	80.62	82.44	78.85	90.21	83.61	57.68‡
22 Fraser North	78.84	83.22*	74.55	91.55†	82.38	46.56‡
33 North Shore/Coast Garibaldi	76.83	77.79	75.92	85.35	81.21	51.96‡
21 Fraser East	75.83	76.04	75.63	83.15	80.33	49.52‡
23 Fraser South	75.74	76.33	75.17	87.39	79.79	42.63‡
51 Northwest	73.26	72.07	74.53	80.58	76.86	41.86E‡
53 Northeast	72.21	73.87	70.43	75.09	74.71	47.03‡
41 South Vancouver Island	71.90	72.10	71.73	89.53†	76.34	44.91‡
43 North Vancouver Island	70.34	71.71	69.02	90.72†	74.14	40.10‡
42 Central Vancouver Island	68.14	68.70	67.60	91.94†	70.87	46.63‡
11 East Kootenay	67.98	69.17	66.77	90.92†	71.18	39.27‡
52 Northern Interior	67.39	69.21	65.48	80.90	70.26	34.23‡
14 Thompson Cariboo Shuswap	67.14	67.68	66.61	83.35	69.94	44.62‡
13 Okanagan	65.59	67.78	63.52	87.37†	70.40	38.86‡
12 Kootenay Boundary	63.29	64.70	61.83	81.65	62.87	53.60
British Columbia (2007/8)	**74.28**	**75.65***	**72.95**	**87.53†**	**78.13**	**46.60‡**
British Columbia (2005)	**75.57**	**76.74**	**74.42**	**86.82†**	**79.09**	**49.82‡**

⊠ Crosshatching beside the 2007/8 provincial rate indicates it is significantly different than the 2005 rate, while crosshatched HSDAs are significantly different than the 2007/8 provincial rate.
E interpret data with caution (16.67 ≤ coefficient of variation ≤ 33.3).

* Males differ significantly from females.
† 12-19 age cohort differs significantly from the 20-64 age cohort.
‡ 65+ age cohort differs significantly from the 20-64 age cohort.
F data suppressed (n < 10, or coefficient of variation > 33.3).

British Columbia/Canada Cohort Comparison 2007/2008

Canada ■   British Columbia ▨
⊥ 95% confidence limits of estimate

Chronic conditions often render people unable to carry out regular activities without enduring pain or restriction. The CCHS asked respondents if they *"have any difficulty hearing, seeing, communicating, walking, climbing stairs, bending, learning, or doing any similar activities (sometimes, often, never)."* More than seven in every ten BC respondents (74.28%) indicated they never had difficulty with regular activities. Respondents in Fraser North, Richmond, and Vancouver (all over 78%) indicated significantly higher rates of never having difficulty with regular activities, whereas East Kootenay, Kootenay Boundary, Okanagan, Thompson Cariboo Shuswap, Central Vancouver Island, and Northern Interior respondents (all below 69%) had significantly lower averages.

Provincially, males (75.65%) were significantly more likely than females (72.95%) to have no difficulties with regular activities. Male respondents in Fraser North had a significantly higher average than females.

Among HSDAs, males in Fraser North and Vancouver (both above 82%) were significantly higher than the provincial average for males, while those in Kootenay Boundary, Okanagan, Thompson Cariboo Shuswap, and Central Vancouver Island (all below 69%) were significantly lower. For females, respondents in Richmond and Vancouver (both above 78%) were significantly higher than the provincial female average, while those in East Kootenay, Kootenay Boundary, Okanagan, and Thompson Cariboo Shuswap (all below 67%) were significantly lower.

For youth in BC, 87.53% of respondents had no difficulty

with regular activity, significantly higher than the provincial average for the mid-age cohort, and youth had significantly higher values than their mid-age counterparts in East Kootenay, Okanagan, Fraser North, South Vancouver Island, Central Vancouver Island, and North Vancouver Island.

For older respondents, the provincial average of 46.60% was significantly below the mid-age provincial average, as was the case for every HSDA, except Kootenay Boundary. Among older respondents, Vancouver (57.68%) was significantly higher than the provincial average for seniors, while Northern Interior (34.23%) was significantly lower.

The 15 to 20 percentage point spread among HSDAs indicated geographical variation within the province. Patterns were very similar for all respondents–males, females, the mid-age cohort, and, to a lesser extent, older respondents–with higher averages in the urban south west and lower averages in the interior and south eastern regions of BC. Youth, with only a 10 percentage point spread, had a cluster of higher values on Vancouver Island, with lower averages in the north.

There were no significant differences for any BC cohorts between 2005 and 2007/8. When compared to national averages, British Columbians had no significant differences from other Canadians, except BC seniors had a significantly lower average of being free of difficulties with regular activities.

Does not have difficulty with regular activities

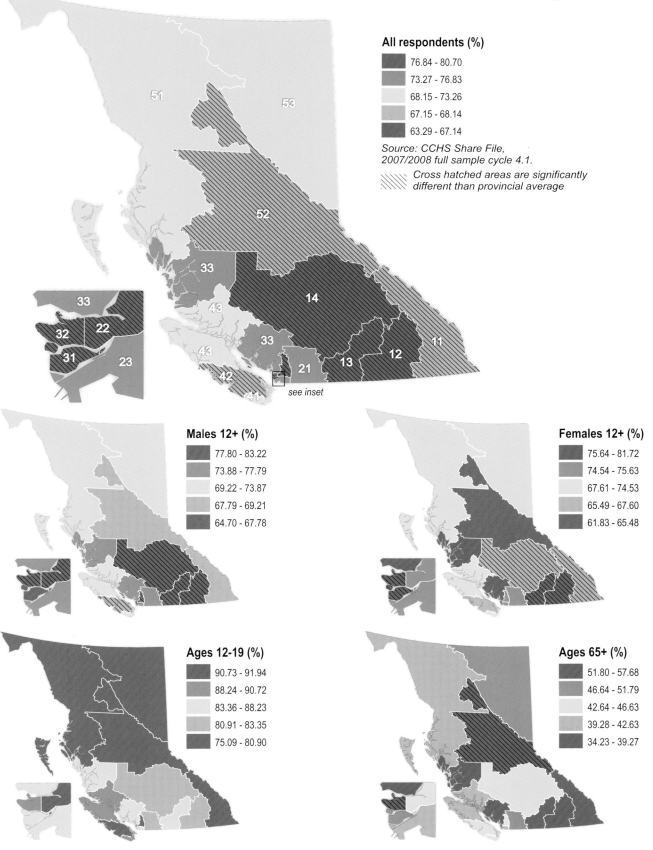

All respondents (%)

- 76.84 - 80.70
- 73.27 - 76.83
- 68.15 - 73.26
- 67.15 - 68.14
- 63.29 - 67.14

Source: CCHS Share File, 2007/2008 full sample cycle 4.1.

Cross hatched areas are significantly different than provincial average

Males 12+ (%)

- 77.80 - 83.22
- 73.88 - 77.79
- 69.22 - 73.87
- 67.79 - 69.21
- 64.70 - 67.78

Females 12+ (%)

- 75.64 - 81.72
- 74.54 - 75.63
- 67.61 - 74.53
- 65.49 - 67.60
- 61.83 - 65.48

Ages 12-19 (%)

- 90.73 - 91.94
- 88.24 - 90.72
- 83.36 - 88.23
- 80.91 - 83.35
- 75.09 - 80.90

Ages 65+ (%)

- 51.80 - 57.68
- 46.64 - 51.79
- 42.64 - 46.63
- 39.28 - 42.63
- 34.23 - 39.27

No long term physical, mental, or health condition that reduces activity at home

Health Service Delivery Area	All respondents 12+ (%)	Males 12+ (%)	Females 12+ (%)	Ages 12-19 (%)	Ages 20-64 (%)	Ages 65+ (%)
31 Richmond	85.96	88.85	83.24	92.21	89.33	64.74‡
32 Vancouver	85.27	87.87	82.72	95.21†	87.02	69.37‡
33 North Shore/Coast Garibaldi	84.83	85.78	83.91	97.27†	86.13	70.32‡
53 Northeast	83.30	86.77	79.54	91.98	83.90	64.88
22 Fraser North	82.67	86.72*	78.72	96.58†	84.25	60.78‡
23 Fraser South	82.32	84.43	80.25	93.02	84.96	57.76‡
21 Fraser East	82.16	83.34	80.99	93.03	83.99	64.83‡
51 Northwest	82.15	84.84	79.27	93.69†	83.10	61.96‡
52 Northern Interior	78.36	79.67	77.00	93.26†	79.76	51.88‡
41 South Vancouver Island	77.74	79.12	76.48	93.27†	79.78	61.29‡
11 East Kootenay	77.51	80.34	74.62	91.12†	78.09	65.90‡
43 North Vancouver Island	77.39	81.25	73.67	94.85†	80.55	51.96‡
12 Kootenay Boundary	75.69	78.04	73.26	93.44†	75.29	66.31
14 Thompson Cariboo Shuswap	75.11	75.92	74.30	89.58†	76.33	60.33‡
42 Central Vancouver Island	75.02	76.31	73.76	93.39†	76.01	61.43‡
13 Okanagan	71.67	76.37	67.23	95.29†	72.19	57.63‡
British Columbia (2007/8)	80.62	83.08*	78.23	94.05†	82.49	62.06‡
British Columbia (2005)	81.68	84.30*	79.13	93.73†	82.94	66.17‡

Crosshatching beside the 2007/8 provincial rate indicates it is significantly different than the 2005 rate, while crosshatched HSDAs are significantly different than the 2007/8 provincial rate.
E interpret data with caution (16.67 ≤ coefficient of variation ≤ 33.3).

* Males differ significantly from females.
† 12-19 age cohort differs significantly from the 20-64 age cohort.
‡ 65+ age cohort differs significantly from the 20-64 age cohort.
F data suppressed (n < 10, or coefficient of variation > 33.3).

British Columbia/Canada Cohort Comparison 2007/2008

Canada ■   British Columbia ▨
⊥ 95% confidence limits of estimate

Chronic conditions can render people unable to perform activities within the home. The CCHS asked respondents if they had a "*long-term physical condition or mental condition or health problem*" that reduces the amount or kind of activity they can do at home." These results reflect the number of people who were never limited at home by any long-term conditions.

Provincially, eight in every ten (80.62%) of all respondents did not have any physical, mental, or health condition that reduced activity at home. Richmond, Vancouver, and North Shore/Coast Garibaldi (all above 84%) had significantly higher values, while Okanagan, Thompson Cariboo Shuswap, and Central Vancouver Island (all below 76%) had significantly lower values than the provincial average.

BC males (83.08%) were significantly more likely than females (78.23%) to have no long-term condition affecting activity at home. Fraser North was the only HSDA in which males had a significantly higher value than their female counterparts. Among HSDA males, respondents in Richmond and Vancouver (both above 87%) had significantly higher values, and Thompson Cariboo Shuswap and Okanagan (both below 77%) had significantly lower values than the provincial average for males. Females in Richmond and North Shore/Coast Garibaldi (both above 83%) had significantly higher values, while Okanagan (67.23%) had significantly lower values than the provincial average for females.

Among youth in BC, 94.05% of respondents reported having no conditions that limited their activity at home,

significantly higher than the provincial average for the mid-age cohort. In almost every HSDA, youth had significantly higher values than their mid-age counterparts. No HSDA was significantly different from the provincial average for the youth cohort.

For older respondents, 62.06% reported having no conditions that would limit activity at home, a significantly lower average than the mid-age cohort. Almost every HSDA had a significantly lower value for older respondents in comparison to mid-age respondents. Comparing HSDA values to the provincial average for this cohort, only North Shore/Coast Garibaldi stood out, with a significantly higher than average value of 70.32%.

Differences were modest and varied, between 8 and 16 percentage points, among the cohorts. Geographically, lower values were clustered mostly in the southern interior and parts of Vancouver Island, while higher values were more likely in the urban south west of BC.

Between 2005 and 2007/8, the older age BC cohort was significantly lower in 2007/8. Compared to the national averages for this variable in 2007/8, all BC respondents were significantly more likely than other Canadians to have long-term conditions that limited activity at home. Among specific cohorts, only the BC older cohort had a significantly lower value than the Canadian average for that cohort.

No long term physical, mental, or health condition that reduces activity at home

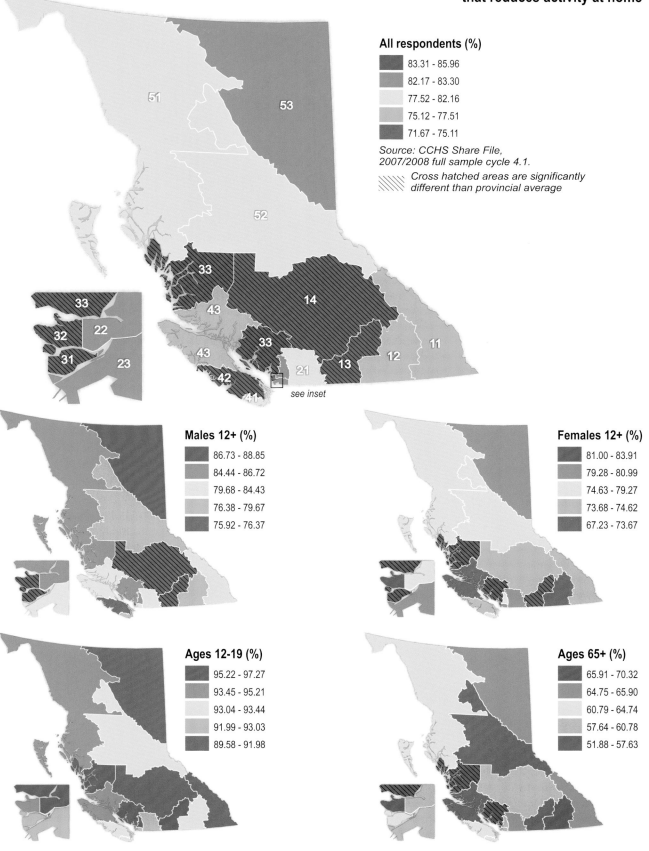

All respondents (%)

- 83.31 - 85.96
- 82.17 - 83.30
- 77.52 - 82.16
- 75.12 - 77.51
- 71.67 - 75.11

Source: CCHS Share File, 2007/2008 full sample cycle 4.1.

Cross hatched areas are significantly different than provincial average

Males 12+ (%)

- 86.73 - 88.85
- 84.44 - 86.72
- 79.68 - 84.43
- 76.38 - 79.67
- 75.92 - 76.37

Females 12+ (%)

- 81.00 - 83.91
- 79.28 - 80.99
- 74.63 - 79.27
- 73.68 - 74.62
- 67.23 - 73.67

Ages 12-19 (%)

- 95.22 - 97.27
- 93.45 - 95.21
- 93.04 - 93.44
- 91.99 - 93.03
- 89.58 - 91.98

Ages 65+ (%)

- 65.91 - 70.32
- 64.75 - 65.90
- 60.79 - 64.74
- 57.64 - 60.78
- 51.88 - 57.63

No long term physical, mental, or health condition that reduces activity outside the home

Health Service Delivery Area	All respondents 12+ (%)	Males 12+ (%)	Females 12+ (%)	Ages 12-19 (%)	Ages 20-64 (%)	Ages 65+ (%)
31 Richmond	86.27	87.14	85.46	92.40	88.04	73.03‡
51 Northwest	83.70	85.08	82.23	92.76	84.50	67.54
32 Vancouver	83.65	83.61	83.69	97.66†	84.13	72.54‡
53 Northeast	83.64	87.38	79.60	89.58	84.06	70.98
22 Fraser North	82.95	87.52*	78.48	97.12†	84.15	63.08‡
23 Fraser South	82.71	83.15	82.27	90.76	83.81	68.98‡
33 North Shore/Coast Garibaldi	82.54	84.56	80.60	97.09†	83.61	67.39‡
21 Fraser East	80.99	79.24	82.71	91.32	82.12	67.38‡
52 Northern Interior	79.26	80.74	77.72	93.60†	79.32	62.26‡
11 East Kootenay	78.95	80.79	77.06	91.55†	79.97	66.25‡
43 North Vancouver Island	78.43	82.89	74.12	89.53	80.51	61.99
14 Thompson Cariboo Shuswap	77.89	77.27	78.51	87.02	77.18	74.49
41 South Vancouver Island	76.14	77.42	74.98	88.72†	77.50	63.91‡
12 Kootenay Boundary	75.57	78.43	72.62	94.70†	75.28	64.97
42 Central Vancouver Island	75.50	76.54	74.50	85.47	74.94	71.76
13 Okanagan	74.93	77.88	72.14	90.42†	75.51	64.96
British Columbia (2007/8)	**80.68**	**82.13***	**79.26**	**92.35†**	**81.60**	**67.83‡**
British Columbia (2005)	**80.93**	**82.86***	**79.05**	**91.99†**	**81.73**	**68.35‡**

Crosshatching beside the 2007/8 provincial rate indicates it is significantly different than the 2005 rate, while crosshatched HSDAs are significantly different than the 2007/8 provincial rate.
E interpret data with caution (16.67 ≤ coefficient of variation ≤ 33.3).

* Males differ significantly from females.
† 12-19 age cohort differs significantly from the 20-64 age cohort.
‡ 65+ age cohort differs significantly from the 20-64 age cohort.
F data suppressed (n < 10, or coefficient of variation > 33.3).

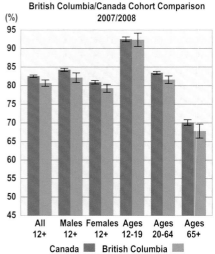

British Columbia/Canada Cohort Comparison 2007/2008

Canada ■ British Columbia ▨
I 95% confidence limits of estimate

The ability to function well for certain activities outside the home can enable an individual to be an active member of the community, and is an important wellness asset. The CCHS found that more than eight out of ten (80.68%) British Columbians were able to carry out regular daily activities outside of the home (including transportation and leisure activities) without restriction from long-term physical, mental, or health conditions. Compared to the provincial average, Richmond had significantly more respondents (86.27%) who were unrestricted by long-term conditions, while South Vancouver Island (76.14%) and Okanagan (74.93%) had significantly fewer.

In BC, male respondents (82.13%) were significantly more likely than female respondents (79.26%) to be free of restrictive long-term conditions. Males in Fraser North (87.52%) were also significantly higher than their female counterparts, and for males, it was also the only HSDA with a significantly higher value than the provincial average for males. For females, Richmond and Vancouver (both above 83%) had significantly higher values than the provincial female average, while Okanagan (72.14%) had a significantly lower value.

As might be expected, youth in BC (92.35%) were more likely to be free from restrictive long-term conditions than the mid-age cohort. There were also eight individual HSDAs in which the youth cohort had significantly higher rates than their mid-age counterparts. Youth respondents in Fraser North and Vancouver (both above 97%) were significantly more likely than the youth provincial average to be free from restrictive long-term conditions.

Older respondents (67.83%) had significantly lower levels of being free from long-term restrictions when compared with the mid-age cohort, and this significant difference was also evident in nine HSDAs across the province. There were no HSDAs that showed a significant difference when compared to the senior provincial average.

Geographically, there was a spread of more than 11 percentage points between HSDAs for all age cohorts. For each of the cohorts, consistently higher values were clustered in the southwest mainland, with a couple of exceptions (Fraser East and North Shore/Coast Garibaldi). Lower values for all respondents and males were clustered in south central BC, while for females there was a cluster of lower values in the southeast.

There were no significant differences for BC respondents between 2005 and 2007/8. British Columbians in all cohorts, except for youth and older respondents, had significantly lower values than their Canadian peers in 2007/8.

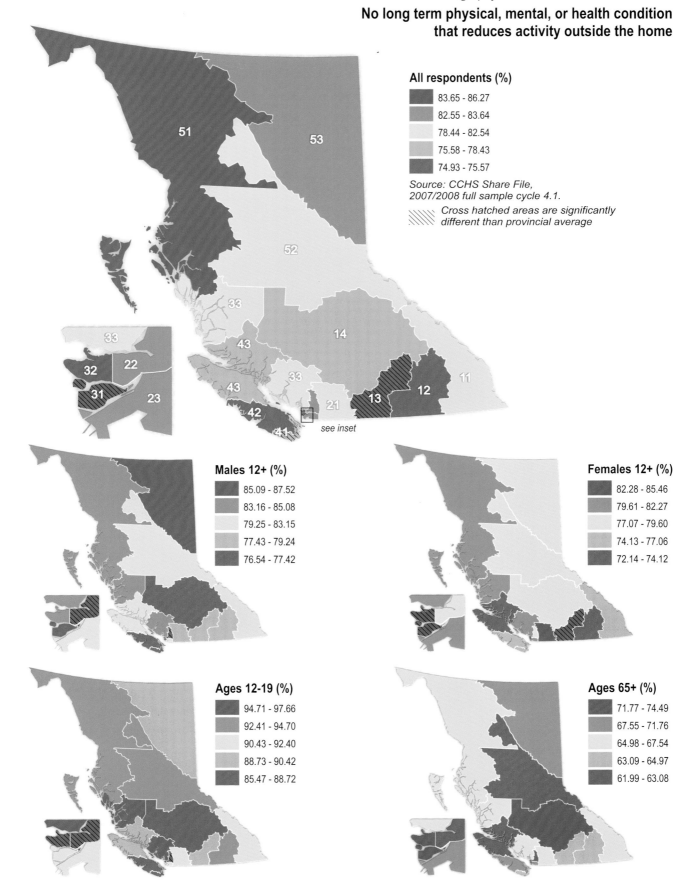

No long term physical, mental, or health condition that reduces activity outside the home

All respondents (%)

- 83.65 - 86.27
- 82.55 - 83.64
- 78.44 - 82.54
- 75.58 - 78.43
- 74.93 - 75.57

Source: CCHS Share File, 2007/2008 full sample cycle 4.1.

Cross hatched areas are significantly different than provincial average

Males 12+ (%)

- 85.09 - 87.52
- 83.16 - 85.08
- 79.25 - 83.15
- 77.43 - 79.24
- 76.54 - 77.42

Females 12+ (%)

- 82.28 - 85.46
- 79.61 - 82.27
- 77.07 - 79.60
- 74.13 - 77.06
- 72.14 - 74.12

Ages 12-19 (%)

- 94.71 - 97.66
- 92.41 - 94.70
- 90.43 - 92.40
- 88.73 - 90.42
- 85.47 - 88.72

Ages 65+ (%)

- 71.77 - 74.49
- 67.55 - 71.76
- 64.98 - 67.54
- 63.09 - 64.97
- 61.99 - 63.08

Never been diagnosed with high blood pressure

Health Service Delivery Area	All respondents 12+ (%)	Males 12+ (%)	Females 12+ (%)	Ages 35-49 (%)	Ages 50-64 (%)	Ages 65+ (%)
32 Vancouver	84.61	83.09	86.09	90.00†	77.38	45.31‡
23 Fraser South	83.98	85.95	82.05	90.11†	73.80	50.90‡
53 Northeast	83.23	82.94	83.55	84.91	82.10	39.93E‡
52 Northern Interior	82.07	83.76	80.31	85.64	72.63	45.09‡
21 Fraser East	82.01	84.83	79.24	90.45†	68.35	53.34
33 North Shore/Coast Garibaldi	81.58	82.58	80.63	86.94†	74.32	57.50‡
31 Richmond	79.80	82.04	77.68	88.98†	69.01	40.14‡
13 Okanagan	79.79	80.04	79.56	90.00†	69.04	55.59
41 South Vancouver Island	79.75	80.46	79.10	89.34†	68.55	53.98‡
22 Fraser North	79.67	79.21	80.12	86.78†	67.35	41.15‡
14 Thompson Cariboo Shuswap	79.39	78.19	80.59	88.66†	69.15	48.90‡
43 North Vancouver Island	78.24	82.09	74.54	86.06	71.14	52.17‡
11 East Kootenay	76.19	75.69	76.70	87.13†	59.31	47.12
12 Kootenay Boundary	76.03	75.62	76.45	73.47	73.68	51.53‡
51 Northwest	75.73	73.92	77.66	85.01†	56.05	44.16
42 Central Vancouver Island	74.93	74.49	75.35	85.01†	63.06	49.87
British Columbia (2007/8)	**80.94**	**81.39**	**80.50**	**88.24†**	**70.47**	**49.50‡**
British Columbia (2005)	**81.93**	**83.38***	**80.51**	**89.45†**	**70.93**	**50.59‡**

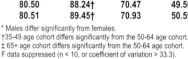

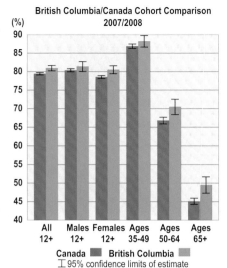

British Columbia/Canada Cohort Comparison 2007/2008

Canada ■   British Columbia ▨
⊥ 95% confidence limits of estimate

▨ Crosshatching beside the 2007/8 provincial rate indicates it is significantly different than the 2005 rate, while crosshatched HSDAs are significantly different than the 2007/8 provincial rate.
E interpret data with caution (16.67 ≤ coefficient of variation ≤ 33.3).

* Males differ significantly from females.
†35-49 age cohort differs significantly from the 50-64 age cohort.
‡ 65+ age cohort differs significantly from the 50-64 age cohort.
F data suppressed (n < 10, or coefficient of variation > 33.3).

High blood pressure is related to strokes, heart attacks, and cardiac arrest. High stress levels, eating foods high in fat and salt, consuming several alcoholic drinks daily, and smoking can raise blood pressure (Heart and Stroke Foundation of Canada, 2010). Results presented here analyse CCHS respondents who indicated that they had never been diagnosed with high blood pressure. Because high blood pressure is age-related, age cohorts used are different than the standard cohorts. It should be noted that high blood pressure is underestimated by about one-third in the Canadian population (Wilkins et al., 2010). This is a new indicator for the Atlas.

Four in every five (80.94%) respondents had never had a diagnosis of high blood pressure. Vancouver (84.61%) and Fraser South (83.98%) were both significantly higher, while East Kootenay, Northwest, and Central Vancouver Island (all 76% or lower) were significantly lower than the BC average. Males (81.39%) were more likely to have not had a high blood pressure diagnosis than females (80.50%), but the difference was not significant.

Among males, Fraser South (85.95%) was significantly higher, and Central Vancouver Island (74.49%) and Northwest (73.92%) were significantly lower than the BC male average. For females, Vancouver (86.09%) and North Vancouver Island (74.54%) were respectively significantly higher and lower than the BC average for females.

The younger (35 - 49 years) cohort was significantly higher (88.24%) than the 50 - 64 years mid-age cohort (70.47%); this significant difference was reflected in all but

four of the HSDAs. The seniors cohort was significantly lower than the mid-age cohort, and 11 individual HSDAs were significantly lower also. Fraser North (41.15%) and Richmond (40.14%) were both significantly lower than the average for seniors.

The percentage points spread among HSDAs ranged from 10 to more than 20. The mid-age group had the greatest spread, with Northeast, 82.10% compared with East Kootenay and Northwest both below 60%.

Geographically, patterns were varied. For all respondents and males and females cohorts, higher values occurred in parts of the lower mainland and the north, but this pattern was not always reflected for the different age cohorts. For the senior cohort, lower values were found in these same HSDAs, while many of the southern interior and southern and central coastal areas had higher than average values.

All BC cohorts had marginally lower values in 2007/8 than in 2005, but none of the differences were significant. For the 2007/8 samples, BC had higher values than Canada for every cohort, with significant differences for all respondents, females, and the age 50 - 64 and senior cohorts.

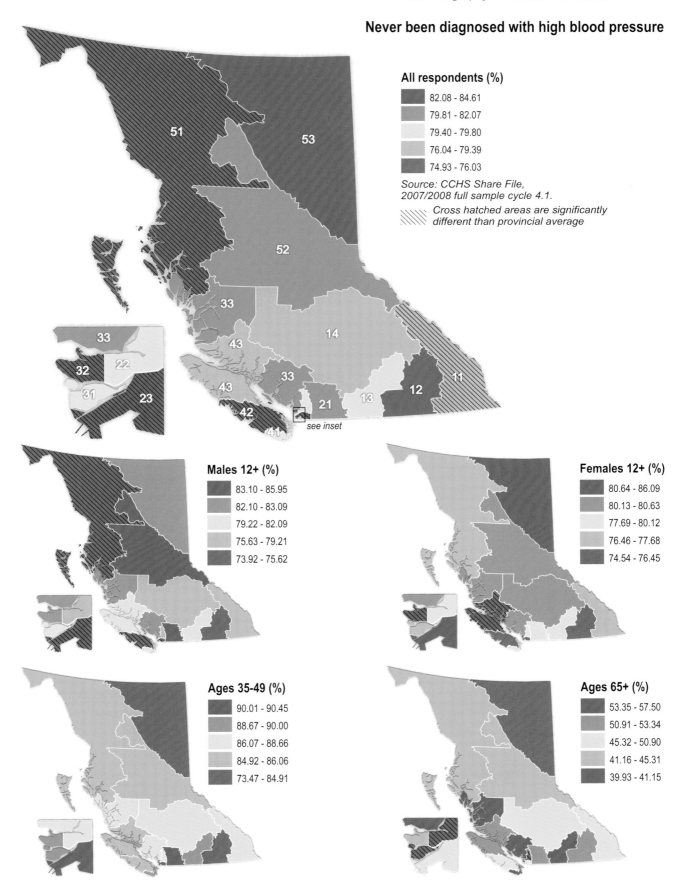

Never been diagnosed with high blood pressure

All respondents (%)

- 82.08 - 84.61
- 79.81 - 82.07
- 79.40 - 79.80
- 76.04 - 79.39
- 74.93 - 76.03

Source: CCHS Share File, 2007/2008 full sample cycle 4.1.

Cross hatched areas are significantly different than provincial average

Males 12+ (%)

- 83.10 - 85.95
- 82.10 - 83.09
- 79.22 - 82.09
- 75.63 - 79.21
- 73.92 - 75.62

Females 12+ (%)

- 80.64 - 86.09
- 80.13 - 80.63
- 77.69 - 80.12
- 76.46 - 77.68
- 74.54 - 76.45

Ages 35-49 (%)

- 90.01 - 90.45
- 88.67 - 90.00
- 86.07 - 88.66
- 84.92 - 86.06
- 73.47 - 84.91

Ages 65+ (%)

- 53.35 - 57.50
- 50.91 - 53.34
- 45.32 - 50.90
- 41.16 - 45.31
- 39.93 - 41.15

Never been diagnosed with cancer

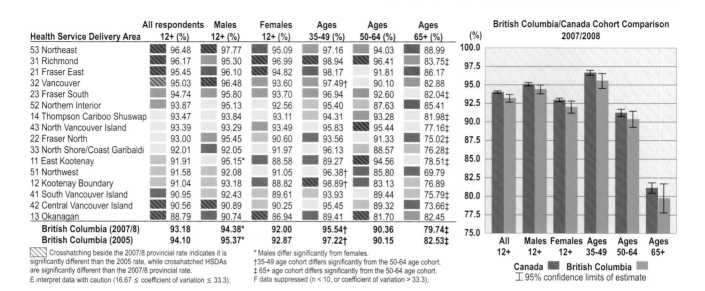

Health Service Delivery Area	All respondents 12+ (%)	Males 12+ (%)	Females 12+ (%)	Ages 35-49 (%)	Ages 50-64 (%)	Ages 65+ (%)
53 Northeast	96.48	97.77	95.09	97.16	94.03	88.99
31 Richmond	96.17	95.30	96.99	98.94	96.41	83.75‡
21 Fraser East	95.45	96.10	94.82	98.17	91.81	86.17
32 Vancouver	95.03	96.48	93.60	97.49†	90.10	82.88
23 Fraser South	94.74	95.80	93.70	96.94	92.60	82.04‡
52 Northern Interior	93.87	95.13	92.56	95.40	87.63	85.41
14 Thompson Cariboo Shuswap	93.47	93.84	93.11	94.31	93.28	81.98‡
43 North Vancouver Island	93.39	93.29	93.49	95.83	95.44	77.16‡
22 Fraser North	93.00	95.45	90.60	93.56	91.33	75.02‡
33 North Shore/Coast Garibaldi	92.01	92.05	91.97	96.13	88.57	76.28‡
11 East Kootenay	91.91	95.15*	88.58	89.27	94.56	78.51‡
51 Northwest	91.58	92.08	91.05	96.38†	85.80	69.79
12 Kootenay Boundary	91.04	93.18	88.82	98.89†	83.13	76.89
41 South Vancouver Island	90.95	92.43	89.61	93.93	89.44	75.79‡
42 Central Vancouver Island	90.56	90.89	90.25	95.45	89.32	73.66‡
13 Okanagan	88.79	90.74	86.94	89.41	81.70	82.45
British Columbia (2007/8)	**93.18**	**94.38***	**92.00**	**95.54†**	**90.36**	**79.74‡**
British Columbia (2005)	**94.10**	**95.37***	**92.87**	**97.22†**	**90.15**	**82.53‡**

Crosshatching beside the 2007/8 provincial rate indicates it is significantly different than the 2005 rate, while crosshatched HSDAs are significantly different than the 2007/8 provincial rate.
E interpret data with caution (16.67 ≤ coefficient of variation ≤ 33.3).

* Males differ significantly from females.
†35-49 age cohort differs significantly from the 50-64 age cohort.
‡ 65+ age cohort differs significantly from the 50-64 age cohort.
F data suppressed (n < 10, or coefficient of variation > 33.3).

Cancer is a chronic condition that is, in most cases, associated with older age. It is related to numerous factors, including lifestyle factors (e.g., smoking, heavy alcohol consumption) and environmental factors, among other things. In 2009, more than 8,900 people died in BC from cancer (Vital Statistics, 2010). Because this disease is primarily age-related, different age cohorts have been used, and we report those CCHS respondents who indicated that they had never been diagnosed with cancer. This is a new indicator for the Atlas.

More than nine in every ten (93.18%) respondents had never been diagnosed with cancer. Northeast, Richmond, Fraser East, and Vancouver (all more than 95%) were significantly higher than the provincial average, while Central Vancouver Island (90.56%) and Okanagan (88.79%) were significantly lower.

Male respondents (94.38%) were significantly more likely never to have been diagnosed with cancer than females (92.00%), but only East Kootenay, had a significantly higher value for males than females. Among male respondents, Northeast (97.77%) and Vancouver (96.48%) were significantly higher than the male average, while Central Vancouver Island (90.89%) was significantly lower. For females, Richmond (96.99%) and Fraser East (94.82%) were significantly higher, while Okanagan was significantly lower than the female average.

The 35 - 49 age cohort provincial average (95.54%) was significantly higher than the 50 to 64 age cohort average (90.36%), although only three individual HSDAs (Vancouver, Northwest, and Kootenay Boundary) were

significantly higher than their 50 - 64 age cohort counterparts. In the 35 - 49 age cohort, Richmond and Kootenay Boundary (both close to 99%) were significantly higher than the provincial average.

For the seniors cohort (age 65 and over), nearly eight in every ten respondents (79.74%) had never been diagnosed with cancer, significantly lower than the average for the 50 to 64 age cohort, and this significant different was also found in nine of the individual HSDAs. No HSDA for seniors was significantly different from the provincial average for seniors.

Geographically, there was not much consistency among cohorts by HSDA. Generally, the southern half of Vancouver Island had consistently low values, while the southeast part of the province also had lower values, although this was not always consistent. Parts of the lower mainland had high values, especially Richmond, as did Northeast, which was an outlier in the north.

Compared to the 2005 CCHS sample, each cohort of the 2007/8 sample had a lower value, except for the 50 - 64 age cohort, but no difference was significant. Compared to the Canadian 2007/8 sample, BC cohorts were lower, but the difference was significant only for the all respondents cohort.

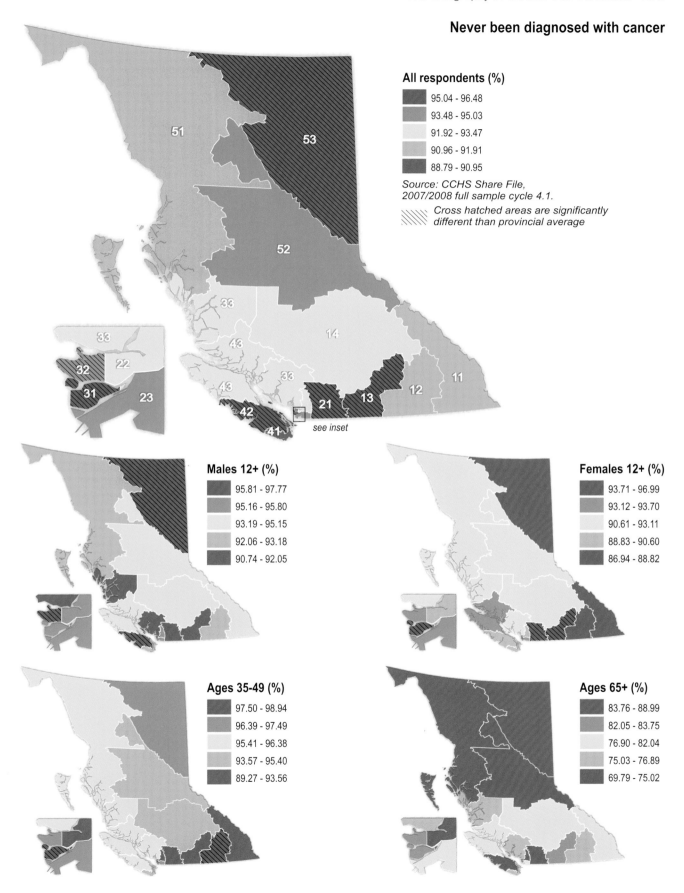

Never been diagnosed with cancer

All respondents (%)

- 95.04 - 96.48
- 93.48 - 95.03
- 91.92 - 93.47
- 90.96 - 91.91
- 88.79 - 90.95

Source: CCHS Share File, 2007/2008 full sample cycle 4.1.

Cross hatched areas are significantly different than provincial average

Males 12+ (%)

- 95.81 - 97.77
- 95.16 - 95.80
- 93.19 - 95.15
- 92.06 - 93.18
- 90.74 - 92.05

Females 12+ (%)

- 93.71 - 96.99
- 93.12 - 93.70
- 90.61 - 93.11
- 88.83 - 90.60
- 86.94 - 88.82

Ages 35-49 (%)

- 97.50 - 98.94
- 96.39 - 97.49
- 95.41 - 96.38
- 93.57 - 95.40
- 89.27 - 93.56

Ages 65+ (%)

- 83.76 - 88.99
- 82.05 - 83.75
- 76.90 - 82.04
- 75.03 - 76.89
- 69.79 - 75.02

Without arthritis or rheumatism

Health Service Delivery Area	All respondents 12+ (%)	Males 12+ (%)	Females 12+ (%)	Ages 35-49 (%)	Ages 50-64 (%)	Ages 65+ (%)
31 Richmond	89.85	93.18*	86.70	96.23†	83.89	65.69‡
32 Vancouver	88.09	90.55	85.62	95.59†	77.98	58.21‡
22 Fraser North	87.87	90.83*	84.99	90.52	84.04	62.68‡
23 Fraser South	87.04	90.30*	83.85	92.00†	79.21	59.74‡
33 North Shore/Coast Garibaldi	86.06	88.23	83.97	89.45	78.28	68.30
12 Kootenay Boundary	84.70	88.03	81.23	93.37†	70.03	69.60
52 Northern Interior	84.65	84.89	84.40	90.63†	73.04	51.05‡
53 Northeast	84.65	88.15	80.86	85.45†	64.94	67.83
21 Fraser East	84.19	87.28	81.14	89.30†	74.11	56.91‡
14 Thompson Cariboo Shuswap	83.89	86.31	81.47	86.19	77.94	63.71‡
41 South Vancouver Island	83.23	84.37	82.19	92.17†	73.79	58.50‡
51 Northwest	81.66	84.12	79.01	80.53	73.94	59.96
42 Central Vancouver Island	81.35	86.48*	76.39	90.47†	74.51	59.67‡
43 North Vancouver Island	79.98	81.40	78.62	89.63†	69.49	52.37
11 East Kootenay	77.69	81.53	73.77	87.97†	61.92	55.00
13 Okanagan	77.34	81.16	73.70	83.82†	60.60	56.08
British Columbia (2007/8)	**85.01**	**87.84***	**82.24**	**90.87†**	**75.91**	**59.97‡**
British Columbia (2005)	**84.31**	**87.93***	**80.78**	**88.70†**	**74.97**	**57.67‡**

Crosshatching beside the 2007/8 provincial rate indicates it is significantly different than the 2005 rate, while crosshatched HSDAs are significantly different than the 2007/8 provincial rate.
E interpret data with caution (16.67 ≤ coefficient of variation ≤ 33.3).

* Males differ significantly from females.
†35-49 age cohort differs significantly from the 50-64 age cohort.
‡ 65+ age cohort differs significantly from the 50-64 age cohort.
F data suppressed (n < 10, or coefficient of variation > 33.3).

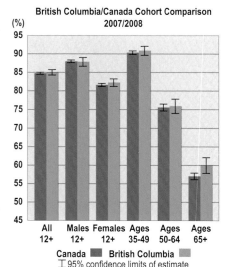

British Columbia/Canada Cohort Comparison 2007/2008

Canada ■ British Columbia ▨
⊥ 95% confidence limits of estimate

Arthritis symptoms include pain, joint inflammation, and swelling. Causes include injury, metabolic abnormalities, hereditary factors, the direct and indirect effect of infections, and a misdirected immune system with autoimmunity (such as in rheumatoid arthritis). Because this condition is age-related, different age cohorts are used in this analysis. Data presented here are based on CCHS respondents who indicated that they were not diagnosed with arthritis or rheumatism. This is a new indicator for the Atlas.

In BC, 85.01% of all respondents indicated they were not diagnosed with arthritis or rheumatism. Among HSDAs, Richmond (89.85%) and Vancouver (88.09%) had significantly higher values than average, while Central Vancouver Island (81.66%), North Vancouver Island (79.98%), East Kootenay (77.69%), and Okanagan (77.34%) all were significantly lower. Males (87.84%) were significantly more likely than females (82.24%) to have no such diagnosis, and this higher value for males occurred for each individual HSDA, although it was only significant in four HSDAs.

For males, Richmond (93.18%) was significantly higher, while East Kootenay, North Vancouver Island, and Okanagan (all below 82%) were significantly lower than the BC average. For females, Central Vancouver Island (76.39%) and East Kootenay and Okanagan (both below 74%) were significantly lower than average.

Not being diagnosed with arthritis or rheumatism fell with age. The younger age cohort (35 - 49 years) was significantly more likely to not be diagnosed (90.87%) than

the mid-age cohort (75.91%). Every HSDA had a higher value for the younger age cohort, and the difference was significant for 12 of the HSDAs. Significantly higher values for the younger age cohort were found in Richmond and Vancouver (both above 95%).

Among seniors (age 65 and over), fewer than six in ten (59.97%) respondents were not diagnosed, and this was significantly lower than the mid-age cohort. Each HSDA had a lower value for seniors than the mid-age cohort, and the difference was significant for nine HSDAs. There were no significant differences among HSDAs for seniors.

Geographically, there were major differences among HSDAs, with variations between 12 and 25 percentage points. Higher values were found in the urban lower mainland, especially Richmond, while lower values were seen in East Kootenay, Okanagan, Northwest, and parts of Vancouver Island.

All cohorts in BC had higher values in 2007/8 than 2005, with the exception of all males, but none of the differences were significant. For the 2007/8 samples, the values for BC and Canada were similar (except for seniors), and there were no significant differences for any of the cohorts.

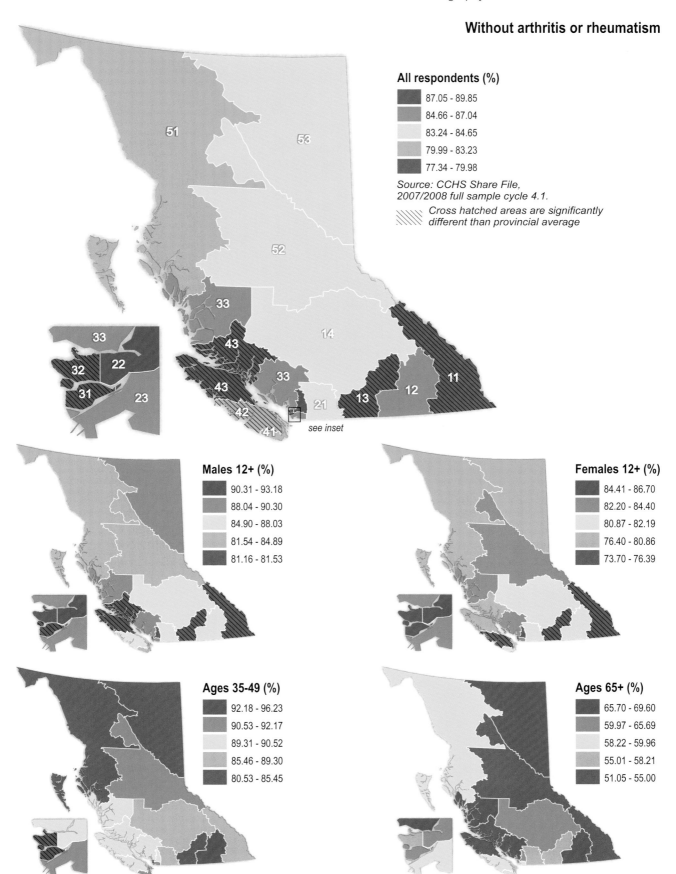

Without arthritis or rheumatism

All respondents (%)

- 87.05 - 89.85
- 84.66 - 87.04
- 83.24 - 84.65
- 79.99 - 83.23
- 77.34 - 79.98

Source: CCHS Share File, 2007/2008 full sample cycle 4.1.

Cross hatched areas are significantly different than provincial average

see inset

Males 12+ (%)

- 90.31 - 93.18
- 88.04 - 90.30
- 84.90 - 88.03
- 81.54 - 84.89
- 81.16 - 81.53

Females 12+ (%)

- 84.41 - 86.70
- 82.20 - 84.40
- 80.87 - 82.19
- 76.40 - 80.86
- 73.70 - 76.39

Ages 35-49 (%)

- 92.18 - 96.23
- 90.53 - 92.17
- 89.31 - 90.52
- 85.46 - 89.30
- 80.53 - 85.45

Ages 65+ (%)

- 65.70 - 69.60
- 59.97 - 65.69
- 58.22 - 59.96
- 55.01 - 58.21
- 51.05 - 55.00

Without asthma

Health Service Delivery Area	All respondents 12+ (%)	Males 12+ (%)	Females 12+ (%)	Ages 12-19 (%)	Ages 20-64 (%)	Ages 65+ (%)
31 Richmond	95.55	95.59	95.52	94.50	95.76	95.32
23 Fraser South	94.60	94.85	94.35	93.33	95.14	92.87
32 Vancouver	94.22	94.86	93.60	92.89	94.09	95.79
33 North Shore/Coast Garibaldi	93.55	93.86	93.24	97.22	92.33	96.20
13 Okanagan	93.53	94.71	92.40	92.40	93.06	95.59
22 Fraser North	93.20	92.89	93.50	98.92†	92.02	94.87
21 Fraser East	92.49	94.95	90.08	92.93	92.27	93.11
51 Northwest	92.19	93.70	90.57	88.52	92.08	97.41
11 East Kootenay	91.94	93.97	89.85	80.76	92.71	96.28
42 Central Vancouver Island	91.89	93.46	90.37	91.67	92.92	88.64
41 South Vancouver Island	91.80	90.42	93.05	84.81	91.48	96.89‡
12 Kootenay Boundary	91.75	90.61	92.93	92.16	90.50	96.26
14 Thompson Cariboo Shuswap	91.67	91.99	91.35	92.04	91.67	91.43
52 Northern Interior	91.29	94.67*	87.76	93.40	91.45	87.90
53 Northeast	89.85	91.16	88.44	93.14	89.21	90.16
43 North Vancouver Island	89.81	92.46	87.25	84.58	91.86	85.34
British Columbia (2007/8)	**93.13**	**93.72**	**92.55**	**92.84**	**93.01**	**93.90**
British Columbia (2005)	**91.84**	**93.06***	**90.65**	**89.58†**	**92.05**	**92.58**

Crosshatching beside the 2007/8 provincial rate indicates it is significantly different than the 2005 rate, while crosshatched HSDAs are significantly different than the 2007/8 provincial rate.
E interpret data with caution (16.67 ≤ coefficient of variation ≤ 33.3).

* Males differ significantly from females.
†12-19 age cohort differs significantly from the 20-64 age cohort.
‡ 65+ age cohort differs significantly from the 20-64 age cohort.
F data suppressed (n < 10, or coefficient of variation > 33.3).

British Columbia/Canada Cohort Comparison 2007/2008

Canada █   British Columbia ▒
⊥ 95% confidence limits of estimate

Asthma is a chronic inflammatory disease that can cause shortness of breath, tightness in the chest, coughing, and wheezing. Asthma can first be diagnosed at any age, but often starts in childhood. The table and maps opposite show the results of those CCHS respondents who indicated that they were not diagnosed with asthma. This is a new indicator for the Atlas.

Overall, 93.13% of BC respondents were not diagnosed with asthma. Richmond (95.55%) was significantly higher than average, while North Vancouver Island (89.81%) was significantly lower. Males (93.72%) were not significantly different than females (92.55%). This differed from 2005, when males were significantly higher. For the 2007/8 results, male respondents in Northern Interior had a significantly higher value than their female counterparts.

There was little variation among HSDAs for male respondents. For females, Richmond (95.52%) was significantly higher, while Northern Interior (87.76%) was significantly lower than the female average for BC.

While not being diagnosed with asthma increased with age, the differences were not significant, unlike for the 2005 sample, when the youth cohort was significantly lower than the mid-age cohort. Provincially, 92.84% of youth in 2007/8 were not diagnosed with asthma. Fraser North (98.92%) had a significantly higher value than the provincial average, and youth in this HSDA had a significantly higher value than the mid-age group.

Among seniors, 93.90% of respondents were not diagnosed with asthma, and no HSDA was significantly

different from the seniors' provincial average. South Vancouver Island seniors had a significantly higher value than their mid-age counterparts.

Geographically, the spread in values among HSDAs varied between 5 and 14 percentage points. The youth cohort showed the biggest variation. There were no consistent overall geographic patterns, although males and females had fairly similar patterns: lower mainland HSDAs tended to have higher than average values, while North Vancouver Island and Northeast had relatively low values. For youth, some lower mainland HSDAs had high values, along with some northern HSDAs, while Vancouver Island had low values, as did Northwest, Thompson Cariboo Shuswap, and East Kootenay. In contrast, the highest values for seniors were found in South Vancouver Island, East Kootenay, and Northwest, while the lowest values occurred on the rest of Vancouver Island and the Northern Interior. Northeast, Thompson Cariboo Shuswap, and South Fraser also had low values.

In comparison to 2005 CCHS samples, all BC cohorts had higher values in 2007/8, and these differences were significant for all respondents, females, and youth cohorts. For the 2007/8 samples, BC respondents had higher values than their Canadian counterparts for all cohorts, and these differences were significant for all respondents, females, and youth cohorts.

Without asthma

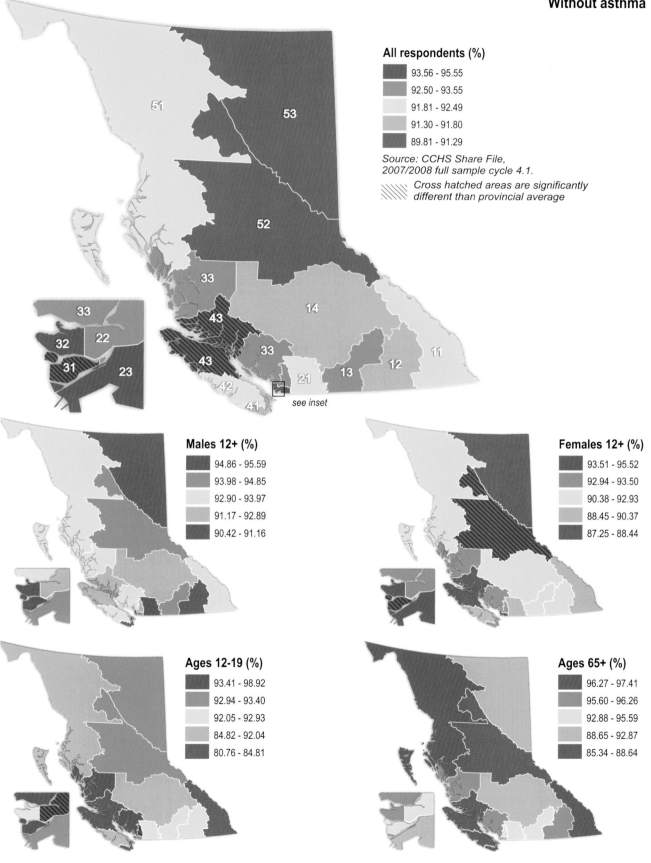

All respondents (%)

- 93.56 - 95.55
- 92.50 - 93.55
- 91.81 - 92.49
- 91.30 - 91.80
- 89.81 - 91.29

*Source: CCHS Share File,
2007/2008 full sample cycle 4.1.*

Cross hatched areas are significantly
different than provincial average

see inset

Males 12+ (%)

- 94.86 - 95.59
- 93.98 - 94.85
- 92.90 - 93.97
- 91.17 - 92.89
- 90.42 - 91.16

Females 12+ (%)

- 93.51 - 95.52
- 92.94 - 93.50
- 90.38 - 92.93
- 88.45 - 90.37
- 87.25 - 88.44

Ages 12-19 (%)

- 93.41 - 98.92
- 92.94 - 93.40
- 92.05 - 92.93
- 84.82 - 92.04
- 80.76 - 84.81

Ages 65+ (%)

- 96.27 - 97.41
- 95.60 - 96.26
- 92.88 - 95.59
- 88.65 - 92.87
- 85.34 - 88.64

Without back problems

Health Service Delivery Area	All respondents 12+ (%)	Males 12+ (%)	Females 12+ (%)	Ages 12-19 (%)	Ages 20-64 (%)	Ages 65+ (%)
31 Richmond	82.74	83.57	81.96	96.42†	83.32	69.97‡
32 Vancouver	80.76	81.70	79.84	91.05†	80.78	74.52
33 North Shore/Coast Garibaldi	80.39	79.74	81.01	88.38	81.55	69.68‡
22 Fraser North	79.23	81.50	77.02	95.04†	77.63	74.22
21 Fraser East	78.92	82.04	75.88	90.43†	77.48	75.52
14 Thompson Cariboo Shuswap	78.32	77.96	78.69	93.32†	79.45	63.59‡
51 Northwest	77.86	80.42	75.11	96.36†	76.54	63.14‡
23 Fraser South	76.41	76.95	75.89	90.58†	75.89	65.74‡
42 Central Vancouver Island	75.79	77.19	74.44	84.89	75.26	72.42
53 Northeast	75.38	75.84	74.88	89.21†	72.31	79.59
52 Northern Interior	74.74	74.01	75.50	88.76†	73.68	65.56
41 South Vancouver Island	73.39	74.62	72.28	94.35†	71.74	68.29
43 North Vancouver Island	73.07	73.40	72.75	83.69	72.17	68.98
11 East Kootenay	72.73	74.85	70.55	85.48	73.66	60.28
13 Okanagan	71.67	72.35	71.02	87.23†	69.92	69.07
12 Kootenay Boundary	70.70	74.85	66.42	81.46	69.25	69.71
British Columbia (2007/8)	77.22	78.31	76.16	90.70†	76.65	70.03‡
British Columbia (2005)	80.16	81.23	79.11	92.42†	79.18	75.29‡

Crosshatching beside the 2007/8 provincial rate indicates it is significantly different than the 2005 rate, while crosshatched HSDAs are significantly different than the 2007/8 provincial rate.
E interpret data with caution (16.67 ≤ coefficient of variation ≤ 33.3).

* Males differ significantly from females.
† 12-19 age cohort differs significantly from the 20-64 age cohort.
‡ 65+ age cohort differs significantly from the 20-64 age cohort.
F data suppressed (n < 10, or coefficient of variation > 33.3).

British Columbia/Canada Cohort Comparison 2007/2008

Canada   British Columbia
95% confidence limits of estimate

Chronic back problems can be very painful and can limit participation in a wide variety of basic activities, as well as interfere with life's enjoyment. CCHS participants were asked if they had any back problems, excluding arthritis and fibromyalgia. In British Columbia, almost eight in every ten (77.22%) of all respondents reported being free of back problems. Respondents in Richmond and Vancouver (both above 80%) were significantly more likely to be free from back problems than average, while those in Okanagan and Kootenay Boundary (both below 72%) were significantly less likely than the provincial average to be free of back problems.

Comparing males (78.31%) to females (76.16%) in the province, there were no significant differences at the provincial or HSDA levels. Comparing the provincial average to HSDA values for both females and males also showed no significant differences, except in East Kootenay where females (70.55%) were significantly less likely than their peers provincially to be free of back problems.

Youth in the province (90.70%) were significantly more likely than their mid-age counterparts to be free of back problems, and the same significant difference was apparent in 11 HSDAs. Comparing individual HSDA youth average responses to the provincial average for youth indicated that there were no significant differences.

For older respondents, the provincial average of 70.03% was significantly lower than that of the mid-age cohort, and five HSDAs also had significantly lower values for older respondents when compared with their mid-age

counterparts. There were also no significant differences between HSDA and provincial rates for older respondents.

The difference among HSDAs for all cohorts was 10 to 15 percentage points. Geographically, lower values of being free from back problems were more likely in the southeast and southern interior of the province, while higher average values were seen in the urban south west, especially Richmond, Vancouver, and parts of the Fraser valley.

The BC sample of respondents was consistently lower for all cohorts for 2007/8 when compared with 2005, and these differences were significant for all cohorts except males and youth. When British Columbians were compared to the national averages, they appeared to be particularly prone to back problems, as respondents in every cohort except the youth cohort were significantly less likely to be free of back problems than their Canadian counterparts in 2007/8.

Without back problems

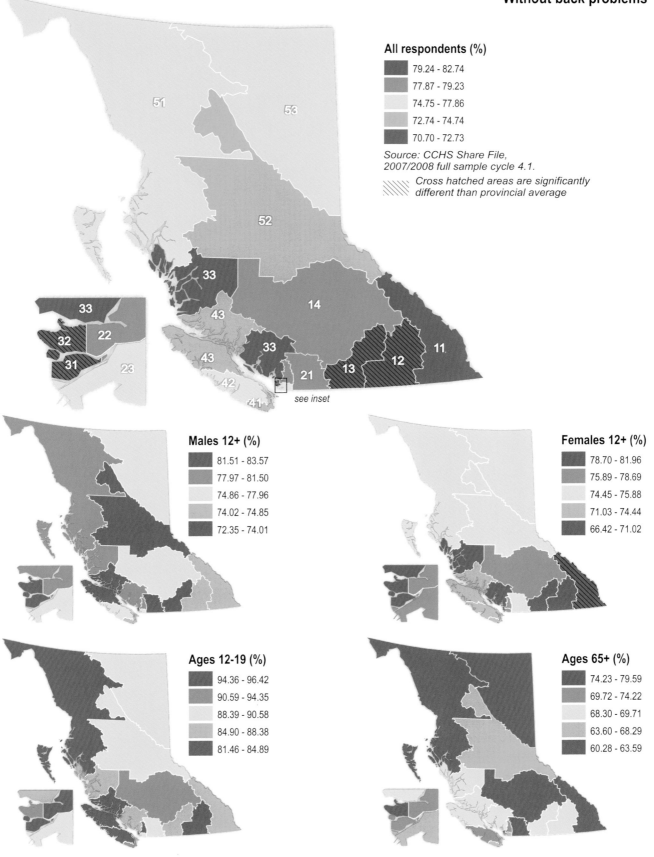

All respondents (%)

- 79.24 - 82.74
- 77.87 - 79.23
- 74.75 - 77.86
- 72.74 - 74.74
- 70.70 - 72.73

Source: CCHS Share File, 2007/2008 full sample cycle 4.1.

Cross hatched areas are significantly different than provincial average

see inset

Males 12+ (%)

- 81.51 - 83.57
- 77.97 - 81.50
- 74.86 - 77.96
- 74.02 - 74.85
- 72.35 - 74.01

Females 12+ (%)

- 78.70 - 81.96
- 75.89 - 78.69
- 74.45 - 75.88
- 71.03 - 74.44
- 66.42 - 71.02

Ages 12-19 (%)

- 94.36 - 96.42
- 90.59 - 94.35
- 88.39 - 90.58
- 84.90 - 88.38
- 81.46 - 84.89

Ages 65+ (%)

- 74.23 - 79.59
- 69.72 - 74.22
- 68.30 - 69.71
- 63.60 - 68.29
- 60.28 - 63.59

Without diabetes

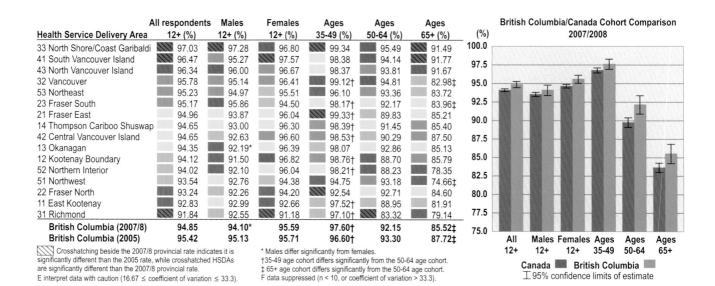

Health Service Delivery Area	All respondents 12+ (%)	Males 12+ (%)	Females 12+ (%)	Ages 35-49 (%)	Ages 50-64 (%)	Ages 65+ (%)
33 North Shore/Coast Garibaldi	97.03	97.28	96.80	99.34	95.49	91.49
41 South Vancouver Island	96.47	95.27	97.57	98.38	94.14	91.77
43 North Vancouver Island	96.34	96.00	96.67	98.37	93.81	91.67
32 Vancouver	95.78	95.14	96.41	99.12†	94.81	82.98‡
53 Northeast	95.23	94.97	95.51	96.10	93.36	83.72
23 Fraser South	95.17	95.86	94.50	98.17†	92.17	83.96‡
21 Fraser East	94.96	93.87	96.04	99.33†	89.83	85.21
14 Thompson Cariboo Shuswap	94.65	93.00	96.30	98.39†	91.45	85.40
42 Central Vancouver Island	94.65	92.63	96.60	98.53†	90.29	87.50
13 Okanagan	94.35	92.19*	96.39	98.07	92.86	85.13
12 Kootenay Boundary	94.12	91.50	96.82	98.76†	88.70	85.79
52 Northern Interior	94.02	92.10	96.04	98.21†	88.23	78.35
51 Northwest	93.54	92.76	94.38	94.75	93.18	74.66‡
22 Fraser North	93.24	92.26	94.20	92.54	92.71	84.60
11 East Kootenay	92.83	92.99	92.66	97.52†	88.95	81.91
31 Richmond	91.84	92.55	91.18	97.10†	83.32	79.14
British Columbia (2007/8)	94.85	94.10*	95.59	97.60†	92.15	85.52‡
British Columbia (2005)	95.42	95.13	95.71	96.60†	93.30	87.72‡

Crosshatching beside the 2007/8 provincial rate indicates it is significantly different than the 2005 rate, while crosshatched HSDAs are significantly different than the 2007/8 provincial rate.
E interpret data with caution (16.67 ≤ coefficient of variation ≤ 33.3).

* Males differ significantly from females.
† 35-49 age cohort differs significantly from the 50-64 age cohort.
‡ 65+ age cohort differs significantly from the 50-64 age cohort.
F data suppressed (n < 10, or coefficient of variation > 33.3).

Diabetes is often associated with poor nutrition and lack of exercise resulting in unhealthy weight. Most diabetes is age-related, although type 1 diabetes is often diagnosed in much younger people, and gestational diabetes is a temporary condition associated with pregnancy. Because this chronic disease is mainly age-related, different age cohorts have been used in this analysis, which focuses on those CCHS respondents who indicated that they were not diagnosed with diabetes. This is a new indicator for the Atlas.

In BC, 94.85% of CCHS respondents (age 12 and over) indicated they were not diagnosed with diabetes. North Shore/Coast Garibaldi (97.03%) and South Vancouver Island (96.47%) were significantly higher than the provincial average, while Richmond (91.84%) was significantly lower. Provincially, male respondents (94.10%) were significantly less likely to not be diagnosed with diabetes than females (95.59%), but this significant difference was only reflected at the individual HSDA level in Okanagan.

For male respondents, North Shore/Coast Garibaldi (97.28%) was significantly higher than average. For females, South Vancouver Island (97.57%) was significantly higher, while Richmond (91.18%) was significantly lower than the BC average for females.

For the younger cohort (35 - 49 years), 97.60% were not diagnosed, significantly higher than the 92.15% for the 50 - 64 age cohort. This higher value was consistent for all but one HSDA (Fraser North), and was significant for nine HSDAs. For the 35 - 49 age cohort, North Shore/Coast

Garibaldi (99.34%) and Fraser East (99.33%) were significantly higher than the provincial average, while Fraser North (92.54%) was significantly lower.

Among seniors, 85.52% were not diagnosed, significantly lower than the 50 - 64 age cohort. This difference was also significant for Vancouver, Fraser South, and Northwest. Older respondents in South Vancouver Island (91.77%) and North Shore/Coast Garibaldi (91.49%) were both significantly higher than the provincial average for seniors.

Throughout the province, there was little geographical variation (a range of 4 to 6 percentage points), except for the two higher age cohorts, which had a range of 14 to 16 percentage points. Higher values, however, were consistently found on parts of Vancouver Island and North Shore/Coast Garibaldi, with lower values in Richmond, and to some extent in East Kootenay.

All cohorts in BC were marginally lower in 2007/8 than in 2005, except for the 35 - 49 age cohort, but none was significantly so. Compared to Canada for 2007/8, BC had higher values, and differences were significant for all respondents, females, and the 50 - 64 age cohorts.

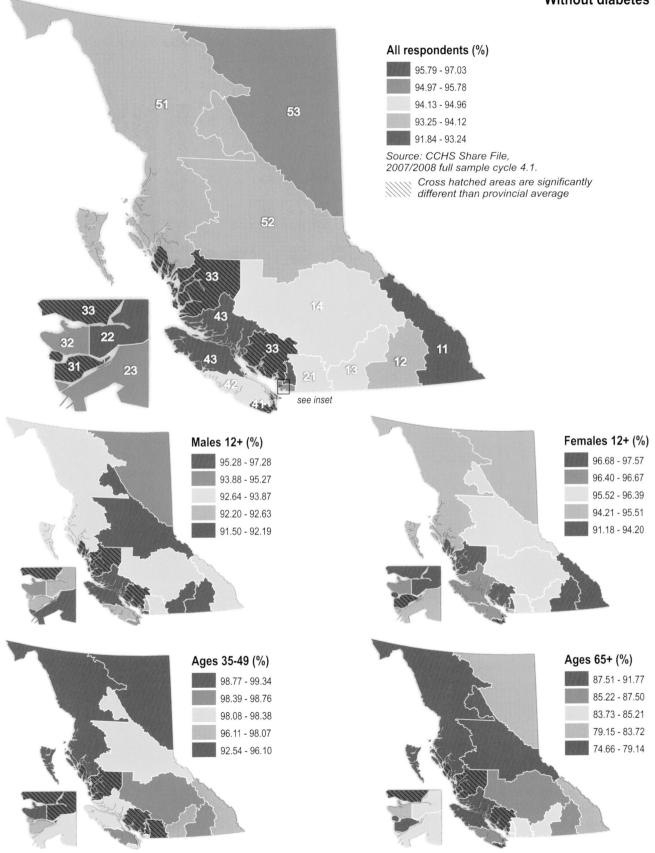

Without diabetes

All respondents (%)

- 95.79 - 97.03
- 94.97 - 95.78
- 94.13 - 94.96
- 93.25 - 94.12
- 91.84 - 93.24

Source: CCHS Share File, 2007/2008 full sample cycle 4.1.

Cross hatched areas are significantly different than provincial average

Males 12+ (%)

- 95.28 - 97.28
- 93.88 - 95.27
- 92.64 - 93.87
- 92.20 - 92.63
- 91.50 - 92.19

Females 12+ (%)

- 96.68 - 97.57
- 96.40 - 96.67
- 95.52 - 96.39
- 94.21 - 95.51
- 91.18 - 94.20

Ages 35-49 (%)

- 98.77 - 99.34
- 98.39 - 98.76
- 98.08 - 98.38
- 96.11 - 98.07
- 92.54 - 96.10

Ages 65+ (%)

- 87.51 - 91.77
- 85.22 - 87.50
- 83.73 - 85.21
- 79.15 - 83.72
- 74.66 - 79.14

Without heart disease

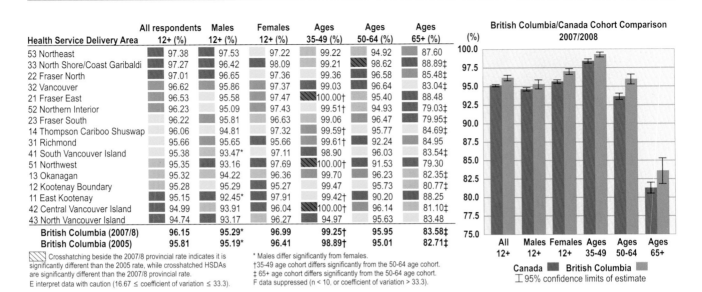

Health Service Delivery Area	All respondents 12+ (%)	Males 12+ (%)	Females 12+ (%)	Ages 35-49 (%)	Ages 50-64 (%)	Ages 65+ (%)
53 Northeast	97.38	97.53	97.22	99.22	94.92	87.60
33 North Shore/Coast Garibaldi	97.27	96.42	98.09	99.21	98.62	88.89‡
22 Fraser North	97.01	96.65	97.36	99.36	96.58	85.48‡
32 Vancouver	96.62	95.86	97.37	99.03	96.64	83.04‡
21 Fraser East	96.53	95.58	97.47	100.00†	95.40	88.48
52 Northern Interior	96.23	95.09	97.43	99.51†	94.93	79.03‡
23 Fraser South	96.22	95.81	96.63	99.06	96.47	79.95‡
14 Thompson Cariboo Shuswap	96.06	94.81	97.32	99.59†	95.77	84.69‡
31 Richmond	95.66	95.65	95.66	99.61†	92.24	84.95
41 South Vancouver Island	95.38	93.47*	97.11	98.90	96.03	83.54‡
51 Northwest	95.35	93.16	97.69	100.00†	91.53	79.30
13 Okanagan	95.32	94.22	96.36	99.70	96.23	82.35‡
12 Kootenay Boundary	95.28	95.29	95.27	99.47	95.73	80.77‡
11 East Kootenay	95.15	92.45*	97.91	99.42†	90.20	88.25
42 Central Vancouver Island	94.99	93.91	96.04	100.00†	96.14	81.10‡
43 North Vancouver Island	94.74	93.17	96.27	94.97	95.63	83.48
British Columbia (2007/8)	**96.15**	**95.29***	**96.99**	**99.25†**	**95.95**	**83.58‡**
British Columbia (2005)	**95.81**	**95.19***	**96.41**	**98.89†**	**95.01**	**82.71‡**

Crosshatching beside the 2007/8 provincial rate indicates it is significantly different than the 2005 rate, while crosshatched HSDAs are significantly different than the 2007/8 provincial rate.
E interpret data with caution (16.67 ≤ coefficient of variation ≤ 33.3).

* Males differ significantly from females.
†35-49 age cohort differs significantly from the 50-64 age cohort.
‡ 65+ age cohort differs significantly from the 50-64 age cohort.
F data suppressed (n < 10, or coefficient of variation > 33.3).

Heart disease, also called cardiovascular disease, is a common chronic condition, often related to smoking, unhealthy weight, chronic stress, and poor exercise, as well as other factors. In 2009, nearly 6,600 people died from cardiovascular disease (Vital Statistics Agency, 2010). The table and maps opposite show the results of those CCHS respondents who indicated that they were not diagnosed with heart disease. Heart disease, like many chronic diseases, is usually age-related, and so the age cohorts for analysis are different from most of the other CCHS indicators. This is a new indicator for the Atlas.

Overall, 96.15% of respondents (age 12 years and over) in BC indicated that they were not diagnosed with heart disease. There was very little variation among HSDAs, and no HSDA was significantly different from the provincial average. Provincially, the average for all male respondents (95.29%) was significantly lower than for female respondents (96.99%), although in only two HSDAs (South Vancouver Island and East Kootenay) were males significantly lower than females. No HSDA in either gender cohort was significantly different from the provincial average.

In BC, 99.25% of the youngest age cohort (35 - 49 years) indicated they were not diagnosed, significantly higher than those in the 50 - 64 age cohort (95.50%). This significant difference between the two age cohorts was also reflected in seven of the individual HSDAs. Fraser East, Northwest and Central Vancouver Island had no respondents who had ever been diagnosed with heart disease in the youngest age cohort, and these were all

significantly higher than the provincial average for this cohort.

For older respondents (age 65 and older), only 83.58% were not diagnosed with heart disease, significantly lower than the 50 - 64 age cohort. Older respondents in all individual HSDAs were lower than their 50 - 64 age cohort counterparts, and this difference was significant in all but six HSDAs. Among the older respondents cohort, no individual HSDA was significantly different from the provincial average.

Geographically, there was only a 4 to 10 percentage point range among HSDAs, and the range among HSDAs increased with age. There were no clear or consistent geographic patterns for this indicator.

All BC cohorts had marginally higher values of not being diagnosed with heart disease in 2007/8 than in 2005, but none of the differences were significant. When the 2007/8 samples were compared between BC and their Canadian counterparts, BC had higher values for every cohort, and the differences were significant for all cohorts except males and seniors.

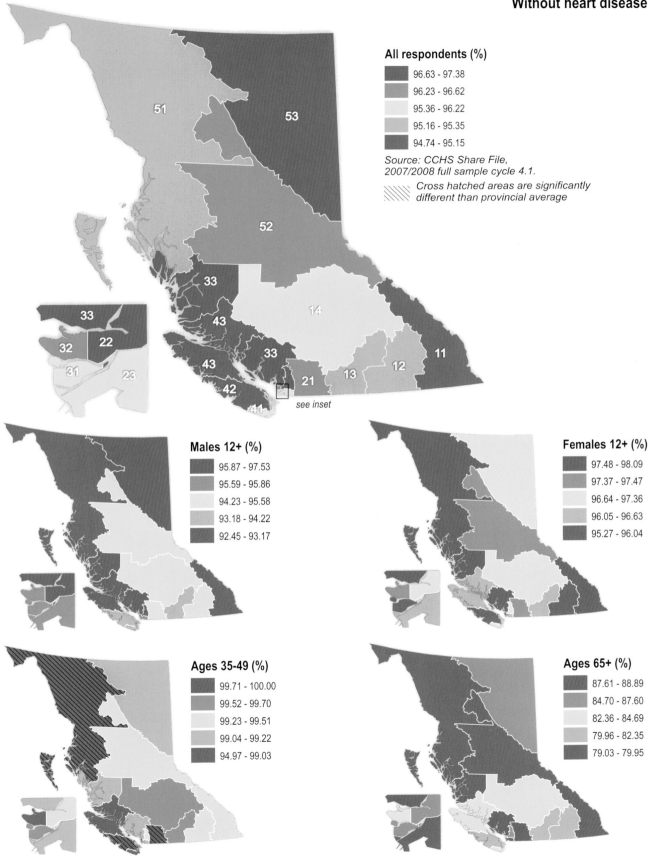

Without heart disease

All respondents (%)
- 96.63 - 97.38
- 96.23 - 96.62
- 95.36 - 96.22
- 95.16 - 95.35
- 94.74 - 95.15

Source: CCHS Share File, 2007/2008 full sample cycle 4.1.

Cross hatched areas are significantly different than provincial average

Males 12+ (%)
- 95.87 - 97.53
- 95.59 - 95.86
- 94.23 - 95.58
- 93.18 - 94.22
- 92.45 - 93.17

Females 12+ (%)
- 97.48 - 98.09
- 97.37 - 97.47
- 96.64 - 97.36
- 96.05 - 96.63
- 95.27 - 96.04

Ages 35-49 (%)
- 99.71 - 100.00
- 99.52 - 99.70
- 99.23 - 99.51
- 99.04 - 99.22
- 94.97 - 99.03

Ages 65+ (%)
- 87.61 - 88.89
- 84.70 - 87.60
- 82.36 - 84.69
- 79.96 - 82.35
- 79.03 - 79.95

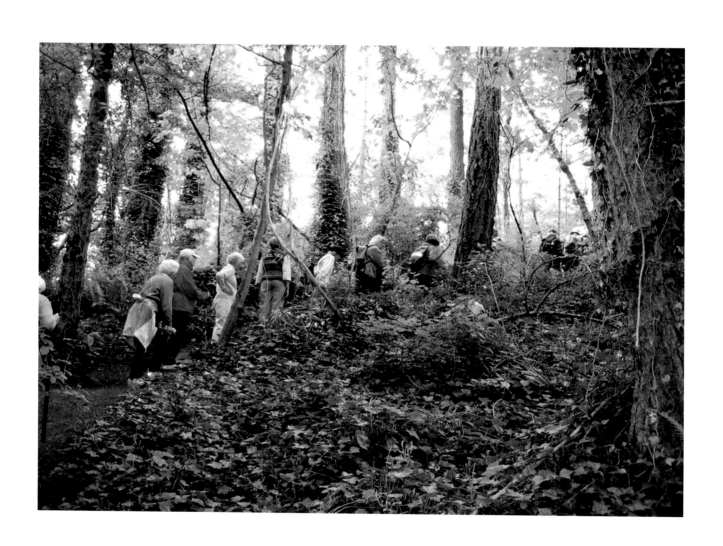

12

The Geography of Wellness Outcomes

This chapter provides a series of health and wellness measures that logically follow from many of those indicators presented earlier. Previous chapters have built upon each other and help determine the wellness outcomes mapped in this chapter.

There are 39 maps in total, most of which are based on survey data from CCHS 4.1 and McCreary AHS IV. Again, we use the half-full or asset approach, rather than focusing on deficits. As noted earlier, wellness is often viewed as personal and subjective. Given this subjectivity, we feel that using information mainly from questionnaire surveys is a good way to measure wellness outcomes. Five of the nine indicators are presented using the five map model used throughout this Atlas for CCHS-derived indicators, and give wellness outcomes for total BC respondents, males and females separately, and for the young and seniors cohorts at the HSDA level.

The first 15 maps look at self-reported health, mental health, and oral health. Self-rated health has been shown in numerous studies to be a good predictor of health and mortality internationally (Idler & Benyamini, 1997; Idler et al., 2000) and healthy behaviours for specific sub-groups of the population (Haddock et al., 2006), and is a common measure of health and wellness. Self-rated mental health has also been shown to be a good indicator of the general mental health of the population, when compared to mental morbidity in the Canadian population (Mawani & Gilmour, 2010). Oral health is important for overall health and for appearance and sense of well-being. Health Canada's website also notes that research "shows the connection between poor oral health and systemic disease such as diabetes in people of all ages and respiratory diseases particularly among elderly people. Research also points to possible connections between oral health and other systemic conditions such as heart disease" (Health Canada, 2009).

The next five maps look at self-rated daily stress. Stress is very personal in nature and can be caused by a variety of factors in daily life, as well as by major events. The negative effects of excessive stress can cause major unwellness, including heart disease, some types of bowel disease, herpes, and mental illness. Stress is also a major risk factor for alcohol and substance abuse. Having largely stress-free days is an important wellness outcome (Health Canada, 2008).

Following these are eight maps that focus on being injury-free. Data from both CCHS 4.1 and McCreary AHS IV are provided. Injuries can be responsible for reductions in activities, and can create chronic conditions affecting life's enjoyment, satisfaction, and well-being. The next five maps focus on the geography of life satisfaction overall. Self-rated satisfaction with life is a key individual wellness outcome indicator, and is based on individual feelings of well-being related to overall quality of life. Some caution in interpreting the results of some of the self-rated indicators is required as the data were collected between 2007 and 2008, mostly before the global recession had major impacts in Canada. It is possible that life satisfaction in particular, as well as stress and perhaps mental health, may have fallen from the results reported here because of the financial crisis and the major uncertainty that it brought to Canada and other countries (Graham, 2008). Evidence certainly shows a reduction in life satisfaction in European countries between 2007 and 2009 (Anderson, Mikulic, & Sandor, 2010).

The final six maps measure life expectancy at birth and also at age 65 years. Life expectancy is a widely accepted key indicator internationally of health and wellness of a population. Data are provided for the total BC population, and for males and females separately at the HSDA level.

Self-rated health is good to excellent

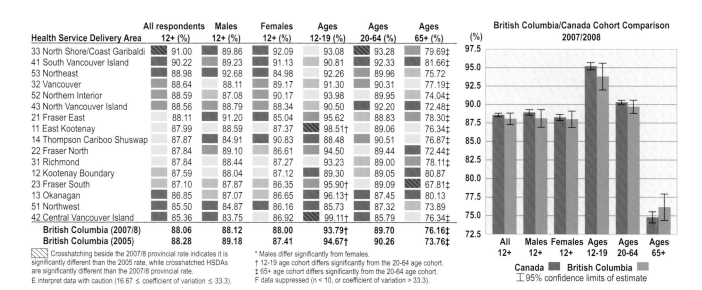

Health Service Delivery Area	All respondents 12+ (%)	Males 12+ (%)	Females 12+ (%)	Ages 12-19 (%)	Ages 20-64 (%)	Ages 65+ (%)
33 North Shore/Coast Garibaldi	91.00	89.86	92.09	93.08	93.28	79.69‡
41 South Vancouver Island	90.22	89.23	91.13	90.81	92.33	81.66‡
53 Northeast	88.98	92.68	84.98	92.26	89.96	75.72
32 Vancouver	88.64	88.11	89.17	91.30	90.31	77.19‡
52 Northern Interior	88.59	87.08	90.17	93.98	89.95	74.04‡
43 North Vancouver Island	88.56	88.79	88.34	90.50	92.20	72.48‡
21 Fraser East	88.11	91.20	85.04	95.62	88.83	78.30‡
11 East Kootenay	87.99	88.59	87.37	98.51†	89.06	76.34‡
14 Thompson Cariboo Shuswap	87.87	84.91	90.83	88.48	90.51	76.87‡
22 Fraser North	87.84	89.10	86.61	94.50	89.44	72.44‡
31 Richmond	87.84	88.44	87.27	93.23	89.00	78.11‡
12 Kootenay Boundary	87.59	88.04	87.12	89.30	89.05	80.87
23 Fraser South	87.10	87.87	86.35	95.90†	89.09	67.81‡
13 Okanagan	86.85	87.07	86.65	96.13†	87.45	80.13
51 Northwest	85.50	84.87	86.16	85.73	87.32	73.89
42 Central Vancouver Island	85.36	83.75	86.92	99.11†	85.79	76.34‡
British Columbia (2007/8)	**88.06**	**88.12**	**88.00**	**93.79†**	**89.70**	**76.16‡**
British Columbia (2005)	**88.28**	**89.18**	**87.41**	**94.67†**	**90.26**	**73.76‡**

Crosshatching beside the 2007/8 provincial rate indicates it is significantly different than the 2005 rate, while crosshatched HSDAs are significantly different than the 2007/8 provincial rate.

E interpret data with caution (16.67 ≤ coefficient of variation ≤ 33.3).

* Males differ significantly from females.
† 12-19 age cohort differs significantly from the 20-64 age cohort.
‡ 65+ age cohort differs significantly from the 20-64 age cohort.
F data suppressed (n < 10, or coefficient of variation > 33.3).

As noted earlier, individual perception of health is an important wellness asset. The CCHS asked respondents *"In general would you say your health is excellent, very good, good, fair or poor?"*. The following represents the number of respondents who reported having good to excellent health.

In BC, nearly nine out of every ten (88.06%) respondents felt their health was good to excellent. At 91%, North Shore/Coast Garibaldi had significantly more respondents with good to excellent self-reported health than the provincial average.

Males (88.12%) and females (88%) reported similar levels of good to excellent health at the provincial level, with no significant differences between the genders in any HSDA. Northeast had the highest value for males at 92.68% and Central Vancouver Island had the lowest at 83.75%, but these were not significantly different from the provincial average. For females, North Shore/Coast Garibaldi had the highest percentage at 92.09% and Northeast had the lowest at 84.98%, but again, these were not significantly different from the provincial average.

In BC, youth (93.79%) were significantly more likely to perceive their health as being good to excellent than the mid-age cohort. Within every HSDA, youth were either as likely as or more likely than the mid-age cohort to report self-perceived health as good to excellent, with significantly higher youth values recorded for East Kootenay, Okanagan, Fraser South, and Central Vancouver Island. Youth respondents in East Kootenay and Central Vancouver Island (above 98%) had

significantly higher values than the provincial average, and there were no regions with significantly lower values.

Overall, older respondents (76.16%) were significantly less likely to report good to excellent health than the mid-age cohort. This was also the case for 12 of 16 HSDAs. For older respondents, Fraser South (67.81%) was significantly low when compared to the provincial average.

There was a very modest 7 to 14 percentage point spread among HSDAs for all cohorts. Nevertheless, there was a high degree of geographical variation. For males, there was a cluster of high values in the south and central coastal regions, while low values were clustered in the southern and central interior and northern coast. For females, there was a cluster of high values along the central coast and inland through the central interior regions. High values for older respondents in this variable were also found in Kootenay Boundary and Okanagan along the southern border of the province. For youth, there were very few high value regions, and these were scattered throughout the province.

There were no significant differences for BC respondents between 2005 and 2007/8. Compared to the national average for good to excellent self-rated health, there was no significant difference for any cohort for 2007/8.

Self-rated health is good to excellent

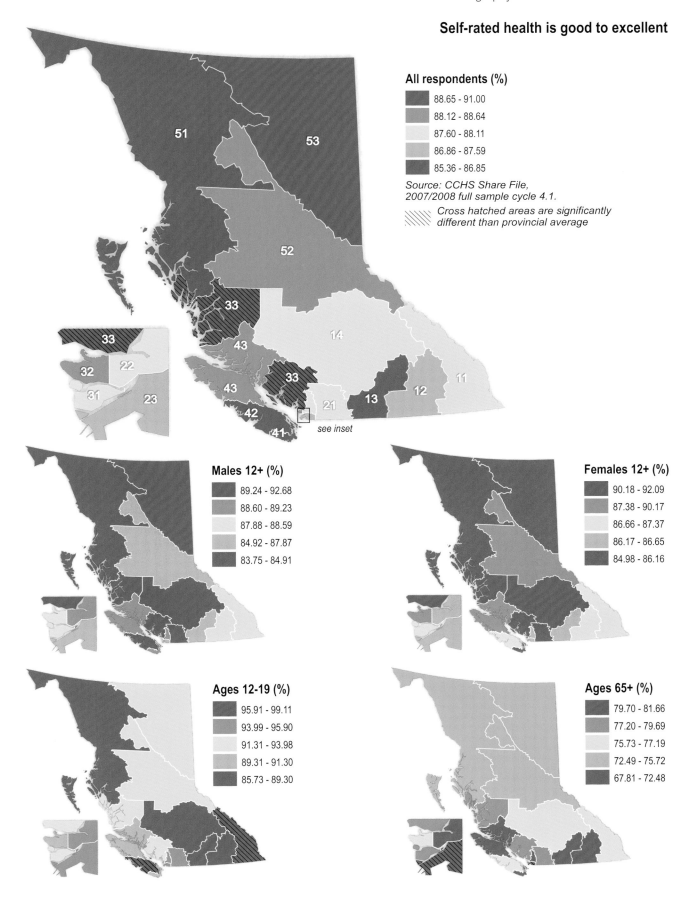

All respondents (%)

- 88.65 - 91.00
- 88.12 - 88.64
- 87.60 - 88.11
- 86.86 - 87.59
- 85.36 - 86.85

Source: CCHS Share File, 2007/2008 full sample cycle 4.1.

Cross hatched areas are significantly different than provincial average

Males 12+ (%)

- 89.24 - 92.68
- 88.60 - 89.23
- 87.88 - 88.59
- 84.92 - 87.87
- 83.75 - 84.91

Females 12+ (%)

- 90.18 - 92.09
- 87.38 - 90.17
- 86.66 - 87.37
- 86.17 - 86.65
- 84.98 - 86.16

Ages 12-19 (%)

- 95.91 - 99.11
- 93.99 - 95.90
- 91.31 - 93.98
- 89.31 - 91.30
- 85.73 - 89.30

Ages 65+ (%)

- 79.70 - 81.66
- 77.20 - 79.69
- 75.73 - 77.19
- 72.49 - 75.72
- 67.81 - 72.48

Self-rated mental health is good to excellent

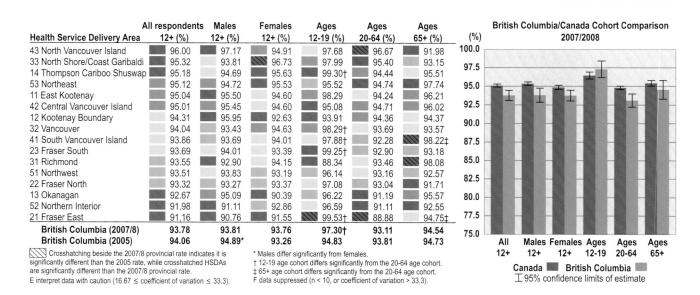

Health Service Delivery Area	All respondents 12+ (%)	Males 12+ (%)	Females 12+ (%)	Ages 12-19 (%)	Ages 20-64 (%)	Ages 65+ (%)
43 North Vancouver Island	96.00	97.17	94.91	97.68	96.67	91.98
33 North Shore/Coast Garibaldi	95.32	93.81	96.73	97.99	95.40	93.15
14 Thompson Cariboo Shuswap	95.18	94.69	95.63	99.30†	94.44	95.51
53 Northeast	95.12	94.72	95.53	95.52	94.74	97.74
11 East Kootenay	95.04	95.50	94.60	98.29	94.24	96.21
42 Central Vancouver Island	95.01	95.45	94.60	95.08	94.71	96.02
12 Kootenay Boundary	94.31	95.95	92.63	93.91	94.36	94.37
32 Vancouver	94.04	93.43	94.63	98.29†	93.69	93.57
41 South Vancouver Island	93.86	93.69	94.01	97.88†	92.28	98.22‡
23 Fraser South	93.69	94.01	93.39	99.25†	92.90	93.18
31 Richmond	93.55	92.90	94.15	88.34	93.46	98.08
51 Northwest	93.51	93.83	93.19	96.14	93.16	92.57
22 Fraser North	93.32	93.27	93.37	97.08	93.04	91.71
13 Okanagan	92.67	95.09	90.39	96.22	91.19	95.57
52 Northern Interior	91.98	91.11	92.86	96.59	91.11	92.55
21 Fraser East	91.16	90.76	91.55	99.53†	88.88	94.75‡
British Columbia (2007/8)	**93.78**	**93.81**	**93.76**	**97.30†**	**93.11**	**94.54**
British Columbia (2005)	**94.06**	**94.89***	**93.26**	**94.83**	**93.81**	**94.73**

Crosshatching beside the 2007/8 provincial rate indicates it is significantly different than the 2005 rate, while crosshatched HSDAs are significantly different than the 2007/8 provincial rate.
E interpret data with caution (16.67 ≤ coefficient of variation ≤ 33.3).

* Males differ significantly from females.
† 12-19 age cohort differs significantly from the 20-64 age cohort.
‡ 65+ age cohort differs significantly from the 20-64 age cohort.
F data suppressed (n < 10, or coefficient of variation > 33.3).

British Columbia/Canada Cohort Comparison 2007/2008

Canada ■   British Columbia ▨
⊥ 95% confidence limits of estimate

An individual's perspective on his or her own mental health is an important indicator of personal wellness. The CCHS asked respondents *"In general, would you say your mental health is: excellent, very good, good, fair or poor?"*. The following represents the percentage of respondents who indicated their mental health was good to excellent. More than nine out of every ten (93.78%) respondents in BC perceived their mental health as being good to excellent, and no HSDA was significantly higher or lower than the provincial average.

Males (93.81%) and females (93.76%) in BC reported very similar values for good to excellent self-reported mental health, with no significant differences between genders in any HSDA. Provincially, for 2005, males had a significantly higher value than females. For males, no HSDA was significantly higher or lower than the provincial average. Females in North Shore/Garibaldi (96.73%) were significantly more likely to report good to excellent mental health when compared to the provincial female average.

In BC, youth (97.3%) were significantly higher than the mid-age cohort. Within every region, youth were more likely than the mid-age cohort to report self-perceived mental health as good to excellent, with significantly higher values recorded for Thompson Cariboo Shuswap, Fraser East, Fraser South, Vancouver, and South Vancouver Island. Youth in Fraser East (99.53%) also had significantly higher values than the provincial average for youth.

Provincially, older respondents (94.54%) were not

significantly different than the mid-age cohort, although Fraser East and South Vancouver Island older respondents were significantly more likely to perceive their mental health as good to excellent when compared to their mid-age counterparts. Richmond and South Vancouver Island (both above 98%) had significantly higher values than the average for older respondents provincially.

There was a very modest nine or less percentage point spread among all the cohorts. Geographically for all respondents, the highest values were found in Northern Vancouver Island, North Shore/Coast Garibaldi, and Thompson Cariboo Shuswap, while the lowest values were found in Okanagan, Northern Interior, and Fraser East. There was a cluster of high values for males in the southeast, with a few low value HSDAs scattered throughout the province. For females, low values were clustered along the southern border of the province in Kootenay Boundary, Okanagan, and Fraser East, while high values were seen along the central coast and inland to Thompson Cariboo Shuswap.

There were no significant differences for BC respondents between 2005 and 2007/8, although the youth cohort had improved the most. Compared to the 2007/8 national averages for this indicator, most cohorts had significantly poorer self-rated mental health, with significantly lower values seen for all respondents, females, males, and the mid-age cohort.

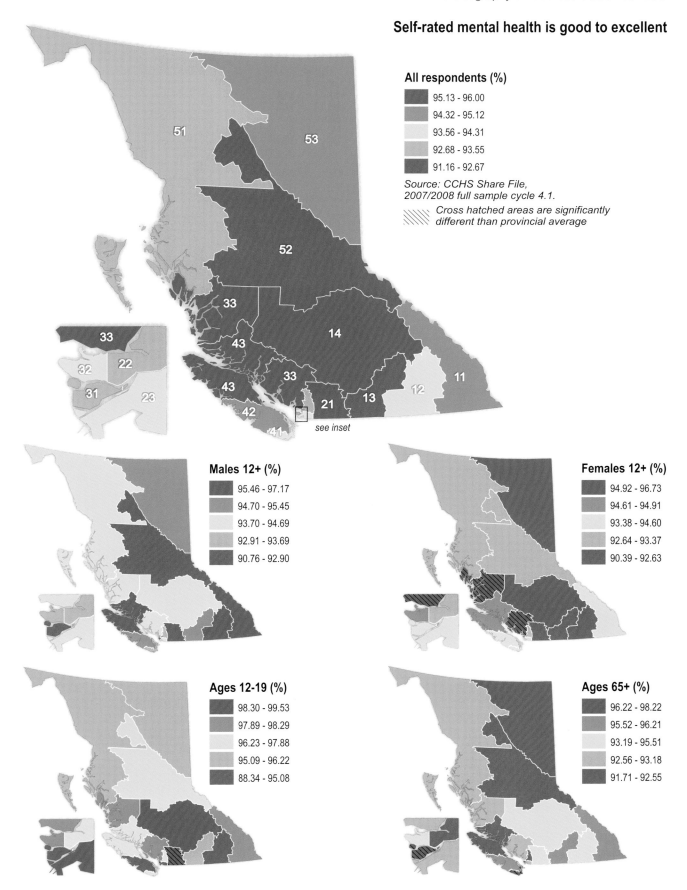

Self-rated mental health is good to excellent

All respondents (%)

- 95.13 - 96.00
- 94.32 - 95.12
- 93.56 - 94.31
- 92.68 - 93.55
- 91.16 - 92.67

Source: CCHS Share File, 2007/2008 full sample cycle 4.1.

Cross hatched areas are significantly different than provincial average

Males 12+ (%)

- 95.46 - 97.17
- 94.70 - 95.45
- 93.70 - 94.69
- 92.91 - 93.69
- 90.76 - 92.90

Females 12+ (%)

- 94.92 - 96.73
- 94.61 - 94.91
- 93.38 - 94.60
- 92.64 - 93.37
- 90.39 - 92.63

Ages 12-19 (%)

- 98.30 - 99.53
- 97.89 - 98.29
- 96.23 - 97.88
- 95.09 - 96.22
- 88.34 - 95.08

Ages 65+ (%)

- 96.22 - 98.22
- 95.52 - 96.21
- 93.19 - 95.51
- 92.56 - 93.18
- 91.71 - 92.55

Self-rated oral health is good to excellent

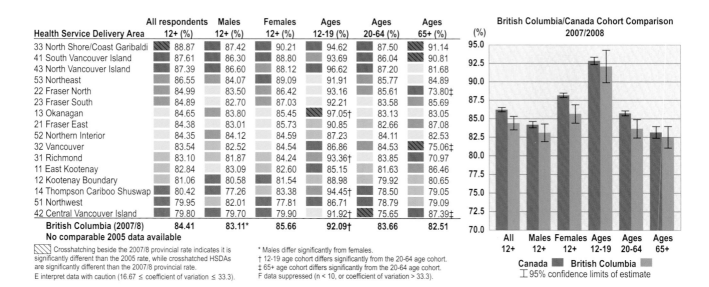

Health Service Delivery Area	All respondents 12+ (%)	Males 12+ (%)	Females 12+ (%)	Ages 12-19 (%)	Ages 20-64 (%)	Ages 65+ (%)
33 North Shore/Coast Garibaldi	88.87	87.42	90.21	94.62	87.50	91.14
41 South Vancouver Island	87.61	86.30	88.80	93.69	86.04	90.81
43 North Vancouver Island	87.39	86.60	88.12	96.62	87.20	81.68
53 Northeast	86.55	84.07	89.09	91.91	85.77	84.89
22 Fraser North	84.99	83.50	86.42	93.16	85.61	73.80‡
23 Fraser South	84.89	82.70	87.03	92.21	83.58	85.69
13 Okanagan	84.65	83.80	85.45	97.05†	83.13	83.05
21 Fraser East	84.38	83.01	85.73	90.85	82.66	87.08
52 Northern Interior	84.35	84.12	84.59	87.23	84.11	82.53
32 Vancouver	83.54	82.52	84.54	86.86	84.53	75.06‡
31 Richmond	83.10	81.87	84.24	93.36†	83.85	70.97
11 East Kootenay	82.84	83.09	82.60	85.15	81.63	86.46
12 Kootenay Boundary	81.06	80.58	81.54	88.98	79.92	80.65
14 Thompson Cariboo Shuswap	80.42	77.26	83.38	94.45†	78.50	79.05
51 Northwest	79.95	82.01	77.81	86.71	78.79	79.09
42 Central Vancouver Island	79.80	79.70	79.90	91.92†	75.65	87.39‡
British Columbia (2007/8)	**84.41**	**83.11***	**85.66**	**92.09†**	**83.66**	**82.51**

No comparable 2005 data available

Crosshatching beside the 2007/8 provincial rate indicates it is significantly different than the 2005 rate, while crosshatched HSDAs are significantly different than the 2007/8 provincial rate.
E interpret data with caution (16.67 ≤ coefficient of variation ≤ 33.3).

* Males differ significantly from females.
† 12-19 age cohort differs significantly from the 20-64 age cohort.
‡ 65+ age cohort differs significantly from the 20-64 age cohort.
F data suppressed (n < 10, or coefficient of variation > 33.3).

Oral health not only influences an individual's sense of well-being, it can also be a determinant of susceptibility to infection and other serious conditions, such as diabetes and respiratory illness. The CCHS asked respondents:, *"In general, would you say the health of your teeth and mouth is: excellent, very good, good, fair, poor?"*. The following represents the percentage of respondents who indicated their oral health was good to excellent. More than eight out of every ten (84.41%) respondents in BC reported their oral health was good to excellent. Only North Shore/Coast Garibaldi (88.87%) had a significantly higher value than the provincial average for this cohort.

Males (83.11%) in BC were significantly less likely than females (85.66%) to report good to excellent oral health at the provincial level; however, there were no significant differences between genders at the individual HSDA level. There were no HSDAs in either gender cohort with a significant difference from the provincial average.

Self-perceived good to excellent oral health decreased consistently with age. In BC, 92.09% of youth indicated they had good to excellent oral health, which was significantly higher than their mid-age counterparts. This significant difference between the youth and mid-age cohorts was also evident in Okanagan, Thompson Cariboo Shuswap, Richmond, and Central Vancouver Island. At the HSDA level, Okanagan (97.05%) was significantly higher than the provincial average for youth.

For older respondents, 82.51% reported having good to excellent oral health. At the HSDA level, older respondents in Central Vancouver Island were significantly

more likely to report good to excellent oral health when compared with the mid-age cohort, while those in Fraser North and Vancouver were significantly less likely to do so. Comparing HSDAs to the provincial average for this cohort, older respondents in North Shore/Coast Garibaldi and South Vancouver Island (both above 90%) had significantly higher values for good to excellent oral health, while those in Vancouver (75.06%) had a significantly lower value.

Geographically, there was a spread of 9 to 20 percentage points among cohorts, with the largest variation occurring in the oldest cohort. Higher values tended to be clustered around the southern and central coastal regions of the province, with lower values seen in the interior regions. Generally, however, there was a large degree of geographical variation among cohorts for this indicator.

There are no comparable data from the 2005 CCHS survey available for this variable. For the 2007/8 sample, compared to Canadians as a whole, British Columbians had lower values in all cohorts with regard to self-perceived oral health, with significantly lower values for all respondents, females, and the mid-age cohorts.

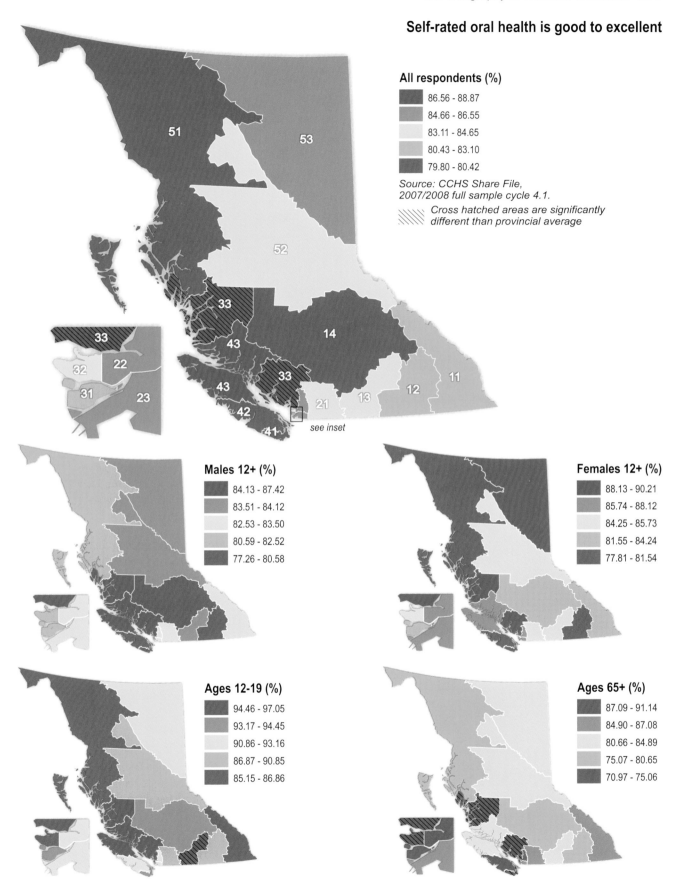

Self-rated oral health is good to excellent

All respondents (%)

- 86.56 - 88.87
- 84.66 - 86.55
- 83.11 - 84.65
- 80.43 - 83.10
- 79.80 - 80.42

Source: CCHS Share File, 2007/2008 full sample cycle 4.1.

Cross hatched areas are significantly different than provincial average

Males 12+ (%)

- 84.13 - 87.42
- 83.51 - 84.12
- 82.53 - 83.50
- 80.59 - 82.52
- 77.26 - 80.58

Females 12+ (%)

- 88.13 - 90.21
- 85.74 - 88.12
- 84.25 - 85.73
- 81.55 - 84.24
- 77.81 - 81.54

Ages 12-19 (%)

- 94.46 - 97.05
- 93.17 - 94.45
- 90.86 - 93.16
- 86.87 - 90.85
- 85.15 - 86.86

Ages 65+ (%)

- 87.09 - 91.14
- 84.90 - 87.08
- 80.66 - 84.89
- 75.07 - 80.65
- 70.97 - 75.06

Most days are not at all stressful

Health Service Delivery Area	All respondents 15+ (%)	Males 15+ (%)	Females 15+ (%)	Ages 15-19 (%)	Ages 20-64 (%)	Ages 65+ (%)
43 North Vancouver Island	44.99	49.26	40.82	40.33E	41.61	60.79
41 South Vancouver Island	41.27	43.81	39.00	50.77†	34.02	65.80‡
11 East Kootenay	40.72	42.40	39.06	25.36E	36.82	64.96‡
14 Thompson Cariboo Shuswap	39.65	44.04	35.24	48.67	33.09	61.69‡
32 Vancouver	39.25	40.76	37.76	31.84E	35.29	64.80‡
42 Central Vancouver Island	38.54	40.03	37.08	46.33E	31.45	59.59‡
23 Fraser South	38.46	37.89	39.01	51.35†	33.02	61.28‡
31 Richmond	38.34	36.32	40.15	38.30E	32.90	65.07‡
12 Kootenay Boundary	38.27	40.41	35.99	40.96E	31.08	65.23‡
51 Northwest	38.25	40.12	36.23	60.18†	32.63	57.75‡
53 Northeast	37.85	40.21	35.23	59.97†	31.39	70.03‡
13 Okanagan	37.78	37.38	38.15	40.97E	30.33	60.55‡
21 Fraser East	36.14	41.76	30.69	45.13	28.60	65.26‡
22 Fraser North	35.81	36.96	34.69	51.01†	31.67	51.88‡
33 North Shore/Coast Garibaldi	35.67	38.75	32.87	25.49E	31.90	55.99‡
52 Northern Interior	35.20	37.82	32.56	42.56	31.99	50.35‡
British Columbia (2007/8)	**38.26**	**39.81**	**36.75**	**44.30†**	**32.85**	**60.93‡**
British Columbia (2005)	**38.06**	**39.81***	**36.38**	**42.30†**	**32.12**	**64.63‡**

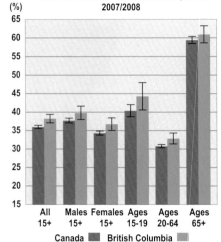

British Columbia/Canada Cohort Comparison 2007/2008

Canada ■   British Columbia ▨
⊥ 95% confidence limits of estimate

▨ Crosshatching beside the 2007/8 provincial rate indicates it is significantly different than the 2005 rate, while crosshatched HSDAs are significantly different than the 2007/8 provincial rate.
E interpret data with caution (16.67 ≤ coefficient of variation ≤ 33.3).

* Males differ significantly from females.
† 12-19 age cohort differs significantly from the 20-64 age cohort.
‡ 65+ age cohort differs significantly from the 20-64 age cohort.
F data suppressed (n < 10, or coefficient of variation > 33.3).

Stress can take its toll on health and well-being, and there is increasing concern around the level of stress that people experience in their day-to-day lives. The CCHS asked respondents: *"Thinking about the amount of stress in your life, would you say that most days are: not at all stressful, not very stressful, quite a bit stressful or extremely stressful?"* The following table and maps represent the percentage of respondents who indicated that most days were not at all stressful.

For all BC respondents (age 15 and over), less than four out of every ten respondents (38.26%) reported having mostly stress-free days, with no significant differences evident in any of the individual HSDAs. Further, there were no significant differences between male (39.81%) and female (36.75%) respondents provincially, or for any individual HSDA. This differs from 2005, when males were significantly higher than females. Among male respondents, no HSDA was significantly different than the male provincial average. Similarly for females, no HSDA was significantly different than the provincial average for female respondents.

In looking at the different age cohorts, some significant differences appear. At 44.3%, younger respondents (age 15 - 19 years) were significantly more likely to have mostly stress-free days than the mid-age cohort (32.85%). This significant difference was also evident for five individual HSDAs. Further, East Kootenay and North Shore/Coast Garibaldi youth (both below 26%) had significantly lower values than the provincial average for youth. However, caution in interpretation is required because half of the

HSDAs had small sample sizes or high coefficients of variation for the youth cohort.

The most profound differences for this indicator were evident for older age respondents, who were significantly more likely (60.93%) than the mid-age cohort to have mostly stress-free days. This significant difference was apparent in all but one HSDA (North Vancouver Island). No individual HSDA was significantly different from the provincial average for this cohort.

For the mid-age cohort, it is worth noting that North Vancouver Island (41.61%) was significantly higher than the provincial average for this age cohort.

Geographically, there was a high degree of variation from cohort to cohort, and there was a 10 to 35 percentage point spread among cohorts. South Vancouver Island was the only HSDA with consistently higher values than average for all cohorts, while North Shore Coast Garibaldi had consistently lower values than the average for all cohorts.

For BC respondents, CCHS results for 2005 and 2007/8 were very similar for all cohorts. For 2007/8, BC respondents had consistently higher values of being mostly stress free than their Canadian peers, and this difference was significant for the all respondent, female, and mid-age cohorts.

Most days are not at all stressful

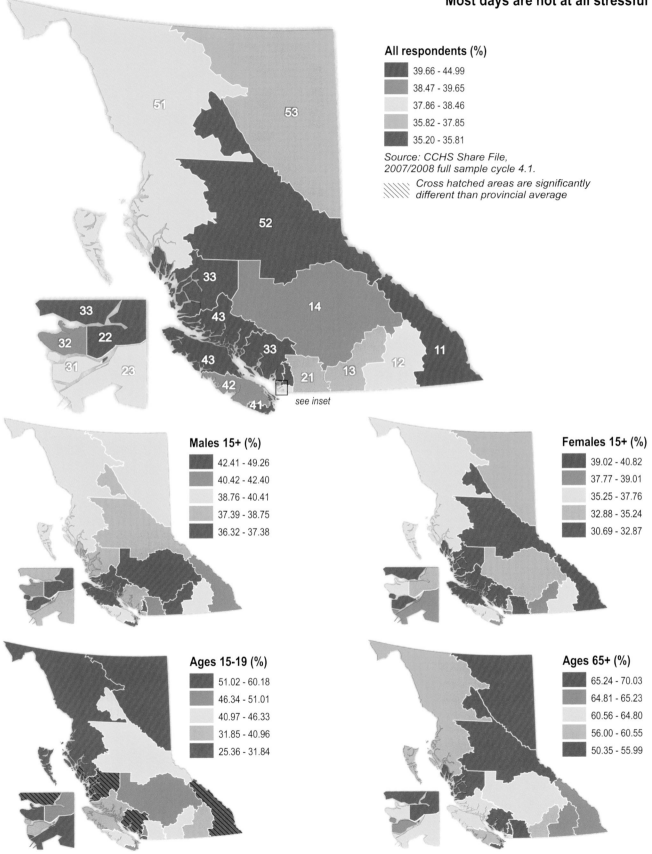

All respondents (%)

- 39.66 - 44.99
- 38.47 - 39.65
- 37.86 - 38.46
- 35.82 - 37.85
- 35.20 - 35.81

Source: CCHS Share File, 2007/2008 full sample cycle 4.1.

Cross hatched areas are significantly different than provincial average

see inset

Males 15+ (%)

- 42.41 - 49.26
- 40.42 - 42.40
- 38.76 - 40.41
- 37.39 - 38.75
- 36.32 - 37.38

Females 15+ (%)

- 39.02 - 40.82
- 37.77 - 39.01
- 35.25 - 37.76
- 32.88 - 35.24
- 30.69 - 32.87

Ages 15-19 (%)

- 51.02 - 60.18
- 46.34 - 51.01
- 40.97 - 46.33
- 31.85 - 40.96
- 25.36 - 31.84

Ages 65+ (%)

- 65.24 - 70.03
- 64.81 - 65.23
- 60.56 - 64.80
- 56.00 - 60.55
- 50.35 - 55.99

Injury-free in the past 12 months

Health Service Delivery Area	All respondents 12+ (%)	Males 12+ (%)	Females 12+ (%)	Ages 12-19 (%)	Ages 20-64 (%)	Ages 65+ (%)
31 Richmond	90.91	89.16	92.57	84.17	91.42	93.21
22 Fraser North	89.15	89.15	89.14	87.72	89.09	90.79
21 Fraser East	88.65	86.10	91.15	83.53	88.73	92.69
32 Vancouver	88.50	87.47	89.51	85.37	87.60	95.59‡
23 Fraser South	86.94	85.01	88.83	80.49	87.73	88.79
43 North Vancouver Island	86.86	86.82	86.90	75.26	88.47	88.78
51 Northwest	84.86	83.49	86.33	73.41	85.63	94.07
13 Okanagan	84.83	82.79	86.77	70.54†	85.65	89.70
14 Thompson Cariboo Shuswap	84.68	85.25	84.11	70.94	85.91	89.11
33 North Shore/Coast Garibaldi	84.43	83.18	85.62	73.50	85.82	86.16
53 Northeast	83.97	79.94	88.33	73.31	85.44	88.19
11 East Kootenay	83.52	83.05	84.00	87.06	80.63	93.16‡
42 Central Vancouver Island	83.40	81.81	84.94	67.61	83.06	93.33‡
52 Northern Interior	82.98	78.97	87.19	77.72	83.99	82.61
41 South Vancouver Island	78.61	75.88	81.09	68.79	78.62	84.00
12 Kootenay Boundary	78.55	78.31	78.79	56.92	80.11	85.80
British Columbia (2007/8)	**85.97**	**84.55***	**87.35**	**78.15†**	**86.31**	**90.06‡**
British Columbia (2005)	**83.49**	**80.46***	**86.43**	**71.56†**	**84.07**	**90.13‡**

Crosshatching beside the 2007/8 provincial rate indicates it is significantly different than the 2005 rate, while crosshatched HSDAs are significantly different than the 2007/8 provincial rate.
E interpret data with caution (16.67 ≤ coefficient of variation ≤ 33.3).
** Only NS and BC opted for this question.

* Males differ significantly from females.
† 12-19 age cohort differs significantly from the 20-64 age cohort.
‡ 65+ age cohort differs significantly from the 20-64 age cohort.
F data suppressed (n < 10, or coefficient of variation > 33.3).

Injuries are responsible for a wide range of temporary or longer lasting chronic conditions that can interfere with life's enjoyment, and therefore wellness. The CCHS asked respondents if they had been injured in the past 12 months (not including repetitive strain injuries). British Columbian respondents indicated that 85.97% had been injury-free in the past year. Respondents in Richmond and Fraser North (both above 89%) were significantly more likely to be injury-free in this period of time than the provincial average, while those in South Vancouver Island and Kootenay Boundary (both below 79%) were significantly less likely to be injury-free.

BC males (84.55%) were significantly less likely than females (87.35%) to be injury-free overall, although there was no particular HSDA in which the average for males was significantly different from that of females. When comparing the provincial average to the HSDA averages for males, only South Vancouver Island was significantly different from the provincial average, with a low value of 75.88%. For females, Richmond (92.57%) stood out with a significantly higher average, while Kootenay Boundary and South Vancouver Island (both below 82%) were significantly lower than the provincial average for females.

BC youth (78.15%) were significantly less likely to be injury-free in comparison to the mid-age cohort, and those in Okanagan were significantly more injury prone compared to their mid-age counterparts in that HSDA. In comparison to the provincial average for youth, respondents in Fraser North (87.72%) were significantly above average for freedom from injury, and respondents in

Kootenay Boundary (56.92%) were significantly below average.

BC seniors (90.06%) were significantly more likely to be injury-free than the mid-age cohort. East Kootenay, Vancouver, and Central Vancouver Island HSDAs all had significantly higher injury-free status for older respondents in comparison to their mid-age counterparts. Vancouver (95.59%) was significantly higher than the average provincial value for older respondents, while South Vancouver Island (84%) was significantly lower.

Overall, there was a modest 10 to 15 percentage points spread among HSDAs for all cohorts, except for youth, which had a 30 percentage point spread. Geographically, higher injury-free values were seen in the lower mainland and Fraser Valley HSDAs for most respondent groups, with low rates seen fairly consistently in South and Central Vancouver Island regions. Lower average values also tended to be found in the central parts of the province.

Between 2005 and 2007/8, all BC cohorts except those for females and older respondents had significantly better injury-free results. BC was one of only two provinces/territories opting for this module, thus comparisons with Canada are not possible.

Injury-free in the past 12 months

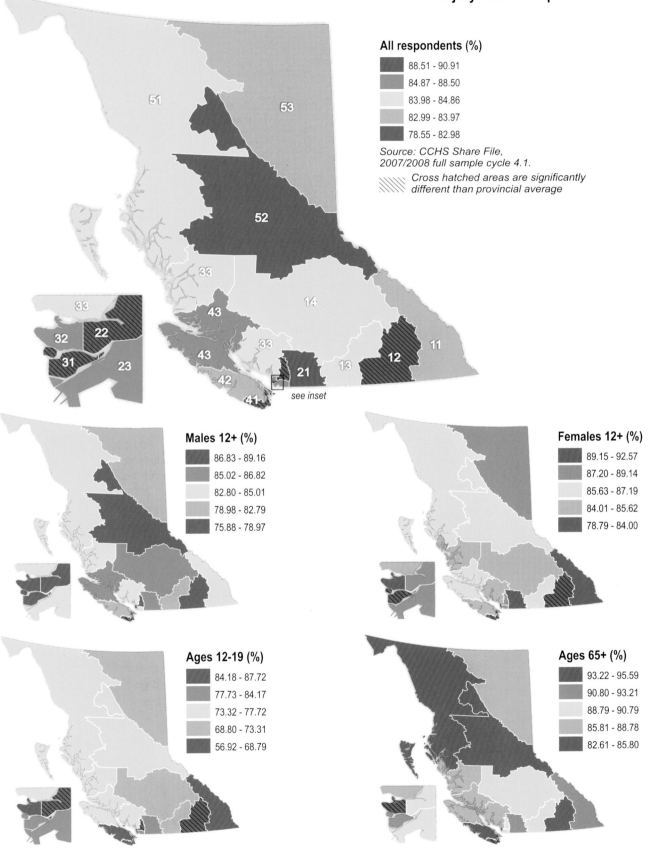

All respondents (%)

- 88.51 - 90.91
- 84.87 - 88.50
- 83.98 - 84.86
- 82.99 - 83.97
- 78.55 - 82.98

*Source: CCHS Share File,
2007/2008 full sample cycle 4.1.*

*Cross hatched areas are significantly
different than provincial average*

see inset

Males 12+ (%)

- 86.83 - 89.16
- 85.02 - 86.82
- 82.80 - 85.01
- 78.98 - 82.79
- 75.88 - 78.97

Females 12+ (%)

- 89.15 - 92.57
- 87.20 - 89.14
- 85.63 - 87.19
- 84.01 - 85.62
- 78.79 - 84.00

Ages 12-19 (%)

- 84.18 - 87.72
- 77.73 - 84.17
- 73.32 - 77.72
- 68.80 - 73.31
- 56.92 - 68.79

Ages 65+ (%)

- 93.22 - 95.59
- 90.80 - 93.21
- 88.79 - 90.79
- 85.81 - 88.78
- 82.61 - 85.80

Youth who were never injured seriously enough to need medical attention in the past 12 months

As noted previously, young people in particular are less likely to be injury-free than older age cohorts. To a large degree, this is associated with the fact that youth are more likely to participate in sports, physical exercise, and hobbies or other leisure time activities that result in injuries. Analysis of 2007/8 CCHS data has shown that 45% of most serious injuries occurred as a result of these activities (Foster, 2009). Many injuries are minor and do not require medical attention, but others are more severe requiring treatment.

The McCreary AHS IV asked students: *"In the past 12 months, how many times were you injured seriously enough that you required medical attention?"* Students indicated that, on average, more than seven in ten (71.27%) did not require any medical attention for any of their injuries in the past 12 months. There were, however, major geographical variations, and most HSDAs were significantly different from the provincial average. Richmond, at 82.14%, had the highest proportion of students who indicated that they had not needed medical treatment for any injury. At the other extreme, East Kootenay students indicated that only 61.56% of respondents had not needed medical treatment because of an injury.

Richmond, Vancouver, and Fraser North (all more than 74%) were significantly higher than the provincial student average. All were in the urban lower mainland part of the province. Fraser South/Fraser East was also above the provincial average, but not significantly so. North Shore/Coast Garibaldi was the only HSDA in the lower mainland that was below the provincial average, and it was significantly lower than the average. All other HSDAs were also significantly below the provincial average for students who had not required medical treatment for an injury in the past 12 months.

There were major significant differences at the provincial level between genders. Female student respondents (75.34%) were significantly more likely to have not required medical treatment because of an injury than male students (66.83%). This differential was consistent for every HSDA, and was significant for 11 of the HSDAs.

Male students had a large difference between the highest and lowest value HSDAs. Vancouver (78.38%) had the highest percentage of students not requiring medical treatment because of an injury, while at the other extreme, East Kootenay (56.2%) had the lowest. Again, Vancouver,

Health Service Delivery Area	All students (%)	Males (%)	Females (%)
31 Richmond	82.14	78.38†	85.94
32 Vancouver	81.90	78.98	84.08
22 Fraser North	74.43	71.34†	77.40
21 Fraser South/Fraser East	73.08	68.76†	76.89
43 North Vancouver Island	67.93	60.17†	74.44
33 North Shore/Coast Garibaldi	67.78	64.22†	71.27
41 South Vancouver Island	67.63	64.43†	70.70
13 Okanagan	67.49	60.36†	73.82
12 Kootenay Boundary	66.23	63.06	69.00
14 Thompson Cariboo Shuswap	65.83	59.71†	71.74
42 Central Vancouver Island	65.16	59.79†	70.60
52 Northern Interior	65.01	60.44†	69.63
51 Northwest	62.54	59.09	65.66
11 East Kootenay	61.56	56.27†	66.28
53 Northeast	N/A	N/A	N/A
British Columbia	**71.27**	**66.83†**	**75.34**

† Male rate is significantly different than female rate.
Crosshatched HSDAs are significantly different than the provincial average.
N/A: No data

Richmond, and Fraser North (all above 71%) were significantly higher than the provincial average, while Fraser South/Fraser East was higher than the provincial average, but not significantly so. All of the remaining HSDAs were lower than the provincial average for male students, and North Shore/Coast Garibaldi, South Vancouver Island, and Kootenay Boundary were the only HSDAs not significantly lower.

The patterns and trends for female respondents were quite similar overall to those for male students. The spread among HSDAs was a little less than 20 percentage points, with Richmond (85.94%) and Vancouver (84.08%) both significantly higher than the average for female students as a whole, and Fraser North and Fraser South/Fraser East also above average. All remaining HSDAs were below the provincial average for female students, and all were significantly so, except for North Vancouver Island, Okanagan, and Thompson Cariboo Shuswap. Northwest (65.66%) had the lowest value among HSDAs for female students.

Results consistently show that the most densely populated HSDAs in the lower mainland were the ones most likely to not have required medical attention in the past 12 months because of an injury.

Youth who were never injured seriously enough to need medical attention in the past 12 months

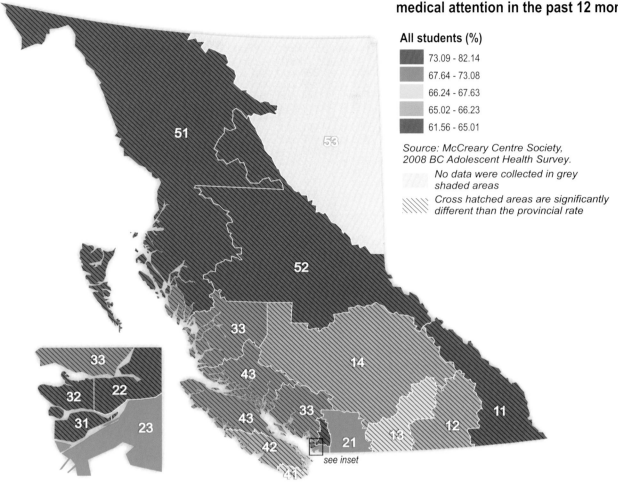

All students (%)

- 73.09 - 82.14
- 67.64 - 73.08
- 66.24 - 67.63
- 65.02 - 66.23
- 61.56 - 65.01

*Source: McCreary Centre Society,
2008 BC Adolescent Health Survey.*

*No data were collected in grey
shaded areas*

*Cross hatched areas are significantly
different than the provincial rate*

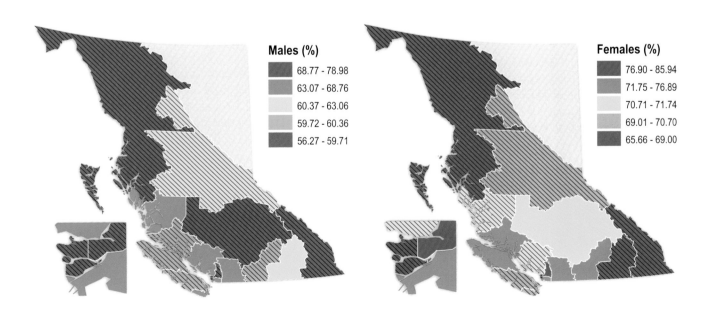

Males (%)

- 68.77 - 78.98
- 63.07 - 68.76
- 60.37 - 63.06
- 59.72 - 60.36
- 56.27 - 59.71

Females (%)

- 76.90 - 85.94
- 71.75 - 76.89
- 70.71 - 71.74
- 69.01 - 70.70
- 65.66 - 69.00

Satisfied with life

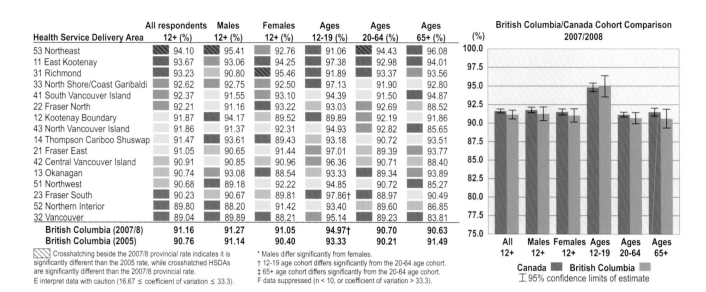

Health Service Delivery Area	All respondents 12+ (%)	Males 12+ (%)	Females 12+ (%)	Ages 12-19 (%)	Ages 20-64 (%)	Ages 65+ (%)
53 Northeast	94.10	95.41	92.76	91.06	94.43	96.08
11 East Kootenay	93.67	93.06	94.25	97.38	92.98	94.01
31 Richmond	93.23	90.80	95.46	91.89	93.37	93.56
33 North Shore/Coast Garibaldi	92.62	92.75	92.50	97.13	91.90	92.80
41 South Vancouver Island	92.37	91.55	93.10	94.39	91.50	94.87
22 Fraser North	92.21	91.16	93.22	93.03	92.69	88.52
12 Kootenay Boundary	91.87	94.17	89.52	89.89	92.19	91.86
43 North Vancouver Island	91.86	91.37	92.31	94.93	92.82	85.65
14 Thompson Cariboo Shuswap	91.47	93.61	89.43	93.18	90.72	93.51
21 Fraser East	91.05	90.65	91.44	97.01	89.39	93.77
42 Central Vancouver Island	90.91	90.85	90.96	96.36	90.71	88.40
13 Okanagan	90.74	93.08	88.54	93.33	89.34	93.89
51 Northwest	90.68	89.18	92.22	94.85	90.72	85.27
23 Fraser South	90.23	90.67	89.81	97.86†	88.97	90.49
52 Northern Interior	89.80	88.20	91.42	93.40	89.60	86.85
32 Vancouver	89.04	89.89	88.21	95.14	89.23	83.81
British Columbia (2007/8)	**91.16**	**91.27**	**91.05**	**94.97†**	**90.70**	**90.63**
British Columbia (2005)	**90.76**	**91.14**	**90.40**	**93.33**	**90.21**	**91.49**

Crosshatching beside the 2007/8 provincial rate indicates it is significantly different than the 2005 rate, while crosshatched HSDAs are significantly different than the 2007/8 provincial rate.
E interpret data with caution (16.67 ≤ coefficient of variation ≤ 33.3).

* Males differ significantly from females.
† 12-19 age cohort differs significantly from the 20-64 age cohort.
‡ 65+ age cohort differs significantly from the 20-64 age cohort.
F data suppressed (n < 10, or coefficient of variation > 33.3).

Life satisfaction is one the most important indicators of wellness as it gives an overall sense of one's happiness and well-being. The CCHS asked respondents: *"How satisfied are you with your life in general: very satisfied, satisfied, neither satisfied nor dissatisfied, dissatisfied or very dissatisfied?"* The results presented here represent the percentage of respondents who identified as being satisfied or very satisfied with life. In BC, more than nine out of every ten (91.16%) respondents reported they were satisfied with life. Northeast had a significantly high level of life satisfaction at 94.10%, and there were no HSDAs with a significantly low level of satisfaction when compared to the provincial average.

Provincially, both males and females had approximately 91% of respondents reporting satisfaction with life, with no significant differences between male and female respondents at the HSDA level. Male respondents in Northeast (95.41%) had significantly higher levels of life satisfaction than the overall male provincial average, while Richmond (95.46%) was the only HSDA that was significantly higher than the provincial average for female respondents.

Provincially, the youth cohort (94.97%) had significantly more respondents reporting satisfaction with life when compared to the mid-age group, but at the HSDA level only Fraser South youth were significantly higher than their mid-age counterparts. For the youth cohort, there were no HSDAs that were significantly lower or higher than the provincial average for youth.

For older respondents (90.63%), there was no significant

difference when compared to the mid-age cohort, nor were there any significant differences between individual HSDAs and the provincial average for the older age cohort. For the mid-age cohort, respondents in Northeast (94.43%) were significantly more likely to be satisfied with life than the provincial average for this cohort.

Geographically, there was a small spread of five or more percentage points for each of the age cohorts, with the greatest variation occurring in the oldest cohort (over 12 percentage points). This indicator showed a high degree of variation, with high and low values scattered around the province for every cohort. A large cluster of higher values was evident in the southwest of the province for the male cohort, and there were clusters of lower values in the south central region of the province for both female and youth respondents.

There were no significant differences for BC respondents between 2005 and 2007/8. In comparison to the national averages for the 2007/8 samples, British Columbians were not significantly different in any age or gender cohort.

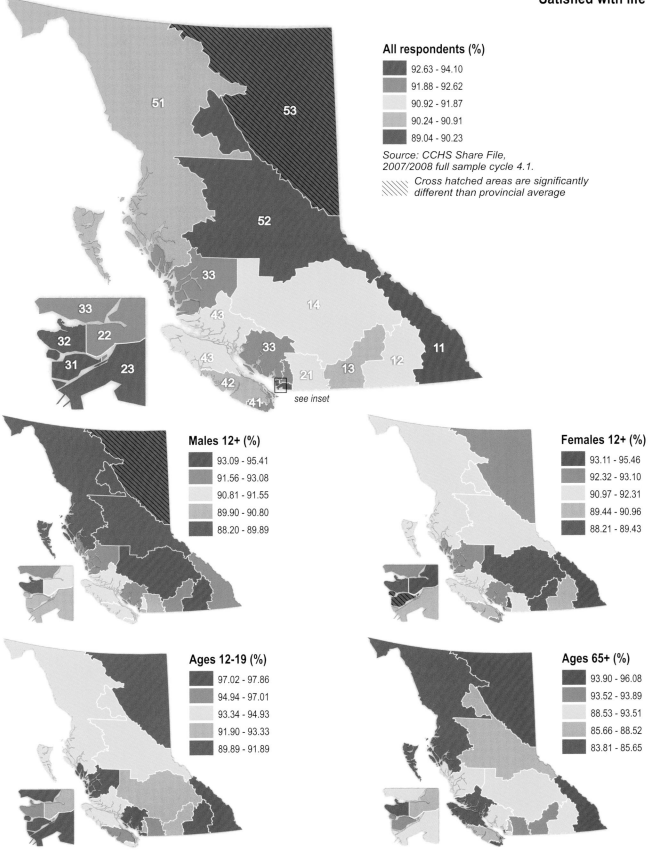

Satisfied with life

All respondents (%)
- 92.63 - 94.10
- 91.88 - 92.62
- 90.92 - 91.87
- 90.24 - 90.91
- 89.04 - 90.23

Source: CCHS Share File, 2007/2008 full sample cycle 4.1.

Cross hatched areas are significantly different than provincial average

Males 12+ (%)
- 93.09 - 95.41
- 91.56 - 93.08
- 90.81 - 91.55
- 89.90 - 90.80
- 88.20 - 89.89

Females 12+ (%)
- 93.11 - 95.46
- 92.32 - 93.10
- 90.97 - 92.31
- 89.44 - 90.96
- 88.21 - 89.43

Ages 12-19 (%)
- 97.02 - 97.86
- 94.94 - 97.01
- 93.34 - 94.93
- 91.90 - 93.33
- 89.89 - 91.89

Ages 65+ (%)
- 93.90 - 96.08
- 93.52 - 93.89
- 88.53 - 93.51
- 85.66 - 88.52
- 83.81 - 85.65

Life expectancy at birth

One of the key international comparative indicators of health and wellness is life expectancy at birth. This is an outcome of several of the indicators already provided in this Atlas. Data for the 5 year average from 2005 to 2009 inclusive are provided in the table and three maps opposite for both sexes combined, and individually for males and for females.

Life expectancy for both sexes

The average life expectancy at birth for the total population in the 2005 to 2009 period was 81.4 years. This is an increase from the 2001 to 2005 average of 80.8 years provided in the original Atlas. The latest comparative data for Canada (2005 to 2007 average) was 80.7 years, and BC had the highest life expectancy in the country (Statistics Canada, 2010). The range among HSDAs was 6.4 years, and varied from a high of 84.9 years for Richmond to a low of 78.5 years for Northwest. Richmond had a 2.3 year longer life expectancy when compared to Vancouver and North Shore/Coast Garibaldi (both at 82.6 years), the next highest HSDAs. Not all HSDAs shared in an increase in life expectancy: Northeast, Northwest, Thompson Cariboo Shuswap, and East Kootenay all had marginal reductions in life expectancy from the earlier 5 year average time period. The largest increase in life expectancy, 0.9 years, was recorded by South Vancouver Island.

Life expectancy for males

BC males had an average life expectancy of 79.2 years for the period 2005 to 2009. This was an increase over the 2001 to 2005 average of 78.5 years. Again, Richmond had the highest life expectancy at 82.9 years, a full 2.3 years more than the next highest, North Shore/Coast Garibaldi (80.6 years). At the other extreme, Northern Interior (76.3 years) and Northwest (76.4 years) had the lowest male life expectancies. While most HSDAs showed increases in life expectancy, East Kootenay, Northern Interior, and Northwest all showed marginal reductions. South Vancouver had the largest increase in life expectancy of 0.9 years from the 2001 to 2005 period.

Life expectancy for females

Female average life expectancy in BC for the period 2005 to 2009 was 83.6 years, 4.4 years higher than that for males, and an increase from 83.0 years for the 2001 to 2005 average. Richmond again had the highest life expectancy (86.7 years), 2.6 years more than the next highest HSDA, which was Vancouver at 85.1 years. At the

Health Service Delivery Area	Total (years)		Male (years)		Female (years)	
31 Richmond		84.9		82.9		86.7
32 Vancouver		82.6		80.0		85.1
33 North Shore/Coast Garibaldi		82.6		80.6		84.4
22 Fraser North		82.0		79.8		84.0
41 South Vancouver Island		82.0		79.8		84.0
23 Fraser South		81.6		79.5		83.5
13 Okanagan		80.9		78.5		83.3
11 East Kootenay		80.8		78.5		83.3
42 Central Vancouver Island		80.3		78.0		82.6
21 Fraser East		80.2		77.9		82.5
43 North Vancouver Island		80.1		77.8		82.5
12 Kootenay Boundary		79.9		77.8		82.0
14 Thompson Cariboo Shuswap		79.5		77.2		81.9
53 Northeast		79.1		76.8		81.6
52 Northern Interior		78.6		76.3		81.1
51 Northwest		78.5		76.4		80.9
British Columbia		**81.4**		**79.2**		**83.6**

other extreme, Northwest had the lowest 5 year average life expectancy of 80.9 years. While most HSDAs witnessed increases in female life expectancy between the 2001 to 2005 and 2005 to 2009 periods, three saw a marginal decrease: Kootenay Boundary, Northeast, and East Kootenay. The largest increase in life expectancy occurred in South Vancouver Island, with a full 1 year increase.

Summary

Overall, geographical patterns were similar for all three cohorts, and there were clear differences throughout the province. The highest life expectancies were found in the southwest lower mainland and South Vancouver Island regions of the province; life expectancies were lower in the interior of the province and the central and northern part of Vancouver Island, and lowest in the northern half of the province. The higher life expectancies of females were consistent for every HSDA, but the greatest difference between genders was 5.1 years for Vancouver. The increase in life expectancies was higher for males on average than for females, confirming a continuing trend of narrowing the gap between genders (Provincial Health Service Authority, 2007; Statistics Canada, 2010).

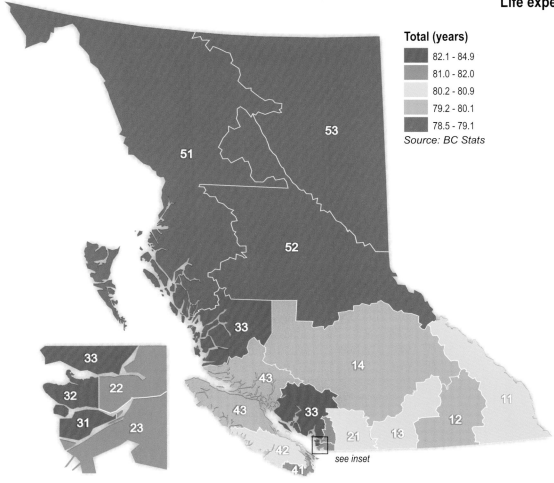

Life expectancy at birth

Total (years)

- 82.1 - 84.9
- 81.0 - 82.0
- 80.2 - 80.9
- 79.2 - 80.1
- 78.5 - 79.1

Source: BC Stats

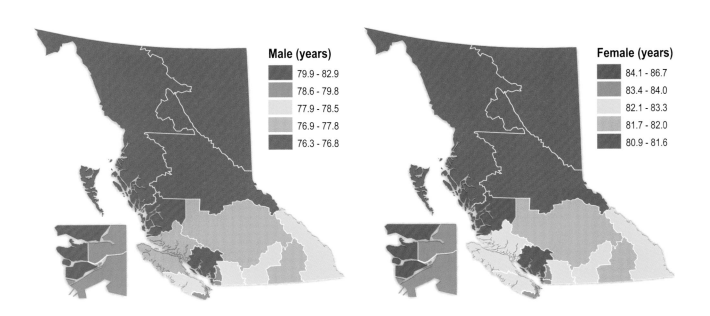

Male (years)

- 79.9 - 82.9
- 78.6 - 79.8
- 77.9 - 78.5
- 76.9 - 77.8
- 76.3 - 76.8

Female (years)

- 84.1 - 86.7
- 83.4 - 84.0
- 82.1 - 83.3
- 81.7 - 82.0
- 80.9 - 81.6

Life expectancy at age 65

Most of the recent gains in life expectancy (about 70%) in Canada have come about as a result of the gains in life expectancy among seniors (Statistics Canada, 2010). Improved lifestyles, including better nutrition and exercise and reductions in smoking, are partly responsible, along with improvements in medical interventions. Life expectancy at age 65 years is a new indicator for the Atlas, and the table and maps opposite show the average results for BC based on data from BC Stats for the 5 year period 2005 to 2009.

Total life expectancy at age 65

Seniors in BC could expect to live an additional 20.45 years beyond age 65, based on the 2005 to 2009 average data. This compared with the Canada average of 19.8 years for the 2005 to 2007 period, the most recent comparative data available (Statistics Canada, 2010). The range among HSDAs was just over 4 years. Richmond had the longest life expectancy, with 22.47 years after age 65, almost a full year more than the next highest, while Northwest had the lowest with only 18.46 years, followed closely by Northern Interior and Northeast, both below 19 years beyond age 65.

Male life expectancy at age 65

The life expectancy for male seniors was an additional 18.97 years beyond age 65, with a range among HSDAs of just over 4 years, and again Richmond had the highest number at 21.00 years. This was greater than a full year more than the next highest, Vancouver, with 19.83 additional years after age 65. At the other extreme, Northwest had the lowest value, with an additional life expectancy of only 16.96 years, again followed by Northern Interior and Northeast, both below 17.5 years.

Female life expectancy at age 65

Senior females in BC could expect to live an additional 21.77 years beyond age 65 on average, based on the 5 year average data for 2005 to 2009, with a range among HSDAs of less than 4 years. As for males, Richmond had an additional life expectancy of 23.68 years after age 65, while Northern Interior at 19.92 years had the lowest value.

Summary

Geographically, the pattern among HSDAs was very similar for all three cohorts, and, not unexpectedly, resembled those for life expectancy at birth. The urban

Health Service Delivery Area	Total (years)	Male (years)	Female (years)
31 Richmond	22.47	21.00	23.68
32 Vancouver	21.51	19.83	23.00
41 South Vancouver Island	21.05	19.49	22.32
33 North Shore/Coast Garibaldi	20.91	19.55	22.08
23 Fraser South	20.41	19.02	21.58
22 Fraser North	20.35	18.78	21.66
13 Okanagan	20.34	18.94	21.67
42 Central Vancouver Island	20.22	18.86	21.54
11 East Kootenay	19.93	18.68	21.16
43 North Vancouver Island	19.78	18.55	20.97
21 Fraser East	19.73	18.31	21.06
14 Thompson Cariboo Shuswap	19.48	18.27	20.68
12 Kootenay Boundary	19.32	18.04	20.50
53 Northeast	18.86	17.34	20.45
52 Northern Interior	18.48	17.15	19.92
51 Northwest	18.46	16.96	20.15
British Columbia	**20.45**	**18.97**	**21.77**

lower mainland HSDAs in the southwest of the province, along with South Vancouver Island had the greatest additional life expectancy at age 65, followed by interior HSDAs and Central and North Vancouver Island. The shortest additional life expectancies were dominated by the HSDAs in the northern half of the province. Again, senior females had longer additional life expectancies than senior males, 2.8 years on average, and higher female life expectancies occurred for every individual HSDA. The greatest difference between genders was 3.19 years for Northwest, followed closely by Vancouver (3.17 years).

Life expectancy at age 65

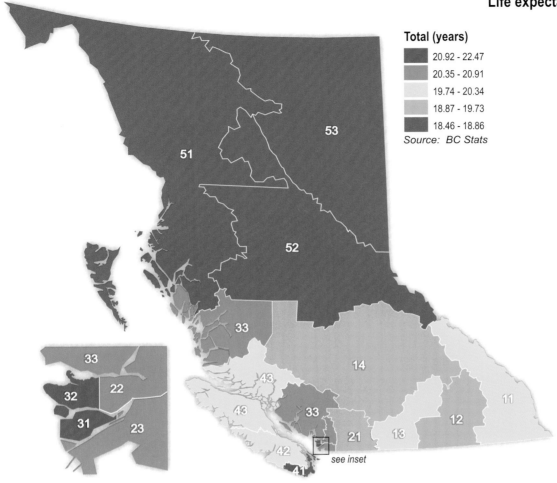

Total (years)
- 20.92 - 22.47
- 20.35 - 20.91
- 19.74 - 20.34
- 18.87 - 19.73
- 18.46 - 18.86

Source: BC Stats

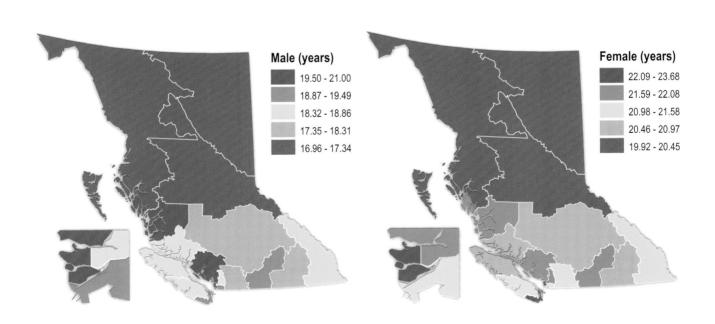

Male (years)
- 19.50 - 21.00
- 18.87 - 19.49
- 18.32 - 18.86
- 17.35 - 18.31
- 16.96 - 17.34

Female (years)
- 22.09 - 23.68
- 21.59 - 22.08
- 20.98 - 21.58
- 20.46 - 20.97
- 19.92 - 20.45

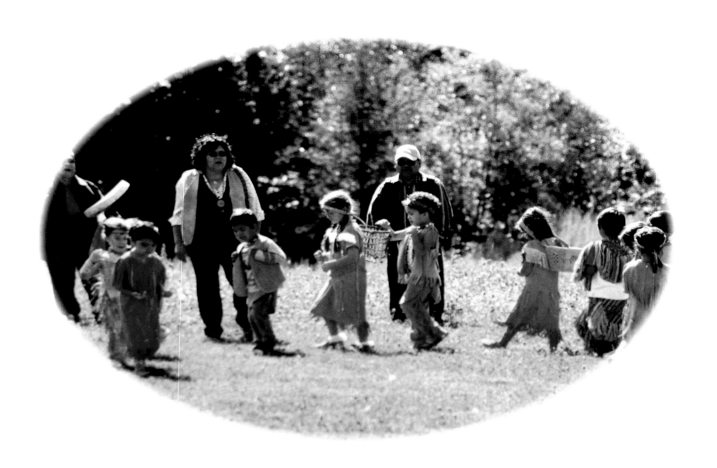

13

Summary and Conclusions

Introduction

This chapter provides summary maps and tables that assist us in giving a final commentary on the geography of wellness in BC. We developed a very simple, easy-to-use ranking system of regions to give an overall geographical picture based on a composite index of wellness in BC. In total there are over 400 maps and approximately 160 different indicators in the Atlas. One of the key challenges that we faced was gathering readily available and relevant data for the province to show geographical variations in wellness. Not all the indicators have the same geographical administrative unit, so it is challenging to combine and summarize all the information we have presented.

However, a majority of indicators were available for the Health Service Delivery Area (HSDA) administrative unit, of which there are 16 in the province, so we focused on this unit as the basis for combining and summarizing results and geographical patterns. This included a total of 90 indicators (56% of all indicators) as follows: 29 for assets; 7 for smoke-free environments and behaviours; 13 for food security and nutrition; 8 for physical activity; 4 for healthy weights; 10 for healthy pregnancies; 10 for chronic-free conditions; and 9 for wellness outcomes. These groupings and their general patterns are described in the following pages.

The second part of the chapter provides summaries based on gender and age, and maps and descriptions based on a combination of all of these indicators together to provide an overall composite picture of wellness in BC. It should be noted, however, that not all 90 indicators were available for gender and age cohort breakdowns, so composite pictures are developed only with those data that were available.

Developing average ranks

Developing an average rank is similar to developing a composite index. A composite indicator is useful in measuring and communicating the overall pattern of a variety of individual indicators in one measure (Vandivere & McPhee, 2008). Developing such a composite indicator of wellness or its sub-components tends to be reflective of overall health and well-being (Profit et al., 2010). A composite index reduces the complexity of many single measures and can be effective in communicating overall patterns, but using a simple average ranking does have disadvantages as many indicators may be closely correlated, or high values of one indicator may offset low values of another (Nardo et al., 2008). Nevertheless, because of its simplicity and ready understandability, we use average ranks as a basis to help describe the overall wellness patterns of the key chapters.

Each indicator for which data were available at the HSDA level was included in the average ranking system that is used in the following summaries. The HSDAs were ranked 1 to 16, with 1 being the best wellness value (percentage, rate, median, or average) and 16 being the poorest. Table 13.1.1 gives an example based on the smoke-free environment and behaviour indicators contained in Chapter 6.

The seven individual indicators were ranked from 1 to 16, and then ranks were summed for each HSDA to give an average rank. Averages based on those indicators that were available at the HSDA level were developed in this manner for each of Chapters 5 to 12 inclusive, for total population, for males and females separately, and for younger respondents and older respondents. Tables 13.1.2 to 13.1.6 give the average ranks for the relevant chapters and cohorts.

Table 13.1.1 Constructing Average Ranks

Health Service Delivery Area	Smoke-free in public places	Smoke-free workplace	Smoke-free vehicle	Smoke-free home	Smoke restricted home	Youth in smoke-free environment	Presently non-smoker	Average Rank
31 Richmond	2	1	2	4	13	1	1	3.43
41 South Vancouver Island	7	6	3	3	4	5	2	4.29
33 North Shore/Coast Garibaldi	15	2	9	1	1	2	3	4.71
23 Fraser South	3	5	7	5	7	6	7	5.71
21 Fraser East	4	8	5	10	6	6	6	6.43
22 Fraser North	10	4	6	6	10	4	5	6.43
43 North Vancouver Island	5	11	1	7	2	10	9	6.43
32 Vancouver	14	3	4	2	16	3	4	6.57
13 Okanagan	6	10	8	8	3	7	10	7.43
42 Central Vancouver Island	1	9	13	9	5	8	14	8.43
12 Kootenay Boundary	13	7	12	11	8	9	13	10.43
51 Northwest	8	13	10	12	11	11	11	10.86
11 East Kootenay	12	12	11	15	12	14	8	12.00
14 Thompson Cariboo Shuswap	11	16	14	14	9	12	15	13.00
52 Northern Interior	16	14	15	13	14	13	12	13.86
53 Northeast	9	15	16	16	15	N/A	16	14.50

N/A: No data were available for this indicator for the Northeast (average is based on only 6 indicators)

Table 13.1.2 Summary of Total Cohort

	Chapter 5	Chapter 6	Chapter 7	Chapter 8	Chapter 9	Chapter 10	Chapter 11	Chapter 12	***Average Rank Score
33 North Shore/Coast Garibaldi	5.59	4.71	3.85	6.88	3.25	8.40	4.50	5.00	5.41
31 Richmond	7.38	3.43	4.15	14.63	6.75	4.70	4.00	5.22	6.33
41 South Vancouver Island	6.24	4.29	5.46	4.38	5.75	9.40	10.10	5.44	6.49
32 Vancouver	8.69	6.57	6.08	12.25	4.00	9.20	2.70	6.00	7.38
12 Kootenay Boundary	5.45	10.43	8.38	3.00	6.75	7.00	12.80	10.89	7.63
22 Fraser North	7.66	6.43	4.92	14.38	6.50	9.20	6.20	7.22	7.68
23 Fraser South	7.97	5.71	8.08	13.38	6.25	7.80	5.20	7.78	7.87
13 Okanagan	7.90	7.43	7.00	6.38	5.25	6.80	12.90	9.89	8.11
21 Fraser East	10.10	6.43	8.69	12.13	8.50	6.60	6.10	9.11	8.79
53 Northeast	8.61	14.50	12.64	8.00	15.00	5.60	5.80	7.75	8.90
11 East Kootenay	7.97	12.00	11.62	5.25	9.25	7.40	12.40	8.11	9.07
43 North Vancouver Island	10.17	6.43	8.38	8.25	10.00	10.90	11.50	5.67	9.22
42 Central Vancouver Island	8.79	8.43	10.85	7.00	10.75	12.50	12.70	10.67	10.02
14 Thompson Cariboo Shuswap	10.10	13.00	10.31	6.88	10.00	11.30	10.40	9.22	10.14
52 Northern Interior	10.00	13.86	12.38	5.25	12.50	8.80	9.20	12.89	10.40
51 Northwest	10.31	10.86	11.31	8.00	12.50	10.40	9.50	13.00	10.58

***Average Rank Score is calculated by weighting each chapter's score by the number of indicators used to calculate that score.

Table 13.1.3 Summary of Male Cohort

		Chapter 5	Chapter 6	Chapter 7	Chapter 8	Chapter 9	Chapter 10	Chapter 11	Chapter 12	***Average Rank Score
33	North Shore/Coast Garibaldi	5.50	5.57	3.54	5.63	6.00		5.70	5.67	5.21
41	South Vancouver Island	5.25	4.86	7.46	5.00	6.50		11.30	6.33	6.83
32	Vancouver	8.33	6.00	7.23	11.50	5.25		3.40	6.78	7.05
13	Okanagan	5.75	7.29	5.62	4.88	3.50	Not Applicable*	12.90	8.33	7.14
23	Fraser South	7.50	6.43	7.15	12.63	5.00		4.90	8.33	7.51
22	Fraser North	9.33	5.29	5.38	14.25	7.25		5.40	7.44	7.67
31	Richmond	11.08	4.00	5.31	13.75	8.50		4.20	7.44	7.67
12	Kootenay Boundary	4.25	11.14	8.00	3.25	8.25		12.40	9.11	7.90
43	North Vancouver Island	9.92	6.43	7.38	9.38	10.75		10.20	5.89	8.46
21	Fraser East	9.25	7.14	9.46	13.38	7.00		5.60	8.33	8.73
53	Northeast	7.50	12.83	12.00	9.50	14.00		5.50	7.75	9.31
42	Central Vancouver Island	8.00	8.00	10.92	7.13	9.00		12.40	10.44	9.60
11	East Kootenay	10.25	11.71	11.69	6.25	8.75		10.80	7.56	9.81
14	Thompson Cariboo Shuswap	7.33	13.43	10.38	8.63	8.00		11.50	9.44	9.81
52	Northern Interior	8.08	14.57	12.00	4.38	10.00		9.80	12.56	10.17
51	Northwest	10.17	9.57	10.69	6.50	13.75		10.00	12.44	10.27

   * Not Applicable: Chapter 10 dealt only with pregnancy and birth outcomes which are considered in the total cohort summary in Table 13.2.1
*** Average Rank Score is calculated by weighting each chapter's score by the number of indicators used to calculate that score.

Table 13.1.4 Summary of Female Cohort

		Chapter 5	Chapter 6	Chapter 7	Chapter 8	Chapter 9	Chapter 10	Chapter 11	Chapter 12	***Average Rank Score
33	North Shore/Coast Garibaldi	5.50	4.29	5.23	7.63	2.75		3.90	5.44	5.14
41	South Vancouver Island	5.17	3.86	5.38	4.88	5.50		9.00	6.00	5.78
31	Richmond	9.50	4.43	3.85	14.25	5.50		5.00	3.78	6.59
32	Vancouver	9.83	7.00	6.69	12.63	4.25		3.30	5.78	7.25
12	Kootenay Boundary	3.08	7.57	8.92	3.13	7.50	Not Applicable*	12.40	12.56	7.90
22	Fraser North	8.83	8.71	5.31	13.38	5.50		7.40	7.00	7.97
21	Fraser East	9.92	5.29	6.62	10.25	9.25		6.50	9.89	8.17
23	Fraser South	9.33	5.29	8.69	13.25	6.75		5.80	7.33	8.24
14	Thompson Cariboo Shuswap	7.67	12.00	9.08	5.13	11.25		8.20	9.67	8.71
13	Okanagan	5.92	7.86	9.15	8.13	7.25		12.80	9.22	8.73
43	North Vancouver Island	10.33	7.14	9.62	7.38	9.00		11.80	6.22	9.02
42	Central Vancouver Island	6.92	9.57	10.23	8.00	10.00		11.90	10.00	9.46
11	East Kootenay	8.50	11.71	11.31	5.25	9.00		12.20	8.33	9.62
53	Northeast	10.50	14.50	12.45	6.50	15.50		8.10	9.00	10.25
51	Northwest	8.33	12.14	11.46	10.00	10.25		8.80	12.67	10.43
52	Northern Interior	10.33	13.14	12.31	6.25	13.50		8.90	11.11	10.62

   * Not Applicable: Chapter 10 dealt only with pregnancy and birth outcomes which are considered in the total cohort summary in Table 13.2.1
*** Average Rank Score is calculated by weighting each chapter's score by the number of indicators used to calculate that score.

Table 13.1.5 Summary of Younger Cohort

		Chapter 5	Chapter 6	Chapter 7	Chapter 8	Chapter 9	Chapter 10	Chapter 11	Chapter 12	***Average Rank Score
32	Vancouver	5.77	5.29	5.00	13.29	7.75		5.10	7.86	6.67
33	North Shore/Coast Garibaldi	6.69	5.14	8.00	8.14	4.50		6.70	7.29	6.89
41	South Vancouver Island	6.31	5.86	8.31	6.71	5.50		9.10	8.43	7.38
22	Fraser North	8.23	8.29	4.00	13.71	8.75		6.70	6.14	7.51
21	Fraser East	8.67	7.00	8.15	7.83	9.00		6.50	5.43	7.54
13	Okanagan	6.77	7.71	9.08	6.00	3.50	Not Applicable*	9.20	8.14	7.62
31	Richmond	7.33	6.14	7.54	12.17	10.00		5.70	8.86	7.81
43	North Vancouver Island	9.92	5.86	4.54	5.60	11.75		10.50	7.86	7.83
23	Fraser South	8.85	6.43	8.85	11.57	6.75		7.80	4.14	8.03
12	Kootenay Boundary	7.17	9.57	9.08	4.33	4.25		8.30	13.29	8.31
14	Thompson Cariboo Shuswap	6.62	13.29	8.00	6.00	9.00		10.20	8.71	8.59
11	East Kootenay	9.33	8.43	9.00	5.17	7.50		11.20	8.00	8.76
52	Northern Interior	7.83	10.57	10.00	6.83	11.25		8.80	9.71	9.15
42	Central Vancouver Island	11.15	8.71	10.69	6.00	9.50		8.90	8.86	9.44
53	Northeast	8.29	13.67	9.67	6.29	13.50		11.60	10.17	10.11
51	Northwest	7.69	12.43	12.31	9.29	9.75		9.70	10.71	10.21

  * Not Applicable: Chapter 10 dealt only with pregnancy and birth outcomes which are considered in the total cohort summary in Table 13.2.1
*** Average Rank Score is calculated by weighting each chapter's score by the number of indicators used to calculate that score.

Table 13.1.6 Summary of Older Cohort

		Chapter 5	Chapter 6	Chapter 7	Chapter 8	Chapter 9	Chapter 10	Chapter 11	Chapter 12	***Average Rank Score
33	North Shore/Coast Garibaldi	6.43	8.33	3.45	5.00	6.50		4.40	8.00	5.62
41	South Vancouver Island	8.57	4.33	7.55	3.29	6.00		8.00	3.71	6.20
13	Okanagan	6.43	7.33	4.82	4.29	8.00		9.70	6.71	6.64
31	Richmond	10.00	7.67	7.18	7.83	1.50		7.00	5.71	7.24
21	Fraser East	10.86	3.50	8.55	12.33	8.00		5.90	6.00	7.80
32	Vancouver	11.00	9.83	7.64	7.43	1.50	Not Applicable*	6.40	8.14	7.92
12	Kootenay Boundary	8.00	13.00	9.18	4.00	11.50		6.30	8.86	8.31
53	Northeast	6.43	10.83	9.82	10.20	14.50		6.50	7.00	8.58
42	Central Vancouver Island	6.86	8.67	11.73	7.29	8.00		8.70	7.57	8.72
14	Thompson Cariboo Shuswap	5.86	11.50	10.91	7.00	11.00		8.40	9.14	9.02
11	East Kootenay	9.29	11.67	10.36	5.83	13.50		9.60	5.86	9.14
22	Fraser North	10.29	5.67	7.18	12.83	4.00		9.40	12.14	9.16
23	Fraser South	7.57	5.67	10.45	11.43	8.00		9.90	9.57	9.28
43	North Vancouver Island	12.71	6.83	9.18	9.00	9.50		11.10	12.00	10.18
51	Northwest	7.29	8.67	10.45	12.40	9.50		11.00	12.00	10.27
52	Northern Interior	8.43	12.50	7.55	9.80	15.00		13.70	13.57	11.00

  * Not Applicable: Chapter 10 dealt only with pregnancy and birth outcomes which are considered in the total cohort summary in Table 13.2.1
*** Average Rank Score is calculated by weighting each chapter's score by the number of indicators used to calculate that score.

The geography of wellness assets in BC

The maps in this group provided more than 60 indicators, of which 29 were at the HSDA level. They presented a variety of wellness-related assets of individuals, families, and communities. Some were based on the traditional "determinants of health," while others focused specifically on initiatives that supported ActNow BC. Some were new to this edition of the Atlas, while others were updates of indicators presented in the original Atlas so that changes over time could be assessed. Overall, these maps provided an important context for the chapters that followed.

When considering family, income, and housing assets, the HSDAs with the best overall results were Northeast and Fraser South, two very different regions of the province. These were followed by Fraser North, Richmond, and South Vancouver Island in the urban southwest of the province, Northern Interior, and East Kootenay in the extreme southeast of the province. The HSDAs with poorest values were North and Central Vancouver Island and Northwest, all in the western part of the province.

For connectedness assets, North Shore/Coast Garibaldi had the best overall results, followed by Kootenay Boundary, Fraser South, South Vancouver Island, and Fraser North, all in the urban southwest of the province. At the other extreme, Northern Interior had the poorest connectedness values, followed by Northwest, also in the northern half of the province, Northern Vancouver Island, and Vancouver. Only Vancouver is in the urban part of BC.

The assets related to health improvements were most prominent in South Vancouver Island and Kootenay Boundary, followed by Central Vancouver Island, Vancouver, and Okanagan. The HSDAs with the poorest results were Fraser North, Fraser South, and Fraser East.

For education, culture, arts, and volunteerism assets, Vancouver and North Shore/Coast Garibaldi had by far the best overall results, followed by Richmond, South Vancouver Island, Kootenay Boundary, and Fraser North. At the other extreme, the three northern HSDAs, Northeast, Northern Interior, and Northwest, as well as Fraser East had the poorest results. Generally, there was a regional split between the urban southwest HSDAs and the northern part of the province, and this reflected, to some extent, the patterns for lifelong learning as demonstrated by the composite learning index.

The last group of assets related to safety. There were two groups with the best safety results: parts of the urban southwest, including North Shore/Coast Garibaldi,

Richmond, and South Vancouver Island; and the southeast part of the province, including Kootenay Boundary and East Kootenay. Those with the poorest safety results included the three northern HSDAs, along with Vancouver in the southwest and Thompson Cariboo Shuswap in the interior of the province.

The geography of smoke-free environments and behaviours in BC

In total, there were nine indicators in this group, eight of which were at the HSDA level. Results from youth non-smoking behaviour were available from two surveys; however, only those from the CCHS 4.1 were used in the average rank calculation.

There were several significant differences between genders and age cohorts. Females were more likely to have a smoke-free environment, have restrictions against smoking in the home, and be non-smokers. Generally, smoke-free environments and behaviours were more prevalent as age increased, except for restrictions against smoking cigarettes at home, when the mid-age cohort was higher than the youth and senior cohorts, and for non-smoking behaviour, when the mid-age cohort was lower than the other two cohorts. However, among grade students, non-smoking decreased as grade increased. Although younger respondents had higher levels of non-smoking, what is worrisome is that youth had lower levels of smoke-free environments, making them susceptible to initiating smoking and to second-hand smoke.

Overall, Richmond, South Vancouver Island, and North Shore/Coast Garibaldi had the best overall results for smoke-free environments and behaviours, followed by Fraser South, Fraser East, and Fraser North. The HSDAs with the poorest results were Northeast, Northern Interior, Thompson Cariboo Shuswap, East Kootenay, Northwest, and Kootenay Boundary. This showed a clear regional pattern, with the southwest part of the province having the best results, and the north and interior parts of the province having relatively poor results.

This pattern was generally repeated for both males and females separately. Among youth, North Vancouver Island, Vancouver, and North Shore/Coast Garibaldi had the best results on average, much higher than for the all respondents cohort, while youth in East Kootenay also had much higher average results. However, Richmond and Fraser North fared more poorly than for the all respondents cohort. Among seniors, Fraser East, South Vancouver Island, and Fraser North and Fraser South had the best values, while Richmond and Kootenay Boundary had lower values than for all respondents.

Comparisons with Canadian averages showed that BC cohorts generally had better smoke-free characteristics, except in the work environment, and to a lesser extent in public places.

The geography of food security and nutrition in BC

The first part of this summary deals with the potential resources for generating healthy, land-based foods in BC. The second part focuses on those indicators that were available at the HSDA level. Of the more than 30 indicators included in this group, 13 were at the HSDA level.

Two basic natural resources for producing food are climate and land. Generally, climatic conditions favour the southern and western parts of the province, the Okanagan Valley, and the Peace River area of the northeast. Farming is concentrated in these regions. A large number of small farms are found particularly in the southwest of the province on the Agricultural Land Reserve. Much larger farms are found in the interior and northeastern part of BC where land and climate conditions are not as favourable as in the south.

The key types of farming are beef cattle ranching and farming, including feedlots; fruit and tree nut farming; and horse and other equine production. Dairy cattle and milk production are important in the lower Fraser Valley in the southwest. Many farms have developed greenhouse production capacity, especially those close to the major population centres in the south. Some of this capacity is taken up by floriculture rather than food production, but has the potential to generate food products if required. Organic fruit and vegetable production is important in the south, while organic animal production is important in the interior and parts of Vancouver Island. One of the major challenges is the pressure between agriculture and housing development, especially in the southwest of the province where most of the population growth has occurred (Katz, 2009).

There were some major gender differences in responses related to nutrition and food security. Females were consistently more likely to avoid certain foods because of concern and knowledge about content (mainly in relation to salt, cholesterol, calories, and fat) compared to males. Females ate more fruit and vegetable servings and engaged in less binge drinking than males. This gender difference was observed across most HSDAs and age cohorts. The three key food security indicators – the derived food security variable, enough of the kinds of food wanted, and always able to afford balanced meals –

improved with age of respondent. Further, youth were less likely to avoid food for content reasons when compared to older age cohorts, and only about half of student respondents always ate breakfast on every school day, a rather disturbing result given the importance of the breakfast meal for learning. These results suggest that the youngest respondents are more vulnerable to food insecurity and poor nutrition.

Those HSDAs with the best results for food security and nutrition based on an average ranking were found in the urban lower mainland of BC. These were North Shore/Coast Garibaldi, followed by Richmond and Fraser North. The poorest overall values for nutrition and food security were found in the north and extreme southeast of BC. These were Northeast, Northern Interior, East Kootenay, and Northwest. These patterns were generally consistent for males and females, separately. For the youth cohort, the pattern was somewhat different, with Fraser North, North Vancouver Island, and Vancouver displaying the best results, while Northwest followed by Central Vancouver Island, Kootenay Boundary, and Northeast had the poorest results. For seniors, North Shore/Coast Garibaldi had by far the best result and Central Vancouver Island had the poorest.

For those indicators where Canadian comparisons could be made, there were no notable differences, except for one indicator: BC respondents were less likely to binge drink.

The geography of physical activity in BC

There were more than 25 indicators in this group, of which 21 were at the HSDA level. However, only 8 were included in the average ranking exercise because many were related to specific types of sports club memberships, and we chose to only include total sports club memberships in the average ranking procedure. Nevertheless, the first part of this summary provides a brief overview of the different sports.

Overall, males were more likely to be members of sports clubs, but there were certain sports for which this was not the case. For example, membership in athletics clubs was quite similar between genders, while artistic gymnastics was dominated by female members, as was equestrian, softball, and figure skating club membership. Female membership was also higher for cross-country skiing. Generally, club membership diminished with age, although golf and curling had a higher number of members in older age groups.

For actual physical activities, males were more likely to have undertaken gardening or yard work and bicycling than females, while females were more likely to have walked and exercised at home than males. It is interesting to note that females that worked outside the home were more likely to have access to health-related programs at or near their workplace. These differences generally occurred at both the provincial and individual HSDA levels. Youth were more likely to have gone swimming or bicycling than the older age cohorts, but the opposite was the case for walking and gardening or doing yard work. Based on data from the Student Satisfaction Survey, vigorous physical activity declined as grade increased, a result recently confirmed in BC using the McCreary AHS IV data (Smith et al., 2011), and the location of physical activity was almost equally divided between school and out-of-school settings. Leisure time physical activity based on the derived Physical Activity Index indicated that males were more active than females, and that physical activity decreased with age.

Overall, based on an average ranking for club membership (only the total sports club membership data were used, as noted above) and physical activities, Kootenay Boundary, South Vancouver Island, East Kootenay, and Northern Interior were the most physically active HSDAs, while HSDAs in the southwest urban lower mainland, with the exception of North Shore/Coast Garibaldi, were the least physically active. With the key exception of South Vancouver Island, there was a clear division between more active individuals in rural HSDAs compared to less physically active individuals in urban HSDAs. This differential has been noted elsewhere for youth in BC (Smith et al., 2011).

These patterns were quite similar for both males and females separately, although females in Thompson Cariboo Shuswap were ranked much higher than males, and for the total population as a whole. Patterns were also similar for the youth and seniors cohorts, with a couple of exceptions. For youth, both North and Central Vancouver Island were more physically active than other age cohorts, and South Vancouver Island less so, while for seniors, North Shore/Coast Garibaldi did better and Northwest poorer than for other age cohorts.

The geography of healthy weight in BC

Only four indicators, all at the HSDA level, were included in this group. Healthy weight tended to fall with age. While females had a healthier BMI than males, males were more likely to perceive their weight as just about right. BC cohorts had healthier BMIs than their Canadian counterparts.

The best healthy weight results for all respondents were found in North Shore/Coast Garibaldi and Vancouver,

followed by Okanagan and South Vancouver Island. The three northern HSDAs, Northeast, Northern Interior, and Northwest, had the poorest results. Generally, the urban southwest HSDAs had the best results, while the north, along with parts of Vancouver Island and some interior HSDAs, had the poorest results for healthy weights. The geographical pattern was quite similar for males and females separately, although Okanagan females had a poorer result than for the total population in that HSDA, while males had the best result among all HSDAs in the province. In addition, while North Shore/Coast Garibaldi females had the best results in the province, males in that HSDA did not do as well as for the total population.

The patterns were somewhat different for the youth and seniors cohorts. For youth, Okanagan had the best result, followed by Kootenay Boundary, North Shore/Coast Garibaldi, and South Vancouver Island, while Northeast, North Vancouver Island, and Northern Interior had the poorest results. For seniors, Richmond, Vancouver, and Fraser North had the best results, while Northern Interior, Northeast, East Kootenay, Kootenay Boundary, and Thompson Cariboo Shuswap had the poorest results. Generally, the poorest results occurred in the north and interior of the province.

The geography of healthy pregnancy and birth in BC

There were 10 indicators in this group, all of which were at the HSDA level. Overall, Richmond and Northeast had the best results based on average rankings for healthy pregnancy and birth. At the other end of the spectrum, Central Vancouver Island had the poorest results, followed by Thompson Cariboo Shuswap, North Vancouver Island, and Northwest. There are a couple of clear regional groupings. With the exception of Richmond in the urban southwest, the best values occurred in the southern interior and eastern parts of the province. The poorest values occurred on Vancouver Island, and the northwest and central interior of BC.

A couple of key points are worthy of comment. There were large variations throughout the province among the different indicators, and no individual HSDA did consistently well, nor poorly, on all indicators. For example, Richmond was in the top quintile for some indicators, but in the lowest quintile for mother's age; Fraser North was in the bottom quintile for a couple of indicators, while it was in the top quintile for infant mortality; North Vancouver Island was in the bottom quintile for several indicators, but in the top quintile for full-term delivery. Among the HSDAs, only South Vancouver Island had no rankings in either the top or bottom quintiles for any of the indicators.

The second important point refers to changes over time when compared to results reported in the previous Atlas. When the same data sources were used, results and patterns were very similar between the two sets of time periods used for the indicators.

Finally, as noted previously, caution in interpreting results is necessary for the northeast and southeast HSDAs because of proximity to Alberta, where some birth events to BC mothers would have occurred.

The geography of chronic-free conditions in BC

There were 10 indicators in this group, all of which were at the HSDA level. As expected, values for every chronic-free measure decreased as age increased. Further, there were gender differences for all but back problems, high blood pressure, and asthma. Males were significantly more likely than females to be free of difficulties with regular activities in general, and for both inside the home and outside activities. Males were also more likely than females to have never been diagnosed with cancer and arthritis or rheumatism. On the other hand, females were more likely than males to have never been diagnosed with heart problems or diabetes.

When the average ranks were calculated based on all of the indicators, there were some clear geographical differences throughout the province. Vancouver had the best overall value for chronic-free conditions, followed by Richmond, North Shore/Coast Garibaldi, Fraser South, and Northeast. With the exception of the latter, these HSDAs were all in the urban lower mainland of BC. At the other extreme, there were two groups with relatively low levels of chronic-free conditions: North, Central, and South Vancouver Island; and the interior HSDAs of Okanagan, Kootenay Boundary, East Kootenay, and Thompson Shuswap Cariboo. These patterns were also evident for males and females separately, with a couple of exceptions. For males, North Shore/Coast Garibaldi dropped in overall ranking while Fraser North improved, although the actual average ranked scores were not that dissimilar. For females, Northeast dropped overall while Fraser East improved.

There were some key differences for the younger and senior cohorts when compared to the patterns for the all respondents cohort. For the younger cohort, the best overall results were still evident in the lower mainland part of BC, Northeast had the poorest overall result, while South and Central Vancouver Island and Kootenay Boundary in particular were improved relative to the all

respondents cohort. For the senior cohort, North Shore/Coast Garibaldi had the best overall results, other lower mainland HSDAs did less well than for other cohorts, while Kootenay Boundary had much better results. At the other extreme, Northern Interior, North Vancouver Island, and Northwest had the poorest results.

In comparing BC to Canadian average values, Canadians as a whole were more likely to be free of back problems, and less likely to have reductions in activity outside the home. Further, Canadian respondents were more likely to have never been diagnosed with cancer than those in BC. However, BC respondents were much more likely to have never been diagnosed with diabetes, high blood pressure, asthma, and heart disease than their Canadian counterparts.

The geography of wellness outcomes in BC

There were nine indicators in this group, all of which were at the HSDA level. Some differences in wellness outcomes were seen based on gender and age. Females generally had better results for wellness outcomes, especially for self-rated oral health and being injury-free, and they had longer life expectancies than males. Wellness outcomes were generally much better for youth than the mid-age and senior cohorts, except for being injury-free. However, seniors had the best result for stress-free days. In comparison to results for Canadian respondents as a whole, BC had poorer values for mental health and oral health for the majority of cohorts, but results were better than their Canadian counterparts for stress-free days.

Based on an average ranking of each of the indicators, North Shore/Coast Garibaldi had the best overall wellness outcomes result, followed by Richmond, South Vancouver Island, North Vancouver Island, and Vancouver. The HSDAs with the poorest results for wellness outcomes were Northwest, Northern Interior, Kootenay Boundary, and Central Vancouver Island. With the exception of North Vancouver Island, the best results for overall wellness outcomes occurred in the urban southwest of the province, including South Vancouver Island, while poorer results were evident in the north (with the exception of Northeast) and interior parts of the province. Central Vancouver Island was an outlier on Vancouver Island, with much poorer results than the other two island HSDAs. Both male and female respondents individually had similar geographical patterns to those for the all respondents cohort, although Richmond males had relatively poorer results while females in Richmond had the best results of all HSDAs in the province.

There were very different patterns evident for the youth and senior cohorts in comparison to the previously described cohorts. For youth, the best results were found in Fraser South, Fraser East, and Fraser North, while much poorer results were evident in Kootenay Boundary, Northwest, and Northeast. For seniors, the best wellness outcomes overall occurred in South Vancouver Island, followed by Richmond, East Kootenay, and Fraser East, while at the other extreme, much poorer wellness outcomes were found in Northern Interior, Fraser North, Northwest, and North Vancouver Island.

A summary of gender differences in wellness

Based on the above summaries of the 63 indicators available separately for males and females, there are some general conclusions we can make about the differences between genders at the provincial average level in terms of wellness. While we include administrative and survey data in terms of this analysis, we include only those survey data in which there was a statistically significant difference in results between genders.

For Chapter 5 (Assets), where gender differences occurred, females had better wellness assets than males. While males did better in terms of income, family connectedness, and having meals with family, females did better in terms of school connectedness, emotional supports, made improvements to health in the past 12 months, and intended to improve health in the coming 12 months. Females were also more likely to have had better access to health programs at or near work, and volunteered more than males. For Chapter 6 (Smoke-free Environments and Behaviours), females did better than males with respect to smoke-free workplaces, restrictions on smoking in the home, and being non-smokers. There were no indicators in this category for which males did better than females.

For Chapter 7 (Food Security and Nutrition), females did better than males on avoiding a variety of foods based on their content, and were more likely to eat healthy portions of fruits and vegetables on a daily basis, and less likely to binge drink. In contrast, males were less likely to have gone to bed hungry and more likely to have eaten breakfast on a school day. For leisure time physical activity (Chapter 8), males were more likely to have participated in gardening or yard work, bicycled, been a member of a sports club, and had a higher healthy leisure time Physical Activity Index than females. However, females were more likely to have walked, exercised at home, and had access to a gym or physical fitness facility at or close to their work than their male counterparts. With

respect to healthy weight issues (Chapter 9), females were more likely to report a healthy BMI, while males were more likely to have considered their weight to be about right.

Based on Chapter 11 (Chronic-free Conditions), males did better overall than females. Males were more likely to have been free of difficulty in performing regular activities, and had no long-term conditions that affected activities either inside or out of the home. Further, males were less likely than females to have been diagnosed with cancer and arthritis or rheumatism. However, females were less likely than males to have been diagnosed with diabetes or heart disease. For wellness outcomes (Chapter 12), females were more likely to have had good oral health, have been injury-free, and had higher life expectancies both at birth and at age 65 years than their male counterparts.

A summary of age differences in wellness

Data were available to make age comparisons at the provincial level for 48 wellness indicators. Younger age (usually 12-19 years) cohorts and senior cohorts (usually 65 years and older) were compared with the mid-age cohort (usually 20-64 years). Only CCHS data were available for this summary.

Younger compared to mid-age

For assets (Chapter 5), younger age respondents were more closely connected to their local communities, and more likely to have done something to improve health in the past 12 months, but responded they would be less likely to do so in the coming 12 months than their mid-age counterparts. However, for smoke-free environments and behaviour (Chapter 6), younger people were less likely to have frequented smoke-free public places, had smoke-free work environments, ridden in smoke-free vehicles, or lived in a home that restricted or did not allow smoking, when compared to the mid-age cohort. On the other hand, younger people were less likely to smoke than the mid-age cohort respondents.

For food security and nutrition (Chapter 7), the younger age cohort was less likely to have responded that they were food secure, or that they had avoided foods because of contents such as calories, cholesterol, fat, or salt, but they were more likely to have eaten healthy amounts of fruits and vegetables, and less likely to have participated in binge drinking than their mid-age counterparts. With respect to physical activities (Chapter 8), younger respondents were less likely to have walked or done gardening or yard work in their leisure time, but more likely to have gone swimming or bicycled and, overall, had a higher healthy Physical Activity Index than the mid-age cohort. For healthy weight issues (Chapter 9), younger people were more likely to have indicated a healthy BMI and perceived their weight to have been just about right.

As expected for chronic-free conditions (Chapter 11), younger age cohorts had much better results than their mid-age counterparts for all chronic conditions except asthma, for which there was no difference. For wellness outcomes (Chapter 12), again younger people had better results than their mid-age counterparts for all comparative indicators, except for injuries, where younger people were more likely to have responded that they had suffered an injury.

Older compared to mid-age

For the assets indicators (Chapter 5), at the provincial level, senior respondents had a stronger connection to their local community, but were less likely to have done something in the past 12 months to improve their health, or planned to improve their health in the next 12 months, when compared to the mid-age cohort. In the smoke-free environments and behaviours (Chapter 6) category, seniors were more likely to have frequented smoke-free environments, travelled in smoke-free vehicles, had smoke-free homes, and been non-smokers than their mid-age counterparts. However, they were less likely to have had smoking restrictions in their residence.

Seniors indicated that they were more food secure (Chapter 7), always had enough of the kinds of food they wanted to eat, and were more likely to have always been able to afford balanced meals in the past 12 months when compared with their mid-age counterparts. Seniors were also more likely to have avoided food because of its contents, particularly cholesterol and salt, but they were less likely to have done so because of the calorie content. Seniors were less likely to have participated in binge drinking and more likely to have had healthy servings of fruits and vegetables than the mid-age cohort. With respect to physical activity (Chapter 8), seniors as a whole were less likely to have gone swimming, cycled, or exercised at home, and seniors also had a lower leisure time Physical Activity Index than the mid-age cohort. There were no differences between the two cohorts for healthy weight indicators (Chapter 9).

Given that chronic conditions generally develop over time, seniors had poorer values than their mid-age counterparts for all chronic-free conditions (Chapter 10), except for asthma, for which there was no difference. However, for wellness outcomes (Chapter 12), seniors indicated they had been less likely to be stressed on a daily basis or to have been injured in the past 12 months when compared

with the mid-age cohort. Overall, though, seniors had poorer self-rated health.

Developing a composite picture of wellness for BC

In order to give a general, overall wellness picture for the province, we combined all of the indicators into an average rank. While the summaries just presented were based on average ranks for the groups of indicators available by *chapter*, this composite picture is based on the rankings for *all* the indicators available at the HSDA level to construct the average rank for each HSDA.

There are many methods available to develop a composite score or index, but our approach is probably the simplest. There are a number of limitations in our approach. First, it assumes that each indicator has the same influence on wellness. Second, the difference in values between ranks can vary substantially. Third, there is also some double counting because one indicator is derived in part from data from another indicator also included in the index. Fourth, we used data from different years. What we are doing is processing information to look at overall *patterns* of wellness within BC, not the *actual values* of wellness. Users can construct their own composite picture by choosing the indicators that they feel are important.

A five map model is used to provide wellness pictures for the total population in the province, for males and females separately, and for younger and older cohorts. In a few cases, the age ranges vary, as noted previously. The number of indicators also varies by cohort. While there were 90 variables for the total cohort, there were fewer for other cohorts. The indicators in Chapter 10 on healthy pregnancy and birth are only used in the total cohort picture. A few indicators for which there are several gaps in data for HSDAs, usually because of small sample sizes, are dropped for those cohorts. The number of variables used for each of the five cohorts is included in the table on the next page. HSDA values in this table guide us in describing overall wellness patterns in BC.

We have no intention to derive actual composite values for wellness. Rather, our focus is to provide overall *relative* comparisons among HSDAs in order to map patterns of overall wellness within BC. The weighted average ranks of each cohort is used to map the summary. The theoretical range of average ranking is from 1 (all indicators in the HSDA ranked 1) to 16 (all ranked 16). Both these scenarios are highly unlikely in practice because of the large number of indicators used to assess the various dimensions of wellness.

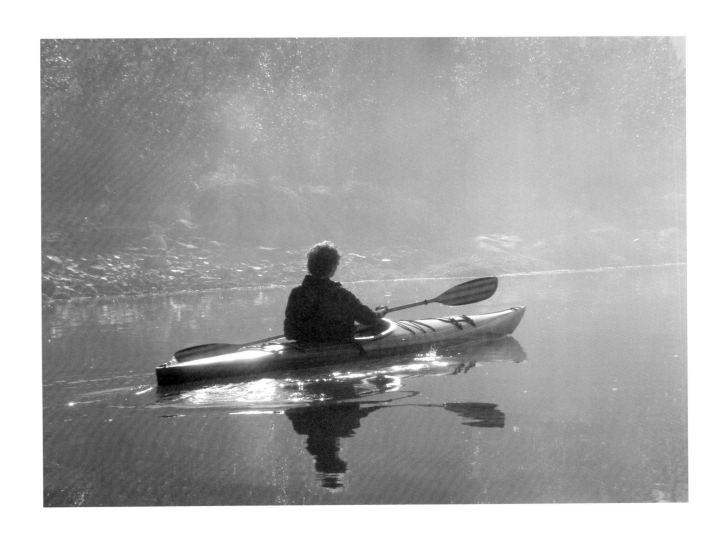

Cohort summary by weighted average value

Health Service Delivery Area	Total	Male	Female	Younger	Older
33 North Shore/Coast Garibaldi	5.41	5.21	5.14	6.89	5.62
31 Richmond	6.33	7.67	6.59	7.81	7.24
41 South Vancouver Island	6.49	6.83	5.78	7.38	6.20
32 Vancouver	7.38	7.05	7.25	6.67	7.92
12 Kootenay Boundary	7.63	7.90	7.90	8.31	8.31
22 Fraser North	7.68	7.67	7.97	7.51	9.16
23 Fraser South	7.87	7.51	8.24	8.03	9.28
13 Okanagan	8.11	7.14	8.73	7.62	6.64
21 Fraser East	8.79	8.73	8.17	7.54	7.80
53 Northeast	8.90	9.31	10.25	10.11	8.58
11 East Kootenay	9.07	9.81	9.62	8.76	9.14
43 North Vancouver Island	9.22	8.46	9.02	7.83	10.18
42 Central Vancouver Island	10.02	9.60	9.46	9.44	8.72
14 Thompson Cariboo Shuswap	10.14	9.81	8.71	8.59	9.02
52 Northern Interior	10.40	10.17	10.62	9.15	11.00
51 Northwest	10.58	10.27	10.43	10.21	10.27
Number of Indicators	**90**	**63**	**63**	**59**	**48**

Total cohort

Based on 90 wellness indicators, North Shore/Coast Garibaldi has the best overall average wellness rank, followed by Richmond and South Vancouver Island. The poorest average wellness ranks occurred in Northwest, Northern Interior, Thompson Cariboo Shuswap, and Central Vancouver Island. The general geographical pattern shows that the urban HSDAs in the southwest of the province, including Southern Vancouver Island, have much better wellness characteristics than the more rural northern and interior HSDAs. A couple of points worth noting are the relatively good average rank for the interior HSDA of Kootenay Boundary, which is marginally better than both Fraser North and Fraser South in the urban lower mainland of the province, and the relatively poor showing of Central Vancouver Island compared to its southern neighbour, South Vancouver Island.

Male cohort

Based on 63 wellness indicators, North Shore/Coast Garibaldi had the best overall average wellness rank, followed by South Vancouver Island. At the other extreme, Northwest, Northern Interior and Northeast had the poorest average ranks. General geographical patterns again showed higher average wellness characteristics for the urban southwest part of the province, and much poorer characteristics for the north and interior HSDAs. In the urban lower mainland region, Richmond did not do as well, while Okanagan, in the interior, did better than for the population as a whole.

Female cohort

Based on 63 wellness indicators (no pregnancy or birth indicators were included as they formed part of the total population cohort characteristics), North Shore/Coast Garibaldi and South Vancouver Island again both had the best overall average wellness rankings, along with Richmond, while the three northern HSDAs, Northern Interior, Northwest, and Northeast, each had relatively poor average wellness characteristics.

Younger cohort

This category includes some relatively older respondents (35-49 years) when chronic-free conditions are included, rather than the 12-19 year cohort used for most indicators. Based on 59 wellness indicators, Vancouver, North Shore/Coast Garibaldi, and South Vancouver Island, all urban areas in the southwest of the province, had the best average wellness ranks, while at the other extreme, Northwest had the poorest, followed by Northeast, Central Vancouver Island and Northern Interior.

Older cohort

Based on 48 wellness indicators, North Shore/Coast Garibaldi had the best average wellness characteristics, followed by South Vancouver Island, and Okanagan in the interior. The HSDA with the poorest average wellness characteristics was Northern Interior, followed by Northwest and North Vancouver Island, all more remote and rural HSDAs. What is quite different for seniors is that Fraser North and Fraser South, both urban HSDAs in the lower mainland, also had relatively poor wellness characteristics.

Cohort summary by weighted average value

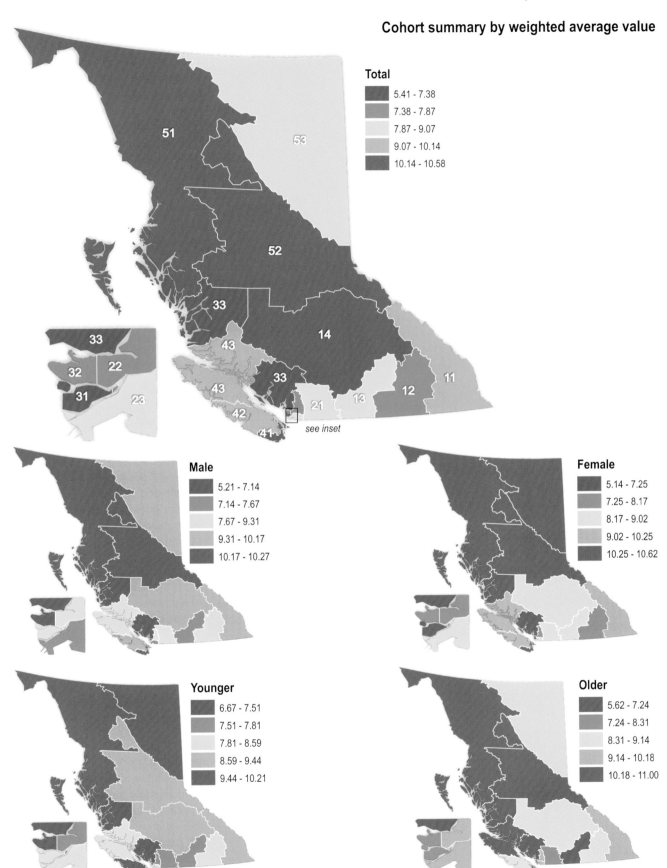

Total
- 5.41 - 7.38
- 7.38 - 7.87
- 7.87 - 9.07
- 9.07 - 10.14
- 10.14 - 10.58

Male
- 5.21 - 7.14
- 7.14 - 7.67
- 7.67 - 9.31
- 9.31 - 10.17
- 10.17 - 10.27

Female
- 5.14 - 7.25
- 7.25 - 8.17
- 8.17 - 9.02
- 9.02 - 10.25
- 10.25 - 10.62

Younger
- 6.67 - 7.51
- 7.51 - 7.81
- 7.81 - 8.59
- 8.59 - 9.44
- 9.44 - 10.21

Older
- 5.62 - 7.24
- 7.24 - 8.31
- 8.31 - 9.14
- 9.14 - 10.18
- 10.18 - 11.00

Developing benchmarks

Average wellness ranks for the total population ranged from 5.41 to 10.58, indicating major geographical differences overall in the province. With one or two minor exceptions, the urban southwest HSDAs, including South Vancouver Island, had relatively better overall wellness indicators in BC, while the more rural and northern HSDAs had much poorer wellness indicators. The urban-rural split is quite noticeable for many of the individual indicators noted in earlier chapters, as well as based on this average ranking approach. Further, it is important to note that the younger cohort had the smallest range (6.67 to 10.21) in ranks among HSDAs, showing the least geographical variation, while seniors, with the highest range (5.62 to 11.00) among HSDAs, had the greatest geographical variation. While part of these differences may be related to the number of indicators included in the average ranking process, this is not the case for the difference between genders: males had a smaller range (5.21 to 10.27) of average ranks than did females (5.14 to 10.62), indicating less geographical variability for males than females.

North Shore/Coast Garibaldi and South Vancouver Island were the only two HSDAs that were consistently in the best quintile for all five cohorts. At the other extreme, Northwest had the poorest overall wellness ranking and was consistently in the lowest quintile for all cohorts, followed by Northern Interior, which was in the lowest quintile for four of the five cohorts, and in the second lowest quintile for the fifth cohort. As an interior, rural HSDA, Kootenay Boundary did relatively well overall, while Okanagan did relatively well for males and for seniors: it had the fourth best rank for males and the third best rank for seniors among all HSDAs.

If users of this Atlas wish to look for potential benchmarks to study further, to discover which HSDAs have good wellness assets, the results of our simple exercise indicate that North Shore/Coast Garibaldi and South Vancouver Island can be viewed as benchmarks worthy of further examination to look at the key characteristics that make them the "best" in BC for wellness. For younger age groups, Vancouver could be studied in more detail, while for seniors, North Shore/Coast Garibaldi could be viewed as the benchmark HSDA for study.

Concluding statement

This Atlas provides approximately 160 different indicators related to wellness, some providing distinctions between gender and age, and over 400 maps showing how these indicators vary within BC. One of the aims of the Atlas was to demonstrate how various indicators showing different components of wellness are distributed throughout the province. While each map is accompanied by a brief description providing salient and significant points, the intention was always to let the "maps speak for themselves" in order to generate discussions about whether or not the geographical differences are important and, if so, what might or should be done to lessen the "inequities" in wellness between regions of the province. Understanding the reasons for the inequities is a job best left to those who live in communities within the administrative units that have been used for mapping purposes.

Examining the values of the various wellness indicators provides an opportunity to determine the "best" HSDA for any particular indicator. Other regions that are below that value can set themselves a target of matching or even improving upon the "best" or benchmark HSDA indicator value. Those areas with a lower value can also look to learn from those that have achieved the "best" result, and examine why they are doing as well as they are: What are the characteristics that make a difference? Are there specific assets in those communities that encourage wellness, such as community gardens, or special facilities such as seniors' parks, or by-laws that are more stringent than provincial standards to encourage wellness behaviours? Are neighbourhoods safe and do they encourage walking and cycling? Are there accessible activity centres and recreation and sport clubs? Are there accessible stores selling fresh fruits and vegetables? At school, are students learning how to be and stay healthy? These are just some of the questions that can be asked, but there are many more.

This chapter has provided summaries of all the key wellness dimensions that we have focused upon, and indicated which HSDAs do best for specific components of wellness, and which do best overall and can be considered as benchmarks for others to learn from. Further, benchmark HSDAs are noted for males and females, separately, as well as for the total population, and benchmark HSDAs are suggested for younger and senior age cohorts, based on a very simple average ranking scheme.

The data, tables, and maps produced in this Atlas give users enough information to ask themselves a variety of questions about their community and region with a view to improving local wellness, which in turn will contribute to improved wellness overall in the province. While our approach has been to use clusters of indicators, users can construct their own composite index using fewer, but perhaps locally agreed upon strategic indicators, or can add more indicators as they see fit. We see this Atlas as a basis for understanding geographical variations in wellness throughout the province, and as a way to provide information visually to users and assist in knowledge development and transfer. We have taken available data that can be updated over time, and combined indicators to develop benchmark HSDAs. There will undoubtedly be better results at a smaller community level. There will be geographical "highs" and "lows" within all of the HSDAs because they cover large geographical areas and/or have large, diverse populations.

The 2010 Olympic and Paralympic Games have been and gone. Internationally, the World Health Organization has recognized ActNow BC as a promising practice for health promotion and chronic disease prevention, as have the Public Health Association of Canada, the Conference Board of Canada, and the Health Council of Canada within Canada. Smoking reduction and healthier pregnancy targets have been met at the provincial level, and while ActNow BC has been "reformatted," health promotion and chronic disease prevention strategies will be continued under the Healthy Families BC Strategy. Goals still need to be achieved to improve the wellness of the citizenry. As demonstrated in this Atlas, major geographical inequities remain such that not all regions have shared in provincial improvements in wellness, and these differences need to be addressed.

We hope that this second edition of the *BC Atlas of Wellness* will contribute to the continuing discussion of why some regions are more "well" than others and what might be done about it, and how efforts and resources can be targeted to reduce inequities and achieve overall improvements in the health and wellness of people in British Columbia.

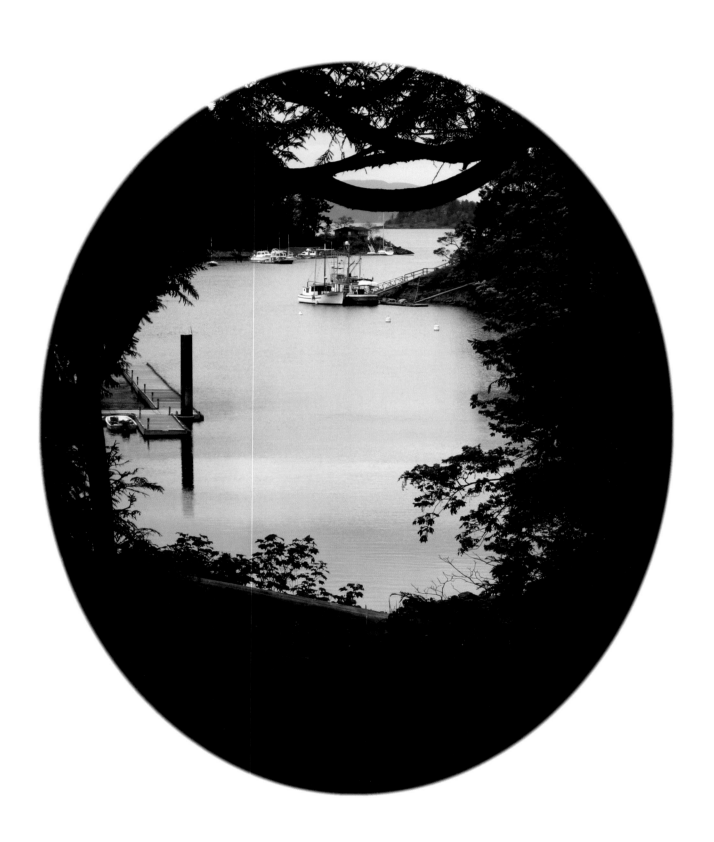

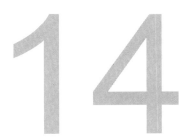

References

2010 Legacies Now. (nd). *Cultural mapping toolkit.* 2010 Legacies Now and Creative City Network of Canada, Partnership. http://www.2010legaciesnow.com/fileadmin/user_upload/ExploreArts/Toolkits/CultureMapping.pdf. Accessed: 25 April, 2010.

Active Healthy Kids Canada. (2010). *Healthy habits start earlier than you think: The Active Healthy Kids Canada Report Card on physical activity for children and youth 2010.* http://www.activehealthykids.ca/ecms.ashx/2010ActiveHealthyKidsCanadaReportCard-shortform.pdf. Accessed: 7 September, 2010.

Active Healthy Kids Canada. (2011). *Don't let this be the most physical activity our kids get after school: The Active Healthy Kids Canada Report Card on physical activity for children and youth 2011.* http://www.activehealthykids.ca/ReportCard/2011ReportCardOverview.aspx. Accessed: 26 April, 2011.

ActNow BC. (2006). *Measuring our success: Baseline Report.* Victoria: ActNow BC. http://www.actnowbc.ca/additional_resources/measuring_our_success. Accessed: 3 January, 2011.

ActNow BC. (2008). *Measuring our success: Progress Report I.* Victoria: ActNow BC. http://www.actnowbc.ca/additional_resources/measuring_our_success. Accessed: 3 January, 2011.

ActNow BC. (2009). *Creating a healthy workplace environment: Workbook and toolkit.* Victoria: Ministry of Healthy Living and Sport.

ActNow BC. (2010). *Measuring our success: Progress Report II.* Victoria: ActNow BC.

Adams, T., Bezner, J., & Steinhardt, M. (1997). The conceptualization and measurement of perceived wellness: Integrating balance across and within dimensions. *American Journal of Health Promotion*, 11: 208-218.

Agricultural Land Commission. (2009). *Annual Report 2008-2009.* Burnaby: Agricultural Land Commission.

Alcoe, J. (2010). *The heart of well-being: Seven tools for surviving and thriving.* London, UK: The Janki Foundation for Global Health Care and the British Holistic Medical Association.

Anderson, R., Mikulic, B., & Sandor, E. (2010). Quality of life in the EU: Trends in key dimensions 2003-2009. Presented at 96th Directors General of the National Statistical Institutes Conference, Measuring progress, well-being and sustainable development. Sofia, 30th September. http://www.dgins-sofia2010.eu/pagebg.php?P=10. Accessed: 2 May, 2011.

Anspaugh, D., Hamrick, M., & Rosato, F. (2004). *Wellness: Concepts and applications (6th edition).* Boston: McGraw Hill. Cited in: G. Miller and L. Foster (2010). A brief summary of holistic wellness literature. *Journal of Holistic Healthcare*, 7(1): 4-8.

Antonovsky, A. (1996). The salutogenic model as a theory to guide health promotion. *Health Promotion International*, 11(1): 11-18.

Armstrong, D. (2000). A survey of community gardens in upstate New York: Implications for health promotion and community development. *Health and Place*, 6(4): 319-327.

Australian Bureau of Statistics. (2010). *Measures of Australia's progress*, 2010. http://www.abs.gov.au/ausstats/abs@.nsf/mf/1370.0. Accessed: 11 February, 2011.

Baber, L.M., & Frongillo, E.A. 2003. Family and seller interaction in farmers' markets in upstate New York. *American Journal of Alternative Agriculture*, 18(2): 87-94.

Baldrey, A., & Farrington, D. (2007). Effectiveness of programs to prevent school bullying. *Victims & Offenders,* 2: 183-204.

Baliunas, D., Patra, J., Rehm, J., Popova, S., Kaiserman, M., & Taylor, B. (2007). Smoking-attributable mortality and expected years of life lost in Canada 2002: Conclusions for prevention and policy. *Chronic Diseases in Canada,* 27(4): 154-162.

BC Association of Farmers' Markets (2010). http://www.bcfarmersmarkets.ca. Accessed: 16 November 2010.

BC Agriculture Council. (2007). *The facts about British Columbia's greenhouse agriculture.* September. Kelowna, BC: BC Agriculture Council.

BC Centre for Disease Control. (2011). *Food and your health: Meat.* http://www.bccdc.ca/foodhealth/meat/default.htm. Accessed: 15 February, 2011.

BC Greenhouse Growers' Association. (2007). *Agricultural advantage: BC's greenhouse vegetables.* Surrey, BC: BC Greenhouse Growers' Association. http://www.bcgreenhouse.ca/publications.htm. Accessed: 15 February, 2011.

BC Healthy Living Alliance. (2005a). *The winning legacy: A plan for improving the health of British Columbians by 2010.* Vancouver: Author.

BC Healthy Living Alliance. (2005b). *Risk factor interventions: An overview of their effectiveness.* Vancouver: Author.

BC Healthy Living Alliance. (2007a). *BC Healthy Living Alliance Community Capacity Building Strategy.* Vancouver: Author.

BC Healthy Living Alliance. (2007b). *BC Healthy Living Alliance Healthy Eating Strategy.* Vancouver: Author.

BC Healthy Living Alliance. (2007c). *BC Healthy Living Alliance Physical Activity Strategy.* Vancouver: Author.

BC Healthy Living Alliance. (2007d). *BC Healthy Living Alliance Tobacco Reduction Strategy.* Vancouver: Author.

BC Healthy Living Alliance. (2009). *Healthy futures for BC families: Policy recommendations for improving the health of British Columbians.* Vancouver: Author.

BC Healthy Living Alliance. (2010*). Leading British Columbia Towards a Healthy Future.* Vancouver: Author.

BC Progress Board. (2002). *2001 Report.* Vancouver, BC: Author.

BC Progress Board. (2008). *8th Annual Benchmark Report.* Vancouver, BC http://www.bcprogressboard.com/benchmarking_reps.html. Accessed: 2 December, 2010.

BC Progress Board. (2010). *10th Annual Benchmark Report.* Vancouver, BC. http://www.bcprogressboard.com/benchmarking_reps.html. Accessed: 2 December, 2010.

BC Reproductive Care Program. (2008). *British Columbia Perinatal Database Registry Annual Report 2007.* Vancouver, BC.

BC Recreation and Parks Association. (nd). *Sports and recreation in Aboriginal communities.*

BC Select Standing Committee on Health. (2004). *The path to health and wellness: Making British Columbians healthier by 2010.* Select Standing Committee on Health first report. Victoria, BC: Legislative Assembly, Select Standing Committee on Health.

BC Select Standing Committee on Health. (2006). *A strategy for combating childhood obesity and physical inactivity in British Columbia*. Select Standing Committee on Health first report. November. Victoria, BC: Legislative Assembly, Select Standing Committee on Health.

BC Stats. (2010a). *Mapping and geography: Interactive atlas*. Ministry of Citizens Services. Victoria. http://www.bcstats.gov.bc.ca/data/pop/georef/geopage.asp. Accessed: 28 December, 2010.

BC Stats. (2010b). Population and demographics. Ministry of Citizens' Services. Victoria, BC. http://www.bcstats.gov.bc.ca/data/pop/popstart.asp. Accessed: 28 December, 2010.

Bellows, A.C., & Hamm, M.W. (2003). International origins of community food security policies and practices in the US. *Critical Public Health,* 13(2): 107-123.

Billings, J., & Hashem, F. (2009). Literature review: Salutogenesis and the promotion of positive mental health in older people. Conference: "Mental Health and Well-being in Older People - Making it Happen," April 2010. Madrid: European Communities.

Blair, D., Giesecke, C., & Sherman, S. (1991). A dietary social and economic evaluation of the Philadelphia Urban Gardening Project. *Journal of Nutrition and Education*, 23(4): 161-167.

Blake, A., & Cloutier-Fisher, D. (2009). Backyard bounty: exploring the benefits and challenges of backyard garden sharing projects. *Local Environment*, 14(9): 797-807.

Boelhouwer, J. (2010). *Wellbeing in the Netherlands: The SCP life situation index since 1974.* The Netherlands Institute for Social Research: The Hague.

Breakfast for Learning. (2007). *Still not making the grade. 2007 report card on nutrition for school children.* http://www.breakfastforlearning.ca/en/services-a-information/research/report-card. Accessed: 10 April, 2011.

Bridge, J., & Turpin, B. (2004). *The cost of smoking in British Columbia and the economics of tobacco control.* Ottawa: Health Canada.

Brien, S.E., Ronskley, P.E., , Turner, B.J., Mukamal, K.J., & Ghali, W.A. (2011). Effect of alcohol consumption on biological markers associated with risk of coronary heart disease: Systematic review and meta-analysis of interventional studies. *British Medical Journal,* 342: d636.

Brewis, A., Wutich, A., Falletta-Cowden, A., & Rodriguez-Soto, I. (2011). Body norms and fat stigma in global perspective. *Current Anthropology*, 52(2): April.

Brown, C., & Alcoe, J. (2010). The heart of wellbeing: A self-help approach to recovering, sustaining and improving wellbeing. *Journal of Holistic Healthcare*, 7(1): 24-28.

Brown, C., & Miller, S. (2008). The impacts of local markets: A review of research on farmers markets and community supported agriculture. *American Journal of Agricultural Economics*, 90 (5): 1296–1302.

Brown, K. & Jameton, A. (2000). Public health implications of urban agriculture. *Journal of Public Health Policy*, 21(1): 20-39.

Bryan, S., & Katzmarzyk, P.T. (2011). The association between meeting physical activity guidelines and chronic diseases among Canadian adults. *Journal of Physical Activity and Health,* 8: 10-17.

Bryant, T. (2009). Housing and health: More than bricks and mortar. In D. Raphael (Ed.), *Social determinants of health: Canadian perspectives* (pp. 235-249). 2nd edition. Toronto: Canadian Scholars' Press.

Butler, G.P., Orpana, H.M., & Wiens, A.J. (2007). By your own two feet: Factors associated with active transportation in Canada. *Canadian Journal of Public Health,* 98(4): 259-263.

Campbell, D.E. (2006). What is education's impact on civic and social engagement? In R. Desjardins and T. Schuller (Eds.), *Proceedings of the Copenhagen Symposium: Measuring the effects of education on health and civic engagement* (pp. 25-108). Paris: Organisation for Economic Co-operation and Development.

Canadian Cancer Society, BC and Yukon Division. (2010). Medical community debunks myths and urges BC Government to act on pesticides. Vancouver, BC. http://www.newswire.ca/en/releases/archive/June2010/04/c2060.html. Accessed: 19 December, 2010.

Canadian Council on Learning. (2010a). *The 2010 Composite Learning Index: Five years of measuring Canada's progress in lifelong learning.* Ottawa: Canada Council on Learning.

Canadian Council on Learning. (2010b). Canada's score on annual learning index stalls. *News Release.* May 20. http://www.cli-ica.ca/en/about/media/2010release.aspx. Accessed: 15 February, 2011.

Canadian Council on Learning. (2010c). *Learning and the arts: Can Mozart make you smarter?* http://www.ccl-cca.ca/CCL/Reports/LessonsInLearning/LinL2010Motzart.html. Accessed: 15 February, 2011.

Canadian Fitness and Lifestyle Research Institute. (2007a). *Changing the Canadian landscape one step at a time: Results of the Physical Activity Monitor.* http://www.cflri.ca/eng/publications/index.php. Accessed: 4 April, 2011.

Canadian Fitness and Lifestyle Research Institute. (2007b). Working to become more active – Increasing physical activity in the Canadian workplace. *Bulletin* No. 6 (April). http://www.cflri.ca/eng/publications/index.php. Accessed: 4 April, 2011.

Canadian Index of Wellbeing. (2010a). *Measuring what matters.* http://www.ciw.ca/en/TheCanadianIndexOfWellbeing.aspx. Accessed: 13 December, 2010.

Canadian Index of Wellbeing. (2010b). *Leisure and culture: A report of the Canadian Index of Wellbeing (CIW).* http://www.ciw.ca/en/TheCanadianIndexOfWellbeing.aspx. Accessed: 13 December, 2010.

Canadian Population Health Initiative. (2004). Improving the health of Canadians. Ottawa: Canadian Institute for Health Information.

Canadian Population Health Initiative. (2006). *Improving the health of Canadians: An introduction to health in urban places.* Ottawa: Canadian Institute for Health Information.

Canadian Population Health Initiative. (2008a). *Mentally healthy communities: A collection of papers.* Ottawa: Canadian Institute for Health Information.

Canadian Population Health Initiative. (2008b). *Reducing gaps in health: A focus on socio-economic status.* Ottawa: Canadian Institute for Health Information.

Canadian Population Health Initiative. (2009). *Development and application of community health indicators.* Ottawa: Canadian Institute for Health Information.

Carson, R. (1961). *Silent spring.* Boston: Houghton Mifflin.

Central Mortgage and Housing Corporation. (2011). *Housing in Canada online: Definitions of variables.* http://cmhc.beyond2020.com/HiCODefinitions_EN.html#_Age. Accessed: 27 February, 2011.

Charities Aid Foundation. (2010). *The World Giving Index 2010.* http://www.cafonline.org/pdf/0882A_WorldGivingReport_Interactive_070910.pdf. Accessed: 7 September, 2010.

Chen, W., Bottorff, J.L., Johnson, J.L., Saewyc, E.M., & Zumbo, B.D. (2007). Susceptibility to smoking among White and Chinese nonsmoking adolescents in Canada. *Public Health Nursing,* 25(1): 18–27.

Chronic Disease Prevention Alliance of Canada. (2009). Obesity and the impact of marketing on children: Developing an intersectoral policy consensus conference. http://www.ohpe.ca/10712. Accessed: 2 April, 2011.

Clark, W. (2008). Kids' sports. *Canadian Social Trends.* Statistics Canada. http://www.statcan.gc.ca/pub/11-008-x/11-008-x2008001-eng.htm. Accessed: 4 April, 2011.

Coish, D. (2004). *Trends and conditions in metropolitan areas. Census metropolitan areas as culture clusters.* Ottawa: Statistics Canada.

Cole, T.J., Bellizzi, M.C., Flegal, K.M., & Dietz, W.H. (2000). Establishing a standard definition for child overweight and obesity worldwide: International survey. *British Medical Journal,* 320: 1-6.

Colley, R.C., Garriguet, D., Janssen, I., Craig, C.L., Clarke, J., & Tremblay, M.S. (2011a). Physical activity of Canadian adults: Accelerometer results from the 2007 to 2009 Canadian Health Measures Survey. *Health Reports*, 22(1): March.

Colley, R.C., Garriguet, D., Janssen, I., Craig, C.L., Clarke, J., & Tremblay, M.S. (2011b). Physical activity of Canadian children and youth: Accelerometer results from the 2007 to 2009 Canadian Health Measures Survey. *Health Reports*, Vol. 22(1): March.

Commission on the Social Determinants of Health (CSDH). (2008). *Closing the gap in a generation: Health equity through action on the social determinants of health.* Final Report of the Commission on Social Determinants of Health. Geneva: World Health Organization.

Conference Board of Canada. (2011). *A report card on Canada.* http://www.conferenceboard.ca/hcp/default.aspx. Accessed: 1 March, 2011.

Connell, D.J., Taggart, T., Hillman, K., & Humphrey, A. (2006). *Economic and community impacts of farmers markets in British Columbia.* BC Association of Farmers Market & University of Northern British Columbia School of Environmental Planning.

Copestake, J. (2007). *Is wellbeing relevant to international development policy and practice?* James Copestake (WeD) Wellbeing in Developing Countries Research Group at University of Bath, UK. http://www.welldev.org.uk/conference2007/final-papers/plenary/JGC-WeD-plenary-d2-paper.pdf. Accessed: 13 December, 2010.

Cox, W., & Pavletich, H. (2011). *7th Annual Demographia International Housing Affordability Survey: 2011.* Winnipeg: Frontier Centre for Public Policy.

Cragg, S., Cameron C., & Craig, C.L. (2006). *2004 National Transportation Survey.* Ottawa: Canadian Fitness and Lifestyle Research Institute.

Crose, R., Nicholas, D.R., Gobble, D.C., & Frank, B. (1992). Gender and wellness: A multidimensional systems model for counseling. *Journal of Counseling and Development*, 77: 149-156.

Cummins, R., Woerner, J., Gibson, A., Lai, L., Weinberg, M., & Collard, J. (2008). *Australian Unity Wellbeing Index Survey 19.* The School of Psychology and The Australian Centre on Quality of Life, Deakin University; and Australian Unity Limited.

De Propris, L, Chapain, C., Cooke, P., MacNeill, S., & Mateos-Garcia, J. (2009). *The geography of creativity.* National Endowment for Science, Technology and the Arts. London, UK.

Dieticians of Canada & Community Nutritionists Council of BC. (2009). *The cost of eating in British Columbia.* http://www.dietitians.ca/bccostofeating. Accessed: 10 April, 2011.

Dockery, A.M. (2009). *Culture and well-being: The case of indigenous Australians.* Perth: Centre for Labour Market Research, Curtin University of Technology.

Drabsch, T. (2010). *Health, Education & Community Indicators for NSW: Statistical Indicators 3/10.* Australia: NSW Parliamentary Library Research Service.

Dunleavy, J., & Dunning, P. (2009). *ArtsSmarts' impact on student engagement: First Research Report 2007-2009.* Ottawa: ArtsSmarts.

Dunn, H. (1961). *High level wellness.* Arlington, VA: Beatty Press.

Durlak, J. (2000). Health promotion as a strategy in primary prevention. In D. Cicchetti, J. Rappaport, I. Sandler, & R. Weissberg (Eds.), *The promotion of wellness in children and adolescents* (pp. 221–241). Washington, DC: Child Welfare League Association Press.

Edmunds, S. (2010). Wellbeing: Conceptual issues and implications for interdisciplinary work. *Journal of Holistic Healthcare*, 7(1): 9-12.

Eisenberg, M.E., Olson, M.S., Neumark-Sztainer, D., Story, M., & Bearinger, L.H. (2004). Correlations between family meals and psychosocial well-being among adolescents. *Archives of Pediatrics and Adolescent Medicine*, 158: 792-796.

Elgar, F.J., & Stewart, J.M. (2008). Validity of self-report screening for overweight and obesity. *Canadian Journal of Public Health,* 99(5): 423-427.

Elliott, S., & Foster, L. (2005). Mind-body-place: A geography of Aboriginal health in British Columbia. In P. Stephenson, S. Elliott, L.T. Foster, & J. Harris (Eds.), *A persistent spirit: Towards understanding Aboriginal health in British Columbia* (pp. 94-127). Western Geographical Series, Vol. 31. Victoria, BC: Western Geographical Press, University of Victoria.

Eriksson, M., and Lindstrom, B. (2008). A salutogenic interpretation of the Ottawa Charter. *Health Promotion International*, 23(2): 190-199.

Ermisch, J., Iacovou, M., & Skew, A. (2011). Family relationships. In S.L. McFall & C. Garrington (Eds.), *Early findings from the first wave of the UK's household longitudinal study* (pp. 7-14). Colchester: Institute for Social and Economic Research, University of Essex.

Ewing, R. (2010). *The arts and Australian education: Realising the potential*. Victoria: Australian Council for Educational Research.

Exeter, D. (2009). Review of the BC Atlas of Wellness 1ˢᵗ Edition. *New Zealand Geographer,* 65: 241-242.

Feagan, R. Morris D., & Krog K. (2004). Niagara region farmers' markets: local food systems and sustainability considerations. *Local Environment*, 9(3): 235-254.

Federation of Canadian Municipalities. (1999). *The FCM Quality of Life Reporting System: Quality of life in Canadian communities*. Ottawa: Federation of Canadian Municipalities. http://www.fcm.ca//CMFiles/qol19991VSO-3272008-6325.pdf. Accessed: 5 November, 2010.

Federation of Canadian Municipalities. (2009). Immigration and diversity in Canadian cities and communities. *Theme Report* No. 5. http://www.fcm.ca/english/View.asp?x=1. Accessed: 5 November, 2010.

Federation of Canadian Municipalities. (2010). *What is the Quality of Life Reporting System (QOLRS)?* http://www.fcm.ca/english/View.asp?mp=1237&x=1115. Accessed: 5 November, 2010.

Ferdjani, J. (2010). Improving global wellbeing, improving personal wellbeing. *Journal of Holistic Healthcare*, 7(1): 33-35.

Field, J. (2009). *Well-being and happiness. Inquiry into the Future of Lifelong Learning.* IFLL Thematic paper 4. Leicester, UK: National Institute of Adult Continuing Education.

Fieldhouse, P. (2007). Eating together: The culture of the family meal. *Transition,* 37(4): 3-6.

Fisher A. (1999). *Hot peppers and parking lot peaches: Evaluating farmers' markets in low income communities*. Community Food Security Coalition. Venice, CA.

Florida, R. (2003). *The rise of the creative class: And how it is transforming work, leisure, community and everyday life*. New York: Basic Books.

Food and Agricultural Organization. (1996). *Report of the World Food Summit (WFS)*. Rome: Food and Agricultural Organization.

Food Security Standing Committee. (2004). *Making the connection: Food security and public health*. Vancouver: Community Nutritionists' Council of BC.

Foster, L.T. (2009). Social determinants of health and injuries. Presentation to the BC Injuries Prevention Research Unit, November, 19.

Foster, L.T., & Keller, C.P. (2007). *British Columbia Atlas of Wellness, 1st Edition*. Western Geographical Series: Department of Geography, University of Victoria, BC. http://www.geog.uvic.ca/wellness. Accessed: 28 June, 2010.

Foster, L.T., & Wharf, B. (2007). *People, politics and child welfare in British Columbia*. Vancouver: University of British Columbia Press.

Franko, D.L., Thompson, D., Affenito, S.G., Barton, B.A., & Striegel-Moore, R.H. (2008). What mediates the relationship between family meals and adolescent health issues? *Health Psychology,* 27(2 Supplement): S109-S117.

Gallup & Healthways. (2011). *The Gallup-Healthways Well-Being Index®.* http://well-beingindex.com. Accessed: 28 February, 2011.

Gainer, A., Lamman, C., & Veldhuis, N. (2010). *Generosity in Canada and the United States: The 2010 Generosity Index.* Vancouver: Fraser Institute.

Geneau, R., Fraser, G., Legowski, B., & Stachenko, S. (2009). *The Case of ActNowBC in British Columbia, Canada.* World Health Organization Collaborating Centre on Chronic Non-communicable Diseases Policy. Geneva: WHO. http://www.phacaspc.gc.ca/publicat/2009/ActNowBC/index-eng.php. Accessed: 8 January, 2011.

Giles, P. (2004). Low income measurement in Canada. *Income Paper Research Series.* Statistics Canada. Ottawa: Ministry of Industry.

Gilmour, H. (2007). Physically active Canadians. *Health Reports,* 18(3): August.

Giovannini, E., & Hall, J. (2008). Measuring the Progress of Societies. *Newsletter,* Issue 3, November. Paris: OECD.

Government of British Columbia. (2006). *Strategic Plan 2006/07 – 2008/09.* http://www.bcbudget.gov.bc.ca/2006/stplan/. Accessed: 10 December, 2010.

Government of Newfoundland and Labrador. (2009). Provincial Community Accounts Endorsed by Senate Committee. *News Release,* June 29. St. Johns: Department of Finance. http://www.releases.gov.nl.ca/releases/2009/fin/0629n02.htm. Accessed: 4 December, 2010.

Graham, C. (2008). *The financial crisis and pursuing happiness.* http://www.brookings.edu/interviews/2008/1125_happiness_graham.aspx. Accessed: 2 May, 2011.

Grieves, V. (2009). Aboriginal spirituality: Aboriginal philosophy, the basis of Aboriginal social and emotional wellbeing, *Discussion Paper* No. 9, Cooperative Research Centre for Aboriginal Health, Darwin.

Grimm, R., Spring, K., & Dietz, N. (2007). *The health benefits of volunteering: A review of recent research.* Office of research and Policy Development. Washington: Corporation for National and Community Service.

Gushulak, B. (2007). Healthier on arrival? Further insight into the "healthy immigrant effect." *Canadian Medical Association. Journal,* 176(10): 1439-1440.

Haddock, C.J., Poston, W.S.C., Pyle, S.A., Klesges, R.C., Vander Weg, M.W., Peterson, A., & Debon, M. (2006). The validity of self-rated health as a measure of health status among young military personnel: Evidence from a cross-sectional survey. *Health and Quality of Life Outcomes,* 4: 57. http://www.hqlo.com/content/4/1/57. Accessed: 1 May, 2011.

Hales, D. (2005). *An invitation to health,* 11th ed. "An Invitation to Health for the Twenty-First Century." Belmont, CA: Thomson & Wadsworth.

Hall, M., Lasby, D., Ayer, S. & Gibbons, W.D. (2009). *Caring Canadians, involved Canadians: Highlights from the 2007 Canada Survey of Giving, Volunteering and Participating.* Imagine Canada. Ottawa: Ministry of Industry.

Hamilton, M., & Redmond, G. (2010). *Conceptualisation of social and emotional wellbeing for children and young people, and policy implications.* A research report for the Australian Research Alliance for Children and Youth and the Australian Institute of Health and Welfare.

Harris, K.C., Kuramoto, L.K., Schulzer, M., & Retallack, J.E. (2009). Effect of school-based physical activity interventions on body mass index in children: A meta analysis. *Canadian Medical Association Journal,* 180(7): 719-26.

Hayes, M. (2007). Defining wellness and its determinants. In L.T. Foster & C.P. Keller (Eds.), *British Columbia Atlas of Wellness* (pp. 17-19). Western Geographical Series, Vol. 42. Victoria, BC: Western Geographical Press, University of Victoria.

Health Canada. (2007). *Food and nutrition atlas of Canada.* Ottawa: Health Canada. http://www.hc-sc.gc.ca/fn-an/surveill/atlas/map-carte/index-eng.php. Accessed: 1 December, 2010.

Health Canada. (2008). *Healthy living: Mental health – coping with stress.* http://www.hc-sc.gc.ca/hl-vs/iyh-vsv/life-vie/stress-eng.php. Accessed: 10 April, 2011.

Health Canada. (2009). *Healthy living: Oral health.* http://www.hc-sc.gc.ca/hl-vs/oral-bucco/index-eng.php. Accessed: 10 April, 2011.

Health Canada. (2011). *Tobacco use statistics.* Ottawa: Health Canada. http://www.hc-sc.gc.ca/hc-ps/tobac-tabac/research-recherche/stat/index-eng.php. Accessed: 3 April, 2011.

Health Council of Canada. (2011). *A citizen's guide to health indicators: A reference guide for Canadians.* Ottawa.

Heart and Stroke Foundation. (2010). http://www.heartandstroke.com/site. Accessed: 15 January, 2011.

Helliwell, J. (2005). *Wellbeing, social capital and public policy: What's new?* Cambridge, MA: National Bureau of Economic Research.

Hettler, B. (1980). Wellness promotion on a university campus. Family and Community Health. *Journal of Health Promotion & Maintenance*, 3: 77-95.

Hill Strategies Research Inc. (2008). Social effects of culture: Exploratory statistical evidence. *Statistical Insights into the Arts*, 6(4), 43 pages. Toronto: Hill Strategies Research Inc.

Hill Strategies Research Inc. (2009). Artists in Canada's provinces and territories based on the 2006 Census. *Statistical Insights into the Arts,* 7(5). Toronto: Hill Strategies Research Inc.

Hofmann, N., Filoso, G., & Schofield, M. (2005). The loss of dependable agricultural land in Canada. *Rural & Small Town Canada Analysis Bulletin,* 6(1): 1-16.

Human Early Learning Partnership (HELP). (2010). *Early Development Instrument.* University of British Columbia. Vancouver. http://www.earlylearning.ubc.ca/research/initiatives/early-development-instrument. Accessed: 28 December, 2010.

Human Resources and Skills Development Canada. (2010). *Indicators of well-being in Canada.* http://www4.hrsdc.gc.ca/h.4m.2@-eng.jsp. Accessed: 2 February, 2011.

Hurst, M. (2009). Who participates in active leisure? *Canadian Social Trends.* Statistics Canada. http://www.statcan.gc.ca/pub/11-008-x/2009001/article/10690-eng.htm. Accessed: 4 April, 2011.

Hutchinson, P.J., Richardson, C.G., & Botorff, J.L. (2008). *Canadian Journal of Public Health,* 99(5): 418-422.

Idler, E.L., & Benyamini, Y. (1997). Self-rated health and mortality: A review of twenty-seven community studies. *Journal of Health & Social Studies*, 38(March): 21-37.

Idler, E.L., Russell, L.B., & Davis, D. (2000). Survival, functional limitations, and self-rated health in the NHANES I Epidemiologic Follow-up Study, 1992. First National Health and Nutrition Examination Survey. American Journal of Epidemiology, 152(9): 874-83.

Ip, F. (2008a). Immigrant population of British Columbia. 2006 Census Fast Facts. *Issue*: 2006:05. Victoria: BC Stats.

Ip, F. (2008b). Mother tongue and home language. 2006 Census Fast Facts. *Issue:* 2006:05. Victoria: BC Stats.

Irwin, J. (1991). Are pesticides killing the boy next door? *Family Practice,* February 9: 10.

Institute of Wellbeing. (2009). *How are Canadians really doing? The First Report of the Institute of Wellbeing.* http://www.ciw.ca/en/TheCanadianIndexOfWellbeing.aspx. Accessed: 13 December, 2010.

Institute of Community Engagement and Policy Alternatives. (2006). *Measuring well-being: Engaging communities. Developing a Community Indicators Framework for Victoria:* The final report of the Victorian Community Indicators Project (VCIP). Melbourne: VCIP. http://www.communityindicators.net.au/data_maps. Accessed: 28 December, 2009.

Janus, M., Brinkman, S., Duku, E., Hertzman, C., Santos, R., Sayers, M., Schroeder, J., & Walsh, C. (2007). *The early development instrument: A population based measure for communities. A handbook on development, properties, and use.* Offord Centre for Child Studies. Hamilton, ON: McMaster University.

Janus, M., & Offord, D. (2007). Development and psychometric properties of the Early Development Instrument (EDI): A measure of children's school readiness. *Canadian Journal of Behavioural Science*, 39: 1-22.

Jensen, P. (2007). Healthiest pregnancies. In L.T. Foster & C.P. Keller. (Eds.), *British Columbia Atlas of Wellness*. Western Geographical Series, Vol. 42. Victoria, BC: Western Geographical Press, University of Victoria.

Kassirer, J., Koswan, S., Spence, K., Morphet, S., Wolnik, C., Goom, S., & Del Matto, T. (2004). *The impact of by-laws and public education programs on reducing the cosmetic/non-essential, residential use of pesticides: A best practices review.* Ottawa: CULLBRIDGE™ and Canadian Centre for Pollution Prevention.

Katz, D. (2009). *The BC Agricultural Land Reserve: A critical assessment.* Studies in Risk and Regulation. Vancouver: Fraser Institute.

Katzmarzyk, P.T., & Janssen, I. (2004). The economic costs associated with physical inactivity and obesity in Canada: An update. *Canadian Journal of Applied Physiology*, 29(1): 90-115.

Keller, P. (1995). Visualizing digital atlas information products and the user perspective. *Cartographic Perspectives,* 20(Winter): 21-26.

Keller, P., & Hystad, P. (2007). Introduction. In L.T. Foster & C.P. Keller (Eds.), *British Columbia Atlas of Wellness* (pp. 3-7). Western Geographical Series, Vol. 42. Victoria, BC: Western Geographical Press, University of Victoria.

Kendall, P.R.W. (2006). *Food health and well-being in British Columbia.* Provincial Health Officer's Annual Report 2005. Victoria, BC: Ministry of Health.

Kendall, P.R.W. (2008a). *An ounce of prevention revisited: A review of health promotion and selected outcomes for children and youth in BC schools.* Provincial Health Officer's Annual Report 2006. Victoria, BC: Ministry of Health.

Kendall, P.R.W. (2008b). *Public health approach to alcohol policy: An updated report from the Provincial Health Officer.* Office of the Provincial Health Officer. Victoria, BC: Ministry of Healthy Living and Sport.

Kendall, P.R.W. (2009). *Pathways to health and healing – 2ⁿᵈ report on the health and well-being of Aboriginal people in British Columbia.* Provincial Health Officer's Annual Report 2007. Victoria, BC: Ministry of Healthy Living and Sport.

Keon, W.J., & Pepin, L. (2009). *A healthy, productive Canada: A determinant of health approach.* The Standing Senate Committee on Social Affairs, Science and Technology Final Report of Senate Subcommittee on Population Health. Ottawa. http://senate-senat.ca/health-e.asp. Accessed: 10 February, 2011.

Keown, L-A. (2009). *Social networks help Canadians deal with change.* Ottawa: Statistics Canada. http://www.statcan.gc.ca/pub/11-008-x/2009002/article/10891-eng.htm. Accessed: 7 March, 2011.

Kierans, W., Luo, Z-C., Wilkins, R., Taylor-Clapp, S., & Foster, L. (2007). *Infant macrosomia among First Nations in British Columbia: Prevalence, trends and characteristics.* BC Vital Statistics Agency. Victoria, BC: Ministry of Health. http://www.vs.gov.bc.ca/stats/indian/REPORT_Macrosomia.pdf. Accessed: 25 January, 2011.

Kindig, D.A. (2007). Understanding population health terminology. *The Milbank Quarterly,* 85(1): 136-161.

Kravitz, A. (2010). British Columbia. In: *Hunger Count 2010* (pp. 20-21). Food Banks Canada. http://foodbankscanada.ca/HungerCount.htm. Accessed: 4 April, 2011.

Kurtz, H. (2001). Differentiating multiple meanings of garden and community. *Urban Geography*, 22(7): 656–670.

Lalonde, M. (1974). *A new perspective on the health of Canadians: A working document.* Ministry of Supply and Services Canada (1981). Ottawa. http://www.phac-aspc.gc.ca/ph-sp/pdf/perspect-eng.pdf. Accessed: 4 February, 2011.

Langlois, K., Garriguet, D., & Findlay, L. (2009). Diet composition and obesity among Canadian adults. *Health Reports,* 20(4): December.

Larson, J.S. (1999). The conceptualization of health. *Medical Care Research and Review,* 56(2): 123-136.

Larsen, K., & Gilliland, J. (2009). A farmers market in a food desert: Evaluating impacts on the price and availability of healthy food. *Health and Place*, 15: 1158-1162.

Leafgren, F. (1990). Being a man can be hazardous to your health: Life-styles issues. In D. Moore & F. Leafgren (Eds.), *Problem solving strategies and interventions for men in conflict* (pp. 265-311). Alexandria: American Association for Counseling and Development.

Lebel, A., Pampalon, R., Hamel, D., & Theriault, M. (2009). The geography of overweight in Quebec: A multilevel perspective. *Canadian Journal of Public Health,* 100(1): 18-23.

Legatum Institute. (2009). *The 2009 Legatum Prosperity Index: An Inquiry into Global Wealth and Wellbeing.* http://www.prosperity.com/index2009.aspx. Accessed: 12 November, 2010

Lepper, J., & McAndrew, S. (2008). Developments in the economics of well-being. *Treasury Economic Working Paper* No. 4. Richmond: HM Treasury. http://www.hm-treasury.gov.uk/d/workingpager4_031108.pdf. Accessed: 28 February, 2011.

Lightman, E., Mitchell, A., & Wilson, B. (2008). *Poverty is making us sick: A comprehensive survey of health and income in Canada.* Toronto: Wellesley Institute.

Lindstrom, B., & Eriksson, M. (2009). The salutogenic approach to the making of HiAP/healthy public policy: Illustrated by a case study. *Global Health Promotion,* 16(1): 17-28.

Lu, O.F. (2010). Quick facts about British Columbia. BC Stats, November 4. Victoria.

MacKenzie, P., Callahan, M., Brown, L., & Whittington, B. (2009). The multiple layers of mothering work: Grandparents raising grandchildren. In D. Cloutier-Fisher, L.T. Foster, & D. Hultsch (Eds), *Health and aging in British Columbia: Vulnerability and resilience* (pp. 165-180). Western Geographical Series, Vol. 43. Victoria, BC: Western Geographical Press, University of Victoria.

Mawani, F.N., & Gilmour, H. (2010). Validation of self-rated mental health. *Health Reports,* 21(3). http://www.statcan.gc.ca/pub/82-003-x/2010003/article/11288-eng.pdf. Accessed: 4 April, 2011.

May, D. (2007). *Determinants of well-being.* Memorial University of Newfoundland and Newfoundland and Labrador Statistics Agency.

McDonald, J.T., & Kennedy, S. (2004). Insights into the 'healthy immigrant effect': Health status and health service use of immigrants to Canada. *Social Science &. Medicine,* 59: 1613-1627.

McCreary Centre Society. (2010). http://www.mcs.bc.ca/. Accessed: 20 February, 2011.

McEwan, A., Tsey, K., & The Empowerment Research Team. (2008). The role of spirituality in social and emotional wellbeing initiatives: The Family Wellbeing Program at Yarrabah, *Discussion Paper* No. 7, Cooperative Research Centre for Aboriginal Health, Darwin.

McIntosh, C.N., Fines, P., Wilkins, R., & Wolfson, M.C. (2009). Income disparities in health-adjusted life expectancy for Canadian adults, 1991 to 2001. *Health Reports,* 20(4), December.

McKee, B., Foster, L.T., & Keller, C.P. (2008). *The British Columbia Atlas of Wellness seniors supplement.* Department of Geography, University of Victoria, BC. http://www.geog.uvic.ca/wellness. Accessed: 28 June, 2010.

McKee, B., Foster, L.T., Keller, C.P., Blake, A., & Ostry, A. (2009a). *The Geography of Wellness and Well-being Across Canada.* Department of Geography, University of Victoria, BC. http://www.geog.uvic.ca/wellness. Accessed: 28 June, 2010.

McKee, B., Foster, L.T., Keller, C.P., Blake, A., & Ostry, A. (2009b). *The Geography of Wellness and Well-being Across British Columbia.* Department of Geography, University of Victoria, BC. http://www.geog.uvic.ca/wellness. Accessed: 28 June, 2010.

Melbourne Charter. (2008). *The Melbourne Charter for promoting mental health and preventing mental and behavioural disorders.* 5th World Conference on the Promotion of Mental Health and the Prevention of Mental and Behavioural Disorders. Melbourne, Australia. http://www.gesundheitsfoerderung.ch/pdf_doc_xls/e/BGF/Melboure_Charter_final.pdf. Accessed: 13 December, 2010.

Merrill, R.M., Aldana, S.G., Pope, J.E., Anderson, D.R., Coberley, C.R., Vyhlida, T.P., Howe, G., & Whitmer, R.W. (2011). Evaluation of a best-practice worksite wellness program in a small-employer setting using selected well-being indices. *Journal of Occupational and Environmental Medicine,* 53(4): 448-454.

Mikkonen, J., & Raphael, D. (2010). *Social determinants of health: The Canadian facts.* Toronto: York University School of Health Policy and Management.

Millar, J., & Hull, C. (1997). Measuring human wellness. *Social Indicators Research*, 40: 147-158.

Miller, G., & Foster, L. (2006). *A critical synthesis of wellness literature.* School of Child and Youth Care and Department of Geography, University of Victoria. Updated in 2010. http://www.geog.uvic.ca/wellness. Accessed: 13 December, 2010.

Miller, G., & Foster, L. (2010). A brief summary of holistic wellness literature. *Journal of Holistic Healthcare*, 7(1): 4-8.

Miller, J.W. (2005). Wellness: The history and development of a concept. *Spektrum Freizeit*, 27: 84-106.

Milligan, C., Gatrell, A., & Bingley, A. (2004). "Cultivating health": therapeutic landscapes and older people in northern England. *Social Science and Medicine*, 58(9): 1781-1793.

Ministry of Agriculture and Lands. (2006). *BC's food self reliance. Can BC's farmers feed our growing population?* http://www.agf.gov.bc.ca/resmgmt/Food_Self_Reliance/BCFoodSelfReliance_Report.pdf. Accessed: 4 April, 2011.

Ministry of Agriculture and Lands & Ministry of Healthy Living and Sport. (2009). Produce availability plan supports remote communities. *News Release,* November 3. http://www2.news.gov.bc.ca/news_releases_2009-2013/2009AL0019-000569.htm. Accessed: 5 April, 2011.

Ministry of Agriculture, Food and Fisheries. (2003). *An overview of the BC greenhouse vegetable industry.* Industry Competitiveness Branch, November. Abbotsford, BC: Ministry of Agriculture, Food and Fisheries.

Ministry of Children and family Development. (2010). *About fetal alcohol syndrome disorder.* http://www.mcf.gov.bc.ca/fasd/index.htm. Accessed 3 November, 2010.

Ministry of Community, Aboriginal and Women's Services. (2004). *Libraries without walls: The world within your reach. A vision for public libraries in British Columbia.* http://www.bced.gov.bc.ca/pls/library_strategic_plan.pdf. Accessed: 17 November, 2010.

Ministry of Community and Rural Development. (2008). BC Spirit Squares: Creating a lasting legacy. http://www.spiritsquares.gov.bc.ca. Accessed: 11 October, 2010.

Ministry of Community and Rural Development. (2010a). *Towns for tomorrow funding.* October 15, *News Release.* Ministry of Community and Rural Development. http://www.townsfortomorrow.gov.bc.ca/. Accessed: 15 December, 2010.

Ministry of Community and Rural Development. (2010b). *Towns for tomorrow: Funding program progress report.* July 2010. Ministry of Community and Rural Development. http://www.townsfortomorrow.gov.bc.ca/docs/progress_report_july_16_2010_combined.pdf. Accessed: 15 December, 2010.

Ministry of Community and Rural Development. (2010c). *Trees for tomorrow.* BC Ministry of Community and Rural Development. http://www.treesfortomorrow.gov.bc.ca/. Accessed: 13 December, 2010.

Ministry of Education. (2008). *Safe, caring and orderly schools: A guide.* BC Ministry of Education. Victoria.

Ministry of Education. (2010a). *StrongStart BC.* Ministry of Education. Victoria. http://www.bced.gov.bc.ca/early_learning/strongstart_bc. Accessed: 10 December, 2010.

Ministry of Education. (2010b). *Guidelines for food and beverage sales in BC schools.* August. Victoria: Ministry of Education and Ministry of Healthy Living and Sport.

Ministry of Education. (2010c). *Provincial reports.* http://www.bced.gov.bc.ca/reporting/. Accessed: 5 February, 2011.

Ministry of Education. (2010d). *Public library services.* http://www.bced.gov.bc.ca/pls/. Accessed: 17 November, 2010.

Ministry of Education & ActNow BC. (2008). *Program guide for daily physical activity: Kindergarten to grade 12*. Victoria: BC Ministry of Education.

Ministry of Education & Ministry of Healthy Living and Sport. (2010). *Food and beverage sales in BC schools*. http://www.bced.gov.bc.ca/health/healthy_eating/food_guidelines/. Accessed: 2 April, 2011.

Ministry of Environment. (2007). *Environmental trends in British Columbia*. http://www.env.gov.bc.ca/soe/. Accessed: 2 April, 2011.

Ministry of Healthy Living and Sport. (2010). Enhanced regulations support local meat sales. *News Release*, April 23. http://www2.news.gov.bc.ca/news_releases_2009-2013/2010HLS0024-000457.htm. Accessed: 15 February, 2011.

Ministry of Health Services. (2011). Join the conversation on childhood obesity. *News Release*. March 8. http://www2.news.gov.bc.ca/news_releases_2009-2013/2011HSERV0012-000202.htm. Accessed: 10 March 2011.

Ministry of Social Development Te Manatu Whakahiato Ora. (2008). *Children and young people: Indicators of wellbeing in New Zealand 2008*. Wellington: New Zealand.

Ministry of Culture and Heritage Te Manato Taonga. (2009). *Cultural indicators for New Zealand*. Wellington: New Zealand.

Mitton, C., MacNab, Y.C., Smith, N., & Foster, L. (2008). Transferring injury data to decision makers in British Columbia: A short report. *International. Journal of Injury Control & Safety Promotion,* 15(1): 41-43.

Mitton, C., MacNab, Y.C., Smith, N., & Foster, L. (2009). Injury data in British Columbia: Policy maker perspectives. *Chronic Diseases in Canada,* 29(2): 70-79.

Møller, L., Stöver, H., Jürgens, R., Gatherer, A., & Nikogosian, H. (2007). *Health in prisons: A WHO guide to the essentials in prison health*. Copenhagen: WHO Regional Office for Europe.

Morgan, A., & Ziglio, E. (2007). Revitalising the evidence base for public health: An assets model. *Promotion & Education,* Supplement (2): 17-22.

Murphy, J.M. (2007). Breakfast and learning: An updated review. *Current Nutrition & Food Science,* 3: 3-36.

Myers, M. (1998). Empowerment and community building through a gardening project. *Psychiatric Rehabilitation Journal,* 22(2):181-183.

National Collaborating Centre for Aboriginal Health. (2009). *Culture and language as social determinants of First Nations, Inuit and Metis health*. Prince George: University of Northern British Columbia.

Natural Resources Canada. (2006). *The Atlas of Canada*. http://atlas.nrcan.gc.ca/site/index.html. Accessed: 10 December, 2010.

New Economics Foundation. (2004). *A well-being manifesto for a flourishing society: The power of well-being*. London, UK: NEF.

New Economics Foundation. (2009a). *The Happy Planet Index 2.0*. London, UK: NEF. http://www.happyplanetindex.org/learn/download-report.html. Accessed: 20 December, 2010.

New Economics Foundation. (2009b). *National accounts of well-being: Bringing real wealth onto the balance sheet*. London, UK: NEF.

Neilson, E. (1988). Health values: Achieving high level wellness – origins, philosophy, purpose. *Health Values,* 12: 3-5.

Ng, E., Wilkins, R., Gendron, F., & Berthelot, J-M. (2005). Dynamics of immigrants' health in Canada: Evidence from the National Population Health Survey. Ottawa: Statistics Canada.

Non-Smokers' Rights Association. (2011). *Compendium of 100% smoke-free municipal bylaws* (Winter update). http://www.nsra-adnf.ca/cms/page1421.cfm. Accessed: 3 April, 2011.

Nord, M., & Hopwood, H. (2008). A comparison of household food security in Canada and the United States. *Economic Research Report* No. 67. Economic Research Service. Washington: US Department of Agriculture.

Norton, J. (2008). *Aboriginal life on/off reserve: Census 2006.* Census Fast Facts, Issue 2006:07. BC Stats. Victoria.

Nutbeam, D. (1998) Health promotion glossary. *Health Promotion International*, 13(4): 349-364.

Oberholtzer, L., & Grow, S. (2003). *Producer-only farmers' markets in the Mid-Atlantic region: A survey of market managers.* Arlington,VA: Henry A.Wallace Center for Agricultural and Environmental Policy at Winrock International.

Office for National Statistics (ONS). (2010). *Consultation: Measuring national well-being.* Newport, Wales: ONS.

Oregon Progress Board. (1991). *Oregon Benchmarks: Setting measurable standards for progress.* Report to 1991 Legislature. http://www.oregon.gov/DAS/OPB/docs/1991_Oregon_Benchmark_Progress_Report.pdf. Accessed: 15 December, 2010. Achieving the Oregon Shines Vision.

Oregon Progress Board. (2009). *Highlights: 2009 Benchmark Report to the people of Oregon.* http://www.oregon.gov/DAS/OPB/docs/2009Report/2009_Benchmark_Highlights.pdf. Accessed: 15 December, 2010.

Organization for Economic Cooperation and Development. (2011a). *Compendium of OECD well-being indicators.* OECD Better Life Initiative. Paris: OECD.

Organization for Economic Cooperation and Development. (2011b). *Create your Better Life Index.* OECD Better Life Initiative. http://www.oecdbetterlifeindex.org/ Accessed 29 May, 2011.

Organisation for Economic Co-operation and Development. (2008). *OECD Health Working Paper No.32: The prevention of lifestyle-related chronic diseases: An economic framework.*

Osberg, L. (2009). *Measuring economic security in insecure times: New perspectives, new events, and the Index of Economic Well-being.* Centre for the Study of Living Standards.

Ostry, A. (2005). The early development of nutrition policy in Canada: Impacts on mothers and children. In C. Warsh (Ed.), *Children's health issues in historical perspective* (pp. 191-208). Waterloo, ON: Wilfrid Laurier Press.

Ostry, A. (2006). *Nutrition policy in Canada, 1870-1939.* Vancouver: University of British Columbia Press.

Ostry, A. (2010a). *Food for thought: The issues and challenges for food security.* Report prepared for the Population and Public Health Program. Vancouver: Provincial Health Services Authority.

Ostry, A. (2010b). *Final report: PHSA/Working Group on Food Recommendations for Obesity Reduction in BC.* Vancouver: Provincial Health Sevices Authority.

Panelli, R., & Tipa, G., (2007). Placing well-being: A Maori case study of cultural and environmental specificity. *EcoHealth*, 4: 445-460.

Park, J. (2009). Obesity on the job. *Perspectives*, February: 14-22.

Patra, J., Taylor, B., Rehm, J.T., Baliunas, D., & Popova, S. (2007). Substance-attributable morbidity and mortality changes to Canada's epidemiological profile. *Canadian Journal of Public Health,* 98(3): 228-234.

Pederson, S. (2006). Evidence review: *Food security. Core public health functions for BC.* Population Health and Wellness. Victoria, BC: Ministry of Health.

Pennock, M.N. (2009). Measuring the progress of communities: Applying the Gross National Happiness Index. *Measuring the Progress of Societies.* Newsletter, Issue 6, September: 9-10.

Pesticide Free BC. (2010). http://www.pesticidefreebc.org/. Accessed: 5 May, 2010, and 19 December, 2010.

Petrick, L.M., Svidovsky, A., & Dubowski, Y. (2011). Thirdhand smoke: Heterogeneous oxidation of nicotine and secondary aerosol formation in the indoor environment. *Environmental Science & Technolology,* 45: 328–333.

Pouliou, T., & Elliott, S.J. (2009). An exploratory spatial analysis of overweight and obesity in Canada. *Preventive Medicine,* 48: 362-367.

Powell, J. (2010). *StrongStart BC early learning programs.* October, BC Ministry of Education. Victoria, BC.

Probart, A.W., Tremblay, M.S., & Gorber, S.C. (2008). Desk potatoes: The importance of occupational physical activity on health. *Canadian Journal of Public Health,* 99(4): 311-8.

Profit, J., Typpo, K.V., Hysong, S.J., Woodward, L.D., Kallen, M.A., & Petersen, L.A. (2010). Improving benchmarking by using an explicit framework for the development of composite indicators: an example using pediatric quality of care. *Implementation Science,* 5:13.

Provincial Health Services Authority. (2007). *Life expectancy as a measure of population health: Comparing British Columbia with other Olympic and paralympic winter games host jurisdictions.* Summary report. Vancouver: PHSA.

Provincial Health Services Authority. (2008a). *Population and Public Health Indicators for British Columbia.* Vancouver.

Provincial Health Services Authority. (2008b). *Indicators for a Healthy Build Environment in BC.* Vancouver.

Public Health Agency of Canada. (2003). *What determines health?* http://www.phac-aspc.gc.ca/ph-sp/determinants/index-eng.php. Accessed: 1 February, 2011.

Public Health Agency of Canada. (2006). *Healthy Aging in Canada.* Ottawa.

Public Health Agency of Canada. (2007). *Business case for active living at work: Executive summary.* http://www.phac-aspc.gc.ca/alw-vat/execsum-resumexec-eng.php. Accessed: 13 October, 2009.

Public Health Agency of Canada. (2009a). *The 2007 Report on the Integrated Pan-Canadian Healthy Living Strategy.* Ottawa. http://www.phac-aspc.gc.ca/hp-ps/hl-mvs/ipchls-spimmvs/2007/index-eng.php. Accessed: 7 July, 2010.

Public Health Agency of Canada. (2009b). *Obesity in Canada: Snapshot.* Ottawa. http://www.phac-aspc.gc.ca/publicat/2009/oc/index-eng.php. Accessed: 4 April, 2011.

Public Health Agency of Canada. (2009c). *What mothers say: The Canadian Maternity Experiences Survey.* Ottawa.

Public Health Agency of Canada. (2011a). *Healthy pregnancy: Alcohol and pregnancy.* http://www.phac-aspc.gc.ca/hp-gs/know-savoir/alc-eng.php. Accessed: 2 February, 2011.

Public Health Agency of Canada. (2011b). *Healthy pregnancy: Smoking and pregnancy.* http://www.phac-aspc.gc.ca/hp-gs/know-savoir/smoke-fumer-eng.php. Accessed: 2 February, 2011.

Public Health Agency of Canada & Canadian Institute for Health Information. (2011). *Obesity in Canada.* A joint report from the Public Health Agency of Canada and the Canadian Institute for Health Information. Ottawa.

Ramage-Morin, P.L., Shields, M., & Martel, L. (2010). Health- promoting factors and good health among Canadians in mid- to late life. *Health Reports,* 21(3): September.

Renger, R.F., Midyett, S.J., Mas, F.G., Erin, T.E., McDermott, H.M., Papenfuss, R.L., Eichling, P.S., Baker, D.H., Johnson, K.A., & Hewitt, M.J. (2000). Optimal living profile: An inventory to assess health and wellness. *American Journal of Health Promotion,* 24(6): 403-412.

Rideout, K., and Ostry, A. (2006). A conceptual model for developing food security indicators for use by regional health authorities. *Canadian Journal of Public Health,* 97(3): 233-236.

Ronskley, P.E., Brien, S.E., Turner, B.J., Mukamal, K.J., & Ghali, W.A. (2011). Association of alcohol consumption with selected cardiovascular disease outcomes: A systematic review and meta-analysis. *British Medical Journal,* 342: d671.

Royal Bank of Canada. (2011). *Higher costs for gas, food impacting BC budgets.* RBC Canadian Consumer Outlook Index. April 12, Toronto.

Ryan, R.M., & Deci, E.L. (2001). On happiness and human potentials: A review of research on hedonic and eudaemonic well-being. *Annual Review of Psychology,* 52: 141-166.

Ryff, C.D., and Singer, B.H. (2006). Best news yet on the six-factor model of well-being. *Social Science Research,* 35: 1103-1119.

Saewyc, E., Wang, N., Chittenden, M., Murphy, A., & The McCreary Centre Society. (2006). *Building resilience in vulnerable youth.* Vancouver, BC: The McCreary Centre Society.

Saltman, D., Hitchman, S.C., Sendzik, T., & Fong, G.T. (2010). The current status of bans on smoking in vehicles carrying children. In: Cancer Advocacy Coalition of Canada, *Report Card on Cancer in Canada,* Volume 12, Winter 2009-10: 5-9.

Sassi, F., Devaux, M., Church, J., Ceccini, M., & Borggonovi, F. (2009). Education and obesity in four OECD countries. *OECD Health Working Papers* No, 46. Paris: Organisation for Economic Co-operation and Development.

Sauve, R. (2010). *The current state of Canadian family finances: 2010 Report.* Ottawa: The Vanier Institute of the Family.

Save the Children. (2008). *Child Development Index: Holding governments to account for children's wellbeing.* London, UK: Save the Children Fund.

Schrier, D. (2009). Low income cut-offs are a poor measure of poverty. *Earnings and Employment Trends.* BC Stats, November.

Sharratt, M., & Hearst, W. (2007). Canada's physical activity guides: Background, process and development. *Canadian Journal Public Health,* 23: S9-S15.

Shields, M. (2006). Overweight and obesity among children and youth. *Health Reports,* 17(3): August.

Shields, M. (2007). Smoking – Prevalence, bans and exposure to second-hand smoke. *Health Reports,* 18(3): August.

Shields, M., Gorber, S.C., & Tremblay, M.S. (2008). Effects of measurement on obesity and morbidity. Sedentary behaviour and obesity. *Health Reports,* 19(2): June.

Shields, M., & Tremblay, M.S. (2008). Sedentary behaviour and obesity. *Health Reports,* 19(2): June.

Shillington, R., & Stapleton, J. (2010). *Cutting through the fog: Why is it so hard to make sense of poverty measures?* Toronto: Metcalf Foundation.

SmartGrowth BC. (nd). *Agricultural land.* http://www.smartgrowth.bc.ca/AboutUs/Issues/AgriculturalLand/tabid/111/Default.aspx. Accessed: 4 April, 2011.

Smith, B.E. (1998). *Planning for agriculture.* Vancouver: Provincial Agricultural Land Commission. http://www.alc.gov.bc.ca/Publications/planning/Planning_for_Agriculture/index.htm. Accessed: 4 April, 2011.

Smith, A., Stewart, D., Peled, M., Poon, C., Saewyc, E., & the McCreary Centre Society. (2009). *A picture of health: Highlights from the 2008 BC Adolescent Health Survey.* Vancouver, BC: McCreary Centre Society.

Smith, A., Stewart, D., Poon, C., Saewyc, E., & the McCreary Centre Society. (2011). *Moving in the right direction: Physical activity among BC youth.* Vancouver, BC: McCreary Centre Society.

Sodium Working Group. (2010). *Sodium reduction strategy for Canada.* Recommendations of the Sodium Working Group. Nutrition Evaluation Division. Ottawa: Health Canada.

Sorhaindo, A., & Feinstein, L. (2006). What is the relationship between child nutrition and school outcomes? *Wider Benefits of Learning Research Report* No. 18. London: Centre for Research on the Wider Benefits of Learning.

SRI International. (2010). *Spas and the Global Wellness Market: Synergies and opportunities.* Global Spa Summit. http://csted.sri.com/projects/spas-and-global-wellness-market-synergies-and-opportunities. Accessed: 3 November, 2010.

State of Oregon. (2009). Oregon Progress Board. http://www.oregon.gov/DAS/OPB/. Accessed 1 March, 2011.

Statistics Canada. (nd). *Canadian Community Health Survey CCHS), 2008 (Annual component) and 2007-2008. Derived Variable (DV) Specifications: Master and Share Files.* Ottawa: Statistics Canada.

Statistics Canada. (2008). *Health indicators: Thematic maps.* Ottawa: Statistics Canada. http://www.statcan.gc.ca/pub/82-221-x/2008001/tmaps-tcartes/5202140-eng.htm#hr. Accessed: 10 December, 2010.

Statistics Canada. (2009). *Canadian Community Health Survey (CCHS) – Annual component. User guide 2007 -2008 microdata files.* Ottawa: Statistics Canada.

Statistics Canada. (2010). Deaths. *The Daily,* February, 23. http://www.statcan.gc.ca/daily-quotidien/100223/dq100223a-eng.htm. Accessed: 12 January, 2011.

Statistics Canada. (2011a). *National Household Survey.* http://www.statcan.gc.ca/survey-enquete/household-menages/5178-eng.htm. Accessed: 10 February, 2011.

Statistics Canada. (2011b). *2006 Census of Agriculture.* http://www.statcan.gc.ca/ca-ra2006/index-eng.htm. Accessed: 15 February, 2011.

Stiglitz, J.E., Sen, A., & Fitoussi, J-P. (2009a). *Report by the Commission on the Measurement of Economic Performance and Social Progress.* Paris: Commission on the Measurement of Economic Performance and Social Progress. http://www.stiglitz-sen-fitoussi.fr/en/index.htm. Accessed: 12 December, 2010.

Stiglitz, J.E., Sen, A., & Fitoussi, J-P. (2009b). *The measurement of economic performance and social progress revisited: Reflections and overview.* Working Paper, September 16. Paris: Commission on the Measurement of Economic Performance and Social Progress. http://www.stiglitz-sen-fitoussi.fr/documents/overview-eng.pdf. Accessed: 12 December, 2010.

Studar, D.T. (2007). Ideas, institutions and diffusion: What explains tobacco control policy in Australia, Canada and New Zealand? *Commonwealth & Comparative Politics,* 45(2): 164-184.

Suhrcke, M., & de Paz Nieves, C. (2011). *The impact of health and health behaviours on educational outcomes in high income countries: A review of the evidence.* Copenhagen: WHO Regional Office for Europe.

Sustainable Society Foundation. (2010). The Hague: SSF. http://www.ssfindex.com/. Accessed: 20 February, 2011.

The Centre for Bhutan Studies (2008). *Gross National Happiness. Explanation of GNH Index.* http://www.grossnationalhappiness.com/gnhIndex/intruductionGNH.aspx. Accessed: 12 December, 2010.

Thomas, J., & Evans, J. (2010). There's more to life than GDP but how can we measure it? *Economic & Labour Market Review,* 4(9): 29-36.

Torjman, S. (2004). *Culture and recreation: Links to well-being.* Ottawa: Caledon Institute of Social Policy.

Toronto Community Foundation. (2010). *Toronto's Vital Signs 2010: Full report.* http://www.tcf.ca/vitalinitiatives/TVS10FullReport.pdf. Accessed: 10 February, 2011.

Travis, J. & Callander, M. (2010). *Beyond ordinary wellness: Full-spectrum wellness – a work in progress.* Personal correspondence with J. Travis, 31 October, 2010.

Tremblay, M.S., Shields, M., Laviolette, M., Craig, C.L., Janssen, I., & Connor Gorber, S. (2010). Fitness of Canadian children and youth: results from the 2007-2009 Canadian Health Measures Survey. *Health Reports,* 21(1): March.

Trichopoulou, A., Bamia, C., & Trichopoulos, D. (2009). Anatomy of health effects of Mediterranean diet: Greek EPIC prospective cohort study. *British Medical Journal,* 338: b2337.

Turcotte, M., & Schellenberg, G. (2007). *A portrait of seniors in Canada.* Ottawa: Statistics Canada.

Turpell-Lafond, M.E. (2010). *No short cuts to safety – Doing better for children living with extended family.* Victoria, BC: Office of the Representative for Children and Youth.

Turpell-Lafond, M.E., & Kendall, P.R.W. (2007). *Health and well-being of children in care in British Columbia: Educational experience and outcomes.* Victoria, BC: Office of the Representative for Children and Youth and Office of the Provincial Health Officer.

Turpell-Lafond, M.E., & Kendall, P.R.W. (2010). *Growing up in British Columbia.* Victoria, BC: Office of the Representative for Children and Youth and Office of the Provincial Health Officer.

Twiss, J., Dickinson, J., Duma, S., Kleinman, T., Paulsen, H., & Rilveria, L. (2003). Community gardens: lessons learned from California healthy cities and communities. American Journal of Public Health, 93:9: 1435-1438.

UNESCO. (2009). *The 2009 UNESCO framework for cultural statistics (FCS).* Paris: UNESCO Institute of Statistics 35 C/INF.20, 16 September 2009. Cited in: Canadian Index of Wellbeing. (2010). *Leisure and Culture: A report of the Canadian Index of Wellbeing (CIW).*

United Nations Development Programme. (2010). *The real wealth of nations: Pathways to human development. Human Development Report 2010.* http://hdr.indp.org. Accessed: 10 February, 2011.

UnitedHealthcare. (2010). *Survey results show health benefits of volunteering.* http://74.125.155.132/scholar?q=cache:Jx8vbXE-heIJ:scholar.google.com/+volunteerism+and+wellness&hl=en&as_sdt=0,5. Accessed: 2 April, 2011.

US Department of Health and Human Services. (2011). *The Surgeon General's Call to Action to Support Breastfeeding.* Washington, DC: US Department of Health and Human Services, Office of the Surgeon General.

US Office of the Surgeon General. (2006). *The Health Consequences of Involuntary Exposure to Tobacco Smoke:* A Report of the Surgeon General. http://www.surgeongeneral.gov/library/secondhandsmoke/. Accessed: 5 August, 2010.

van der Kerk, G., & Manuel, A. (2010). *Sustainable Society Index: SSI-2010.* The Hague: Sustainable Society Foundation.

Vanasse, A., Demers, M., Hemiari, A., & Cousteau, J. (2006). Obesity in Canada: Where and how many? *International Journal of Obesity,* 30: 677-683.

Vandivere, S., & McPhee, C. (2008). Methods of tabulating indices of child well-being and context: An illustration and comparison of performance in 13 American states. *Child Indicators Research,* 1: 251-290.

Vaughan, T., Harris, J., & Caldwell, B.J. (2011). *Bridging the gap in school achievement through the arts: Summary report.* Victoria, BC: The Song Room.

Veenhoven, R. (2008). Healthy happiness: Effects of happiness on physical health and the consequences for preventive health care. *Journal of Happiness Studies,* 9: 449-469.

Virtue, N., McKee, B., Foster, L.T., Blake, A., Cloutier-Fisher, D., Keller, C.P., & Ostry, A. (2010). *The geography of women's wellness and well-being across British Columbia.* Department of Geography, University of Victoria, BC. http://www.geog.uvic.ca/wellness. Accessed: 28 June, 2010.

Vital Statistics Agency. (2010). *Selected vital statistics and health status indicators. Annual report, 2009.* British Columbia Vital Statistics Agency. Victoria, BC: Ministry of Health Services.

VON Canada. (2011). *Let's talk FASD.* http://www.von.ca/fasdonline/default.aspx. Accessed: 2 February, 2011.

Wakefield, S., Yeudall, F., Taron, C., Reynolds, J., & Skinner, A. (2007). Growing urban health: community gardening in south-east Toronto. Health Promotion International, 22(2): 92-101.

Waldron, S. (2010). *Measuring subjective well-being in the UK.* Working Paper, September. Newport, Wales: Office for National Statistics.

Wang, F., Wild, T.C., Kipp, W., Kuhle, S., & Veugelers, P.J. (2009). The influence of childhood obesity on the development of self-esteem. *Health Reports,* 20(2): June.

Wardle, J., Carnell, S., Haworth, C.M.A., & Plomin, R. (2008). Evidence for a strong genetic influence on childhood adiposity despite the force of the obesogenic environment. *American Journal of Clinical Nutrition,* 87(2): 398-404.

Wilkins, K., Campbell, N.R.C., Joffres, M.R., McAlister, F.A., Nichol, M., Quach, S., Johansen, H.L., & Tremblay, M.S. (2010). Blood pressure in Canadian adults. *Health Reports,* 21(1): March.

Wilson, J., & Musick, M.A. (1999). Attachment to volunteering. Sociological Forum, 14(2): 243-272.

World Health Organization. (1948). *Constitution of the World Health Organization.* Geneva: WHO.

World Health Organization. (2000). *Nutrition for health and development.* Geneva: WHO.

World Health Organization. (2007). *Public health mapping and geographic information systems.* http://www.who.int/health_mapping/en/. Accessed: 8 August, 2010.

World Health Organization. (2010). *Global recommendations on physical activity for health.* Geneva, WHO.

Wormley, D. (2010). *Virtual community of support for early learning.* http://www.des.prn.bc.ca/groups/strongstart/. Accessed: 10 December, 2010.

Yang, S., Logan, J., & Coffey, D.L. (1995). Mathematical formulae for calculating the base temperature for growing degree days. *Agricultural & Forest Meteorology*, 74: 61-74.

Young, K., & Katzmarzyk, P. (2007). Physical activity of Aboriginal people in Canada: Issues and challenges. *Canadian Journal of Public Health*, 98 (Supplement 2 E): S148-S160.